MATERNITY NURSING

MATERNITY NURSING Twelfth Edition

Elise Fitzpatrick, R.N., M.A.
*Associate Professor of Nursing, School of Nursing,
University of Wisconsin at Milwaukee;
Formerly Associate Professor of Maternity Nursing,
Francis Payne Bolton School of Nursing,
Case Western Reserve University*

Sharon R. Reeder, R.N., M.S.
*Formerly Assistant Professor of Maternity Nursing,
University of California at Los Angeles*

Luigi Mastroianni, Jr., M.D., F.A.C.S., F.A.C.O.G.
*William Goodell Professor and Chairman,
Department of Obstetrics and Gynecology,
University of Pennsylvania School of Medicine*

J. B. LIPPINCOTT COMPANY
Philadelphia   •   Toronto

Preface

Again, with the 12th edition of this book almost every chapter has been revised, and many have been rewritten extensively.

In the chapter "Orientation to Maternity Nursing" the vital statistics have been updated to reflect current trends. The concept of high-level wellness is introduced because we believe this has particular significance in the care of maternity patients. Health goals to maximize the patient's potential in the environment in which she finds herself are especially important for the care and well-being of essentially healthy patients experiencing normal childbirth, which is a normal physiologic process of the body.

Dimensions of effective nursing care have been enlarged, based on recent research and conceptual developments in nursing practice and related disciplines. The areas of antepartal care, parent education, the conduct of normal labor, care of the full-term and premature infant, nursing in emergency situations and in conditions with complications reflect this current thought.

Although the content on nurse-midwifery has been revised, it would be almost impossible to enlarge this chapter to include all of the expanding facets of this subject in the confines of this book.

Three new chapters have been added to this edition in an effort to include some of the vast amount of knowledge and thinking regarding the reproductive cycle, its participants, and their relationship to society in general at this time.

The focus in the chapter "Patient Teaching" is directed to teaching groups of patients in preparation for childbearing. Some of this content was presented in other sections of previous editions, but as preparation for parenthood programs have become more prevalent throughout the country, this approach is more appropriate. Some important concepts of the teaching-learning process which have particular relevance in patient teaching are introduced, and the student is encouraged to explore the subject more widely.

The chapter "Social Factors in Maternal Care" examines a number of issues related to maternal care, e.g., the meaning of human reproduction in our culture and the consequences it entails for the family as well as the larger society of which they are a part. Concepts of health, illness and the sick role are utilized to encourage the nurse to develop and explore innovations—which seem so necessary in this age of rapid social change—in her thinking and practice.

The entire subject of fetal medicine is relatively new to this generation but has already advanced beyond fetal diagnosis and now includes treatment and genetic assessment as well. In this new chapter some specific fetal problems are examined, and the present status of fetal diagnosis and treatment is reviewed.

The chapter on the care of premature infants has been extensively rewritten to include recent knowledge of the diagnosis and classification of low birth-weight infants, as well as the medical and nursing management of infants with such conditions. The disorders of the newborn and nursing in crises and emergency conditions have also been revised. The history of obstetrics has been enlarged to include the development and the present state of maternity nursing in the United States.

Many new developments and approaches to maternity care have been incorporated into this edition. In order to maintain a happy balance, some previous content has been refined and reorganized. As one example, mental hygiene of pregnancy and childbirth, per se, has been reorganized and mental health concepts have been incorporated throughout the text as an integral part of comprehensive maternity care.

Many new illustrations, both photographs and original drawings, have been added to this edition. The suggested reading lists that accompany each chapter have been brought up to date with references from current professional literature. The conference material and study questions at the end of the various study units, as well as the glossary, have been found essential by our readers and therefore have been retained.

ELISE FITZPATRICK, R.N.
SHARON R. REEDER, R.N.
LUIGI MASTROIANNI, JR., M.D.

Acknowledgments

Since the publication of the 11th edition of this book, our co-author, Nicholson J. Eastman, M.D., has retired from authorship. We wish to acknowledge Dr. Eastman's significant contributions to the development of this book for more than twenty-five years.

We wish to express our gratitude for the help and encouragement of many colleagues and friends in the revision of this text. Specifically, we thank Mrs. Kara Rosenburg, whose valuable assistance in researching the literature is greatly appreciated; Miss Ruth Dehlinger, R.N., C.N.M., for her guidance in preparation of the section "Nurse-Midwifery"; Mrs. Alice Orton, for her help in preparing the manuscript; and Elaine Pierson, M.D., Ph.D., for her valuable suggestions. We are also indebted to Mrs. Ruth Lubic, General Director of Maternity Center Association of New York, for permission to publish the exercises taught by Maternity Center Association in its program "Preparation for Childbirth."

We are indebted to Mr. Wesley Kaswell, Department of Photography, University Hospitals of Cleveland, for his outstanding photography and his cooperation in securing certain special photographs. We wish to express our gratitude also to Mr. Lowell F. Bernard, Director of the Cleveland Health Museum and Education Center, for his contribution. To Michael J. Zugzda, Chief, Statistical Resources Section, Division of Vital Statistics, National Center for Health Statistics, we are indebted for assistance in compiling data for vital statistics.

We wish to acknowledge the assistance of the Rev. Msgr. Francis M. Beres, J.C.D., Milwaukee Archdiocese and Father Donald N. Weber, Executive Director, Milwaukee Archdiocesan Family Life Program, for consultation and guidance concerning teachings of the Roman Catholic Church on family planning.

The authors express their appreciation to colleagues, publishers and organizations for the use of illustrations in this text. We wish to express our gratitude to the nursing students and parents who granted permission for photographs to appear in this book.

Finally, we take this opportunity to thank the J. B. Lippincott Company, particularly Mr. David T. Miller, Miss Mary Dennesaites, Dr. Walter Kahoe and Mr. J. Stuart Freeman, Jr., for their steadfast interest, cooperation and assistance.

THE AUTHORS

Contents

UNIT ONE
Human Reproduction

Orientation to Maternity Nursing
Anatomy Related to the Reproductive System
Physiology in Relation to Human Reproduction
Development and Physiology of the Fetus
Presentations and Positions

Orientation to Maternity Nursing

1

INTRODUCTION

The study of obstetrics and of the nursing care of women during the various phases of childbearing includes the study of anatomic and physiologic adaptations to human reproduction and, in the full meaning, the study of human growth and development and the many interdependent relationships concerned. The vast importance of professional maternity care to mothers, infants and families of our country must be fully understood by all who participate in their care.

This chapter is planned to begin the student's orientation to maternity nursing. Certain basic terminology will be defined. Basic concepts of maternity care will be introduced, as well as the childbearing mother and her infant—all as they form a part of the expanding family found in our society.

The subsequent chapters of this unit survey the anatomy and the physiology related to human reproduction. Knowledge of the anatomy and the physiology of the reproductive organs and of the development of the unborn child from conception to birth is basic to the understandings required of every maternity nurse. The physiologic mechanism by which conception takes place and a new human being develops is not only a fascinating story in itself, but also one that has far-reaching implications for the mother, the child and the family. All that a human being becomes depends on many factors: his heritage, his prenatal environment, his care at birth and his care thereafter throughout infancy and childhood. Thus, it is all the more important that the safety, the health and the well-being of each mother and infant be protected, and, simultaneously, that the highest level of health possible for every childbearing family be achieved in the broader sense of physical, emotional and social well-being.

Unit One concludes with a consideration of the various positions which the fetus in utero may occupy. A clear grasp of the material in this unit is essential to a basic understanding of maternity care. The illustrations should be studied in close correlation with the text.

OBSTETRICS

Obstetrics is defined as that branch of medicine which deals with parturition, its antecedents and its sequels. It is concerned principally, therefore, with the phenomena and the management of pregnancy, labor and the puerperium under both normal and abnormal circumstances.[1]

The etymology of "obstetrics" is mentioned here to serve as basic information. For many students it will undoubtedly arouse curiosity and interest for further study. Briefly, the word "obstetrics" is derived from the Latin *obstetricia* or *obstetrix,* meaning midwife. The verb form *obsto* (*ob,* before, plus *sto,* stand) means "to stand by." Thus, in ancient Rome a person who cared for women at childbirth was known as an *obstetrix,* or a per-

---

[1] Eastman, N. J., and Hellman, L. M.: Williams Obstetrics, ed. 13, p. 1, New York, Appleton, 1966.

son who "stood by" the woman in labor. In both the United States and Great Britain this branch of medicine was called "midwifery" for several centuries—in fact, until the latter part of the 19th century. The term "obstetrics" really came into usage little more than a century ago, although reference to a variety of words of common derivation can be found occasionally in earlier writings. With the use of new terminology that has developed down through the years, it is not unusual to find that from the standpoint of semantics, changes have developed also in the present era. Today, in light of the various changes which have evolved in the total care of childbearing women, the usage of the term "obstetric care" is open to question. In the current frame of reference it seems more appropriate to use the term "maternity care," since this term implies a broader meaning of the care of the mother and her offspring throughout the childbearing experience. Moreover, it focuses attention on the care of a *person,* on the importance of interpersonal relationships—particularly those relationships which are *significant to her*—and the kind of patient care which will assist in promoting the health and the well-being of the expanding family group.

The World Health Organization Expert Committee on Maternity Care has defined maternity care as follows:

> The object of maternity care is to ensure that every expectant and nursing mother maintains good health, learns the art of child care, has a normal delivery, and bears healthy children. Maternity care in the narrower sense consists in the care of the pregnant woman, her safe delivery, her postnatal examination, the care of her newly born infant, and the maintenance of lactation. In the wider sense it begins much earlier in measures aimed to promote the health and well-being of the young people who are potential parents, and to help them develop the right approach to family life and to the place of the family in the community. It should also include guidance in parentcraft and in problems associated with infertility and family planning.[2]

MATERNITY NURSING

Maternity nursing involves direct, personal ministrations to maternity patients and their newborn infants, or related activities on their behalf, during the various phases of the childbearing experience. Maternity nursing differs from the practice of nursing in any of the other areas only in that the clinical focus primarily involves the care of maternity patients (in contrast, for example, with the care of surgical patients or psychiatric patients). How the maternity nurse meets the nursing needs of mothers and their newborn infants cannot be spelled out in stereotyped activities any more than it can in any other situation in which individualized nursing care is the underlying objective. In fact, the nurse may be called on at times to perform what superficially appears to be rather elementary nursing tasks; for example, in relation to body cleanliness. It is *how* the nurse carries out her care of the patient, the depth of problem-solving ability she employs, that makes the difference between truly professional nursing and nursing on a technical level.

In the practice of nursing, the nurse intervenes to relieve or to reduce the patient's problems due to physical, physiologic or psychologic stress. A significant aspect of maternity nursing on the professional level is that patient care involves purposeful, sustained interaction between the nurse and the patient, during which the nurse assesses the patient's problems (i.e., makes a nursing diagnosis as to the nature of the discomfort or the dysfunction) and takes action to relieve the problem if it can be alleviated properly with nursing measures.

Begetting children is a family affair; thus, the nursing care of maternity patients is properly a family-centered activity. In most situations today the maternity patient is a healthy woman involved in the normal physiologic process of childbearing. However, like individuals facing any other new experience in the family life cycle, maternity patients may begin the experience at various stages of preparation for pregnancy and childbirth, with various kinds of stress and at various levels of contentment. It is safe to say that in almost no other normal physiologic process does one find such individual extremes of reactions within a normal context. These individual reactions may be based on events going back to childhood, to certain experiences shared in growing up, or to later happenings. Certainly, they are influenced by the home environment from which the mother comes and to which, a short time after the delivery, she will return with her newborn infant. The level of satisfaction with which the expectant mother leaves the clinic or the level of contentment with which the newly delivered mother leaves the hospital en-

[2] World Health Organization Technical Report Series, No. 51, Geneva, Switzerland, World Health Organization, 1952.

vironment with her baby will be modified somewhat by the interpersonal relationships of those most significant to her in that environment. Thus, the nurse can provide more continuity in the time spent with patients than other professionals and by the nature of her position has it within her ability to make a significant contribution to maternity care.

The usual reference to the maternity patient as a healthy woman involved in the normal physiologic process of childbearing has almost become a cliché. Some nurses acknowledge that they find little challenge in maternity nursing because the majority of the patients are healthy, with similar nursing care problems. Most are also ambulatory soon after delivery and are capable of taking care of their own physical needs.

High-Level Wellness

Good health (i.e., wellness) is not a static condition, but may be manifest in degrees of well-being or overlapping levels of wellness. Providing optimal maternal care requires an explanation of the many facets and factors responsible for the good health of maternity patients. From this point we may then be able to make statements in objective terms about what high-level wellness means for the individual, the family and others who are significant to the patient.

In maternity nursing the concept of high-level wellness is particularly appropriate in the promotion of good health for patients, whether the patient is pregnant, is in the course of labor or is the newly delivered mother with her infant.

"High-level wellness is a term which has been devised to make the person who uses it think about well-being in degrees or levels. High-level wellness for the individual is defined as an integrated method of functioning which is oriented towards maximizing the potential of which the individual is capable. It requires that the individual maintain a continuum of balance and purposeful direction within the environment where he is functioning."[3] Wellness, then, is a direction in progress towards an even higher potential of functioning for the total individual in all of his uniqueness. Dunn has proposed that in order to utilize the goal of high-level wellness it is essential to think in terms of disease and health as a graduated scale.[4] This scale is conceptualized as one axis of the "health grid" (Figure 1-1). The health

---

[3] Dunn, H. L.: High-Level Wellness, pp. 4-5, Arlington, Virginia, R. W. Beatty, 1961.

[4] Dunn, H. L.: High-level wellness for man and society, in Folta, J. R. and Deck, E. S., p. 214. A Sociological Framework for Patient Care. New York, John Wiley and Sons, 1966.

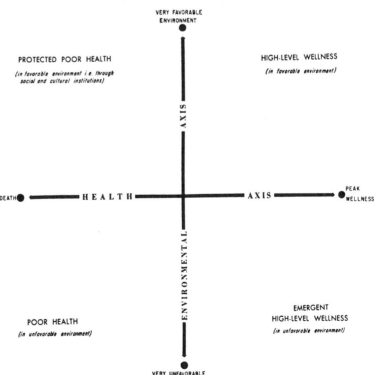

FIG. 1-1. The health grid, its axes and quadrants. (Data from U.S. Department of Health, Education, and Welfare, Public Health Service, National Office of Vital Statistics.) (Dunn, H. L.: High-level wellness for man and society. Am. J. Public Health 49: 220, June, 1959)

grid is made up of (1) the health axis, (2) the environmental axis, and (3) the resulting health and wellness quadrants. The environmental axis includes the physical and biological factors of the environment, as well as the socioeconomic components affecting the health of the individual. The health axis ranges from death at the left extremity to peak wellness at the right.

As one looks at the health grid, with its health axis and its environmental axis, it seems relatively easy to appreciate the extremes from severe illness and death on one side to the maximum or peak wellness on the other side of the axis. Man lives in a very complex environment today and, as with progress, the environment tends to become more complicated. Freeman divides the environment into three major areas: the physical, the biologic, and the social.[5] We are in daily interaction with physical factors (or the "elements" in the environment). Temperature and humidity alone can contribute to the comfort or the extreme discomfort of a pregnant woman. Considering the various aspects of atmospheric pressure, one might consider the changes in altitude; for example, creating a situation comparable to "Mt. Everest in utero." In the biologic environment, there are forces from the plant and animal kingdom constantly interacting with man (e.g., microorganisms), some of which contribute to health rather than illness. The biologic area includes the sources which contribute to our food and clothing. Freeman says that the biologic environmental area provides the major source for physiologic growth and development, and that the social segment of our environment provides the major source for psychological growth and development. As far as the social area of the environment is concerned, we are in constant interaction with people and the culture around us through many avenues of communication, such as the arts, the press, the radio, and television.

When we learn how to diagnose high-level wellness through objective measures we shall probably find that a substantial amount of creative expression and love of daily life is essential in the approach to a high state of well-being. The goal of high-level wellness for man can be achieved. The needs are for clear-cut concepts, for understanding and for a reassessment of our basic

values. "We must dare to dream, for dreams are the seedlings of realities."[6]

MATERNAL AND CHILD HEALTH

Despite the fact that today the use of the term "maternal and child health" seems to imply a relatively new concept of care, it actually was in usage more than 50 years ago. In 1912 the United States Children's Bureau was created by an act of Congress for the purpose of promoting maternal and child health "among all classes of people." It was said to be a public health nurse who first conceived the idea of a Federal bureau of this kind and originally suggested the plan to President Theodore Roosevelt in 1905. The Children's Bureau has continually stressed the importance of public health nursing in maternal and child welfare. Between the years 1921 and 1929, public health nursing consultants were employed by the Bureau, and their services were offered to the states for maternal and infant hygiene. In rural areas throughout the United States, public health nursing services were greatly extended, and 2,978 centers for prenatal and child health work were established.

Since these early beginnings the Children's Bureau has continued to make significant contributions to the promotion of maternal and child health in this country (see Suggested Reading).

Maternal and child health nursing has been interpreted in many different ways, often depending on the individual's frame of reference. To some it means a combination of the traditional courses in maternity and pediatric nursing. To others it is a concept of patient care which takes into consideration the relationship of the mother to the care of a child, or the relationship of the mother and her newborn infant in maternity care. To still others it refers to the care of healthy mothers and children.

The authors of this textbook refer to maternal and child health nursing as a philosophy of patient care rather than a special area of nursing. Whether it concerns maternity nursing, pediatric nursing, the nursing of children or maternal-child health nursing, the patient care involves the nursing of mothers or children. Thus, the crux lies in the care of families. There is a body of knowledge which specifically pertains to maternity nursing, and, likewise, there is a closely related but sepa-

---

[5] B. J. Freeman: Human aspects of health and illness: beyond the germ theory, *in* Folta, J. R., and Deck, E. S.: A Sociological Framework for Patient Care, p. 84, New York, Wiley, 1966.

[6] Dunn, H. L.: High-level wellness for man and society. Am. J. Public Health, 49:219, June, 1959.

rate body of knowledge which pertains to the nursing of children or pediatric nursing. As one develops knowledge, understanding and skills in these areas, a philosophy of maternal and child health also evolves.

This is a philosophy of nursing that is shared by many colleagues. For example, Bruce and Hall have said:

> When maternity and pediatric nurses study and work together in providing nursing care for parents and children, the whole family benefits. . . . The members of each field bring with them their own unique skills and understandings which, when put together, cannot help but enrich the total practice.[7]

EXPANDING FAMILIES IN AMERICA

An awareness of the many facets involved in a changing society, especially as they relate to young childbearing families, should help the maternity nurse to develop an understanding of the forces that these changes exert on family life and, in addition, to see wherein they have implications for maternity care.

[7] Bruce, S. J., and Hall, E. J.: Maternity and pediatric nurses study and work together. Am. J. Nurs. 63:105, March, 1963.

In recent years it has been said repeatedly that family life in the United States is rapidly changing due to the impact of socioeconomic pressures. This is reflected in a change in American family structure, a change in traditional male and female roles, a change in family relationships, and even a change in concepts of maternity care.

The objective of this brief discussion is merely to introduce some observations that concern young childbearing families in our society and to stimulate the student's interest. It is in no way any attempt to pursue the broad and complex subject of trends in American family life.

Young couples today marry at a younger age than their elders did. The average age of the young bride is 20 years, and many brides are in their late teens. The average age of the groom is a little more than 2 years older than his bride. Nearly all young couples establish a household of their own when they marry. In many situations the young bride may still be completing her formal education; if she has been employed, she is likely to continue working outside the home. These couples not only spend more of their leisure time together, but they share in the homemaking responsibilities as well.

Young married couples today appear to be interested in having children, not only more chil-

FIG. 1-2. An expectant family.

dren than their parents did, but having them spaced closer together. The average size family today has 3 or 4 children, and often the last child is born by the time that the wife is 26 years old. When the wife becomes pregnant, the husband and the wife are likely to attend some kind of expectant parents' classes together. He is also likely to accompany his wife on her visits to the obstetrician, if his job requirements and responsibilities make it at all possible. It has become customary for husbands to stay with their wives during labor if they wish to, since the majority of modern maternity hospitals no longer exclude them. And after the baby is born, husbands more

FIG. 1-3 (*Top*). Expectant couples on conducted tour of the maternity hospital. FIG. 1-4 (*Bottom*). Following the walking tour the professional nurse and the expectant couples join for refreshment and informal discussion. (MacDonald House, University Hospitals of Cleveland, Cleveland, Ohio)

often are helping at home with the care of their babies—something which was considered to be strictly the role of the mother in the Victorian era.

As a consequence of the mobility of our population, smaller living quarters and other social changes, the more typical family in an urban industrial community usually consists of the husband, the wife and their children—the so-called "nuclear family." Since they live apart from their original families, there are fewer close relatives near at hand to help out in time of need; for example, when the new baby arrives. Much has been said about the added stress which young couples must cope with because they live by themselves and therefore lack the so-called advantages to be gained from living in the "family" home with the large 3-generation household. One cannot help wondering whether such thinking does not stem from those of the older generation who look at the young pregnant woman through the lens of their own past experiences; for many women of this older generation had to face childbirth with poor preparation for the experiences of childbearing.

From observations of mothers who enter the hospital to have their babies today, the average middle-class young woman is fairly well prepared for the experience. Most of them have done some reading from the current literature for expectant parents, many have attended some kind of parents' classes, and most of them have taken advantage of getting their questions answered by their doctors. And since most of the hospitals now conduct regularly scheduled tours of the maternity unit for maternity patients, the husband and wife are likely to have taken advantage of this sometime during the latter part of pregnancy. Granted, all of this preparation does not always hold true for the majority of women who come from the disadvantaged, low-income families, but it is in evidence as the quality of *total* maternity care in the clinics progresses.

One of the concerns about the 2-generation family found in most of the United States is the need for greater support for young couples who have married early and have children (i.e., there is no one there to help them). From observations it can be said that most of the expectant parents have made some satisfactory arrangements for help upon returning home from the hospital with the new baby. It is not unusual to find that the patient's mother or mother-in-law or a close relative is coming to be with her and to manage the household for a short period of time. Often it is said, "She'll be with me as long as I need her." Even when parents live out of the state, the mobility of the population—so prevalent today—is evident in the ease with which relatives travel great distances when there is a need. Sussman questions the notion that the nuclear family in modern society is the atomistic and isolated unit it has often been reputed to be. Empirical evidence indicates that the nuclear family is functioning today within a network of other nuclear families, particularly with families of orientation and in-law families, and that this network offers services and help of all kinds—during emergencies, on ceremonial occasions, and in everyday situations.[8]

VITAL STATISTICS

With reference to frequency distribution, an examination of the vital statistics reports gives us quantitative data which has been systematically gathered and collated. These data are presented in this chapter because they relate to statistical changes in the large body of people with whom we are concerned—statistics on births, marriages, population, morbidity and mortality.

In this country these data are published officially by the United States Public Health Service, National Center for Health Statistics, Vital Statistics Division. To understand the significance of the vital statistics quoted in the following discussion, the nurse should be familiar with the following terms, explained according to the definitions of the National Center for Health Statistics. Deaths are classified according to the World Health Organization Manual of International Classification of Diseases, Injuries and Causes of Death, based on recommendations of the Seventh Revision Conference, 1955, volume 1, Geneva, Switzerland, 1957.

Birth Rate. The number of births per 1,000 population

Marriage Rate. The number of marriages per 1,000 total population

Fertility Rate. The number of births per 1,000 women aged 15 to 44 years

Neonatal. Pertaining to the first 4 weeks after birth

---

8 Sussman, M. B.: The isolated nuclear family: Fact or fiction? *in* Sussman, M. B. (ed.): Sourcebook in Marriage and the Family. Ed. 3, p. 49, Boston, Houghton, 1968.

TABLE 1-1. LIVE BIRTHS AND POPULATION, UNITED STATES, 1930-1968*

| YEAR | LIVE BIRTHS† | | | BIRTH RATE | POPULATION OF UNITED STATES |
	TOTAL	WHITE	NONWHITE		
1968	3,503,000	2,912,000	589,000	17.5	200,000,000
1967	3,531,000	2,923,000	598,000	17.8	200,000,000
1963	4,098,000	3,326,000	639,000	21.7	189,375,000
1960	4,258,000	3,601,000	657,000	23.7	180,000,000
1954	4,078,000	3,475,000	603,000	25.3	162,409,000
1950	3,632,000	3,108,000	524,000	24.1	151,700,000
1940	2,559,000	2,199,000	360,000	19.4	132,100,000
1930	2,618,000	2,274,000	344,000	21.3	123,100,000

* Beginning 1959, includes Alaska, and beginning 1960, includes Hawaii.

† Refers to births occurring within the United States. Adjusted for underregistration 1930-1957. Figures rounded to nearest thousand.

SOURCES:

Birth Statistics: U.S. Department of Health, Education, and Welfare, Public Health Service, Health Services and Mental Health Administration, National Center for Health Statistics, Division of Vital Statistics.

Total Population: Department of Commerce, Bureau of the Census, Current Population Reports: 1968.

Neonatal Death Rate. The number of neonatal deaths per 1,000 live births

Fetal Death or "Stillbirth." One in which the infant of 20 weeks or more gestational age dies in utero prior to birth

Perinatal Mortality. The sum of deaths of fetuses and infants weighing 1,000 Gm. or over which occur between 28 weeks of gestation and 4 weeks of age (i.e., to the end of the neonatal period)

Infant Mortality Rate. The number of deaths before the first birthday per 1,000 live births

Maternal Mortality Rate. The number of maternal deaths per *100,000* live births

Race and Color.[9] Births in the United States are classified for vital statistics according to the race of the parents in the categories of white, Negro, American Indian, Chinese, Japanese, Aleut and Eskimo combined, Hawaiian and part-Hawaiian combined, and "other nonwhite." In most tables a less detailed classification of "white" and "nonwhite" is used.

The category "white" includes births to parents classified as white, Mexican, Puerto Rican or "not stated." If one parent is Hawaiian and the other is not, the birth is classified as part-Hawaiian. If one parent is Negro, and the other is not Hawaiian, the birth is classified as Negro. In other cases of mixed parentage in which both parents are nonwhite, the child is assigned the father's race; if the father is white, the child is assigned the mother's race.

NATALITY

The number of registered births in the United States has decreased appreciably in the last ten years, from over 4 million live births in 1957 to some 3½ million live births in 1968. The latter figure (for 1968) is at the same level as the total number of live births in 1950, when the population was substantially smaller (see Table 1-1). In 1947, immediately following World War II, there was a sharp rise in births, reaching a birth rate of 25.8, but after this peak the birth rate for the total population declined slightly and remained at about 25.0 during the next decade. The total number of live births in this country began to decline gradually in 1958. In 1963, while there were more than 4 million registered births, the birth rate decreased to 21.7. In 1968 there were less than 4 million live births in this country, with a birth rate of 17.5. At first glance these figures would seem almost unbelievable with the population of the United States almost 200 million in 1968. As in previous years the birth

[9] U. S. Department of Health, Education, and Welfare, Public Health Service, National Center for Health Statistics: Vital Statistics of the United States 1963, vol. 1, Natality, Washington, D. C., U. S. Government Printing Office, 1965.

TABLE 1-2. TOTAL FERTILITY RATES AND BIRTH RATES BY AGE OF MOTHER, BY COLOR: UNITED STATES, 1960-1968

[Total fertility rates are the sums of birth rates by age of mother multiplied by 5. Birth rates are live births per 1,000 women in specified group.]

YEAR AND COLOR	TOTAL FERTILITY RATE	AGE OF MOTHER							
		10-14 YEARS	15-19 YEARS	20-24 YEARS	25-29 YEARS	30-34 YEARS	35-39 YEARS	40-44 YEARS	45-49 YEARS
TOTAL—REGISTERED BIRTHS									
1968	2,476.8	1.0	66.1	167.4	140.3	74.9	35.6	9.6	0.6
1967	2,572.6	0.9	67.9	174.0	142.6	79.3	38.5	10.6	0.7
1966	2,736.1	0.9	70.6	185.9	149.4	85.9	42.2	11.7	0.7
1965	2,928.0	0.8	70.4	196.8	162.5	95.0	46.4	12.8	0.8
1964	3,207.5	0.9	72.8	219.9	179.4	103.9	50.0	13.8	0.8
1963	3,333.2	0.9	76.4	231.2	185.8	106.2	51.3	14.2	0.9
1962	3,473.5	0.8	81.2	243.7	191.7	108.9	52.7	14.8	0.9
1961	3,629.0	0.9	88.0	253.7	197.9	113.3	55.6	15.6	0.9
1960	3,653.6	0.8	89.1	258.1	197.4	112.7	56.2	15.5	0.9
WHITE—REGISTERED BIRTHS									
1968	2,368.4	0.4	55.3	162.2	139.7	72.5	33.8	8.9	0.5
1967	2,453.1	0.3	57.3	168.8	140.7	76.5	36.6	9.8	0.6
1966	2,609.2	0.3	60.8	179.9	146.6	82.7	40.0	10.8	0.7
1965	2,790.3	0.3	60.7	189.8	158.8	91.7	44.1	12.0	0.7
1964	3,073.7	0.3	63.2	213.1	176.2	100.5	47.7	13.0	0.7
1963	3,201.2	0.3	68.1	224.7	151.5	102.6	48.9	13.4	0.8
1962	3,347.5	0.4	73.1	238.0	187.7	105.2	50.2	14.1	0.8
1961	3,501.9	0.4	78.8	247.9	194.4	110.1	53.2	14.8	0.9
1960	3,532.9	0.4	79.4	252.8	194.9	109.6	54.0	14.7	0.8
NONWHITE—REGISTERED BIRTHS									
1968	3,196.9	4.4	133.3	200.8	144.8	91.2	48.6	15.0	1.2
1967	3,385.3	4.1	135.2	212.1	155.9	99.1	52.4	16.8	1.2
1966	3,614.9	4.0	135.5	228.9	169.3	107.9	57.7	18.4	1.4
1965	3,891.4	4.0	136.1	247.3	188.1	118.3	63.8	19.2	1.5
1964	4,153.4	4.0	138.7	268.6	202.0	127.5	67.5	20.9	1.5
1963	4,268.7	4.0	139.9	277.3	211.8	129.3	68.9	21.0	1.5
1962	4,395.8	3.9	144.6	285.7	217.4	132.4	72.0	21.7	1.5
1961	4,532.6	4.0	152.8	292.9	221.9	136.2	74.9	22.3	1.5
1960	4,522.1	4.0	158.2	294.2	214.6	135.6	74.2	22.0	1.7

U.S. Department of Health, Education, and Welfare, Public Health Service: Vital Statistics of the United States, 1968, Vol. I—Natality. Table 1-6, U.S. Government Printing Office, Washington, D.C., 1970.

rate ratios of white and of nonwhite population occur in about the same proportion (i.e., about 5 of every 7 births were white).

An important consideration which influences the number of children being born annually is the size and the age composition of the female population of childbearing age. Although the fertility rate is computed on the basis of births per one thousand women between the ages of 15 and 44, most of the childbearing is concentrated among women in their 20's. In 1968, for example, about three of every five births were to women who were between 20 and 29 years of age. In that same year there were an estimated 40.9 million women between the ages of 15 and 44, with a fertility rate of 85.7. The fertility rate has declined steadily since 1958, dropping from 122.9 births per one thousand women 15 to 44 years of age to a rate of 85.7 in 1966, the lowest since the end of World War II (see Table 1-2).

Another factor which influences the number of infants being born annually is the number of marriages. According to the provisional Vital Statistics for the United States, the total number of marriages in 1968 was 2,059,000, some 334,000 in excess of the 1964 figures. Moreover, this is 7.7 per cent over the total number of marriages in 1965 and explains why the rate of marriages per one thousand population reached 10.3, continuing the riisng trend of the last decade.

The frequency of multiple births is always a subject of great interest and bears mention in this brief discussion of natality. Of the 3,531,000 live births in the United States in 1967, some 68,336 were born in plural deliveries.

Over the years there has been a decline in the frequency of multiple births in the United States. The twin rate of the 1940's and the 1950's, 10.7 per one thousand deliveries, is lower than that of the 1920's and 1930's, and the 1964 twin rate of 10.1 per one thousand deliveries is lower than that of the 1950's. Changes in age and the racial composition of the population may contribute to some of this decline. We know that there are dif-

FIG. 1-5. Certificate of live birth used by Ohio State Department of Health. Similar forms are used by other cities and states.

ferences in the occurrence of twins depending on the age and the race of the mother. Furthermore, the incidence of twins is higher in the Negro population than in the white. There are also differences in the rate of twinning depending on the number of births the mother has had before delivery of the multiple birth. It should also be mentioned that there are differences between the rate of monozygotic, or identical twins, and dizygotic, or fraternal twins. The relative proportions of monozygotic and dizygotic twins are not the same for all races. The incidence of dizygotic twins is cited: white 60 per cent, Negro 70 per cent, Japanese 40 per cent. In the United States the twinning rate varies slightly from one region to another (e.g., the region with the highest rate of 10.5 is in the Northeast; the lowest rate, 9.4, is in the West).[10]

The Birth Certificate

In 1915 the Federal Government began to collect data on registered births and organized birth registration. At first only 10 states and the District of Columbia were included in this method of reporting births, but it gradually expanded so that by 1933 the entire country was included. The dependencies were admitted to the area: the Virgin Islands in 1924, the Territory of Hawaii in 1929, Puerto Rico in 1943 and Alaska in 1950. At the present time all 50 states and the District of Columbia demand that a birth certificate be filled out on every birth, and that it be submitted promptly to the local registrar. After the birth has been registered, the local registrar sends a notification to the parents of the child. Also, a complete report is forwarded from the local registrar to the state authorities, and then to the National Office of Vital Statistics in Washington.

Complete and accurate registration of births is a legal responsibility (see Fig. 1-5). The birth certificate gives evidence of age, citizenship and family relationships and as such often is required for military service, passports and even to collect benefits on retirement. On the basis of birth certificates, information which is essential to those agencies concerned with human reproduction is compiled by the National Office of Vital Statistics. The brief reports of statistics presented in this chapter are only a fraction of the volume of such studies compiled by that office.

POPULATION

The population of the United States more than doubled during the first half of this century, and has continued to grow in tremendous proportions as was predicted. Between the time of the 1950 census and mid-1967, the population of the United States grew from 151 million to over 200 million, the figure indicated by the United States Census Bureau projections for 1970. The predominant growth factor in this addition of some 49 million people in 17 years resulted from natural increases rather than international migration. This growth has required huge expenditures, both public and private, for such basic facilities as shelter, schools, and highways. The high birth rates of the 1940's and the early 1950's first produced pressures for expansion of elementary education, then for the expansion of secondary education facilities and, as we are aware now, for college facilities and jobs.

Three vital factors determine the rate at which population grows: births, deaths and migration. The decline in the death rate that was so apparent in the first half of this century has fluctuated near the same relatively low level (9.7 deaths per 1,000 population) for the last decade. Control of immigration began in this country about a half century ago, and even with recent modifications it still continues to exert an influence on this factor in our population growth. The 1963 report from the National Vital Statistics Division states that "the dynamic factor in population growth in the United States is, and will continue to be, the number of births—births of Native parentage."[11]

One should not be deceived by the falling birth rate, which at first glance gives the impression that there is no need to have any concern about a "population problem" in the United States. The impression left by the tabulation of birth rates is that the number of live births has been relatively stable. However, it must be remembered that the birth rate relates to the number of births *per 1,000 population*. Table 1-1 shows the relationship of live births to population of the United States since 1930. The number of infants added to the population during the 1950's was greater than for any previous decade in the Nation's history. Although the birth rate declined from 23.7 in 1960 to 17.5 in 1968, in those same years, the population increased by some 20,000,000 persons. The slight

[10] U. S. Department of Health, Education, and Welfare, National Center of Health Statistics. Vital and Health Statistics, Series 21, Number 14, Multiple Births, United States, 1964.

[11] U. S. Department of Health, Education, and Welfare, National Vital Statistics Division, Public Health Service: Indicators, March, 1963, Washington, D. C., U. S. Government Printing Office, 1963.

MATERNAL MORTALITY RATES BY COLOR:
BIRTH-REGISTRATION STATES, 1915-67

(Rates per 100,000 live births)

NOTE – Deaths each year are classified according to the International Lists used
at that time; for discussion of comparability, see Technical Appendix.

FIG. 1-6 (*Top*). Causes of maternal mortality, percentage distribution by cause, 1967. (Data from Vital Statistics of the United States, 1967, Vol. II—Mortality, Part A; Table 1-15, United States Department of Health, Education and Welfare, Public Health Service, 1969)

(*Bottom*). Maternal mortality by color: birth-registration states, 1915-1967. Deaths from complications of pregnancy, childbirth and the puerperium per 100,000 live births in the specified groups. (Data from Vital Statistics of the United States, 1967, Vol. II—Mortality, Part A, Table 1-16, United States Department of Health, Education and Welfare, Public Health Service, 1969)

decline in births we experienced in the 1960's is anticipated to continue for perhaps 2 or 3 years.

The decline in the annual number of births is partly related to the age and sex structure of the population. The majority of Americans are young. More than half are under 28 years of age, but the proportion is shifting because of the fluctuating birth rates. The young adult group, those in the age group 18 to 34, is now the fastest growing portion of the population, reflecting the high birth rates which followed World War II. This group, now 22 per cent of the total, will increase to 28.5 per cent of the total by 1980. The 40 to 50 year old segment of the population is not expected to increase proportionately, but moderately large increases are anticipated in the older age groups, that is, 65 years and over.

According to population projections made by the Bureau of the Census, during the next ten years the number of women of childbearing age will probably rise in this country. Further population growth is anticipated for the United States, but how much is uncertain. The population may total between 280 and 360 million by the year 2000, a gain of 80 to 160 million citizens in 33 years. The uncertainty as to how much the population will grow rises from the unpredictable number of children who will be born to contemporary young couples. Though their fertility potential is huge, much will depend upon whether they choose to hold the size of their families to the average of 3.4 children of 1966 or to reduce or increase that average.

MATERNAL MORTALITY

Maternal mortality refers to the deaths which occur as a direct result of childbearing; in other words, the underlying cause of the woman's death is the result of complications of pregnancy, childbirth or the puerperium.

During 1968 a total of 950 maternal deaths was registered in the United States (provisional statistics). It must be noted that the maternal mortality rate was computed in 1960 for the first time on the larger base of 100,000 live births. Prior to 1960, the computation was made on the base of 10,000 live births. The Bureau of Vital Statistics explains that such a change was made (i.e., presenting the rates per 100,000 live births) to facilitate a comparison of the differences in rates from one year to another in the categories in which frequencies are small.

The reduction in maternal mortality rates has been rather consistent since 1915 (Fig. 1-6).

The dramatic decline in these rates began about the mid-30's and continued until 1956. During the next succeeding 5 years the maternal mortality rate declined more slowly, reaching an all-time minimum in 1962. In 1963 the maternal death rate rose slightly to 35.8 per 100,000 live births, but resumed its decline the following year and reached a low rate of 28.0 in 1967.

The risk of maternal death for all mothers is lowest at ages 20 to 24 years (16.6 per 100,000 in 1967). It is slightly higher under 20 years of age, and from 25 years of age on. Increasing age is associated with a steep rise in maternal mortality. At 40 to 44 years of age, the mortality rate is 6 times greater than at 20 to 24. At the oldest age in the reproductive age span, 45 years or older, the mortality is 12½ times greater than the low figure.

The reduction in maternal mortality from the toxemias of pregnancy was the largest single factor responsible for the reduction in the total maternal mortality rate (from 82.7 per 100,000 live births in 1949-51 to a low of 27.4 in 1968). Hemorrhage and sepsis (cases other than abortion) were next in importance as conditions affecting the mortality rate. Subsequently, these three conditions will be discussed in detail, but it is important to stress the fact that deaths from these causes are for the most part preventable. Substantial achievements in maternity care have caused the death rate from puerperal infection and toxemias of pregnancy to fall more dramatically than from hemorrhage. Consequently, hemorrhage has become the predominant cause of death in childbirth. According to the *official classification,* only the direct cause of death is considered, even though the predisposing cause may be an important factor. For example, in a case in which the mother has a massive hemorrhage and then (in her weakened condition) develops a puerperal infection that eventually causes her death, the death is classified as due to puerperal infection. Hemorrhage is often a predisposing factor, and in this manner its toll in maternal mortality probably exceeds all other causes combined.

Puerperal infection is a wound infection of the birth canal after childbirth, which sometimes extends to cause phlebitis or peritonitis. The nurse can play an important role in helping to prevent such infections, not only in terms of flawless technique in performing nursing procedures, but also in protecting the mother from exposure to anyone with an infection.

The toxemias of pregnancy are certain disturbances peculiar to gravid women, characterized mainly by hypertension, edema, albuminuria and in some severe cases by convulsions and coma. Antepartal care plays an important role in prevention or early detection of symptoms, and with suitable treatment the disturbance often can be allayed.

Many factors are responsible for achieving the overall reduction in maternal mortality in this country during the past 25 years. Most important perhaps is the development of widespread training and educational programs in obstetrics which have provided more and better qualified specialists, professional nurses and other personnel in maternity programs. Better hospital facilities, multiple safeguards provided in the modern maternity hospitals and advances in therapy have all played major roles.

The distinct change in attitudes of doctors, nurses and parents also has contributed to this progressive saving of mothers. Childbirth is no longer an event to be awaited helplessly by the expectant mothers with what fortitude she is able to muster; instead, it is the climax of a period of preparation—a true state of preparedness attained through the cooperation of the physician, the nurse and the expectant mother or parents. As indicated before, this preparation for childbirth, based on careful medical and nursing supervision throughout pregnancy, is called antepartal (sometimes termed prenatal) care.

Antepartal care is one of the most important achievements in maternity care during the present century. It will be of interest to the nurse to know that this salutary contribution to the mother's welfare was initiated by the nursing profession. It had its beginning in 1901, when the Instructive Nursing Association in Boston began to pay antepartal visits to some of the expectant mothers who were to be delivered at the Boston Lying-In Hospital. This work gradually spread until, in 1906, all of these women prior to confinement were paid at least one visit by a nurse from the association. By 1912 this association was making about three antepartal visits to each patient. In 1907 another pioneer effort in prenatal work was instituted when George H. F. Schrader gave the Association for Improving the Condition of the Poor, New York City, funds to pay the salary of two nurses to do this work. In 1909 the Committee on Infant Social Service of the Women's Municipal League, Boston, organized an experiment in antepartal work. The pregnant women

TABLE 1-3. PERCENTAGE DISTRIBUTION OF LIVE BIRTHS BY ATTENDANT, BY COLOR:
UNITED STATES, EACH GEOGRAPHIC DIVISION, 1968*

GEOGRAPHIC DIVISION	IN HOSPITAL**	NOT IN HOSPITAL		
		BY PHYSICIAN	BY MIDWIFE	BY OTHER AND NOT SPECIFIED
United States	98.5	0.4	1.1	0.2
New England	99.8	0.2	—	0.0
Middle Atlantic	99.6	0.3	0.0	0.1
East North Central	99.5	0.3	0.0	0.2
West North Central	99.6	0.3	0.1	0.0
South Atlantic	97.3	0.5	2.0	0.2
East South Central	93.7	0.7	5.4	0.2
West South Central	96.8	0.3	2.6	0.2
Mountain	99.1	0.4	0.2	0.3
Pacific***	99.3	0.5	0.0	0.2

* Souce: Department of Health, Education, and Welfare. Vital Statistics of the United States, 1968, Vol. I, Washington, D.C., U.S. Government Printing Office, 1970. Based on data taken from Table 1-23, page 1-21.

** Includes all births in hospitals or institutions and births attended by physicians in clinics. A very large proportion of births in hospitals are attended by physicians.

*** Includes Alaska and Hawaii.

were visited every 10 days—oftener if necessary. Blood pressure readings and urine tests were made at each visit. This important work was limited because of the effort to make it as nearly self-supporting as possible; therefore, only mothers under the care of physicians and hospitals were accepted. Thus began this movement for ante-partal care which has done more than any other single effort to save mothers' lives in our time.

Another important factor in the reduction of maternal mortality has been the development of maternal and child health programs in State Departments of Public Health, particularly the work of public health nurses in maternal hygiene. These nurses visit a large number of the mothers who otherwise would receive little or no medical care, bringing them much-needed aid in pregnancy, labor and the puerperium. This service fills a great need not only in rural areas but also in metropolitan centers.

Still another factor responsible for the decline in maternal mortality is the trend toward hospitalization for childbirth—a trend that is gaining ground every year. In the early years of the century women rarely went to a hospital for such care. In 1935, 37 per cent of live births occurred in hospitals, and in 1963, 97.4 of the live births were attended by physicians in hospitals (see Table 1-3). This means that the percentage of hospital births has increased more than 2½ times during a 25-year period. In our larger cities the vast majority of babies are born in hospitals. This table also shows that in the United States, the great majority of women are attended by physicians in childbirth, some 98.2 per cent in 1963.

INFANT MORTALITY

The two groups of problems in infant mortality which are of chief concern in maternity care are (1) those in which the fetus dies in the uterus prior to birth (so-called stillbirth) and (2) those in which it dies within a short period of time after birth (neonatal death). The phrase *perinatal mortality* often is used to designate all deaths in these two categories.

In May, 1950, in an effort to end confusion arising from usage of a variety of terms such as stillbirth, abortion, miscarriage, etc., the World Health Organization recommended the adoption of the following definition of fetal death:

Fetal death is a death prior to complete expulsion or extraction from its mother of a product of conception, irrespective of duration of pregnancy; the death is indicated by the fact that after such separation, the fetus does not breathe or show any other evidence of life such as beating of the heart, pulsation of the umbilical cord, or definite movement of voluntary muscles.[12]

WHO further defined fetal death by indicating four subgroups, according to gestation age in weeks.

[12] National Summaries: Fetal Deaths, U. S., 1954, National Office of Vital Statistics, vol. 44, No. 11, August 17, 1956.

In the United States in 1963 there was reported a total of 103,390 infant deaths before the first birthday. Approximately 10 per cent of the infant deaths occurred on the first day after birth and 72 per cent under 28 days of age. The great toll taken in the first day of life in this country can be compared with the number of deaths occurring in the rest of the first year (Figs. 1-7—9). The relatively favorable health conditions experienced by the general population of the United States in 1963 were reflected in a decline in the infant mortality rate to the lowest figure on record for this

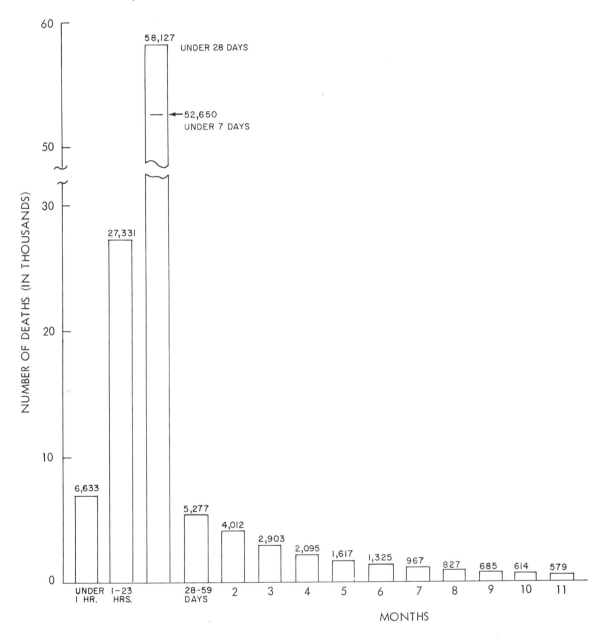

Fig. 1-7. Infant mortality by age, United States, 1967. Note the magnitude of neonatal deaths (under 28 days) as compared with mortality in later months.

In 1968 the total number of registered infant deaths under 1 year was 76,263. (Data from U.S. Department of Health, Education, and Welfare, Public Health Service, Health Services and Mental Health Administration, National Center for Health Statistics, Division of Vital Statistics.)

country. The neonatal mortality rate for 1968 was 16.1, the lowest it ever has been. Despite the fact that the reduction in infant mortality is indeed gratifying, it is not comparable with the fall in maternal mortality in the United States. Moreover, when it is compared with other infant mortality rates throughout the world, the United States ranks 15th.*

---

* The United States dropped to 15th place among 15 modern industrial countries in 1969.

A consideration of the infant losses is incomplete unless the potential lives lost because of fetal death also is considered. In 1968 there were 55,293 fetal deaths (so-called stillbirths) reported. These deaths added to the 56,456 neonatal deaths in 1967 show the overwhelming sum of 111,749 infant losses associated with pregnancy, labor and the early weeks of life.

Many causes are responsible for this staggering infant mortality. The vast number of infant deaths is the result of several main causes: pre-

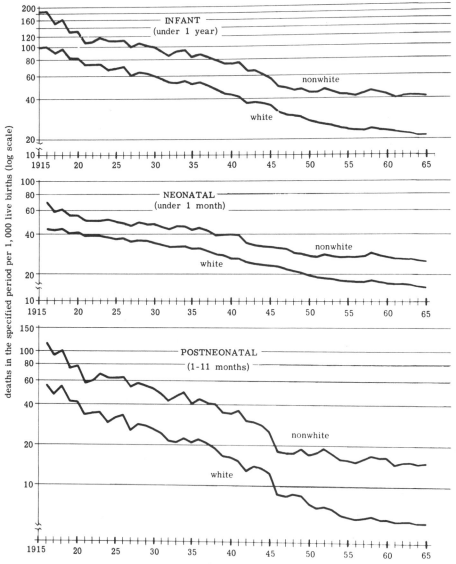

Fig. 1-8. Mortality rate of white and nonwhite infants by age, United States, 1915-1965 (birth registration area). (United States Department of Health, Education, and Welfare, Social and Rehabilitation Service, Children's Bureau. Data from United States Public Health Service, National Center for Health Statistics.) (Nelson, W. E. (ed.): Textbook of Pediatrics. ed. 9, Philadelphia, W. B. Saunders, 1969)

TABLE 1-4. CAUSES OF NEONATAL MORTALITY, UNITED STATES, 1967 *

CAUSE OF DEATH**	NUMBER OF DEATHS		
	TOTAL	WITH IMMATURITY	WITHOUT MENTION OF IMMATURITY
All causes	58,127	. . . .	. . . .
Certain diseases of early infancy:	47,382	. . . .	. . . .
Birth injuries	6,555	4,168	2,387
Postnatal asphyxia and atelectasis	12,536	9,283	3,253
Pneumonia of the newborn	2,219	593	1,626
Diarrhea of the newborn	222	36	186
Other infections of the newborn	817	387	430
Neonatal disorders arising from certain diseases of mother during pregnancy	532	329	203
Hemolytic disease of newborn (erythroblastosis)	1,186	364	822
Hemorrhagic disease of newborn	514	236	278
Ill-defined disease peculiar to early infancy, including nutritional maladjustment	9,821	7,948	1,873
Immaturity with mention of any other subsidiary condition	1,138	. . . .	. . . .
Immaturity, unqualified	11,842	. . . .	. . . .
Congenital malformations	7,850	. . . .	. . . .

* Department of Health, Education, and Welfare: Vital Statistics of the United States, 1967, vol. II, Part A, Table 2-10, Washington, D.C., U.S. Government Printing Office, 1969.

** Classified according to the Seventh Revision of International Lists, 1955.

mature birth, asphyxia and atelectasis, congenital malformations and birth injuries.

During the first 4 weeks of life prematurity is the most important cause of death (Table 1-4). Birth injuries, another of the main causes of infant loss, accounted for almost 7,000 infant deaths in 1967. Almost one third of these deaths were due to intracranial and spinal injury at birth; for example, cerebral injury as a result of anoxia in utero or traumatic injury to the brain suffered in passing through the birth canal. In the vast majority of these cases death occurred under 7 days of life. Congenital malformations was another cause of some 7,850 neonatal deaths in 1967. Subsequently, these conditions will be discussed in detail. It suffices to say that one of the first and most important of them, prematurity, is largely a nursing problem. Indeed, in all the wide range of nursing care there is no area which offers such a challenge to the nurse or such lifesaving possibilities as that of caring for the premature infant.

The welfare of some 4,000,000 babies born annually in the United States is very much the concern of maternity nurses and obstetricians and one of the main objectives of the entire field of maternity care. To reduce the enormous loss of newborn lives, to protect the infant not only at birth, but also in the prenatal period and during the early days of the life of the infant, to lay a solid foundation for his health throughout life—these are the problems and the challenge.

Abortion

The vast number of infants lost by abortion, the spontaneous or artificial termination of pregnancy prior to the period of viability, is a matter of grave importance (see Chap. 19). The abortion rate in this country exceeds stillbirths and neonatal deaths in fetal wastage. About 10 per cent of all pregnancies terminate in spontaneous abortion due to such factors as faulty germ plasm; unsatisfactory environmental conditions, hormonal and otherwise; many unknown etiologic causes; and an unknown number of criminal interruptions.

CURRENT PROBLEMS IN MATERNITY CARE

An orientation to maternity nursing would be incomplete without calling attention to the broad problems in maternity care which reflect on the childbearing potential of families in the United States. In 1965 Dr. Arthur Lesser, the Deputy Chief of the United States Children's Bureau, made the analogy that some of the current problems in maternal and child care are like the old moving pictures shown on TV: "They are old and familiar. The problems which faced us 25 years ago are the same today."[13]

Today the problems for the United States as a whole reflect also a symptom of the far-reaching social changes since the last war. The tremendous reduction in maternal and infant mortality rates presents concrete evidence of the noteworthy progress that has been achieved in maternity care in this country. Nevertheless, the problems of maternity care which are currently a major cause of concern relate to the kind of maternity care that a large segment of our population is receiving. Maternal and infant mortality rates are valuable

[13] Lesser, A. J.: Current problems in maternal and child care. Paper presented at First Ohio Congress, Maternal and Child Health, Columbus, Ohio, March 3, 1965.

in analyzing the current problems; moreover, they help to identify some of the areas in which difficulties exist.

Infant mortality has continued to decrease; in fact, the lowest figure on record for this country was recorded in 1961, when the infant mortality rate reached 25.3 (deaths under 1 year per 1,000 live births). Although the decline in infant mortality during the previous decade was substantial, 11 per cent, the greatest percentage of this decline was achieved between 1950 and 1955. In addition, 7 of the 10 largest cities had significant increases in infant mortality, increases ranging as high as 26.4 per cent, with infant mortality rates exceeding the national average of 26.0. Although the overall maternal mortality has been reduced dramatically in the last 35 years, in 1963 the maternal death rate rose slightly to 35.8 per 100,000 live births—1.7 per cent above the comparable figure for the previous year (Fig. 1-6).

Fig. 1-9. Infant mortality rates by color: United States, 1967. (Data from Vital Statistics of the United States, 1967, Vol. II—Mortality, Part A, United States Department of Health, Education and Welfare, Public Health Service, 1969)

The needs resulting from problems of maternal and child health in rural areas continue today, but what is new and alarming is that now there is a parallel situation in the larger cities.

Since the last war major shifts in population have occurred; urban middle-class families have migrated to suburban areas, whereas large numbers of families from rural areas have moved to the large urban industrial areas. Despite the increase in employment and in income generally, the population still includes a large segment of disadvantaged, low-income families who recently have concentrated in the major cities. With the increased cost of health services in general and the cost of hospital care in particular, these low-income families are straining the local resources of the communities in which they reside. Also, the number of maternity patients in these areas has greatly increased as a result of migration, producing overcrowding of clinics and hospital maternity in-service divisions. To accommodate such large numbers of maternity patients, many of the hospitals with large maternity services have had to resort to limiting the mother's hospital stay, some women being discharged 24 hours after delivery. The most serious problem by far is that many of these women are receiving poor or, often, no antepartal care, due in part to dissatisfaction with the kind of care provided. Inadequate care during pregnancy has been demonstrated to bear a direct relationship to the rate of prematurity (see Chap. 17).

It has been mentioned already that social factors play a role in morbidity and mortality and in fact influence the reproduction efficiency of childbearing women.

Much of the difficulty in providing adequate care is due to a shortage of professional personnel (i.e., there are not enough physicians, nurses and social workers to provide the necessary services for maternity patients). The rapid growth of the population has not been accompanied by a proportionate increase in physicians and nurses. This shortage is compounded by the fact that not enough physicians and nurses are being attracted into this area of specialization. Student nurses might well investigate the reason for this apathy and in good time provide some solution to this problem.

In a previous paper Dr. Arthur Lesser summarized some of the recommendations which were proposed on the national level to alleviate the current problems of maternity care. A part of the summary states:

The problems of maternity care led the President's Panel on Mental Retardation to make them the focus of one of its major recommendations. The Panel urged that a new program be established with Federal funds authorized on a project basis to assist state and local health departments in meeting the costs of administering programs of comprehensive maternity and infant care for women who have problems associated with pregnancy which increase the hazards of childbearing for themselves and for their infants and who are unlikely to receive the care they need because of low income or for other reasons. These programs would make it possible to:

1. increase the number of prenatal and post-natal clinics,

2. bring the prenatal and postpartum clinics close to the population served,

3. establish special clinics for some patients with complications of pregnancy (where more time by obstetricians, nurses, social workers, nutritionists and others can be provided),

4. pay for hospital care not only for the delivery but also during the prenatal period as needed,

5. relieve overcrowding in tax-supported hospitals by paying for care in voluntary hospitals,

6. pay for hospital care of premature infants and other infants needing special attention,

7. provide consultation services.

The Panel also recommended that the Children's Bureau support some comprehensive demonstration programs, including the provision of long-range child health supervision, especially among families which lack motivation, are apathetic and uncooperative.[14]

These and other recommendations related to the work of the Children's Bureau were enacted into legislation in 1963 with the maternal and the child health and the mental retardation amendments to the Social Security Act. The maternity care provisions of this statute authorize grants not only for new programs in preventive service, care, treatment and research but also provide for increased grants to the states for maternal and child health services, beginning in 1964. The funds are granted to the various state health departments or, with their agreement, directly to a local health department. These grants are for support of medical care programs—they are not demonstration projects—and upon request are granted to specific areas where they are most needed (see Suggested Reading).

---

[14] Lesser, A. J.: Current Problems of Maternity Care, pp. 8-9, Washington, D. C., U. S. Department of Health, Education, and Welfare, Welfare Administration, Children's Bureau, 1963.

SUGGESTED READING

Anderson, E. H., and Lesser, A. J.: Maternity care in the United States: gains and gaps. Am. J. Nurs., 66:1539-1544, July, 1966.

Baird, Sir Dugold: The social aspect of obstetric practice. Obstet. Gynec. Survey 20:410-430, June, 1965.

Bruce, S. J., and Hall, E.: Maternity and pediatric nurses study and work together. Am. J. Nurs. 63: 105-108, March, 1963.

Chambers, W.: Nursing diagnosis. Am. J. Nurs. 62: 102-104, November, 1962.

Children's Bureau: Five Decades of Action for Children (Pub. No. 3581). Washington, D. C., U. S. Government Printing Office, 1962.

Children and Youth at the Mid-Decade. Children 12: entire issue, March-April, 1965.

Close, K.: Giving babies a healthy start in life. Children 12, No. 5:179-184, September-October, 1965.

Dunn, H. L.: High-Level Wellness. Arlington, Virginia, R. W. Beatty, 1961.

————: High-level wellness for man and society. Am. J. Public Health, 49:786-792, June, 1959.

Duvall, E. M.: Family Development. ed. 3, Philadelphia, J. B. Lippincott, 1967.

Freeman, V. J.: Human aspects of health and illness: beyond the germ theory, in Folta, J. R. and Deck, E. F.: A Sociological Framework for patient care. New York, John Wiley, 1966, pp. 83-89.

Goodwin, B.: What is Maternity Nursing?, in Jeffries, J. E. (ed.): Can Maternity Nursing Meet Today's Challenge?, Ross Round Table on Maternal and Child Nursing, pp. 45-51. Columbus, Ross Laboratories, 1967.

Harpine, F.: Concepts in maternal and child health. Am. J. Nurs. 63:84-87, March, 1963.

Hendricks, C. H.: Delivery patterns and reproductive efficiency among groups of differing socioeconomic status and ethnic origins. Am. J. Obstet. Gynec. 90:608-624, March 1, 1967.

Herzog, E., and Bernstein, R.: Health Services for Unmarried Mothers. Children's Bureau Publication No. 425, Washington, D. C., U. S. Government Printing Office, 1964.

Hilleboe, H. E.: Public health in the United States in the 1970's. Am. J. Public Health 58:1588, September, 1968.

Hogan, A.: The role of the nurse in meeting needs of the new mother, Nurs. Clin. N. Am. 3:337-344, June, 1968.

Jacobson, H. and Reid, D. E.: A pattern of comprehensive maternal and child care. New Eng. J. Med. 271:243-249, July 30, 1964.

————: A pattern of comprehensive maternal and child care. New Eng. J. Med. 271:302-307, August 6, 1964.

Johnson, D. E.: The nature of a science of nursing, Nurs. Outlook 7:291-294, May, 1959.

————: A philosophy of nursing, Nurs. Outlook 7:198-200, April, 1959.

Keettel, W. Z.: An Appraisal of Maternity Care in Iowa. J.A.M.A. 207:721-723, January 27, 1969.

Kenneth, H. Y.: Community nursing service to the "well Family," in ANA Clinical Sessions. The American Nurses' Association 1968, Dallas, pp. 72-79, New York, Appleton-Century-Crofts, 1968.

Kreuter, F. R.: What is good nursing care? Nurs. Outlook 5:302-304, May, 1957.

Lemat, A.: The public health nurse in maternity service. Nurs. Outlook 12:58-61, October, 1964.

Lesser, A.: Concepts and content of maternal and infant care projects from a national view point, Am. J. Public Health 56:725-733, May, 1966.

Lesser, A. J.: Accent on prevention through improved service. Children 2:13-18, January-February, 1964.

————: Current Problems of Maternity Care, Washington, D. C., U. S. Children's Bureau, 1963.

Lesser, M. S., and Keane, V. R.: Nurse-Patient Relationships in a Hospital Maternity Service. St. Louis, C. V. Mosby, 1956.

Lock, F. R.: The right to be well born: quality versus quantity in obstetrics and gynecology, Am. J. Obstet. Gynec. 105:651-688, November 1, 1969.

Malinowski, B.: Parenthood—the basis of social structure, in Sussman, M. B. (ed.): Sourcebook in Marriage and the Family. pp. 40-48, Boston, Houghton, 1963.

Maternity Center Association: Meeting the Childbearing Needs of Families in a Changing World. New York, [Maternity Center] The Association, 1960.

————: The Forty-Fifth Annual Report, New York, [Maternity Center] The Association, 1965.

Melber, R. B.: An approach for evaluating and improving maternity nursing and care, in ANA Clinical Sessions, The American Nurses' Association 1968, Dallas, pp. 181-189, New York, Appleton-Century-Crofts, 1968.

Monahan, H. B., and Spencer, E. C.: Deterrents to prenatal care. Children 9:114-119, May-June, 1962.

Murray, B. L., McConnell, N., and Claypool, J. M.: Implications for learning: persistent aspects of maternal-child nursing situations. J. Nurs. Ed. 2:5-9, 22-24, February-March, 1963.

Oettinger, K. B.: This Most Profound Challenge, U. S. Department of Health, Education, and Welfare, Welfare Administration, Children's Bureau, 1965.

Peckham, B. M.: Optimal maternal care. Obstet. Gynec. 33:862-868, June, 1969.

Peerboon, P.: Major Trends in Health, Education, and Welfare, in U. S. Department of Health, Education, and Welfare: Health, Education, and Welfare Trends. Part 1, pp. 1-24, National Trends, 1966-67.

Peplau, H. E.: Interpersonal techniques: the crux of psychiatric nursing. Am. J. Nurs. 62:50-54, June, 1962.

Pollak, O.: Some Challenges to the American Family. Children 2:19-20, January-February, 1964.

Reeder, S. J. and Reeder, L. G.: Some correlates of prenatal care among low income and unwed women. Am. J. Obstet. Gynec. 90:1304-1314, December 15, 1964.

Robinson, D.: Obstetrical care and social patterns in metropolitan Boston. Public Health Rep. 82:117, February, 1967.

Roemer, M. I.: Governmental health programs affecting the American family. Journal of Marriage and the Family 29:40-63, February, 1967.

Rosen, M., et al.: The quality of reproduction in an urban indigent population. Obstet. Gynec. 31: 276-282, February, 1968.

Rubin, R.: Maternity care in our society. Nurs. Outlook 11:519-522, July, 1963.

Shapiro, S., Schlesinger, E. R., and Nesbitt, R. E. L., Jr.: Infant, Perinatal, Maternal, and Childhood Mortality in the United States, Cambridge: Harvard University Press, 1968.

Shyne, A. W., et al.: Evaluating public health nursing service to the maternity patient. Nurs. Outlook 11:56-58, January, 1963.

Sussman, M. B.: The isolated nuclear family: fact or fiction? in Sussman, M. B. (ed.): Sourcebook in Marriage and the Family. pp. 48-53, Boston, Houghton, 1963.

Taylor, H. C., Jr.: Once again retrospect and prospect, Am. J. Obstet. Gynec. 87:839-847, December 1, 1963.

U. S. Children's Bureau: It's Your Children's Bureau. Publication No. 357, Washington, D. C., U. S. Department of Health, Education, and Welfare, 1964.

U. S. Department of Commerce, Bureau of the Census: Current Population Reports: Population Estimates, Series P-25, Washington, D. C., U. S. Government Printing Office, 1969.

U. S. Department of Commerce, Bureau of the Census: 200 Million Americans. Washington, D. C., U. S. Government Printing Office, November, 1967.

U. S. Department of Health, Education, and Welfare: Health, Education, and Welfare Trends, 1966-67, Washington, D. C., U. S. Government Printing Office, 1967.

U. S. Department of Health, Education, and Welfare: The President's Panel on Mental Retardation: A Proposed Program for National Action to Combat Mental Retardation; Report to the President, October 1962, Washington, D. C., U. S. Government Printing Office, 1963.

———: Health, Education, and Welfare Trends, 1966-67 ed., Washington, D. C., U. S. Government Printing Office, 1967.

———: Vital Statistics of The United States 1967, Vols. I and II, Washington, D. C., U. S. Government Printing Office, 1969.

———: Vital Statistics of the United States, Vols. I and II, Washington, D. C., U. S. Government Printing Office, 1967.

Wallace, H. M.: Health Services for Mothers and Children. Philadelphia, W. B. Saunders, 1962.

Wessel, M. A.: A physician looks at maternity nursing. Bull. Am. Coll. Nurs. Midwifery 9:44-45, Fall, 1964.

Wooden, H. E.: Impact of the industrial revolution on hospital maternity care. Nurs. Forum 1:90, Winter, 1961-1962.

———: The family-centered approach to maternity care. Nurs. Forum 1:61-77, Spring, 1962.

World Health Organization: Manual of the International Statistical Classification of Diseases, Injuries and Causes of Death, 7th rev. of the Lists of Diseases, Injuries and Causes of Death, Geneva, Switzerland, World Health Organization, 1957.

———: First Report of Expert Committee on Maternity Care, WHO Technical Report Series, No. 51, Geneva, Switzerland, World Health Organization, 1952.

———: Social Aspects in the Teaching of Obstetrics and Gynecology, WHO Technical Report Series, No. 266, Geneva, Switzerland, World Health Organization, 1963.

Anatomy Related to the Reproductive System

2

Pelvis • Female Organs of Reproduction • Mammary Glands
Male Organs of Reproduction

PELVIS

The pelvis, so called from its resemblance to a basin (*pelvis,* a basin), is a bony ring interposed between the trunk and the thighs. The vertebral column, or backbone, passes into it from above, transmitting to it the weight of the upper part of the body, which the pelvis in turn transmits to the lower limbs. From an obstetric point of view, however, we have to consider it as the cavity which contains the generative organs, and particularly as the canal through which the baby must pass during birth.

Structure

The pelvis is made up of four united bones: the two hip bones (*os coxae* or innominate) situated laterally and in front, and the sacrum and the coccyx behind (Figs. 2-1 to 3). Anatomically, the hip bones are divided into three parts: the ilium, the ischium and the pubis. These bones become firmly joined into one by the time the growth of the body is completed (i.e., at about the age of 20 to 25), so that on examining them in the prepared pelvis no trace of the original edges or divisions of these three bones can be discovered. Each of these bones may be roughly described as follows.

The ilium, which is the largest portion of the bones, forms the upper and back part of the pelvis. Its upper flaring border forms the prominence of the hip or crest of the ilium (hip bone). The ischium is the lower part below the hip joint; from it projects the tuberosity of the ischium on

which the body rests when in a sitting posture. The pubis is the front part of the hip bone; it extends from the hip joint to the joint in front between the two hip bones, the symphysis pubis, and then turns down toward the ischial tuberosity, thus forming with the bone of the opposite side the arch below the symphysis, the pubic or subpubic arch. This articulation closes anteriorly the cavity of the pelvis.

The sacrum and the coccyx form the lowest portions of the spinal column. The former is a triangular wedge-shaped bone, consisting of five vertebrae fused together; it serves as the back part of the pelvis. The coccyx forms a tail end to the spine. In the child the coccyx consists of four or five very small, separate vertebrae; in the adult these bones are fused into one. The coccyx is usually movable at its attachment to the sacrum (the sacrococcygeal joint) and may become pressed back during labor to give more room for the passage of the fetal head.

Of special importance is the marked projection which is formed by the junction of the last lumbar vertebra with the sacrum; this is known as the sacral promontory and is one of the most important landmarks in obstetric anatomy.

Articulation and Surfaces

The articulations (joints) of the pelvis, which possess obstetric importance, are 4 in number. Two are behind, between the sacrum and the ilia on either side, and are termed the sacro-iliac articulations (Fig. 2-1 A); one is in front between the two pubic bones and is called the symphysis pubis (Fig. 2-1 B), and the fourth, of little consequence, is between the sacrum and coccyx, the sacrococcygeal articulation (Fig. 2-1 C).

All of these articular surfaces are lined with fibrocartilage, which becomes thickened and softened during pregnancy; likewise, the ligaments which bind the pelvic joints together become softened, and as a result greater mobility of the pelvic bones develops. A certain definite though very limited motion in the joints is desirable for a normal labor; however, there is no change in the actual size of the pelvis. From a practical standpoint, one of the most important facts for the nurse to know about these joints is that the increased mobility which they develop in pregnancy produces a slight "wobbliness" in the pelvis and throws greater strain on the surrounding muscles and ligaments. This accounts in large part for the frequency of backache and legache in the latter months of pregnancy.

The pelvis is lined with muscular tissue which provides a smooth, somewhat cushioned surface over which the fetus has to pass during labor; these muscles also help to support the abdominal contents.

Divisions

Regarded as a whole, the pelvis may be described as a two-storied, bony basin that is divided by a natural line of division (the inlet or brim) into two parts. The upper part is called the false pelvis and the lower part is called the true pelvis (see Fig. 2-4).

The false pelvis, or upper flaring part, is much less concerned with the problems of labor than is the true pelvis, but it is considered in obstetrics because it offers certain landmarks for the practice of pelvimetry or pelvic measurements, and because its shape and inclination aid in estimating the nature of the true pelvis. It also supports the uterus during late pregnancy and directs the fetus into the true pelvis at the proper time.

The true pelvis, or lower part, forms the bony canal through which the baby must pass during parturition; for convenience in description it is divided into three parts: an inlet or brim, a cavity and an outlet.

Pelvic Inlet. Continuous with the sacral promontory and extending along the ilium on each side in circular fashion is a ridge called the linea terminalis (brim). This bounds an area or plane

Fig. 2-1. Pelvis. (A) Sacro-iliac articulations. (B) Symphysis pubis. (C) Sacrococcygeal articulation.

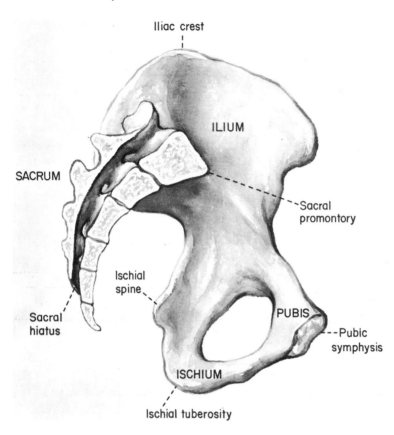

Iliac crest

ILIUM

SACRUM

Sacral
promontory

Ischial
spine

Sacral
hiatus

PUBIS

Pubic
symphysis

ISCHIUM

Ischial tuberosity

FIG. 2-2. Lateral view of left innominate bone showing its 3 constituent parts (erect position).

called the inlet, so named because it is the entry-way or inlet through which the baby's head must pass in order to enter the true pelvis. The pelvic inlet, sometimes also referred to as the pelvic brim or superior strait, divides the false from the true pelvis. It is roughly heart-shaped, the promontory of the sacrum forming a slight projection into it from behind (Fig. 2-5); it is widest from side to side, and narrowest from back to front (i.e., from the sacral promontory to the symphysis). It should be noted particularly that the baby's head enters the inlet with its longest diameter (antero-posterior) in the transverse diameter of the pelvis. In other words, as shown in Figure 2-5, the greatest diameter of the head accommodates itself to the greatest diameter of the inlet. As the inlet is entirely surrounded by bone, it cannot be measured directly with the examining fingers in a living woman. However, the measurements of its anteroposterior diameter can be estimated on the basis of the diagonal conjugate diameter (see Figs. 2-21, 22).

The measurements of these diameters are very important, since variations from the normal (e.g., smaller in size or flattened) may cause grave difficulty at the time of labor (see p. 484).

Pelvic Outlet. When viewed from below, the pelvic outlet is a space bounded in front by the symphysis pubis and the pubic arch, at the sides by the ischial tuberosities, and behind by the coccyx and the greater sacrosciatic ligaments (Fig. 2-6). It requires only a little imagination to see that the front half of the outlet resembles a triangle, the base of which is the distance between the ischial tuberosities, and the other two sides of which are represented by the pubic arch. From an obstetric point of view, this triangle is of great importance, since the baby's head must make use of this space to gain exit from the pelvis and the mother's body (Fig. 2-6). For this reason Nature has provided a wide pubic arch in females, whereas in males it is narrow (see Fig. 2-14). If the pubic arch in women were as narrow as it is in men, natural childbearing would be extremely difficult, since the baby's head, unable to squeeze itself into the narrow anterior triangle of the out-let, would be forced backward against the coccyx and the sacrum, where its progress would be impeded.

As has been stated, the greatest diameter of the inlet is the transverse (from side to side), whereas the greatest diameter of the outlet is the anteroposterior (from front to back) (Fig. 2-7). Moreover, the baby's head, as it emerges from the pelvis, passes through the outlet in the anteroposterior position, again accommodating its greatest diameter to the greatest diameter of the passage. Since the baby's head enters the pelvis in the transverse position and emerges in the anteroposterior, it is obvious that the head must rotate some 90° as it passes through the pelvis. This process of rotation of the baby's head is one of the most important phases of the mechanism of labor and will be discussed in more detail later on pages 222 and 223.

Pelvic Cavity. This is the space between the inlet above, the outlet below and the anterior, the posterior and the lateral walls of the pelvis. The pelvic canal is practically cylindric in shape in its upper portion and curved only in its lower half. It is important to note the axis of the cavity when viewed from the side (Fig. 2-9). It is apparent that during the delivery the head must descend along the downward prolongation of the axis until it nearly reaches the level of the ischial spines and then begins to curve forward. The axis of the cavity determines the direction which the baby takes through the pelvis in the process of delivery. As might be expected, labor is made more complicated by this curvature in the pelvic canal, because the baby has to accommodate itself to the curved path as well as to the variations in the size of the cavity at different levels.

Pelvic Variations

The pelvis presents great individual variations—no two pelves are exactly alike. Even those patients with normal measurements may present differences in contour and muscular development which influence the actual size of the pelvis. These varying differences are due in part

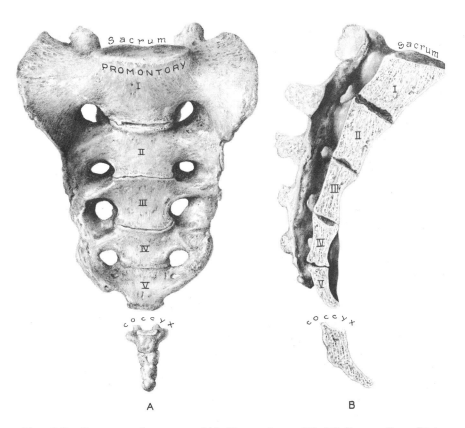

A   B

Fig. 2-3. Sacrum and coccyx. (A) Front view. (B) Median section. Note how promontory of sacrum juts forward.

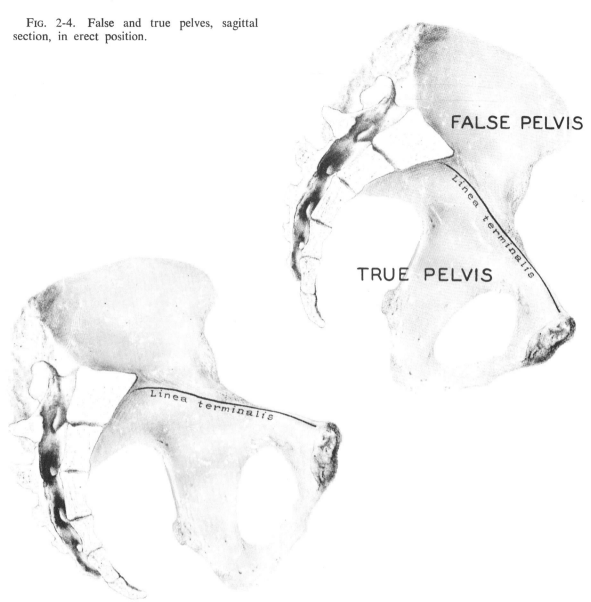

FIG. 2-4. False and true pelves, sagittal section, in erect position.

FALSE PELVIS

TRUE PELVIS

Linea terminalis

Linea terminalis

to heredity, disease, injury and development. Heredity may be responsible for passing on many racial and sexual differences. Such diseases as tuberculosis and rickets cause malformations. Accidents and injuries during childhood or at maturity result in deformities of the pelvis or other parts of the body which affect the pelvis. Adequate nutrition and well-formed habits related to posture and exercise have a very definite influence on the development of the pelvis.

It must be remembered also that the pelvis does not mature until between the ages of 20 and 25 years, and until that time complete ossification has not taken place.

There are many so-called borderline cases of abnormal pelvic development. Such pregnant patients should be supervised closely. At periodic intervals the size of the fetus is estimated (by palpation of the abdomen), and definite arrangements are made for the type of delivery indicated.

There are several **types of pelves.** Even pelves whose measurements are normal differ greatly in the shape of the inlet, in the proximity of the greatest transverse diameter of the inlet to the

FIG. 2-5. Largest diameter of baby's head entering largest diameter of inlet (as viewed from above). Therefore it enters transversely.

FIG. 2-6. Measurements of the inlet of a normal female pelvis, showing the 4 diameters: the anteroposterior, the transverse, and the 2 oblique diameters. The diameters shown with broken lines indicate transverse measurements of the false pelvis.

FIG. 2-7. Largest diameter of baby's head passing through largest diameter of outlet (as viewed from below). Therefore it passes through outlet antero-posteriorly.

FIG. 2-8. Measurement of the outlet, showing transverse diameter in a normal female pelvis.

sacral promontory, in the size of the sacrosciatic notch, and in their general architecture. Dr. H. C. Moloy and the late Dr. W. E. Caldwell, of the Sloane Hospital for Women, New York City, have utilized these characteristics in establishing a classification of pelves which has been of great interest and value to obstetricians. The four main types, according to this classification, are shown in Figures 2-10 to 13. The manner in which the baby passes through the birth canal and, consequently, the type of labor vary considerably in these pelvic types.

In addition, of course, there are many pelvic types which result from abnormal narrowing of one or the other diameters. These contracted pelves will be described in a subsequent chapter (see p. 484).

In comparing the male and the female pelves, several differences will be observed (Fig. 2-14). As already emphasized, the most conspicuous difference is in the pubic arch, which has a much wider angle in women. The symphysis is shorter in women, and the border of the arch probably is more everted. Although the female pelvis is more shallow, it is more capacious than the male, much lighter in structure and smoother. The male pelvis is deep, compact, conical and rougher in texture, particularly at the site of muscle attachments. The findings of Drs. Daniel G. Morton and Charles T. Hayden, of San Francisco, indicate that both males and females start life with pelves which are identical in type, and that the major differences observed in adult male and female pelves do not appear until puberty and are therefore due to the influence of the sex hormones. (For definition and description of the sex hormones, see pp. 58-60, 63.)

Pelvic Measurements

Importance of Pelvic Measurements. The entire problem in childbirth centers on the safe pas-

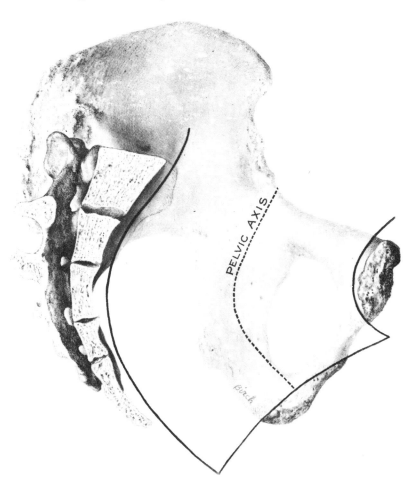

Fig. 2-9. Pelvic cavity. Heavy black line indicates location of soft parts, vagina, etc.

sage of the fully developed fetus through the pelvis of the mother. Slight irregularities in the structure of the pelvis may delay the progress of labor, while any marked deformity may render the delivery by the natural passages impossible. For these reasons the pelvis of every pregnant woman should be measured accurately in the antepartal period to enable the physician to determine before labor begins whether or not there is anything in the condition of the mother's pelvis that may complicate the delivery. This examination is a part of the antepartal examination. In addition to a general physical examination, the pelvic measure-ments are made and compared with the dimensions of the normal pelvis.

Types of Pelvic Measurements. Physicians rely chiefly on internal and external pelvic measurements, made manually, as a means of estimating the size of the pelvis. In occasional instances, however, x-ray pelvimetry may be desirable (see p. 39). In the majority of abnormal pelves the most marked deformity affects the anteroposterior diameter of the inlet. It has long been a practice to determine a number of external measurements of the pelvis (intercristal diameter, interspinous diameter, intertrochanteric diameter, external con-

(*Left*) Fig. 2-10. Gynecoid (normal female) pelvis. Inlet is well rounded in hind- and fore-pelvis (A, B). Sacrosciatic notch is curved, moderate in width and depth (C).

(*Right*) Fig. 2-11. Anthropoid pelvis. Inlet is deep in hind- and fore-pelvis, increased in antero-posterior diameter (A, B). Sacrosciatic notch is broad, shallow (C).

(Roentgenograms from W. E. Caldwell, M.D., and H. C. Moloy, M.D., Sloane Hospital for Women, New York) jugate) with an instrument called a pelvimeter, in the belief that they permit an approximate estimation of the size of the inlet (Figs. 2-15 to 20). Authorities today (among them Greenhill, Thomas, Eastman) consider the transverse external measurements to be of dubious value as methods of measuring the true pelvis. Nevertheless, these measurements are still required on the records in many hospitals and clinics and are used by many experienced obstetricians in the belief that they do possess some value.

The EXTERNAL PELVIC MEASUREMENTS which are used to obtain an approximate idea of the size of the pelvic inlet are taken with a pelvimeter. Those measurements most commonly made are: (1) the intercristal diameter or the distance between the lateral edges of the iliac crests (average, 28 cm.); (2) the interspinous diameter or the distance between the external aspects of the anterosuperior iliac spines (average, 25 cm.); (3) intertrochanteric diameter or the distance between the external aspects of the trochanters of the femurs (average, 31 cm.); (4) the external conjugate (Baudelocque's diameter) or the distance between the anterior aspect of the symphysis pubis in front and the depression below the spine of the

(Left). FIG. 2-12. Platypelloid pelvis. Inlet is a transverse oval, well-curved but decreased in anteroposterior diameter (A, B). Sacrosciatic notch is curved, small (C).

(Right). FIG. 2-13. Android pelvis. Inlet is wedged-shaped with shallow hind-pelvis and pointed fore-pelvis (A, B). Sacrosciatic notch is narrow, deep, pointed (C).

(Roentgenograms from W. E. Caldwell, M.D., and H. C. Moloy, M.D., Sloane Hospital for Women, New York)

5th lumbar vertebra behind (average, 18 to 20 cm.). In addition, some physicians measure the right and the left oblique external diameters. For all the pelvic measurements just described, the patient lies on her side or on her back, according to the diameter to be measured, with the abdomen exposed.

The INTERNAL PELVIC MEASUREMENTS are made to determine the actual diameters of the inlet. The chief internal measurement taken is the *diagonal conjugate*, or the distance between the sacral promontory and the lower margin of the symphysis pubis. The patient should be placed on her back on the examining table with her knees drawn up and her feet supported by stirrups. Two fingers are introduced into the vagina, and, before measuring the diagonal conjugate, some evaluation of the pelvis is made by palpation: the height of

the symphysis pubis and the shape of the pubic arch, the motility of the coccyx, the inclination of the anterior wall of the sacrum and the side walls of the pelvis and the prominence of the ischial spines.

In order to obtain the length of the diagonal conjugate, the two fingers passed into the vagina are pressed inward and upward as far as possible until the middle finger rests on the sacral promontory. The point on the back of the hand just under the symphysis is then marked by putting the index finger of the other hand on the exact point (Fig. 2-21), after which the fingers are withdrawn and measured. The distance from the tip of the middle finger to the point marked represents the *diagonal conjugate measurement*. This distance may be measured with a rigid measuring scale attached to the wall (Fig. 2-22) or with a pel-

FEMALE   **MALE**

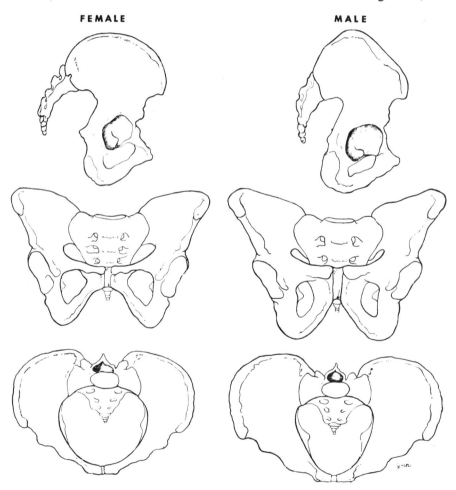

FIG. 2-14. Female pelvis contrasted with male in lateral, front and inlet views.

Fig. 2-15. Method of measuring intercristal diameter.

vimeter (Fig. 2-23), but the former is preferred because there is less chance of error. If the measurement is greater than 11.5 cm., it is justifiable to assume that the pelvic inlet is of adequate size for childbirth. In common medical parlance this measurement is often referred to as the "C.D." (conjugata diagonalis).

An extremely important internal diameter is the *true conjugate* or, in Latin, the conjugata vera (C.V.), which is the distance between the posterior aspect of the symphysis pubis and the promontory of the sacrum. However, direct measurement of this diameter cannot be made except by means of a roentgenogram; consequently, it has to be estimated from the diagonal conjugate measurement. It is believed that if 1.5 to 2 cm., according to the height and the inclination of the symphysis pubis, is deducted from the length of

Fig. 2-16. Intercristal diameter measured on bony pelvis.

FIG. 2-17. Method of measuring inter-spinous diameter.

the diagonal conjugate, the true conjugate is ob-tained. For example, if the diagonal conjugate measures 12.5 cm., and the symphysis pubis is considered to be "average," then the conjugata vera may be estimated as being about 11.0 cm.

In this method the problem consists of estimating the length of one side of a triangle, the conjugata vera; the other two sides, the diagonal conjugate and the height of the symphysis pubis, are known. If the symphysis pubis is high and has a marked

FIG. 2-18. Interspinous diameter measured on bony pelvis.

FIG. 2-19. Method of measuring external conjugate diameter (Baudelocque's diameter).

inclination, the physician takes this into consideration and may deduct 2 cm. The length of the true conjugate, or conjugata vera, is of utmost importance, since it is about the smallest diameter of the inlet through which the baby's head must pass. Indeed, the main purpose in measuring the diagonal conjugate is to give an estimate of the size of the conjugata vera.

Students sometimes are confused when they are confronted with the term "obstetric conjugate." This term identifies a diameter which begins at the sacral promontory and terminates just below

FIG. 2-20. External conjugate diameter measured on bony pelvis.

FIG. 2-21. Method of obtaining diagonal conjugate diameter (solid line). The upper broken line represents the conjugata vera, and the lower broken line represents the obstetric conjugate.

the conjugata vera on the inner surface of the symphysis pubis, a few millimeters below its upper margin (Fig. 2-21). The *obstetric conjugate* is in reality the shortest diameter through which the infant's head must pass as it descends into the true pelvis. A distinction is rarely made between the *conjugata vera* and the *obstetric conjugate*, except in x-ray pelvimetry (pp. 39-40).

Next to the diagonal conjugate measurement the most important clinical dimension of the pelvis is the transverse diameter of the outlet, the diameter between the ischial tuberosities. This is sometimes called the *tuberischii diameter* (often abbreviated T.I.), or biischial diameter, or intertuberous diameter (Fig. 2-8). This measurement is taken with the patient in the lithotomy position, well down on the table and with the legs widely separated. The measurement is taken from the innermost and lowermost aspect of the ischial tuberosities, on a level with the lower border of the anus. The instruments usually employed are the Williams' pelvimeter (Figs. 2-24, 25) or the Thoms'

FIG. 2-22. Method of measuring diagonal conjugate diameter as obtained in Figure 2-21, using wall bracket.

FIG. 2-23. Method of measuring diagonal conjugate diameter as obtained in Figure 2-21, using pelvimeter.

pelvimeter. A diameter in excess of 8 cm. is considered average.

X-ray Pelvimetry

The most accurate means of determining pelvic size is x-ray pelvimetry. This subjects the maternal ovaries and the fetal gonads to a certain amount of irradiation. Although the amount involved is minimal, exposure of pregnant women to irradiation should be avoided unless this procedure is really necessary. Hence, x-ray pelvimetry is used prior to labor only in cases in which there are sound reasons for suspecting pelvic contraction, such as small manual measurements or a history of difficult labor in the past.

Since there is no accurate means to evaluate the size of the presenting part relative to the pelvis, pelvimetry is also indicated when there has been failure to progress normally in labor, to rule out previously unsuspected cephalopelvic disproportion. It is also important to evaluate pelvic size in term breech presentations, since the head is the largest part of the fetus and the adequacy of the pelvis is not really tested until the body has already been delivered. For this reason, many physicians evaluate pelvic size with pelvimetry routinely in the primigravida at term with a breech presentation.

A variety of techniques have been developed. One which has stood the test of time, with minor modifications, is that devised by Dr. Herbert Thoms, a pioneer in this field. For a complete study, two roentgenograms are made as follows:

1. The patient is placed on the x-ray table in a semirecumbent position so that her pelvic inlet is horizontal and as nearly parallel as possible with the plate beneath her (Fig. 2-26). The exact plane in which the patient's inlet lies, both front and back, is now determined and recorded. After an exposure of the film has been made, the patient is removed from the table, and a lead plate or grid containing perforations a centimeter apart is placed in the plane previously occupied by the inlet of the patient. Another exposure now is made on the same film. When the latter is developed, the outline of the inlet is shown, as are also the dots produced by the perforations in the lead plate. Since the projected dots on the film represent centimeters in the plane of the inlet, the diameters of the inlet can be read off directly as centimeters.

2. A somewhat similar procedure is carried out with the patient standing and from the lateral view (Fig. 2-27). Here, however, an upright lead and iron rod, with a centimeter scale notched on its edge, is placed posterior to the patient and close to the gluteal fold. After an exposure has been made, the developed film will show a lateral view of the symphysis pubis, the sacral promontory, other bony landmarks and, in addition, of course, the notched centimeter scale for estab-

FIG. 2-24. Method of measuring tuber-ischii or intertuberous diameter of outlet, using the Williams' pelvimeter. The measurement is made on a line with the lower border of the anus.

lishing the distance between important points. Diameters which may be measured by x-ray pelvimetry are the obstetric conjugate, posterior sagittal at the inlet, midpelvis and outlet, and the anteroposterior diameter at the midpelvis and outlet.

Other techniques entail the use of stereoscopic procedures which allow the physician to view the films with 3-dimensional vision and thus gain a clear image of all pelvic relationships.

When roentgenograms are made late in preg-

FIG. 2-25. Tuberischii or intertuberous diameter measured on bony pelvis.

FIG. 2-26. Pelvic inlet roentgenogram. The scale represents corrected centimeters for various levels of the pelvic canal. The top line is used for measuring the diameters of the inlet. The other levels are established on the lateral roentgenogram. Pelvic morphology is readily established by viewing both lateral and inlet views. Thoms technique.

FIG. 2-27. Lateral roentgenogram. The scale represents corrected centimeters in the midplane of the body. By means of calipers the various diameters may be measured. The lateral morphologic aspects are readily visualized.

nancy by any of these methods, it is possible to secure also an impression of the size of the baby's head. When this is considered in relation to the pelvic picture, helpful information may be obtained in forecasting whether or not this particular pelvis is large enough to allow this particular baby to pass through.

Preventive Care Based on Pelvimetry. The importance of the knowledge gained through skillful performance of external and internal pelvimetry cannot be overestimated. Especially it should never be neglected in the case of a woman pregnant for the first time, or in any case in which the patient has suffered previously from difficult or tedious labors.

FEMALE ORGANS OF REPRODUCTION

The female organs of reproduction are divided into two groups—the external and the internal (Figs. 2-28 to 33).

External Organs

The external female reproductive organs are called the *vulva* (L., covering). This includes everything which is visible externally from the lower margin of the pubis to the perineum, namely, the mons veneris, the labia majora and minora, the clitoris, the vestibule, the hymen, the urethral opening and various glandular and vascular structures (Fig. 2-28). The term "vulva" often has been used to refer simply to the labia majora and minora.

The mons veneris is a firm, cushionlike formation over the symphysis pubis and is covered with crinkly hair.

The labia majora are two prominent longitudinal folds of adipose tissue covered with skin which extend downward and backward from the mons veneris and disappear in forming the anterior border of the perineal body. These two thick folds of

FIG. 2-28. External organs of reproduction.

skin are covered with hair on their outer surfaces after the age of puberty but are smooth and moist on their inner surfaces. At the bottom they fade away into the perineum posteriorly, joining together to form a transverse fold, the posterior commissure, situated directly in front of the fourchet. This fatty tissue is supplied with an abundant plexus of veins which may rupture as the result of injury sustained during labor and give rise to an extravasation of blood or hematoma.

The labia minora are two thin folds of reddish tissue covered entirely with thin membrane and situated between the labia majora, with their outer surfaces in contact with the inner surfaces of the labia majora; the labia minora extend from the clitoris downward and backward on either side of the orifice of the vagina. In the upper extremity each labium minus separates into two branches which when united with those of the opposite side enclose the clitoris. The upper fold forms the prepuce and the lower the frenum of the clitoris.

At the bottom, the labia minora pass almost imperceptibly into the labia majora or blend together as a thin fold of skin forming the anterior edge of the perineum or perineal body. This thin edge is known as the fourchette.

The clitoris is a small, highly sensitive projection composed of erectile tissue, nerves and blood vessels and is covered with a thin epidermis. It is analogous to the penis in the male and is regarded as the chief seat of voluptuous sensation. The clitoris is so situated that it is partially hidden between the anterior ends of the labia minora.

The vestibule is the almond-shaped area which is enclosed by the labia minora and extends from the clitoris to the fourchette. It is perforated by 4 openings: the urethra, the vaginal opening, the ducts of Bartholin's glands and the ducts of Skene's glands. Bartholin's glands are two small glands situated beneath the vestibule on either side of the vaginal opening. During sexual excitement varying amounts of mucoid material are secreted

FIG. 2-29. The vestibule, showing the urethra, the vaginal orifice and Bartholin's glands. Insert shows the orifices of the ducts of Skene's glands, which open just within the urethral meatus.

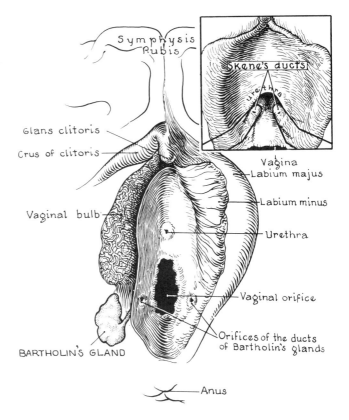

by these glands. In women infected with gonorrhea, these ducts sometimes harbor gonococci, which may cause the glands to suppurate, so that the entire labia become distended by pus. Skene's ducts open upon the vestibule on either side of the urethra (Fig. 2-29).

The hymen marks the division between the internal and the external organs. It is a thin fold of mucous membrane situated at the orifice of the vagina. It may be entirely absent, or it may form a complete septum across the lower end of the vagina. In women who have had children the irregularity of torn edges remains. The hymen presents marked differences in shape and consistency. In the newborn child it projects beyond the surrounding parts. In adult virgins it is a membrane of varying thickness which closes the vaginal opening more or less completely and presents an aperture which varies in size from a pinpoint to one which will readily admit one or even two fingers. The opening is circular or crescentic in shape. In rare instances the hymen may be imperforate and cause retention of menstrual discharge if it occludes the vaginal orifice completely.

The perineum consists of muscles and fascia of the urogenital diaphragm, which lies across the pubic arch, and the pelvic diaphragm, which consists of the coccygeus and the levator ani muscles. The levator ani is the larger and consists of three portions: the iliococcygeus, the pubococcygeus and puborectalis. These muscles form a slinglike support for the pelvic structure, and between them pass the urethra, the vagina and the rectum (Fig. 2-30). Between the anus and the vagina the levator ani is reinforced by a central tendon of the perineum to which 3 pairs of muscles converge: the bulbocavernosus, the superficial transverse muscles of the perineum and the external sphincter ani. These structures constitute the perineal body and form the main support of the perineal floor. They often are lacerated during delivery.

Internal Organs

The internal organs of reproduction are the vagina, the uterus, the fallopian tubes and the ovaries.

Ovaries. The ovaries are 2 small almond-shaped organs situated in the upper part of the pelvic cavity, one on either side of the uterus. Their chief functions are the development and the expulsion of ova and the provision of certain internal secretions (hormones). These organs correspond to the testes in the male. They lie embedded in the posterior fold of the broad ligament of the uterus (Fig. 2-31) and are supported by the suspensory, the ovarian and the mesovarian ligaments.

Each ovary contains in its substance at birth a large number of germ cells or ovules (primordial ova) (p. 55). This huge store of primordial follicles present at birth more than suffices the woman for life. It is usually believed that no more are formed, and that this large initial store is gradually exhausted during the period of sexual maturity. Beginning at about the time of puberty, one (or possibly two) of the follicles which contain the ovules enlarges each month, gradually approaches the surface of the ovary and bursts (Fig. 3-1, see p. 56). The ovum and the fluid content of the follicle are liberated on the exterior of the ovary into the abdominal cavity; then they are swept into the tube and so pass into the uterus. The development and the maturation of the follicles (containing the ova) and the ova continue from puberty to menopause.

The arteries which supply the ovary are four or five branches that arise from the anastomosis of the ovarian artery with the ovarian branch of the uterine (Fig. 2-34). The veins proceeding from the ovary become tributary to both the uterine and the ovarian plexus.

The nerves supplying the ovaries are derived from the craniosacral and the thoracolumbar sympathetic systems. The postganglionic and visceral afferent fibers form a plexus surrounding the ovarian artery, which in turn is formed by contributions from the renal and the aortic plexuses and corresponds to the spermatic plexus in the male.

Fallopian Tubes. The fallopian tubes (Figs. 2-31, 34, 36, 3-1, 4-5) are two trumpet-shaped, thin, flexible, muscular tubes, about 4½ inches long and somewhat thinner than a lead pencil. They extend from the upper angles of the uterus, the cornua, in the upper margin of the broad ligament, toward the sides of the pelvis. They have two openings: one into the uterine cavity and the other into the abdominal cavity. The opening into the uterine cavity is minute and will admit only a

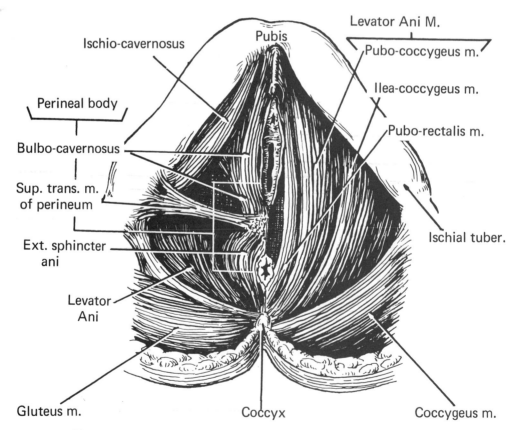

FIG. 2-30. Muscles of the pelvic floor from below. (After Dickinson)

fine bristle. The abdominal opening is somewhat larger and is surrounded by a large number of fine fringes; hence the term "fimbriated end." The fimbriated extremity lies near the ovary, but it is not necessarily in direct contact with it. It is generally believed that the cilia upon the fimbriated end of the tube create a current in the capillary layer of fluid lying between the various pelvic organs. The fallopian tubes convey the discharged ova by peristaltic action from the ovaries to the cavity of the uterus; by their tentaclelike processes the fimbriated ends of the tube draw the escaped ova into the tube. Thus, the function of the fallopian tube is to conduct the ovum along the canal by peristaltic action until it reaches the uterus. The tubes are lined with mucous membrane containing ciliated epithelium. The muscular layer

is made up of longitudinal and circular fibers which provide peristaltic action. The serous membrane covering the tubes is a continuation of the peritoneum, which lines the whole abdominal cavity.

The fallopian tubes receive their blood supply from the ovarian and the uterine arteries (Fig. 2-34). The veins of the tubes follow the course of these arteries and empty into the uterine and the ovarian trunks. The nerves which supply the uterus supply the tubes.

Uterus. The uterus is a hollow thick-walled, muscular organ (Figs. 2-31, 32, 33). It serves two important functions: (1) it is the organ of menstruation and (2) during pregnancy it receives the fertilized ovum and retains and nourishes it

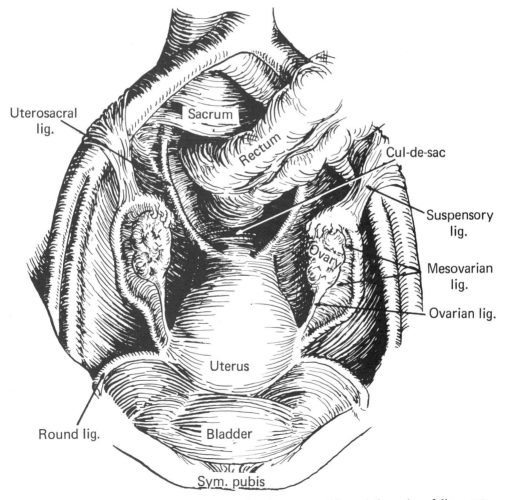

FIG. 2-31. Pelvic contents from above, showing the position of the pairs of ligaments and the relationship to the uterus, the tubes and the ovaries. (After Dickinson)

FIG. 2-32. Pelvic contents in median section with the subject on her back. (Robert L. Dickinson, M.D., New York)

until it expels the products of conception at the time of labor.

The uterus varies in size and shape according to the age of the individual and whether or not she has borne children. The uterus of the adult nullipara weighs approximately 60 Gm. and measures 5.5 to 8 cm. in length. It resembles a flattened pear in appearance and has two divisions: the upper triangular portion, the corpus, and the lower constricted cylindric portion, the cervix, which projects into the vagina. The fallopian tubes extend from the cornu (L., horn) of the uterus at the upper outer margin on either side. The upper rounded portion of the uterus between the points of insertion of the fallopian tubes is called the fundus. (Fig. 2-33).

The nonpregnant uterus is situated in the pelvic cavity between the bladder and the rectum. Almost the entire posterior wall and the upper portion of the anterior wall is covered by peritoneum. The lower portion of the anterior wall is united to the bladder wall by a thick layer of connective tissue. The lower posterior wall of the uterus and the upper portion of the vagina are separated from the rectum by an area called Douglas' cul-de-sac. Due to its muscular composition, the uterus is capable of enlarging to the size of a pumpkin; at the termination of pregnancy it weighs about 2 pounds. It is made up of involuntary muscle fibers arranged in all directions, making expansion possible in every direction to accommodate the products of conception. Due to the nature of this arrangement of the muscle, the uterus is able to expel its contents at the termination of normal labor (Fig. 6-7). Arranged between these muscular layers are many blood vessels, lymphatics and nerves.

The cavity of the uterus is very small and somewhat triangular in shape, being widest at the fundus, between the very small openings into the canals of the fallopian tubes, and narrowest below at the opening into the cervix. The anterior and the posterior walls lie almost in contact, so that if a cross section of the uterus could be examined, the cavity between them would appear as a mere slit. The uterus is lined with mucous membrane (endometrium) and is divided into two parts: the cavity of the body of the uterus and the cavity of the cervix.

The cervix is less freely movable than is the body of the uterus. Its muscular wall is not so thick, and the mucous membrane lining its cavity (cervical endometrium) is different in that it is much folded and contains more glands, which produce mucus and are the chief source of the mucous secretion during pregnancy. The cervix has an upper opening called the internal os, leading from the cavity of the uterine body into the cervical canal, and a lower opening called the external os, opening into the vagina. The cervix is very small in the nonpregnant woman, barely admitting a probe, but at the time of labor it dilates to a size sufficient to permit the passage of the fetus (Fig. 11-6, see p. 219).

LIGAMENTS. The uterus is supported in two ways: by ligaments extending from either half of the uterus (Fig. 2-33) and by the muscles of the pelvic floor (Fig. 2-30). The ligaments which support the uterus in the pelvic cavity are the broad ligaments (2) (Fig. 2-33), the round ligaments (2), and the uterosacral (2). The broad ligaments are two winglike structures which extend from the lateral margins of the uterus to the pelvic walls and serve to divide the pelvic cavity into an anterior and a posterior compartment. Each consists of folds of peritoneum which envelop the fallopian tubes, the ovaries and the round and the ovarian ligaments. Its lower portion, the *cardinal ligament* (Fig. 2-33), is composed of dense connective tissue which is firmly united to the supravaginal portion of the cervix. The median margin is connected with the lateral margin of the uterus and encloses the uterine vessels. The round ligaments are two fibrous cords which are attached on either side of the fundus just below the fallopian tubes. They extend forward through the inguinal canal and terminate in the upper portion of the labia majora. These ligaments aid in holding the

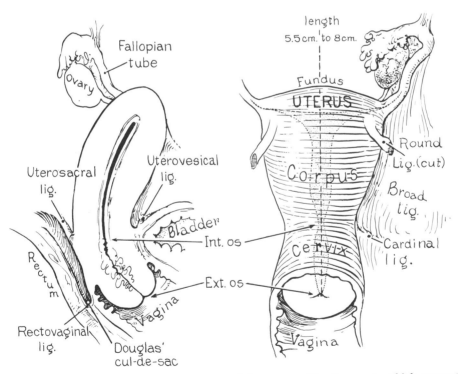

FIG. 2-33. Lateral and anterior views of the uterus. The ligaments which support the uterus in the pelvic cavity are the broad ligaments (2), the round ligaments (2), the uterosacral ligaments (2).

fundus forward. The uterosacral ligaments are two cordlike structures which extend from the posterior cervical portion of the uterus to the sacrum. These aid in supporting the cervix. The uterovesical ligament is merely a fold of the peritoneum which passes over the fundus and extends over the bladder. The rectovaginal ligament is a fold of the peritoneum which passes over the posterior surface of the uterus and is reflected upon the rectum.

UTERINE BLOOD SUPPLY. The uterus receives its blood supply from the ovarian and the uterine arteries (Fig. 2-34). The uterine artery, the principal source, is the main branch of the hypogastric, which enters the base of the broad ligament and makes its way to the side of the uterus. The ovarian artery is a branch of the aorta. It enters the broad ligament and on reaching the ovary breaks up into smaller branches which enter that organ, while its main stem makes its way to the upper

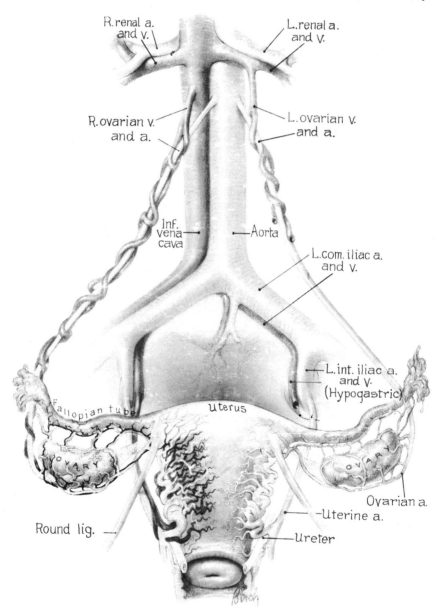

FIG. 2-34. Blood supply of the uterus and the adnexa.

margin of the uterus, where it anastomoses with the ovarian branch of the uterine artery.

The uterovaginal plexus returns the blood from the uterus and the vagina. These veins form a plexus of exceedingly thin-walled vessels which are embedded in the layers of the uterine muscle. Emerging from this plexus, the trunks join the uterine vein, which is a double vein. These veins follow on either side of the uterine artery and eventually form one trunk, emptying into the hypogastric vein, which makes its way into the internal iliac.

UTERINE NERVE SUPPLY. The uterus possesses an abundant nerve supply derived principally from the sympathetic nervous system but partly from the cerebrospinal and parasympathetic system. Both the sympathetic and the parasympathetic nerve supplies contain motor and a few sensory fibers. The functions of the nerve supply of the two systems are in great part antagonistic. The sympathetic causes muscular contraction and vasoconstriction; the parasympathetic inhibits contraction and leads to vasodilatation.

Since the uterus is a freely movable organ suspended in the pelvic cavity between the bladder and the rectum, the position of the uterus may be influenced by a full bladder or rectum, which pushes it backward or forward (see Figs. 2-32, 36). The uterus also changes its position when the patient stands, lies flat or turns on her side. Also, there are abnormalities such as anteflexion, in which the fundus is tipped too far forward (Fig. 2-36); retroversion, in which it is tipped too far backward (Fig. 2-36); and prolapse, due to the relaxation of the muscles of the pelvic floor and the uterine ligaments.

LYMPHATIC VESSELS. The lymphatic vessels drain into the lumbar lymph nodes.

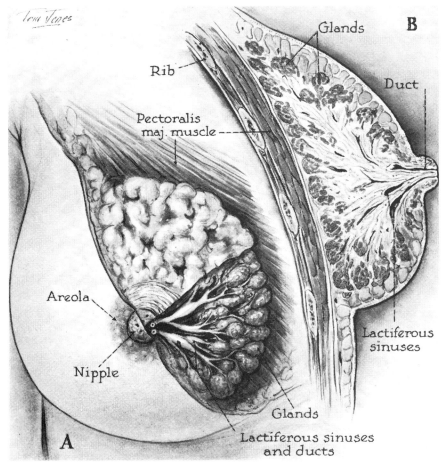

FIG. 2-35. (A) Mammary gland, showing the lactiferous ducts and sinuses. (B) Cross section of the breast.

Fig. 2-36. Female anatomy. (Dickinson, Robert L.: Human Sex Anatomy, Baltimore, Williams & Wilkins)

FIG. 2-37. Male anatomy. (Dickinson: Human Sex Anatomy, Williams & Wilkins)

Vagina. The vagina is a dilatable passage lined with mucous membrane situated between the bladder and the rectum. The vaginal opening occupies the lower portion of the vestibule and in the virgin appears almost completely closed by the hymen. The vagina is from 3 to 5 inches in length, and at the upper end is a blind vault, commonly called the fornix, into which the lower portion of the cervix projects. The fornices (plural of fornix) are divided into four parts for convenience of description. The lateral fornices are the spaces between the vaginal wall on either side and the cervix; the anterior fornix is between the anterior vaginal wall and the cervix; the posterior fornix is between the posterior vaginal wall and the cervix. The posterior fornix is considerably deeper than the anterior since the vagina is attached higher up on the posterior than the anterior wall' of the cervix. The fornices are important because the physician is usually able to palpate the internal pelvic organs through their thin walls. The vagina serves three important functions: it represents the excretory duct of the uterus through which its secretion and the menstrual flow escape, it is the female organ of copulation, and it forms part of the birth canal during labor. Its walls are arranged into thick folds, the columns of the vagina, and in women who have not borne children, numerous ridges or rugae extend outward and almost at right angles to the vaginal columns and give the surface a corrugated appearance. Normally, the anterior and the posterior walls of the vagina lie in contact, but they are capable of stretching to allow marked distention of the passage, as in the process of childbirth. The vagina is kept moist by a small amount of secretion from the uterus.

The vagina receives its abundant blood supply from branches of the uterine, the inferior vesical, the median hemorrhoidal and the internal pudic arteries. The passage is surrounded by a venous plexus; the vessels follow the course of the arteries and eventually empty into the hypogastric veins. The lymphatics empty into the inguinal, the hypogastric and the iliac glands.

Related Pelvic Organs

Bladder. The bladder is a thin, muscular sac which serves as a reservoir for the urine. It is situated in front of the uterus and behind the symphysis pubis. When empty or only moderately distended, it remains entirely in the pelvis, but if it becomes greatly distended, it rises into the abdomen. Urine is conducted into the bladder by the ureters, two small tubes which extend down from the basin of the kidneys over the brim of the pelvis and open into the bladder at about the level of the cervix. The bladder is emptied through the urethra, a short tube which terminates in the meatus (Fig. 2-28). Lying on either side of the urethra and almost parallel with it are two small glands, less than 1 inch long, known as Skene's glands. Their ducts empty into the urethra just above the meatus. Often in cases of gonorrhea, Skene's glands and ducts are involved (see Fig. 2-29).

Anus. The anus is the entrance to the rectal canal. The rectal canal is surrounded at the opening or anus by its sphincter muscle, which binds it to the coccyx behind and to the perineum in front. It is supported by the muscles passing into it (see Fig. 2-30).

The muscles involved are those that aid in supporting the pelvic floor. The rectum is considered here because of the proximity to the field of delivery.

MAMMARY GLANDS

The *breasts*, or mammary glands, are two highly specialized cutaneous glands located on either side of the anterior wall of the chest between the 3rd and the 7th ribs (Fig. 2-35). Because they are abundantly supplied with nerves, formerly it was believed that direct nervous system connection existed between the uterus and the breasts. But the demonstration that lactation can be established after excluding the spinal nervous mechanism by severing all nerves supplying the breasts clearly indicated that some other factor must be involved in the explanation of mammary changes in pregnancy. It is evident that the stimulation to growth of the mammary gland is hormonal and not nervous in origin.

The internal mammary and the intercostal arteries supply the breast gland, and the mammary veins follow these arteries. Also, there are many cutaneous veins which become dilated during lactation. The lymphatics are abundant, especially toward the axilla. These breast glands are present in the male, but only in the rudimentary state, and are not connected by the sympathetic system to the male generative organs.

Internal Structure

The breasts of a woman who never has borne a child are, in general, conic or hemispheric in form, but they vary in size and shape at different ages and in different individuals. In women who have nursed one or more babies they tend to become pendulous. At the termination of lactation, certain exercises aid in restoring the tone of the breast tissue.

The breasts are made up of glandular tissue and fat. Each organ is divided into 15 or 20 lobes, which are separated from each other by fibrous and fatty walls. Each lobe is subdivided into many lobules, and these contain numerous acini cells. The acini are composed of a single layer of epithelium, beneath which is a small amount of connective tissue richly supplied with capillaries. By the process of osmosis the products necessary for the milk are filtered from the blood, but the secretion of the milk really begins in the acini cells. As the ducts leading from the lobules to the lobes and from the lobes approach the nipple, they are dilated to form little reservoirs in which the milk is stored; they narrow again as they pass into the nipple. The size of the breast is dependent on the amount of fatty tissue present and in no way denotes the amount of lactation possible.

External Structure

The external surface of the breasts is divided into three portions. The first is the white, smooth and soft area of skin extending from the circumference of the gland to the areola. The second is the areola, which surrounds the nipple and is of a delicate pinkish hue in blondes and a darker rose color in brunettes. The surface of the areola is more or less roughened by small fine lumps of papillae, known as the glands of Montgomery (Plate 3, *right, bottom*). These enlarged sebaceous glands, white in color and scattered over the areola, become more marked during pregnancy. Under the influence of gestation, the areola becomes darker in shade, and this pigmentation, which is more marked in brunettes than in blondes, in many cases constitutes a helpful sign of pregnancy (Plate 4). The nipple or third portion is largely composed of sensitive, erectile tissue and forms a large conic papilla projecting from the center of the areola and having at its summit the openings of the milk ducts. These openings may be from 3 to 20 in number. The care of the breasts (see Chap. 8) constitutes one of the important phases of the nursing care of the maternity patient throughout pregnancy and the puerperium.

MALE ORGANS OF REPRODUCTION

The male reproductive system consists of the testes and a system of excretory ducts with their accessory structures (Fig. 2-37).

External Organs

The scrotum and the penis are called the external genitalia. The scrotum contains the testes and may be considered as an evagination of the body wall or a continuation of the abdominal cavity. In the adult male the testes have descended into the scrotal sac, and the canal connecting the sac with the abdominal cavity has closed, although it is open in the fetus.

The penis, the male organ of copulation, consists of the cavernous bodies (erectile parts) and a urethra through which the seminal fluid is brought to the female generative tract. The cavernous bodies contain blood spaces which are usually quite empty, and the organ is flaccid. When these spaces fill with blood, the organ becomes turgid. The flow of blood is controlled by the autonomic nervous system (vasodilator fibers) and varies with sexual activity. The enlarged conic structure at the free end of the penis which contains the external orifice of the urethra is called the glans penis. The glans is almost completely enclosed by a fold of skin called the prepuce or foreskin. At circumcision this part of the skin is removed.

Internal Organs

The internal organs consist of the testes and a canal system with accessory structures. Each testis is a compound gland, divided into lobules. These contain the terminal portions of the seminiferous tubules which join repeatedly and eventually form the single much-coiled tube of the epididymis. The epithelium lining the tubules consists of supporting cells and spermatogenetic cells which produce the spermatozoa. In the human testes, spermatogenesis begins at the age of puberty and continues throughout life. However, the seminiferous tubules undergo gradual involution with advancing age.

The blood supply to the testes is derived from the internal spermatic arteries. The arteries and the veins form a part of the spermatic cords.

The lymphatic vessels accompany the blood vessels in the spermatic cord, and eventually the lymphatics empty into the lumbar lymph nodes.

The efferent nerves which supply the testes are derived from the thoracolumbar and sacral divisions of the autonomic system. They are distributed chiefly to the walls of the blood vessels. Afferent fibers convey impulses from these structures to the central nervous system.

The canal system consists of the epididymis (which is made up of numerous seminiferous tubules), the ductus deferens (which passes from the epididymis to the ejaculatory duct), the ejaculatory duct (formed by the union of the ductus deferens and the duct of the seminal vesicle) and the urethra, which is surrounded by the prostate gland and terminates in the penis.

The accessory structures consist of the seminal vesicles (sacculated structures located behind the bladder and in front of the rectum), the prostate gland (which surrounds the base of the urethra and the ejaculatory duct) and the bulbo-urethral glands or Cowper's glands (which lie at the base of the prostate and on either side of the membranous urethra).

SUGGESTED READING

Anthony, C. P.: Textbook of Anatomy and Physiology. ed. 7. St. Louis, C. V. Mosby, 1967.

Caldwell, W. E., and Moloy, H. C.: Anatomical variations in the female pelvis and their effect in labor with a suggested classification. Am. J. Obstet. Gynec. 26:479, 1933.

Chaffee, E. C., and Greisheimer, E. M.: Basic Physiology and Anatomy. ed. 2, Philadelphia, J. B. Lippincott, 1969.

Eastman, N. J., and Hellman, L. M.: Williams Obstetrics. ed. 13, New York, Appleton-Century-Crofts, 1966.

Goss, C. M. (ed.): Gray's Anatomy of the Human Body. ed. 28, Philadelphia, Lea and Febiger, 1966.

Netter, F. H.: Reproductive Systems. Summit, N. J., Ciba Pharmaceutical, 1954.

Physiology in Relation to Human Reproduction

3

Sexual Maturity • Menstrual Cycle • Infertility • Menopause

A general review of reproductive physiology is included here. This should serve as background material for the more practical aspects of maternity nursing. An understanding of physiology is essential, so that the nurse may recognize the special relation of physiology to the problems in obstetrics.

SEXUAL MATURITY

Evidence of sexual maturity in the female begins at the time of puberty, with the onset of dramatic bodily changes. Early in the course of puberty, axillary and pubic hair appear. Shortly thereafter, there is an increase in the size of the external genitalia. The breasts also begin to mature at this time. These changes usually precede the onset of menstruation, referred to as the menarche. Establishment of the menstrual cycle is the most clearly identifiable sign of puberty and serves as an indication that the internal sex organs are approaching maturity. These physical changes are accompanied by emotional changes, as the young girl recognizes these outward signs that she is now approaching womanhood. The whole process of puberty spans about 5 years and culminates with menarche.

Menarche

Menarche usually occurs between the ages of 12 and 16, although heredity, race, state of nutrition, climate and environment may influence its early or late appearance; for example, maturity tends to appear earlier in warm climates and later in cold regions. The reproductive period spans about 35 years, from the beginning of menstrua-tion until its cessation during the menopause at about the age of 45 to 50.

Ovulation and Menstruation

Each month, with considerable regularity, a blisterlike structure about a centimeter in diameter develops on the surface of one or the other ovary. Within this bubble, almost lost in the fluid about it, lies a tiny speck, scarcely visible to the naked eye; a thimble would hold 3 million of them. This little speck is the human ovum—a truly amazing structure. It not only possesses within its diminutive compass the potentialities of developing into a human being, but also embodies the mental as well as the physical traits of the woman and her forebears: perhaps her own brown eyes or her father's tall stature; possibly her mother's love of music or her grandfather's genius at mathematics. These and a million other potentialities are contained in the ovum, which is so small that it is about one fourth the size of the period at the end of this sentence.

In a process known as ovulation, one blister on one ovary bursts at a given time each month and discharges an ovum. The precise day on which ovulation occurs is a matter of no small importance; for instance, since the ovum can only be fertilized (impregnated by the spermatozoon, or male germ cell) within a few hours after its escape from the ovary, the day after ovulation a woman is no longer fertile. However, a person is potentially fertile for a number of days preceding the actual time of ovulation, since the spermatozoa survive in the female reproductive tract for many hours, or even days, awaiting the arrival of the ovum. In a given cycle, the time of ovulation is unpredictable. Even the person who consistently has regular menstrual periods could experience a delayed ovulation, or early ovulation in any one cycle. This possibility of irregularity, combined with the potential for fertility any time prior to ovulation by virtue of the fact that the spermatozoa retain their ability for fertilization, makes it difficult to identify accurately the fertile phase of a given cycle. It should be remembered that ovulation can take place any time in a cycle, and the only really infertile interval is after ovulation has occurred. The time between ovulation and menstruation is very standard; the time between menstruation and ovulation is variable enough that ovulation cannot be predicted from one cycle to the next. It should be assumed that intercourse will result in conception unless some means of contraception is used or the patient is assured, by the use of the temperature chart described later, that she is past ovulation.

Graafian Follicle. In delving further into this process of ovulation, we find that at birth each ovary contains a huge number of undeveloped ova, probably more than 400,000. These are rather large round cells with clear cytoplasm and a good-sized nucleus occupying the center. Each of these ova is surrounded by a layer of a few small, flattened or spindleshaped cells. The whole structure—ovum and surrounding cells—is spoken of as a "follicle," while in its underdeveloped state at birth it is referred to as a "primordial follicle." The formation of primordial follicles ceases at birth or shortly after, and the large number contained in the ovaries of the newborn represents a lifetime's supply. The majority of these disappear before puberty, so that there are then perhaps 30,000 left in each ovary. This disintegration of follicles continues throughout the reproductive period, with the result that usually none is found after the menopause.

Meanwhile, from birth to the menopause a certain few of these primordial follicles show signs of development. The surrounding granular layers of cells begin to multiply rapidly until they are several layers deep, at the same time becoming cuboidal in shape. As this proliferation of cells continues, a very important fluid develops between them, the follicular fluid. After puberty this accumulates in such quantities that the multiplying follicle cells are pushed toward the margin, and the ovum itself is almost surrounded by fluid, being suspended from the periphery of the follicle by only a small neck of cells. The structure is now known as the *graafian follicle*, after Von Graaf, the famous Dutch physician who in 1672 first described it (Figs. 3-1, 2). While increasing in size so enormously, the graafian follicle nat-

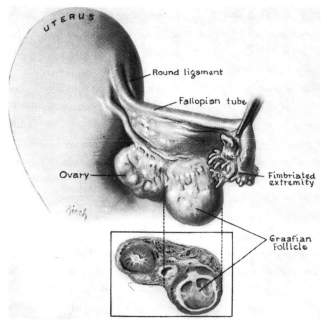

Fig. 3-1. Ovary with graafian follicle.

urally pushes aside other follicles, forming each month, as has been said, a very noticeable, blister-like projection on the surface of the ovary. At one point the follicular capsule becomes thin, and as the ovum reaches full maturity, it breaks free from the few cells attaching it to the periphery and floats in the follicular fluid. The thinned area of the capsule now ruptures, and the ovum is expelled into the peritoneal cavity.

Changes in the Corpus Luteum. After the discharge of the ovum, the ruptured follicle undergoes a change. It becomes filled with large cells containing a special yellow colored matter. The follicle then is known as the corpus luteum or yellow body. If pregnancy does not occur, the corpus luteum reaches full development in about 8 days, then retrogresses and is gradually replaced by fibrous tissue, corpus albicans. If pregnancy does occur, the corpus luteum enlarges somewhat and persists throughout the period of gestation, reaching its maximum size about the 4th or 5th month and retrogressing slowly thereafter. The corpus luteum secretes an extremely important substance, *progesterone,* which will be considered in a later section of this chapter.

In the absence of pregnancy, the corpus luteum remains active for about two weeks. The constancy of progesterone production by the corpus luteum accounts for the relatively standard duration of the postovulatory phase of the menstrual cycle.

MENSTRUAL CYCLE
Menstruation in Relation to Pregnancy

Menstruation is the periodic discharge of blood, mucus, and epithelial cells from the uterus. It usually occurs at monthly intervals throughout the reproductive period, except during pregnancy and lactation, when usually it is suppressed entirely. Accordingly, the span of years during which childbearing is possible—that is, from the age of about 12 to 45—corresponds to the period during which ovulation and, therefore, menstruation occur. In general, a woman who menstruates is able to conceive, whereas one who does not is probably infertile. Ovulation and menstruation are closely interlinked, and since no process of nature is purposeless, menstruation must play some vital and indispensable role in childbearing. What is this role?

If day by day we were privileged to watch the endometrium (or lining membrane of the uterus), we would observe some remarkable alterations. Immediately following the termination of a menstrual period, this membrane is very thin, measuring a few millimeters in depth. Each day thereafter it becomes a trifle thicker and harbors an increasing content of blood, while its glands become more and more active, secreting a rich nutritive substance. About a week before the onset of the next expected period this process reaches its height; the endometrium is now of the thickness of heavy, downy velvet and has become soft and succulent with blood and glandular secretions. At this time the egg, if one has been fertilized, embeds itself into this luxuriant lining.

All these changes have only one purpose: to provide a suitable bed in which the fertilized ovum may rest, secure nourishment and grow. If an egg is not fertilized, these alterations are unnecessary; accordingly, through a mechanism which even today is obscure, the swollen endome-

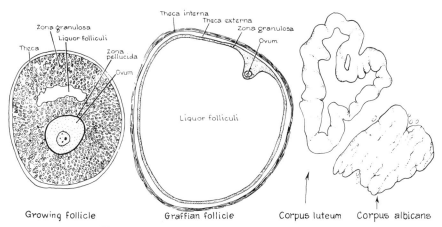

FIG. 3-2. Development of the graafian follicle.

trium disintegrates, and the encased blood and glandular secretions escape into the uterine cavity; passing through the cervix, they flow out through the vagina, carrying the egg with them. In other words, menstruation represents the abrupt termination of a process designed to prepare board and lodging, as it were, for a fertilized ovum; it betokens the breakdown of a bed which was not needed because the "boarder" did not materialize; its purpose then is to clear away the old bed so that a new and fresh one may be created the next month.

Hormonal Control of Menstruation

The menstrual cycle is regulated primarily through the highly coordinated function of the pituitary, the ovaries and the uterus. If, while watching the changes in the endometrium during the menstrual cycle it were possible to inspect the ovaries from day to day, one would note that the uterine alterations are directly related to certain changes that take place in the ovary. If it were possible to look further, one might see that the alterations which occur regularly in the ovarian cycle are directly related to certain phenomena which take place in the anterior pituitary gland and the hypothalamus, a portion of the brain which lies above the pituitary. Thus, the whole sequence represents the harmonious, integrated reactions of several processes within the human organism, all of which are necessary to maintain proper relationships in the menstrual cycle.

Proliferative Phase. Immediately following menstruation, it will be recalled, the endometrium of the uterus is very thin. During the subsequent week or so it proliferates markedly. The cells on the surface become taller, while the glands which dip into the endometrium become longer and wider. As the result of these changes, the thickness of the endometrium increases 6-fold or 8-fold. During this phase of the menstrual cycle (from the 5th to the 14th days, approximately) a graafian follicle each month is approaching its greatest development and is manufacturing increasing amounts of follicular fluid. This fluid contains a most important substance, the estrogenic hormone, called estrogen. The word "hormone" comes from a Greek word which means "I bring about," and in the case of estrogen it brings about (among other things) the thickening of the endometrium described. Each month, then, after the cessation of menstruation, a de-

veloping graafian follicle produces this hormone, estrogen, as an ingredient of the follicular fluid; and estrogen acts on the endometrium to build it up. For this reason this phase of the menstrual cycle is more commonly referred to as the proliferative phase, although it is still sometimes referred to as the follicular or estrogenic phase.

Secretory Phase. Following the release of the ovum from the graafian follicle (ovulation), the cells which form the corpus luteum begin to secrete, in addition to estrogen, another important hormone, progesterone. This supplements the action of estrogen on the endometrium in such a way that the glands become very tortuous or corkscrew in appearance and are greatly dilated. This change is due to the fact that they are swollen with a secretion. Meanwhile, the blood supply of the endometrium is increased; it becomes vascular and succulent. Since these effects are directed at providing a bed for the fertilized ovum, it is easy to understand why the hormone which brings them about is called "progesterone," meaning "for gestation." It is also clear why this phase of the cycle, occupying the last 14 ± 2 days, is commonly called the secretory phase and why occasionally it is referred to as the progestational, luteal or premenstrual phase.

Menstrual Phase. Unless the ovum is fertilized, the corpus luteum is short-lived. Since corpus luteum cells secrete not only progesterone but also estrogen, cessation of corpus luteum activity means a withdrawal of both of these hormones which have been responsible for building up the endometrium. As a result, the endometrium degenerates. This is associated with rupture of countless small blood vessels in the endometrium with innumerable minute hemorrhages. Along with the blood, superficial fragments of the endometrium, together with mucin from the glands, are cast away, and all this constitutes the menstrual discharge (Fig. 3-3). Naturally, this phase of the cycle (the 1st to the 5th days, approximately) is called the menstrual phase.

Role of the Pituitary Gland. The pituitary gland is of considerable importance in the function of the reproductive system. The anterior lobe of the pituitary, the "master clock," releases, among other hormones, the gonadotropins, whose function is to stimulate the ovary. These hormones produce the ovarian alterations associated with ovulation. There are two principal gonadotropins. One is called the follicle-stimulating hormone, sometimes abbreviated as FSH. This, as its name implies, stimulates the development of the follicle. The other is the luteinizing hormone (LH), which has its principal activity during the luteal phase of the cycle.

The release of the gonadotropic hormones by the pituitary is regulated by the hypothalamus—a specialized structure within the brain located just above the pituitary. The hypothalamus has a vascular connection to the pituitary gland. It also has nervous connections with the central nervous system. Indeed, its function can be modified by influences within the central nervous system. Thus, the function of the pituitary gland may be affected by the brain. The cyclic release of gonadotropin is brought about through the influence on the pituitary gland by hormonal agents released by the hypothalamus. These are referred to as releasing factors, since they directly affect the release of both FSH and LH from the pituitary gland.

The posterior lobe of the pituitary gland produces oxytocin, a hormone that has an important role in obstetrics but one that differs altogether from the purposes of the present discussion (see Chaps. 13 and 14).

Other Functions of Estrogen and Progesterone. In addition to their role in controlling menstruation, these two ovarian hormones, estrogen and progesterone, have other far-reaching and important functions. Estrogen is responsible for the development of the secondary sex characteristics, that is, all those distinctive sex manifestations which are not directly concerned with the process of reproduction. Thus, the growth of the breast at puberty, the distribution of body fat, the size of the larynx and its resulting influence on the

FIG. 3-3. Hormonal control of the normal menstrual cycle.

quality of the voice, as well as mating instincts, are all the result of estrogenic action. We may almost say, therefore, that a woman is a woman because of estrogen.

Progesterone, aside from its action on the endometrium, plays a most important role in preserving the life of the embryo during early pregnancy. It also has a relaxing action on the uterine muscle. For these two reasons, it is sometimes employed therapeutically in cases in which there is a tendency to abort, although its efficacy has not been established.

Clinical Aspects of Menstruation

From what has been said concerning the underlying mechanism of menstruation, it is clear that the monthly flow of blood is only one phase of a marvelous cyclic process which not only makes childbearing possible but also profoundly influences both body and mind. For this reason the time of the onset of menstruation is a critical period in the life of a young woman. The term "menarche" is used to indicate the onset of the first menstruation. The term "puberty" has a much broader connotation and refers to the whole transitional stage between childhood and maturity. During this time the appearance of secondary sex characteristics and the development of sex consciousness are other equally important manifestations.

The average age of the onset of menstruation is between 12 and 14 years. It may be as early as the 9th year or as late as the 18th year and still be within normal limits. Although the interval of the menstrual cycle, counting from the beginning of one period to the onset of the next, averages 28 days, there are wide variations even in the same woman. Indeed, there is scarcely a woman who menstruates exactly every 28 or 30 days. This question has been the subject of several studies on normal young women, chiefly student nurses, who have conscientiously recorded the time and the nature of each period. These investigations show that the majority of women (almost 60%) experience variations of at least 5 days in the length of their menstrual cycles; differences in the same woman of even 10 days are not uncommon and may occur without explanation or apparent detriment to health.

Normal menstruation should not be accompanied by pain, although quite often there is some general malaise, together with a feeling of weight and discomfort in the pelvis. Frequent, also, are such disturbances as a sense of fatigue, headache, backache, sensitivity in the breasts and unstable emotional reactions. If there is great irregularity or extremely profuse flow or marked pain, a pathologic condition may be present. Painful menstruation is known as *dysmenorrhea*. Absence of the menses is known as *amenorrhea*. The most common cause of amenorrhea is pregnancy, but sometimes it is brought about by emotional disturbances, such as fear, worry or fatigue, which work through the hypothalamus, or debilitating disease (anemia, tuberculosis).

The cessation of menstrual function usually occurs between the ages of 45 and 50. The period over which this alteration takes place is known as the *menopause, or climacteric,* but generally it is referred to by the laity as the "change of life." About one half of all women cease menstruating between these years, about one fourth stop before 45, and another quarter continue to menstruate until past 50.

Variations in Basal Body Temperature

Beginning about the first year of life, slight daily variations in body temperature occur normally in all human beings. These temperature variations have relation to the time of the day and the nature of the circumstances surrounding the individual. For example, the body temperature is lowest in the morning before breakfast, after a good night's rest, and prior to assuming activity. Then after a day of normal activity the body temperature is usually highest toward afternoon and early evening. The fact that physiologic variations in basal body temperature also occur in relation to the menstrual cycle is important here, because it can be useful in assessing ovarian activity and in establishing the time of ovulation. Such an index becomes extremely important in studies of fertility and sterility.

In the woman who is ovulating, there is normally a rhythmic variation in the basal body temperature curve during the course of the menstrual cycle. The basal temperature is lower during the first part of the menstrual cycle, the proliferative phase. It rises in association with ovulation and remains relatively higher during the luteal phase of the cycle. The rise in the basal temperature occurs as a result of the influence of progesterone, produced by the corpus luteum following ovulation. Progesterone causes this thermogenic effect through its influence on the central nervous system. The basal temper-

Fig. 3-4. Directions for using this chart are given on the following page.

ature rises as much 0.5 of a degree, and a relatively higher temperature is sustained until just before the onset of the menstrual period. This interval occupies the 14 ± 2 terminal days in the cycle. If pregnancy occurs, the levels of progesterone are maintained, and under its influence the basal temperature remains high past the expected time of the period. In the absence of pregnancy, the basal temperature usually drops a day or so before the menstrual period.

THE USE OF THE BASAL TEMPERATURE GRAPH

The basal body temperature is one of the most practical means for the diagnosis of ovulation. It is the relative difference in basal body temperature during the course of the cycle which is the important diagnostic criterion for ovulation. It is only useful in the timing of ovulation retrospectively. Thus, when there is infertility, efforts to time intercourse to coincide with changes in the temperature chart have not proved worthwhile. In fact, such regulation of coital habits is not recommended. However, for the diagnosis of ovulation, the temperature chart has proved valuable. The temperature chart is also useful as an adjunct to the rhythm method of family planning. As suggested earlier, since the ovum has a life of 24 hours or less, intercourse in the postovulatory phase of the menstrual cycle, if it occurs more than 24 hours after ovulation, is relatively safe. Since the basal temperature rise occurs in association with ovulation, a 3-day interval of temperature readings at a higher level than previously recorded provides reasonable assurance that ovulation has passed. Coitus then becomes "safe." We are reasonably sure that the ovum is short-lived, and even if the rise in temperature should precede ovulation by a day or so, an additional 2 days of abstinence provides an adequate safety factor under ordinary circumstances. It should be pointed out that the temperature chart method is no panacea. Any exposure to spermatozoa in the preovulatory phase of the menstrual cycle carries with it the risk of pregnancy. Thus, the patient with irregular ovulation or unusually prolonged cycle must exercise abstinence over long periods of time, if the temperature chart method for rhythm is to be used with reasonable safety. Those patients who are highly motivated and whose cycles are relatively short may use the temperature chart effectively to regulate coitus. For such patients, this method has proved useful as an adjunct to the rhythm method.

Directions

1. The first day of menses is considered to be the first day of the menstrual cycle. The duration of menstrual flow is recorded, beginning on cycle day 1, with X's on the chart (See Fig. 3-4). The date of onset of flow is recorded, and each subsequent date is recorded in the spaces provided. Following cessation of flow, the morning temperature is taken. Oral temperatures are as satisfactory as rectal recordings and are certainly more convenient. The temperature should be taken immediately after waking and before getting out of bed, talking, eating, drinking, or smoking. Ideally, it should be taken at about the same time every morning.

2. The thermometer is read to within 0.1 of a degree, and the reading is recorded on the chart.

3. Any known cause for temperature variation should be noted on the chart, for example, interrupted or shortened sleep, a cold, indigestion, emotional disturbance. If intercourse has occurred, that fact should be recorded with a circle around the recording the following morning.

4. Some women can recognize ovulation by characteristic pain in the lower abdomen, so-called "mittelschmerz." Others have vaginal bleeding or clear preovulatory vaginal discharge. Such manifestations should be recorded on the chart.

INFERTILITY

Although the problem of infertility is considered to be in the field of gynecology, it is a factor which has complicated the childbearing of many women. Thus, the nurse needs to be aware of its implications.

It is estimated that about 10 per cent of couples are involuntarily infertile. Infertility should be looked upon as a symptom which reflects derangement in the anatomy and physiology of the male and/or female reproductive tracts. The problem may occur as a result of deficiencies in the seminal, cervical, tubal and ovarian factors. Coital factors may also play a role. It is generally acknowledged that if conception has failed to occur following a year's unimpeded exposure, an infertility investigation is in order. A variety of factors which might account for infertility should be carefully explored before any definitive treatment is decided upon. The male and the female partner should be given equal attention, and efforts should be made to treat the couple as a unit. A thorough diagnostic survey has become increasingly important, as newer means of treatment have become available. For example, we are now able to treat patients with some forms of failure of ovulation with methods which were unavailable only a few years ago. One of the important features of the diagnostic survey is that through it the physician can give the couple a prognosis. If the cause of the infertility cannot be corrected, the couple can be so advised, so that they can perhaps plan adoption at an early stage in their marriage. However, it is estimated that at least 30 per cent of barren marriages can be rendered fertile, and improved techniques for the treatment of infertility are increasingly available.

MENOPAUSE

The term "menopause" refers to the cessation of menstruation which usually occurs during a woman's middle years, somewhere between the ages of 45 and 50. It has been said that, in general, the earlier puberty occurs in the child, the later the menopause will occur in womanhood. Conversely, the later puberty is experienced, the earlier the menopause will begin. The menopause, which is a normal consequence of aging, takes place as a gradual process. The periods first become scanty, then one may be missed, and finally they cease altogether.

The cause of the natural menopause is due to cessation of ovarian activity. As one considers the normal life cycle of the woman and focuses on the reproductive years, an analogy can be made that as the menarche is associated with puberty, so the menopause is associated with the climacteric. Often the terms "menopause" and "climacteric" are used synonymously, but one can readily understand that this usage is not accurate. The climacteric, a word derived from the Greek, meaning "rung of ladder, critical time in human life," is defined as "the syndrome of endocrine, somatic and psychic changes occurring at the termination of the reproductive period in the female. . . ."[1] Consider briefly the implication that these endocrine changes have for the ovaries. Having for some 30 years performed the function of provid-

ing a mature ovum each month with some degree of regularity, the ovary now regresses and gradually shrivels up into a small, flat organ composed mostly of scar tissue. As a consequence of this, estrogen no longer is produced. This permanent and complete withdrawal of estrogen results in atrophy of the uterus, the fallopian tubes, the vagina and the vulva. Furthermore, the withdrawal of estrogen is likely to produce other symptoms, such as "hot flashes," vague muscle and joint pains, headache, edema, and manifestations of emotional instability—for example, irritability, sudden outbursts of tears, etc. Other evidences of the climacteric may be observed in the dryness of the skin and the hair, which makes the fact that she is aging more apparent to the woman.

"Hot flashes" is a familiar term to most people. Mentioned in association with the menopause down through the years, the expression has been passed along for generations almost like an old wives' tale. But "hot flashes" are no old wives' tale; they are the result of vasomotor instability, just as sweating or sensations of cold are during this time. The term "hot flashes" is descriptive; it says what the patient feels—an abrupt sensation of being very hot that seems momentarily to sweep upward from the body to envelop her to the very top of the head, and most particularly about the face and the neck. The face suddenly becomes very flushed, and she may break out in a sweat, manifestations that will be quite apparent to others. The women so affected may have "hot flashes" at any time and in varying degrees, from very mild to severe.

The menopause may result from other than the natural physiologic alterations of the climacteric. Artificial menopause relates to the cessation of menstruation produced by some artificial means, such as irradiation of the ovaries or surgical operation for the removal of the ovaries (oophorectomy) or the uterus (hysterectomy). Each of these brings about one manifestation in common (i.e., the woman will no longer menstruate). But beyond this the manifestations in the patient are not identical.

Certain misunderstandings based on incorrect interpretation of terminology are rather widespread and should be clarified. The fact that a woman has had a hysterectomy and ceases to menstruate does not mean that her healthy ovaries will now cease to function, because the hysterec-

---

[1] Dorland's Illustrated Medical Dictionary, ed. 24, Philadelphia, Saunders, 1965.

tomy involves only the removal of the uterus. On the other hand, if the ovaries are removed surgically or are treated by irradiation, the source of estrogen is withdrawn abruptly, and thus the symptoms relating to the sudden withdrawal of this hormone will occur.

When severe symptoms are produced by lack of ovarian function resulting from either the normal climacteric or artificial menopause, the patient may find them intolerable and may require hormone therapy to control the symptoms. Estrogen, either as the pure hormone or as one of the several synthetic estrogens, finds its greatest usefulness in alleviating these menopausal disorders. It can be said that the better the woman's general health is as she approaches her middle years, the more she can look forward to an uneventful menopause.

SUGGESTED READING

Goldfarb, A. F. (ed.): Dynamics and abnormalities of puberty. Obstet. Gynec. 11:755-878, 1968.

Israel, S. L.: Diagnosis and treatment of menstrual disorders and sterility. Hoeber Medical Division, New York, Harper and Row, 1967.

Kleegman, S. J., and Kaufmann, S. A.: Infertility in Women. Philadelphia, F. A. Davis, 1966.

Mastroianni, L. (ed.): Ovulation. Clin. Obstet. Gynec. 10:345-417, 1967.

Development and Physiology of the Fetus

Maturation of Ovum and Sperm Cells • Determination of Sex
Fertilization and Changes Following Fertilization • Implantation of the Ovum • Decidua
The Three Germ Layers • Amnion, Chorion and Placenta • Size and Development of the Fetus
Duration of Pregnancy • Calculation of the Expected Date of Confinement
Physiology of the Fetus • Periods of Development • Maternal Impressions

In all Nature's wide universe of miracles there is no process more wondrous, no mechanism more incredibly fantastic, than the one by which a tiny speck of tissue, the human egg, develops into a 7-pound baby. So miraculous did primitive peoples consider this phenomenon that they frequently ascribed it all to superhuman intervention and even overlooked the fact that sexual intercourse was a necessary precursor. Throughout unremembered ages our own primitive ancestors doubtless held similar beliefs, but now we know that pregnancy comes about in only one way: from the union of a female germ cell, the egg or ovum, with a male germ cell, the spermatozoon (Fig. 4-1). These two gametes, ovum and spermatozoon, become fused into one cell or zygote, which contains the characteristics of both the female and the male from which these gametes originated.

MATURATION OF OVUM AND SPERM CELLS

Until about 2 days before ovulation, the ovum remains in a resting stage of development. Its nucleus is large and round and has been described as vesicular, because it resembles a bleb or vesicle. While still in the follicle, the ovum undergoes a process referred to as meiosis, through which it is matured and its genetic material (chromosomes) is prepared for fertilization.

The spermatozoon is fully matured before it is discharged from the tubules in the testis. It, too, has undergone a meiotic process preparatory to fertilization. By the time the gametes (the ovum and the spermatozoon) are matured and ready for union, a number of significant changes already have occurred, as shown in Figure 4-2.

In all human cells, with the exception of the mature sex cells, there are normally 46 chromo-

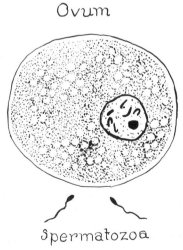

FIG. 4-1. Relative size of spermatozoa and ovum. (After Eastman)

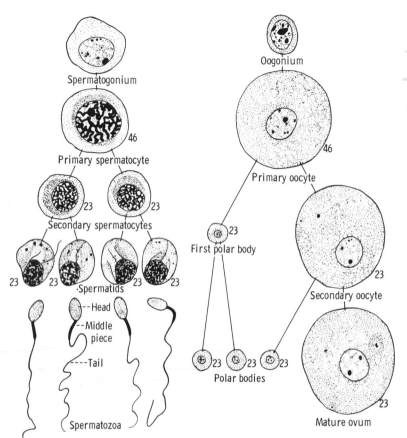

Spermatogonium

Primary spermatocyte

46

Secondary spermatocytes

23   23

23   23   Spermatids   23   23

--Head

--Middle
piece

----Tail

Spermatozoa

Oogonium

Primary oocyte

46

First polar body   23

Secondary oocyte   23

Polar bodies   23   23   23

Mature ovum   23

FIG. 4-2. Diagram of gametogenesis. The various stages of spermatogenesis are indicated on the left; 1 spermatogonium gives rise to 4 spermatozoa. On the right the various stages of oogenesis are indicated. From each oogonium 1 secondary oocyte and 3 polocytes arise. An ovum reaches maturity only if it is fertilized. In gametogenesis the chromosomes are reduced to one half the number characteristic for the general body cells of the species. In man the number in the body cells is 46, and that in the mature spermatozoon (and secondary oocyte) is 23. (Greisheimer, E. M.: Physiology and Anatomy, ed. 8, p. 766, Fig. 401, Philadelphia, Lippincott, 1963)

somes (chroma, color; soma, body). Normally, the chromosomes within each somatic cell are paired. Thus, each cell contains 22 pairs of autosomes (auto, self) and one pair of sex chromosomes. The cells of the female normally contain 2 X chromosomes; male cells normally contain 1 X and 1 Y chromosome. The sex chromosome of the mature ovum is always of the X type. The mature spermatozoon may have either an X chromosome or a Y chromosome. When fertilization occurs with a spermatozoon containing the X chromosome, the resulting product is genetically female. When an ovum is fertilized by a spermatozoon containing a Y chromosome, the resulting product is genetically male. At the completion of the fertilization process, the fertilized ovum contains 46 chromosomes, the number normally present in all somatic cells.

Prior to fertilization, each gamete undergoes a reduction in its total number of chromosomes to half the usual number, the haploid number. This reduction occurs through the process of meiosis, the special arrangement for cell division during

the course of gametogenesis. In the meiotic process, each gamete normally receives only 1 chromosome of each pair. Thus, each mature spermatozoon has 23 chromosomes in its nucleus, and each mature ovum also contains 23 chromosomes, the haploid number. The chromosomes of the ovum have been reduced as a result of extrusion of chromosomal material in the form of a "polar body," so called because it is observed at one pole of the developing ovum. Altogether, two polar bodies are extruded. The first is released prior to ovulation and, as a result of its release, the number of chromosomes is halved. Upon fertilization, a second polar body is released, and the final product, the fertilized ovum, once again contains a set of 46 chromosomes. Thus, the chromosomes of the fertilized ovum are derived from both germ cells (i.e., half from the ovum and half from the spermatozoon that fertilized the ovum).

The chromosomes differ in form and size, ranging from small spherical masses to long rods. By the use of cell culture techniques, it has been pos-

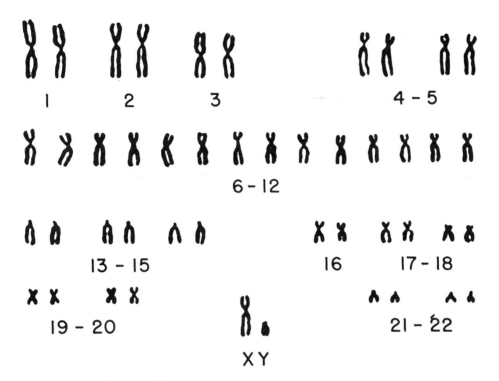

FIG. 4-3. Normal male karyotype. (Dr. M. Neil Macintyre, Department of Anatomy, Western Reserve University School of Medicine)

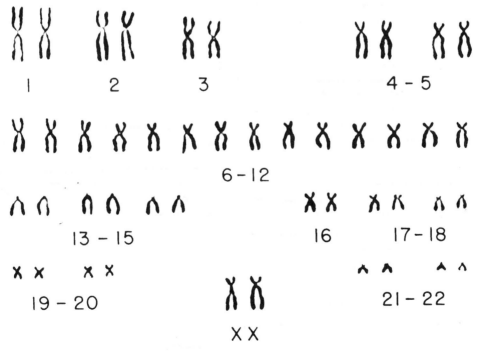

FIG. 4-4. Normal female karyotype. (Dr. M. Neil Macintyre, Department of Anatomy, Western Reserve University School of Medicine)

sible to photograph the individual chromosomes in a given cell. The white blood cell has proven to be the most useful cell for this technique. A sample of blood is taken, and the white blood cells are separated and cultured. After a period of culture, cell division (mitosis) occurs. This division is arrested by the introduction of the drug colchicine into the culture medium. Colchicine causes arrest of cell division in metaphase, a time when the individual chromosomes are separate from one another. The chromosomes are then photographed and the individual chromosomes are cut out and arranged in pairs according to their relative lengths. "Karyotype" is the technical term for the arrangement of the chromosomes of a single cell in this way. The examples of normal karyotypes are shown in Figures 4-3 and 4-4. The 46 chromosomes (greatly magnified) appear as rod-shaped structures split longitudinally into two chromatids, lying side by side and held together at the constricted region, the centromere.

Except for the mature ovum and spermatozoon, which contain the haploid number of chromosomes, each normal cell in the body contains a standard number of chromosomes. After fertilization, the ovum again has its full complement of 46 chromosomes. In every cell division thereafter, throughout the differentiation of all tissues, each cell will have 46 chromosomes. Preparation for the passing on of the requisite number of chromosomes to each of two daughter cells is accomplished by an internal change in the cell before division, the completion of mitosis. Each of the chromosomes replaces itself and splits in half, and each of the two new cells (daughter cells) receives its half of the halved chromosomes. This splitting and halving occurs in all dividing cells until growth ceases.

Within the chromosomes, distributed along the chromosomal threads, are the ultramicroscopic self-perpetuating bodies called genes. When the cell divides into two daughter cells, each daughter cell is an exact duplicate of the other and of the mother cell before division. For the daughter cells to be identical, each must have the same complement of genes in its chromosomes; thus there must be a duplication of genes before cell division occurs. This is accomplished by mitosis.

As division proceeds, then, the mother cell will have identical sets of 46 chromosomes for each daughter cell.

Now consider briefly what happens when the ovum is fertilized and conception takes place. Each gamete, ovum and spermatozoon, comes from a different person with a different ancestral history—and with different genes in its 23 chromosomes. To these genes are attributed such differences as color of hair and eyes, facial characteristics, and body build. Since a single gene may carry more than one character, there may be numerous variable results in the offspring of any two parents. The hereditary possibilities discarded or retained in the mature gametes is a matter of chance, but the nature of the combination of the germ plasm which occurs in each generation when two gametes fuse in fertilization is of great significance. If either parent brings defective germ plasm, the result may affect the zygote and later the characteristics of the child.

Biologists have estimated that at the time of the reduction division some 17 million different combinations are possible due to the interchange of genes. Apparently, there is sufficient stability produced during this intricate interchange process to ensure perpetuation of the characteristics of the progenitors.

Chromosomal Aberrations. The normal development of the embryo depends on the normal complement of chromosomes in the zygote, as well as the proper genetic balance. When this is not the case, developmental abnormalities occur. Malformations may result from alterations in a single gene, or in a number of genes, and from chromosomal abnormalities involving whole chromosomes. Some of these abnormalities are determined before fertilization takes place (during gametogenesis), almost certainly due to nondisjunction or failure of separation of chromosomes in the first reduction division in meiosis. For example, this aberration is now known to be the cause of Down's syndrome (mongolism). Here the zygote has 3 homologous autosomes, and it is trisomic; thus it is sometimes referred to as "trisomy 21."

A number of chromosomal aberrations have been identified in humans, involving both autosomes and sex chromosomes. Because this subject is highly specialized, the student is referred to the current literature on genetics for elaboration on it. A number of excellent references are included in the suggested readings for this chapter.

The Ovum

As described in Chapter 3, ova normally are discharged from the human ovary at the rate of

TABLE 4-1. CHROMOSOMAL ABERRATIONS IN MAN*

I. In all cells of body (presumed to be due to an error occurring prior to conception).
  A. Anomalies of number. (Normal male:—(46) 44 + X + Y; normal female:—(46) 44 + X + X.)
    1. Involving individual chromosomes (aneuploidy).
      (a) Autosomes.
        α Monosomy (45) ♂ 43 + X + Y; ♀ 43 + X + X.
        β Trisomy (47) ♂ 45 + X + Y; ♀ 45 + X + X (mongolism). (Trisomy may involve more than one chromosome. Thus 49 chromosomes in an abnormal child have been interpreted as 46 + X + X + Y; i.e., trisomy of two autosomes and an extra X chromosome.)
      (b) Sex chromosomes (gonosomes).
        α Y absent (45) ♀ 44 + X + O (Turner's syndrome).
        β One X deficient (46) ♀ 44 + X + x (primary amenorrhoea).
        γ Extra X (47) ♀ 44 + X + X + X (sometimes called superfemale).
        δ Extra X (47) ♂ 44 + X + X + Y (Klinefelter's syndrome).
        ε Two extra X (48) ♂ 44 + X + X + X + Y (? Klinefelter's syndrome).
        (Y + O has not been observed; it would almost certainly be lethal.)
    2. Involving chromosome sets. (Normal—two sets diploid.)
      (a) Monoploidy (23) 22 + X; 22 + Y (not known).
      (b) Triploidy (69) ♂ 66 + X + X + Y (one case reported by Böök and Santeson (1960); male with multiple abnormalities). The condition could be regarded as trisomy of every chromosome pair which results in a triploid individual.
      (c) Higher degrees of polyploidy. (Not known.)
  B. Translocations.

II. In certain cells only of body. *Mosaicism* (presumed to be due to error occurring subsequent to conception).
  A. Anomalies of number.
    1. Mosaic of XO and XX (45/46) ♀ 44 + X + O/44 + X + X (Turner's syndrome).
    2. Mosaic of XO and XXX (45/47) ♀ 44 + X + O/44 + X + X + X.
    3. Mosaic of XX and XXY (46/47) ♂ 44 + X + X/44 + X + X + Y (Klinefelter's syndrome).
  B. Translocations.

* Hamilton, W. J., Boyd, J. D., and Mossman, H. W.: Human Embryology, ed. 3, p. 144, Cambridge, England, W. Heffer & Sons Ltd., 1962.

one a month. Under the influence of the gonadotropins, the graafian follicle that is destined to release an ovum has matured. The ovum itself has been pushed to one side of the fluid-filled cavity of the follicle. It is surrounded by a translucent coat, the zona pellucida. Immediately adjacent to the zona pellucida, and connected to it, is a layer of follicular cells, the corona radiata, so named because the cells are arranged in a radial pattern. Peripheral to this is a more loosely arranged layer of cells, the cumulus oophorus. The ovum, surrounded by this entourage of cells, having matured through release of its first polar body, and now containing the haploid number of chromosomes, is released through the process of ovulation. Transfer of the ovum into the fallopian tube, the site of fertilization, occurs relatively rapidly and with great efficiency. At this time, the ovum is a relatively large cell, measuring about 0.2 millimeters (1/25 of an inch) and is barely visible to the naked eye.

Transport Through the Fallopian Tube

The fallopian tube is an important structure which serves a number of functions in reproduction (Fig. 4-5). It is responsible for the transfer of the ovum into its lumen from the rupturing follicle, and for providing a temporary environment for the ovum and the spermatozoon. The fallopian tube also provides the environment

Implantation occurs midway on
rear or front wall
of uterus.

FIG. 4-5. Travel of egg from ovary through implantation, with alterations en route: 3 days in tube, 4 days in uterus before implantation. (Robert L. Dickinson, M.D., New York, adapted from Sellheim, with suggestions from Streeter, Frank and Hartman)

1. Follicle bursts.

2. Ovum with adhering
   granulosa cells.
   First polar body.
   2nd. maturation spindle.

3. Sperm enters egg.
   2nd maturation division.

4. Male and Female pronuclei

5. Pronuclei fusing
   Fertilization accomplished.
   5a. First cleavage division

6-7. Early cleavage

8. Morula.

9-10. Early and later gastrula.

11. Fatty unplanted growing embryo. (Miller.)

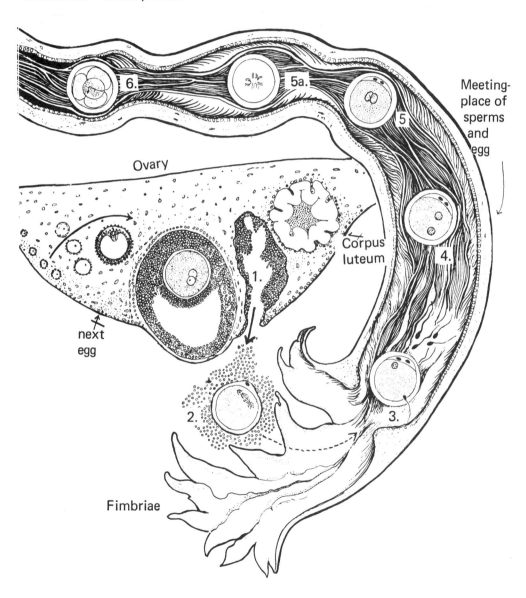

Ovary

Meeting-
place of
sperms
and
egg

Corpus
luteum

next
egg

Fimbriae

in which the fertilization process occurs, and in which the ovum passes through many cell divisions during the early stages of human life. Finally, the tube is responsible for transport of the fertilized, cleaving ovum into the uterus after a 3-day interval.

The tube is uniquely designed anatomically for its various functions. At its ovarian end, it is endowed with specialized structures, the fimbriae. These are arranged in fronds and are lined with hairlike projections, the cilia, which beat in such a manner as to direct any overlying fluid—as well

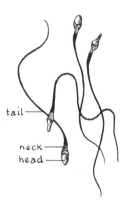

FIG. 4-6. Spermatozoa.

as any particles that float thereon—in the direction of the uterine cavity. The remainder of the fallopian tube is also lined with cilia, and these are important in the transportation of the newly released ovum along the fallopian tube. The cilia create a current which courses along the fallopian tube, and which is partially responsible for the transportation of particles through it. The anatomical arrangement at the fimbriated end of the tube is important in ovum pickup mechanisms. A separate strand of fimbria, the fimbria ovarica, extends from the tube to the ovary to which it is attached. This contains a separate bundle of smooth muscle. At the time of ovulation this muscle contracts, pulling the ovary in the direction of the tubal opening. The remainder of the fimbria are thought to embrace the ovary near the point of ovulation, or over it, and they exercise muscular movement which moves them to and fro over the rupturing follicle. Thus, the cilia lining the fimbriae soon come into contact with the cumulus cells surrounding the ovum. Through these mechanisms an efficient process of ovum transfer is arranged, and ovum pickup is practically assured, in spite of the fact that the ovum itself is miniscule in size. Once the ovum is safely within the tubal ostium, it is transported

FIG. 4-7. The sex of the offspring is determined at the time of fertilization by the combination of the sex chromosome of the spermatozoon (either X or Y) and that of the ovum (X). The ovum fertilized by a sperm cell containing the X chromosome produces a female (44 regular chromosomes + 2 X chromosomes). If it is fertilized by a spermatozoon containing the Y chromosome, the union produces a male (44 regular chromosomes + X + Y).

Note: The structures depicted as chromosomes are diagrammatic only. In this illustration it was not possible to include the total correct number.

rapidly to a point well within the fallopian tube. There, fertilization occurs. The fertilizing spermatozoon has previously been conditioned so that it has acquired the ability to fertilize an ovum. After fertilization, the ovum passes through many cell divisions, during which it is retained in the fallopian tube for approximately 3 days. Eventually it develops into a solid mass of cells called a morula. The mechanism by which the ovum is retained in the tube (in the human) is not as yet clear. However, the importance of the 3-day residence within the tube can be extrapolated from experiments in other mammals. In the rabbit, for example, if the ovum is removed from the tube prematurely, it degenerates and fails to implant. Although for obvious reasons the actual experiment has not been carried out in the human, it is generally accepted that the 3-day residence within the human tube is important. Premature expulsion of the ovum from the tube could result in failure of implantation. Prolonged retention could result in ectopic pregnancy, with implantation into the tube itself and consequent tubal rupture and hemorrhage. The latter condition constitutes a serious obstetrical emergency. The importance of the fallopian tube, a once-neglected organ which bridges the space between the ovary and the uterus, is now quite evident.

Spermatozoa

These minute, wriggling spermatozoa are in some respects even more remarkable than the ova which they fertilize. In appearance they resemble microscopic tadpoles, with oval heads and long, lashing tails about 10 times the length of the head. The human spermatozoon consists of 3 parts: the head, the middlepiece (or neck) and the tail (Fig. 4-6). The nucleus, and consequently the chromatin material, is in the head; the tail serves for propulsion. Spermatozoa are much smaller than ova, their over-all length measuring about one quarter the diameter of the egg, and it has been estimated that the heads of 2 billion of them—enough to regenerate the entire population of the world—could be placed, with room to spare, in the hull of a grain of rice. As a result of the wriggling motion of the tails, spermatozoa swim with a quick vibratory motion and have been "timed" under the microscope at rates as fast as one seventh of an inch a minute. In ascending the uterus and the fallopian tube they must swim against the same currents that waft the ovum downward; in their ascent, they are assisted by the muscular action of the uterus, which propels them upward in the direction of the tube. Spermatozoa have been observed in the fallopian tube within 30 minutes of insemination.

The most amazing feature of spermatozoa is their huge number. At each ejaculation, the climax of intercourse in the male, about 300 million are discharged into the vagina. If each of these could be united with an ovum, the babies which would be created would exceed the total number born in the United States during the past 100 years—all from a single ejaculation. Of the millions of spermatozoa deposited in the vagina during coitus, many are expelled immediately; some remain in the vagina for an interval and are later extruded. Those retained in the vagina lose their motility at the end of about an hour because of the rather hostile acid environment provided by the vagina. Those transferred into the secretions of the cervix find a more favorable environment there and may remain motile for as long as several days. Thousands of spermatozoa

sex chromatin

of infant female

of adult female

not seen in male

FIG. 4-8. Photomicrographs of epithelial cells from the oral mucosa stained with cresyl-echt violet (× 2,000). The upper 2 nuclei have Barr bodies, which are indicated by arrows. (Moore, K. L., and Barr, M. L.: Lancet 2:57, July 9, 1955, *in* Ham, A. W.: Histology, ed. 6, p. 72, Philadelphia, Lippincott, 1969)

FIG. 4-9. 1. Section of a follicular oocyte at the time of recovery. The cytoplasm contains a round, centrally located nucleus with nucleoli. Layers of corona cells are seen outside the zona pellucida. (× 201.) 2. Section of a human follicular oocyte after 24 hours of culture. A granular nucleus is located near the surface of the cytoplasm. Some altered corona cells surround the zona pellucida. (× 400.) 3. Human follicular oocyte cultured for 48 hours. The first polar body has been extruded. Phase-contrast microscopy. (× 102.) 4. Human follicular oocyte displaying metaphase II chromosomes and first polar body. (Lacmoid stained. × 780.) (Mastroianni, L., and Noriega, C.: Observations on human ova and the fertilization process. Am. J. Obstet. Gynec., 107:682-690, 1970)

find their way into the cavity of the uterus; fewer still reach the lumen of the fallopian tube. Only one is afforded the privilege of continued biologic life through fertilization and, at that, only occasionally. The remainder are disposed of in the reproductive tract, and as they degenerate they are phagocytized by the white blood cells in that region. However, it should be remembered, that once the spermatozoon is in the female reproductive tract it may retain its motility and, therefore, its potential ability to fertilize for hours, and even for days. Spermatozoa are conditioned to fertilize an egg after they are exposed to the female reproductive tract, a process referred to as *capacitation*. Within the female reproductive tract they "lie in wait" for the ovum (Fig. 4-5).

DETERMINATION OF SEX

In the human being, age, state of health and natural physical strength have nothing to do with the determination of the sex of the offspring. The sex is determined at the time of fertilization by the spermatozoon—not by the ovum.

Each mature ovum contains 22 regular chromosomes and an X chromosome. Each spermatozoon contains 22 regular chromosomes, and either an X chromosome or a Y chromosome. Spermatozoa are about equally divided between those containing only an X chromosome and those containing only a Y chromosome. If a sperm cell containing 22 chromosomes and an X chromosome fertilizes an ovum, a female will result, because in the union of the sperm and the ovum

Fig. 4-10. (*Left*) Electronmicrograph of a penetrated human ovum showing male and female pronuclei (pn). n = nucleoli. (*Right*) A portion of the penetrating spermatozoon is seen in the cytoplasm of the penetrated human pronuclear ovum. (Zamboni, L., *et al.*: Fine structure of the human ovum in the pronuclear stage. J. Cell Biol. 30:579, 1966)

there will be 44 regular chromosomes and an X chromosome from the ovum and an X chromosome from the spermatozoon. If, on the other hand, a sperm cell containing 22 regular chromosomes and a Y chromosome fertilizes an ovum, a male will result, because in the union there will be 44 regular chromosomes and an X chromosome from the ovum and a Y chromosome from the spermatozoon (Fig. 4-7). It is definitely a matter of chance, as far as is known today, whether a sperm with an X or a Y chromosome will fertilize an ovum. This is evidenced by the fact that almost universally about 94 female babies are born to every 100 male babies in single births.

Recently, cells have been recovered from the amniotic fluid surrounding the fetus in late pregnancy, and their sex chromatin pattern has been used to predict with accuracy the sex of the unborn infant.

Sex Chromatin

In females, from 20 to 90 per cent of the nuclei of the somatic (body) cells contain a small mass of material which stains red with suitable dyes, known as sex chromatin. This is probably formed by an inactive X chromosome, since it is not usually present in the body cells of males. This sex chromatin has proved to be useful in determining the sex of the embryo or fetus in early abortions and under other circumstances in which the generative organs are improperly developed (Fig. 4-8).

FERTILIZATION AND CHANGES FOLLOWING FERTILIZATION

After the ovum is well within the fallopian tube, dispersion of the peripheral layers of cells, the cumulus oophorus, occurs (Fig. 4-9). These cells begin to separate, partly as a result of the influence of the enzyme hyaluronidase contained in the head of the spermatozoon. The spermatozoon makes its way through this peripheral layer of cells, and meanwhile the densely packed layer of cells, the corona radiata, has undergone certain changes. These cells become looser under the influence of tubal fluid, and the spermatozoon then finds its way through this layer to the zona pellucida. It is now thought that the zona pellucida is penetrated by the spermatozoon because of a trypsin-like enzyme which is present in the sperm head. The spermatozoon makes a channel through the zona pellucida. It is then in a position to penetrate the membrane of the ovum itself. As the spermatozoon penetrates the ovum, it brings a portion of its tail with it (Fig. 4-10). Soon after penetration, the nucleus of the spermatozoon and the nucleus of the ovum undergo characteristic changes. They become pronuclei—

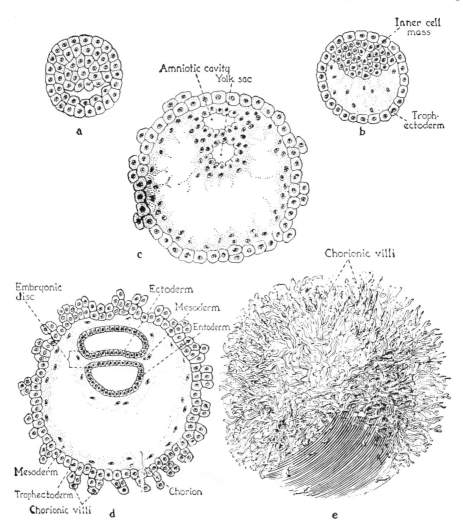

Fig. 4-11. Early stages of development. (a, b) The cells are separated into a peripheral layer and an inner cell mass; the peripheral layer is called the trophoblast or trophectoderm; the entire structure is called a blastodermic vesicle. (c) The formation of the amniotic cavity and yolk sac is indicated. The former is lined by ectoderm; the latter, by entoderm. (d) The location of the embryonic disk and the three germ layers are shown, together with the beginning of the chorionic villi. (e) The external appearance of the developing mass is shown; the chorionic villi are abundant. (Greisheimer, E. M.: Physiology and Anatomy, ed. 8, p. 799, Fig. 416, Philadelphia, Lippincott, 1963)

distinct, clearly identifiable bodies of chromatin. A second polar body is released. The male pronucleus and the female pronucleus then fuse, and the process of fertilization is now biologically complete. The new cell now contains the full complement or diploid number of chromosomes, half from the spermatozoon and half from the ovum. Soon thereafter, the first cell division occurs. In this process, the male and the female chromosomes and their genes are mingled and finally split, forming two sets of 46 chromosomes, one set of 46 going to each of the two new cells. This process is repeated again and again until masses containing 16, 32, and 64 cells are produced successively. These early cell divisions produce a solid ball of cells called the "morula," because they resemble a mulberry. In this stage, the dividing ovum is delivered into the uterus (Fig. 4-5).

Retention in the fallopian tube is believed to occupy about 3 days. The fertilized ovum then spends a period of time some 4 days in the uterine cavity before actual embedding takes place. Thus, a total interval of some 7 days lapses between ovulation and implantation. Meanwhile, important changes are taking place in the internal structure of the fertilized ovum. The cells in the center of the mulberry mass secrete a fluid which pushes the remaining cells to the periphery of the sphere. At the same time it becomes apparent that this external envelope of cells is actually made up of two different layers, an inner and an outer. A specialized portion of the inner layer, after some 260 days, will develop into the long-awaited baby. The outer layer is a sort of foraging unit, called the trophoblast (trophectoderm), which means

Fig. 4-12. Various stages in the process of implantation; the relation of the uterine mucosa to the embryonic vesicle during implantation is shown: (s) decidua basalis, (v) decidua vera, (c) decidua capsularis, and (o) the ovum or embryonic vesicle. (Greisheimer, E. M.: Physiology and Anatomy, ed. 8, p. 809, Fig. 421, Philadelphia, Lippincott, 1963)

"feeding" layer; it is the principal function of these cells to secure food for the embryo (Fig. 4-11).

While the ovum is undergoing these changes, the lining of the uterus, it will be recalled, is making preparations for its reception. Considering that ovulation took place on the 14th day of the menstrual cycle and that the tubal journey and the uterine sojourn required 7 days, 21 days of the cycle will have passed before the ovum has developed its trophoblastic layer of cells. This is the period when the lining of the uterus has reached its greatest thickness and succulence. In other words, the timing has been precisely correct; the bed is prepared, and the ovum has so developed that it is now ready to embed itself.

IMPLANTATION OF THE OVUM

The embedding of the ovum is the work of the outer "foraging" layer of cells, the trophoblast, which possesses the peculiar property of being able to digest or liquefy the tissues with which it comes into contact. This process is carried out by means of enzymes. In this manner these cells not only burrow into the uterine lining and eat out a nest for the ovum, but also digest the walls of the many small blood vessels that they encounter beneath the surface. The mother's blood stream is thus tapped, and presently the ovum finds itself deeply sunk in the lining epithelium of the uterus, with tiny pools of blood around it (Fig. 4-12). Sprouting out from the trophoblastic layer, quivering, fingerlike projections now develop and extend greedily into the blood-filled spaces. Another name for the trophoblast, and one more commonly employed as pregnancy progresses, is the chorion, and the fingerlike projections mentioned above become known as chorionic villi (Fig. 4-11). These chorionic villi contain blood vessels connected with the fetus and are extremely important, because they are the sole means by which oxygen and nourishment are received from the mother. The entire ovum becomes covered with villi, which grow out radially and convert the chorion into a shaggy sac.

DECIDUA

The thickening of the uterine endometrium, which occurs during the premenstrual phase of menstruation, has been described already. If pregnancy ensues, this endometrium becomes even more thickened, the cells enlarge, and the structure becomes known as the decidua. It is simply a direct continuation in exaggerated form of the already modified premenstrual mucosa.

For purposes of description, the decidua has been divided into three portions. That part which lies directly under the embedded ovum is known as the decidua basalis (Fig. 4-12). That portion which is pushed out by the embedded and growing ovum is called the decidua capsularis. The remainder of the decidua, or that portion which is not in immediate contact with the ovum, is known as the decidua vera. As pregnancy advances, the decidua capsularis expands rapidly over the growing embryo and at about the 4th month lies in intimate contact with the decidua vera.

THE THREE GERM LAYERS

With nutritional facilities provided, the cells which are destined to form the baby grow rapidly. At first they all look alike, but soon after embedding, groups of cells here and there assume distinctive characteristics and differentiate into three main groups: an outer covering layer, a middle layer and an internal layer. These are called, respectively, the ectoderm, the mesoderm and the entoderm.

From the *ectoderm* the following structures arise: epithelium of skin, hair, nails, sebaceous glands, sweat glands, epithelium of the nasal and the oral passages, salivary and mucous glands of the mouth and the nose, enamel of the teeth, and

Fig. 4-14. Development of decidua basalis, capsularis and vera; chorion frondosum.

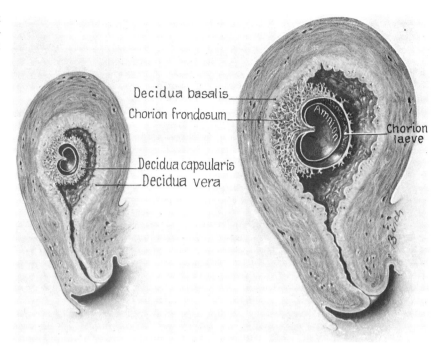

Decidua basalis
Chorion frondosum
Decidua capsularis
Decidua vera
Amnion
Chorion laeve

the nervous system. From the *mesoderm* are derived: muscles, bone, cartilage, dentin of teeth, ligaments, tendons, areolar tissue, kidneys, ureters, ovaries, testes, heart, blood, lymph and blood vessels, and lining of pericardial, pleural and peritoneal cavities. From the *entoderm* arise: the epithelium of the digestive tract, of glands which pour their secretion into the tract, of the respiratory tract and of the bladder, the urethra, the thyroid and the thymus.

AMNION, CHORION AND PLACENTA

Amnion. Even before these structures become evident, however, a fluid-filled space develops about the embryo, a space which is lined with a smooth, slippery, glistening membrane, the amnion. The space is the amniotic cavity; being filled with fluid, often it is spoken of as the bag of waters; in this the fetus floats and moves (Fig. 4-13). At full term this cavity normally contains from 500 to 1,000 cc. of liquor amnii, or the "waters." The amniotic fluid has a number of important functions: it keeps the fetus at an even temperature, cushions it against possible injury and provides a medium in which it can move easily; furthermore, it is known that the fetus drinks this fluid. At the end of the 4th month of pregnancy the amniotic cavity has enlarged to the

size of a large orange and, with the fetus, occupies the entire interior of the uterus.

Chorion. As explained, the early ovum is covered on all sides by shaggy chorionic villi, but very shortly those villi which invade the decidua basalis enlarge and multiply rapidly. This portion of the trophoblast is known as the chorion frondosum (leafy chorion) (Fig. 4-14). Contrariwise, the chorionic villi covering the remainder of the fetal envelope degenerate and almost disappear, leaving only a slightly roughened membrane. This latter is called the chorion laeve (bald chorion). The chorion laeve lies outside of the amnion, of course, with which it is in contact on its inner surface, while its outer surface lies against the decidua vera. The fetus is thus surrounded by two membranes, the amnion and the chorion, and in ordinary clinical discussions these are usually referred to simply as "the membranes."

Placenta. By the 3rd month another important structure, the placenta, has formed. This is a fleshy, disklike organ; late in pregnancy it measures about 8 inches in diameter and 1 inch in thickness. It receives its name from a Latin word meaning cake, which this structure resembles somewhat in shape. The placenta is formed by the union of the chorionic villi and the decidua basalis. An analogous situation is seen when a

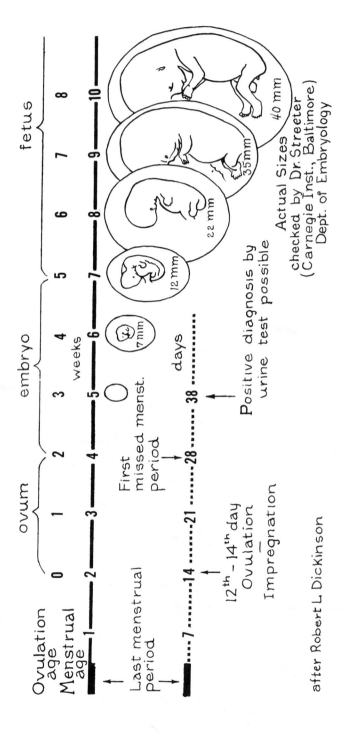

Fig. 4-15. Growth of ovum, embryo and fetus during the early weeks of pregnancy.

FIG. 4-16. Human embryo. Length, 7 mm. C. R. Estimated age, 35 days. (*Top*) In the closed sac. (*Bottom*) In the open sac. (Photos by Wesley Kaswell, University Hospitals of Cleveland)

tree or a plant sends down its roots into a bed of earth for nourishment; when the plant is removed, a certain amount of the earthy bed clings to the interlocking roots. Similarly, a thin layer of the uterine bed clings to the branching projections of chorionic villi, and together they make up this organ which supplies food to the fetus, as the roots and the earth provide nourishment for a plant. At term the placenta weighs about 500 Gm., or 1 pound. Its fetal surface is smooth and glistening, being covered by amnion, and beneath this membrane may be seen a number of large blood vessels (Plates 1 and 2). The maternal surface is red and fleshlike in character and is divided into a number of segments, about an inch in diameter, called cotyledons.

FIG. 4-17. Human embryo photographed by Chester F. Reather. This specimen represents about 40 days' development and is shown in the opened chorion. It is reproduced at a magnification of 1.7. (Carnegie Institution, Washington, D. C.)

The placenta and the fetus are connected by means of the *umbilical cord,* or funis, which is usually about 20 inches in length and about three quarters of an inch in diameter. The cord leaves the placenta near the center and enters the abdominal wall of the fetus at the umbilicus, a trifle below the middle of the median line in front. It contains two arteries and one large vein, which are twisted upon each other and are protected from pressure by a transparent, bluish-white, gelatinous substance called Wharton's jelly.

SIZE AND DEVELOPMENT OF THE FETUS

Size at Various Months

The physician, as well as the nurse, is sometimes called upon to estimate the intra-uterine age of a fetus which has been expelled prematurely.

In general, the length affords a more accurate criterion of the age of the fetus than the weight. Haase's rule suggests that for clinical purposes the length of the embryo in centimeters may be approximated during the first 5 months by squaring the number of the month to which the pregnancy has advanced; in the second half of pregnancy, by multiplying the month by 5. Conversely, the approximate age of the fetus may be obtained by taking the square root of its length in centimeters during the first 5 months, and thereafter by dividing its length in centimeters by 5. For instance, a fetus 16 cm. long is about 4 months old; a 35-cm. fetus is about 7 months old.

Development Month by Month

Most women consider themselves 1 month pregnant at the time of the first missed menstrual

FIG. 4-18. Actual size of fetus at approximately 1 month, 2 months and 3 months, respectively. (Eastman: Expectant Motherhood, Boston, Little)

period, 2 months pregnant at the second missed period, and so on. Since conception does not take place until ovulation, 14 days after the onset of menstruation in a 28-day cycle, it is obvious that an embryo does not attain the age of 1 month until about a fortnight after the first missed period (assuming a 28-day cycle), and its "birthday" by months regularly falls 2 weeks or so after any numerically specified missed period. If the cycle is longer than 28 days, or if ovulation was delayed in the conceptive cycle, the duration of actual pregnancy, relative to the last menstrual period, will be shorter. This should be remembered in reading the month-by-month development of the fetus. Thus, in speaking of the age of a pregnancy in "months," physicians refer to "lunar months," that is, periods of 4 weeks. Since a lunar month corresponds to the usual length of the menstrual cycle, they find it easier to "figure" in this way (Fig. 4-15).

Month by month the development of the fetus is something as follows:

End of First Lunar Month. The embryo is about one quarter of an inch long if measured in a straight line from head to tail—for it does have a tail at this early stage—and recognizable traces of all organs have become differentiated. The backbone is apparent but is so bent upon itself that the head almost touches the tip of the tail. At one end of the backbone the head is extremely prominent, representing almost one third of the entire embryo. (Throughout intra-uterine life the head is always very large in proportion to the body, a relationship which is still present, although to a lesser degree, at birth.) The rudiments of the eyes, the ears and the nose now make their appearance. The tube which will form the future heart has been formed, producing a large, rounded bulge on the body wall; even at this early age this structure is pulsating regularly and propelling

blood through microscopic arteries. The rudiments of the future digestive tract are also discernible—a long, slender tube leading from the mouth to an expansion in the same tube which will become the stomach; connected with the latter the beginnings of the intestines may be seen. The incipient arms and legs are represented by small nubbins that resemble buds (see Fig. 4-16).

End of Second Lunar Month. The fetus, the term used to refer to the product of conception after the 5th week of gestation, now begins to assume human form (Fig. 4-17). Due to the development of the brain, the head becomes disproportionately large so that the nose, the mouth and the ears become relatively less prominent. It has an unmistakably human face and also arms and legs, with fingers, toes, elbows and knees. During the past 4 weeks it has quadrupled in length and measures about 1 inch from head to buttocks; its weight is approximately one thirtieth of an ounce. The external genitalia become apparent, but it is difficult to distinguish between male and female. During the 2nd month the human tail reaches its greatest development, but by the end of the month it is less prominent and then undergoes retrogression.

End of Third Lunar Month. The fetus now measures somewhat over 3 inches in length and weighs almost an ounce. The sex can now be distinguished because the external genitalia are beginning to show definite signs of sex. Centers of ossification have appeared in most bones; the fingers and the toes have become differentiated, and the fingernails and the toenails appear as fine membranes. Early in this month, buds for all the temporary "baby" teeth are present, and sockets for these develop in the jawbone. Rudimentary kidneys have developed and secrete small amounts of urine into the bladder, which in all probability escape later into the amniotic fluid. Movements of the fetus are known to occur at this time, but they are too weak to be felt by the mother (Fig. 4-18).

End of Fourth Lunar Month. The fetus from head to toe is now 6½ inches long and about 4 ounces in weight. The sex as evidenced by the external genital organs is now quite obvious (Fig. 4-19).

End of Fifth Lunar Month. The length of the fetus now approximates 10 inches, while its weight is about 8 ounces. A fine downy growth of hair, *lanugo,* appears on the skin over the entire body. Usually, about this time the mother becomes con-

FIG. 4-19. Actual size of fetus at approximately 4 months.

scious of slight fluttering movements in her abdomen, which are due to movements of the fetus. Their first appearance is referred to as *quickening,* or the perception of life. At this period the physician often is able to hear the fetal heart for the first time. If a fetus is born now, it may make a few efforts to breathe, but its lungs are insufficiently developed to cope with conditions outside the uterus, and it invariably succumbs within a few hours at most (Fig. 4-20).

End of Sixth Lunar Month. The length of the fetus is 12 inches, and its weight is 1½ pounds. It now resembles a miniature baby, with the exception of the skin, which is wrinkled and red with practically no fat beneath it. At this time, however, the skin begins to develop a protective covering called *vernix caseosa,* which means "cheesy varnish." This fatty, cheesy substance adheres to the skin of the fetus and at term may be an eighth of an inch thick. Although a few cases are on record in which fetuses of this size have survived, the outlook must be regarded as practically hopeless.

End of Seventh Lunar Month. The fetus measures about 15 inches in length and weighs approximately 2½ pounds. If born at this time, it has some chance of survival, at least 1 in 10. There is a widespread notion, quite incorrect, that infants born at the 7th month are more likely to survive than those born at the 8th month. This is another of those old superstitions which have descended through more than 2,000 years from the time of the ancient Greek physicians. They believed that the fetus is born by means of its own effort; that is, it pushes with its legs against the upper part of the womb and wriggles out into the world. It was their opinion that the fetus first attempts to escape from the uterus at the 7th month and, if strong, it succeeds. If the attempt fails, it is repeated at the 8th month. However, if it now succeeds, it is so exhausted as the result of the previous attempt that it is more likely to die than if it had been successful in the prior attempt a month earlier. We now know, of course, that the fetus is entirely passive, that it is expelled from the mother's body solely through the muscular action of the uterus, and that this old belief is wholly fallacious. The fetus born at the 8th month stands a much better chance of survival than one born at the 7th.

End of Eighth Lunar Month. The fetus measures about 16.5 inches and weighs some 4 pounds. Its skin is still red and wrinkled, and vernix caseosa and lanugo are still present. In

PLATE 1. Placenta stripped to the main vessels.
Arteries are red; veins, blue. (Life Magazine.
Picture taken by Rudolph Skarda Research
Anatomist, University of California, San Fran-
cisco, Calif.)

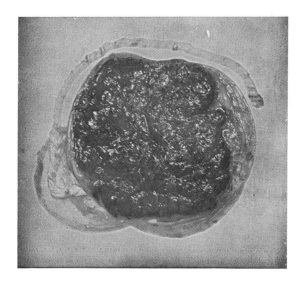

PLATE 2. (*Top*) Fetal surface of placenta.
(*Bottom*) Maternal surface of placenta.

appearance it resembles a little old man. With proper incubator and good nursing care, infants born at the end of the 8th month have better than even chances of survival, possibly as high as 3 chances in 4.

End of Ninth Lunar Month. For all practical purposes the fetus is now a mature infant, measures some 19 inches and weighs around 6 pounds. Due to the deposition of subcutaneous fat, the body has become more rotund and the skin less wrinkled and red. As though to improve its appearance before making its debut into the world, the fetus devotes the last 2 months in the uterus to putting on weight and during this period gains ½ pound a week. Its chances of survival are now quite as good as though born at full term.

Middle of Tenth Lunar Month. Full term has now been reached, and the fetus weighs on an

FIG. 4-20. Actual size of fetus at approximately 5 months.

average about 7 pounds if a girl and 7½ if a boy; its length approximates 20 inches. Its skin is now white or pink and thickly coated with the cheesy vernix. The fine, downy hair which previously covered its body has largely disappeared. The fingernails are firm and protrude beyond the end of the fingers (Fig. 4-21).

DURATION OF PREGNANCY

The length of pregnancy varies greatly; it may range, indeed, between such wide extremes as 240 days and 300 days and yet be entirely normal in every respect. The average duration from the time of conception is 9½ lunar months, that is, 38 weeks or 266 days. From the first day of the last menstrual period its average length is 10 lunar months, that is, 40 weeks or 280 days. That these average figures mean very little, however, is shown by the following facts. Scarcely one pregnancy in 10 terminates exactly 280 days after the beginning of the last period. Less than one half terminate within 1 week of this 280th day.

FIG. 4-21. Full-term fetus in utero, with placental circulation shown in color.

TABLE 4-2. DEVIATION FROM CALCULATED DATE OF CONFINEMENT, ACCORDING TO NAEGELE'S RULE, OF 4,656 BIRTHS OF MATURE INFANTS*

DEVIATION IN DAYS	EARLY DELIVERY	DELIVERY ON CALCULATED DATE	LATE DELIVERY
0	....	189 (4.1)†	....
1– 5	860 (18.5)†	....	773 (16.6)†
6–10	610 (13.1)	....	570 (12.2)
11–20	733 (15.7)	....	459 (9.9)
21–30	211 (4.5)	....	134 (2.9)
31 and over	75 (1.6)	....	42 (0.9)

The menstrual cycles of the mothers were 28 ± 5 days. The infants were at least 47 cm. in length and 2,600 Gm. in weight (Burger and Korompai).

* Eastman, N. J.: Williams Obstetrics, ed. 13, p. 220, New York, Appleton, 1966.

† Numbers in parentheses represent per cent of cases considered.

In 10 per cent of cases birth occurs a week or more before the theoretical end of pregnancy, and in another 10 per cent it takes place more than 2 weeks later than we would expect from the average figures cited above. Indeed, it would appear that some fetuses require a longer time, others a shorter time, in the uterus for full development.

CALCULATION OF THE EXPECTED DATE OF CONFINEMENT

In view of the wide variation in the length of pregnancy, it is obviously impossible to predict the expected day of confinement (often abbreviated EDC) with any degree of precision. The time-honored method, based on the above "average figures," is simple. Count back 3 calendar months from the first day of the last menstrual period and add 7 days (Naegele's rule). For instance, if the last menstrual period began on June 10, we would count back 3 months to March and, adding 7 days, arrive at the date of March 17. An easier way to calculate this is to substitute numbers for the months. Then this example becomes: 6/10 minus 3 months equals 3/10, plus 7 days equals 3/17. Although it may be satisfying to the curiosity to have this date in mind, it must be understood that less than 5 per cent of all pregnant women go into labor on the estimated date of confinement, and in 35 per cent a

deviation of from 1 to 5 days before or after this date may be expected (Table 4-2).

Yet, whether pregnancy terminates a week before or 2 weeks later than the day calculated, the outlook for mother and baby is usually as good as though it had ended at "high noon" on the due date. Actually, women seldom go "overterm"; in most of these cases it is the system of calculation and not Nature which has erred. For example, ovulation and hence conception may have occurred some days later than calculated; this error would make the beginning and the end of pregnancy that many days later. If, in addition to this circumstance, we were dealing with a baby which required a slightly longer stay in the uterus for complete development, it would be clear that the apparent delay was quite normal and for the best.

PHYSIOLOGY OF THE FETUS
Nutrition; Placental Transmission

During the period when the ovum lies unattached in the uterine cavity, its nutriment is provided by an endometrial secretion which is rich in glycogen and has been called "uterine milk." With the burrowing of the ovum into the endometrium, it lies in a lake of fluid representing the broken-down product of endometrial cells and obtains nourishment from this source (Fig. 4-12).

Very early in pregnancy, certainly by the 3rd or the 4th week, the chorionic villi have blood vessels within them (connected with the fetal blood stream), and since these villi have already opened up the maternal blood vessels, nourishment is available from the maternal blood by the process of osmosis. Such substances as oxygen and glucose in the maternal blood must diffuse through several layers of tissue of the chorionic villi to reach the fetus. These layers are the cellular epithelium covering the villus, the loose connective tissue within it and finally the endothelium of the capillary blood vessel in the center of the villus. In this manner oxygen passes into the fetal circulation, while the fetal waste product, carbon dioxide, diffuses in the opposite direction. The placenta thus serves as the "lungs" of the baby in utero. Simple food substances, such as glucose, salt, calcium, phosphorus, iron, amino acids and fatty acids, all diffuse through the chorionic villus to the fetus by this process of osmosis.

It is particularly important to note that most drugs pass readily to the fetus and, if given to the mother very shortly before birth, may affect

FIG. 4-22. Roentgenogram showing fetal and placental circulation at 11 weeks gestation, injected with Thorotrast (a contrast medium) by Charles H. Hendricks, M.D., and Frederick P. Zuspan, M.D. (Department of Obstetrics and Gynecology, Western Reserve University)

the behavior of the newborn baby (p. 227). In addition, it is interesting to observe that maternal estrogen is transmitted to the fetus and produces certain effects in the newborn which may be very striking. First, as the result of the action of this hormone, the breasts of both boy and girl babies may become markedly enlarged during the first few days of life and even secrete milk—the so-called "witch's milk" (Chap. 16, Breast Engorgement). Second, estrogen causes the endometrium of the female fetus to hypertrophy, as it does that of an adult woman. After birth, when this hormone is suddenly withdrawn, the endometrium breaks down, and sometimes bleeding occurs. For this reason perhaps 1 girl baby in every 15 manifests a little spotting on the diaper during the first week of life. This is entirely normal and clears up of itself within a few days.

Fetal Circulation

Since the placenta acts as the intermediary organ of transfer between the mother and the fetus, the fetal circulation differs from that required for extra-uterine existence. The fetus re-
ceives oxygen through the placenta, since the lungs do not function as organs of respiration in utero. To meet this situation the fetal circulation contains certain special vessels (they may be regarded as "bypasses" or "detours") which shunt the blood around the lungs, with only a small amount circulating through them for nutritional purposes (Fig. 4-22).

The oxygenated blood flows up the cord through the umbilical vein and passes into the inferior vena cava; on the way to the inferior vena cava, part of the oxygenated blood has gone through the liver, but most of it has passed through a special fetal structure, the *ductus venosus,* which connects the umbilical vein and the inferior vena cava (Fig. 4-24). The liver is proportionately so large in a newborn infant because it receives a considerable supply of freshly vitalized blood directly from the umbilical vein.

From the inferior vena cava the current flows into the right auricle and goes directly on to the left auricle through a special fetal structure, the *foramen ovale,* passing thence into the left ventricle and out through the aorta. The blood which

TABLE 4-3. CHANGES IN FETAL CIRCULATION AFTER BIRTH*

STRUCTURE	BEFORE BIRTH	AFTER BIRTH
Umbilical vein	Brings arterial blood to liver and heart.	Obliterated. Becomes the round ligament of liver.
Umbilical arteries	Bring arteriovenous blood to the placenta.	Obliterated. Become vesical ligaments on anterior abdominal wall.
Ductus venosus	Shunts arterial blood into inferior vena cava.	Obliterated. Becomes ligamentum venosum.
Ductus arteriosus	Shunts arterial and some venous blood from the pulmonary artery to the aorta.	Obliterated. Becomes ligamentum arteriosum.
Foramen ovale	Connects right and left auricles (atria).	Obliterated usually. At times open.
Lungs	Contain no air and very little blood.	Filled with air and well supplied with blood.
Pulmonary arteries	Bring little blood to lungs.	Bring much blood to lungs.
Aorta	Receives blood from both ventricles.	Receives blood only from left ventricle.
Inferior vena cava	Brings venous blood from body and arterial blood from placenta.	Brings venous blood only to right auricle.

* Williams, J. F.: Anatomy and Physiology, ed. 7, Philadelphia, Saunders.

circulates up the arms and the head returns through the superior vena cava to the right auricle again, but instead of passing through the foramen ovale, as before, the current is deflected downward into the right ventricle and out through the pulmonary arteries, partly to the lungs (for purposes of nutrition only), but mainly into the aorta through the special fetal structure, the ductus arteriosus.

The blood in the aorta, with the exception of that which goes to the head and the upper extremities (this blood has been accounted for), passes downward to supply the trunk and the lower extremities (Fig. 4-23). The greater part of this blood finds its way through the internal iliac, or hypogastric arteries, and so back through the cord to the placenta, where it is again oxygenated; but a small amount passes back into the ascending vena cava to mingle with fresh blood from the umbilical vein and again make the circuit of the entire body.

Circulation Change at Birth

The fetal circulation is so arranged that the passage of blood to the placenta through the umbilical arteries and back through the umbilical vein is possible up to the time of birth, but it ceases entirely the moment the baby breathes and so begins to take its oxygen directly from its own lungs. During intra-uterine life the circulation of

blood through the lungs is for the nourishment of the lungs and not for the purpose of securing oxygen (Figs. 4-23, 24).

In order to understand, even in a general way, the course of the blood current and how it differs from the circulation after birth, it must be borne in mind that in infants after birth, as in the adult, the venous blood passes from the two venae cavae into the right auricle of the heart, thence to the right ventricle and through the pulmonary arteries to the lungs, whence it gives up its waste products and takes up a fresh supply of oxygen. After oxygenation the so-called arterial blood flows from the lungs, through the pulmonary veins to the left auricle, thence to the left ventricle and out through the aorta, to be distributed through the capillaries to all parts of the body and eventually collected, as venous blood, in the venae cavae and discharged again into the right auricle.

Circulation Path After Birth

As soon as the baby is born and breathes, the function of the lungs is established, and the placental circulation ceases (the baby no longer is dependent on his mother's blood for oxygen but is a separate being and breathes to oxygenate his own blood). This change not only alters the character of the blood in many vessels but also makes many of these vessels of no use as such; the umbilical arteries within the baby's body be-

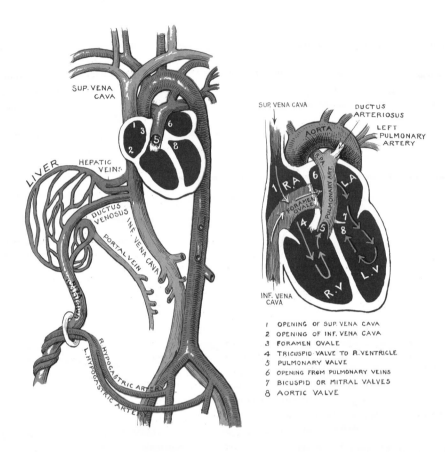

FIG. 4-23 (*Left*). Fetal circulation before birth. The material needed for the nourishment and the develop-ment of the fetus is brought to it from the placenta by way of the umbilical vein. Since the lungs do not func-tion in the exchange of gases, the placenta serves as the respiratory organ in supplying oxygen to the fetus and also serves as an excretory organ for waste products. After the blood is purified in the placenta, it is sent with its nutritive material to the fetus by way of the umbilical vein; this vein divides into two branches after entering he abdominal wall. One of these branches joins directly to the portal vein which empties its blood into the liver, from which it is carried to the inferior vena cava by way of the hepatic veins. The other branch, the ductus venosus, joins directly the inferior vena cava, from which the blood is then carried to the right auricle of the heart. From the right auricle it goes through the foramen ovale to the left auricle and then to the left ventricle to the upper extremity by way of the aorta.

The blood returning from the upper extremity through the superior vena cava enters the right auricle, then the right ventricle, and then goes to the lungs by way of the pulmonary artery. Since the lungs do not function before birth, only a small portion of this blood gains access to them. Most of the blood from the pulmonary artery is diverted through the ductus arteriosus to the aorta and is then carried to the trunk and lower extremities.

FIG. 4-24 (*Right*). Fetal circulation after birth. Pulmonary circulation becomes established with birth. The umbilical cord circulation ceases. The arteries and the vein become obliterated immediately at the body junction. Shortly the hypogastric arteries, which are a continuance of the umbilical arteries after entrance into the body, become obliterated at their distal ends, followed by occlusion and obliteration of the umbilical vein and ductus venosus. The ductus arteriosus and the foramen ovale undergo a slower metamorphosis, finally occluding the circulation through the ductus arteriosus and closure of the foramen ovale. (Philips J. Carter, M.D., Louisiana State University, New Orleans) come filled with clotted blood and ultimately are converted into fibrous cords, and the umbilical vein within the body, after occlusion of the vessel, becomes the round ligament of the liver. After the umbilical cord is tied and separated, the large amount of blood returned to the heart and the lungs, which are now functioning, causes more or less equal pressure in both of the auricles— this pressure causes the foramen ovale to close. The foramen ovale remains closed and eventually disappears, and the ductus arteriosus and the ductus venosus finally shrivel up and are converted into fibrous cords or ligaments in the course of 2 or 3 months. The instantaneous closure of the foramen ovale changes the entire course of the blood current and converts the fetal circulation into the adult type.

The changes in the fetal circulation after birth may be tabulated as given in Table 4-3.

PERIODS OF DEVELOPMENT

Human life may be divided into periods. The successive periods, with the duration of each, are indicated below.

The period of the ovum extends from fertilization to implantation, about the close of the 1st week of prenatal life. (The term "ovum" is used in a strict sense to denote the female germ cell and also to indicate the developing zygote [fertilized ovum] previous to implantation.)

The period of the embryo extends from the 2nd to the 5th weeks of gestation, during which time the various organs are developed, and a definite form is assumed.

The period of the fetus extends from after the 5th week to the time of birth.

The period of the newborn (neonatal) extends from birth to the close of the 1st month of postnatal life.

The period of infancy extends from the close of the 1st month to the close of the 2nd year of life (Nelson's Textbook of Pediatrics, Saunders, 1959).

The period of childhood extends from the close of the 2nd year to about the 14th year in females and to about the 16th year in males. Puberty ends the period of childhood.

The period of adolescence extends from puberty to the last years of the 2nd decade (late teens) in females and to the first years of the 3rd decade (early 20's) in males.

The period of maturity extends from the end of the adolescent period to senility (old age).

Development goes on throughout life; during senility, retrogressive or degenerative changes occur.

MATERNAL IMPRESSIONS

One of the commonest superstitions relating to childbearing is the old belief that the mental condition of the mother may modify the development of the unborn infant or, as people used to say, "mark it." For instance, if a pregnant woman were frightened by some ugly beast, let us say, it used to be thought that when the baby was born, it might be "marked" or distorted in the likeness of the animal. Very often the "marking" took the form of reddish blotches on the skin of the infant, which in the mother's imagination seemed to resemble the beast. Or, sometimes it was thought that the blotch resembled some article of food that the pregnant woman particularly craved.

This belief, like most obstetric superstitions, is of hoary antiquity. The Biblical story of Jacob and the "speckled and spotted" cattle and goats and the "brown" sheep reflects it, and dramatists and novelists from Shakespeare to Dickens have perpetuated the idea in stirring plots. The facts are these: There is no nervous connection between mother and fetus—in other words, no possible pathways along which any such impulses, pleasant or otherwise, could travel. Furthermore, the anlagen for the various organs of the fetus are developed by the 6th week of pregnancy, that is, at a period when most women scarcely realize that they are pregnant; and, almost without exception, the causative mental shock or experience which is alleged to have brought about the "marking" occurred much later, long after the organ in question was in its final state of formation. Finally, all modern experience refutes the belief. Obstetricians of vast experience, as well as maternity hospitals with thousands of deliveries annually, never have reported an authentic case.

How, then, is this age-old superstition to be explained? A number of factors probably contribute to it, chiefly coincidence. Approximately 1 baby in every 200 is born with some kind of blemish. In the event that such a blemish is present—let us say a reddish blotch on the buttocks of the baby—would it not be easy for an introspective mother, who had been told of this legend, to think finally of some object, some animal, or possibly some article of diet that she craved during pregnancy and, in her imagination, correlate it with the little red blotch?

SUGGESTED READING

Behrman, S. J., and Kistner, R. W.: Progress in Infertility. Boston, Little, Brown, 1968.

Hafez, E. S. E., and Blandau, R. J.: The Mammalian Oviduct. Chicago, University of Chicago Press, 1969.

Porter, I. H.: Heredity and Disease. New York, McGraw-Hill, 1968.

Thompson, G. S., and Thompson, M. W.: Genetics in Medicine. Philadelphia, W. B. Saunders, 1966.

Presentations and Positions

Fetal Habitus • Fetal Head • Presentation • Positions • Diagnosis of Fetal Position

FETAL HABITUS

By habitus, or attitude, of the fetus is meant the relation of the fetal parts to one another. The most striking characteristic of the fetal habitus is flexion. The spinal column is bowed forward, the head is flexed with the chin against the sternum, and the arms are flexed and folded against the chest. The lower extremities also are flexed, the thighs on the abdomen and the calves of the lower legs against the posterior aspect of the thighs. In this state of flexion the fetus assumes a roughly ovoid shape, occupies the smallest possible space and conforms to the shape of the uterus. In this attitude it is about half as long as if it were completely stretched out. However, there are times when the fetus assumes many other positions.

FETAL HEAD

From an obstetric viewpoint the head of the fetus is the most important part. If it can pass through the pelvic canal safely, there is usually no difficulty in delivering the rest of the body, although occasionally the shoulders may cause trouble.

The cranium, or skull, is made up of 8 bones. Four of the bones—the sphenoid, the ethmoid and the 2 temporal bones—lie at the base of the cranium, are closely united and are of little obstetric interest. On the other hand, the 4 bones forming the upper part of the cranium are of great importance; these are the frontal, the occipital and the 2 parietal bones. These bones are not knit closely together at the time of birth but are separated by membranous interspaces called *sutures*. The intersections of these sutures are known as *fontanels* (Fig. 5-1).

By means of this formation of the fetal skull the bones can overlap each other somewhat during labor and so diminish materially the size of the head during its passage through the pelvis. This process of overlapping is called "molding," and after a long labor with a large baby and a snug pelvis, the head often is so definitely molded that several days may elapse before it returns to its normal shape.

The most important sutures are: the sagittal, between the 2 parietal bones; the frontal, between the 2 frontal bones; the coronal, between the frontal and the parietal bones; and the lambdoid, between the posterior margins of the parietal bones and the upper margin of the occipital bone. The temporal sutures, which separate the parietal and the temporal bones on either side, are unimportant in obstetrics because they are covered by fat parts and cannot be felt on the living baby.

The fontanels of importance are the anterior and the posterior. The anterior fontanel, large and diamond-shaped, is at the intersection of the sagittal and the coronal sutures, while the small triangular posterior fontanel lies at the junction of the sagittal and the lambdoid suture. The sutures and the posterior fontanel ossify shortly after birth, but the anterior fontanel remains open until the child is over a year old, constituting the familiar "soft spot" just above the forehead of an infant. By feeling or identifying one or another of the sutures or fontanels, and considering its relative position in the pelvis, the physician is enabled to determine accurately the position of the head.

PRESENTATION

The term "presentation" or "presenting part" is used to designate that portion of the infant's body which lies nearest the internal os, or, in other words, that portion which is felt by the examining fingers of the physician when they are introduced into the cervix. When the presenting part is known, by abdominal palpation, it is possible to determine the relation between the long axis of the baby's body and that of the mother.

Head or *cephalic presentations* are the most common, being present in about 97 per cent of all cases at term. Cephalic presentations are divided into groups, according to the relation which the infant's head bears to its body. The most common is the *vertex presentation,* in which the head is sharply flexed so that the chin is in contact with the thorax; then the vertex is the presenting part. The *face presentation,* in which the neck is sharply extended so that the occiput and the back come in contact, is more rarely observed.

Next to the cephalic presentation, *the breech presentation* is the most common, being present, however, in only about 3 per cent of all cases. In breech presentations the thighs may be flexed and the legs extended over the anterior surface of the body (*frank breech presentation*), or the thighs may be flexed on the abdomen and the legs on the thighs (*full breech presentation*), or

one or both feet may be the lowest part (*foot or footling presentation*).

When the fetus lies crosswise in the uterus, the shoulder is the presenting part—*shoulder presentation.* The common causes of a "transverse lie" are: (1) abnormal relaxation of the abdominal walls due to great multiparity, (2) pelvic contraction, and (3) placenta previa. Shoulder presentations are relatively uncommon, and, with very rare exceptions, the spontaneous birth of a fully developed child is impossible in a "persistent transverse lie."

POSITIONS

Beside knowing the presenting part of the baby, it is important to know the exact position of this presenting part in relation to the pelvis. This relationship is determined by finding the position of certain points on the presenting surface with regard to the four imaginary divisions or regions of the pelvis. For this purpose the pelvis is considered to be divided into quadrants: left anterior, left posterior, right anterior and right posterior. These divisions aid the physician in indicating whether the presenting part is directed toward the right or the left side and toward the

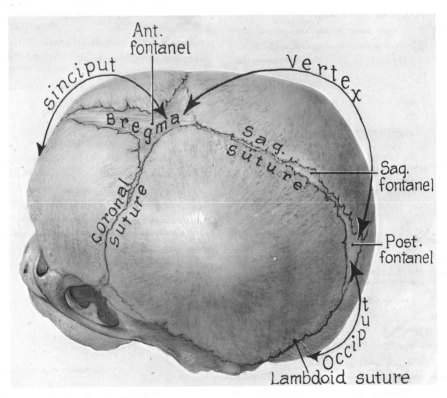

Fig. 5-1. Fetal skull, showing sutures and fontanels.

front or the back of the pelvis. Certain points on the presenting surface of the baby have been arbitrarily chosen as points of direction in determining the exact relation of the presenting part to the quadrants of the pelvis. In vertex presentations the occiput is the guiding point; in face presentations, the chin (mentum); in breech presentations, the sacrum; and in shoulder presentations, the scapula (acromion process).

Position, then, has to do with the relation of some arbitrarily chosen portion of the fetus to the right or the left side of the mother's pelvis. Thus, in a vertex presentation, the back of the head (occiput) may point to the front or to the back of the pelvis. The occiput rarely points directly forward or backward in the median line until the second stage of labor, but usually is directed to one side or the other.

The various positions are usually expressed by abbreviations made up of the first letter of each word which describes the position. Thus, left-occipito-anterior is abbreviated L.O.A. This

POSITIONS OF PRESENTING PARTS

FIG. 5-2. Left-occipito-anterior (L.O.A.).

FIG. 5-4. Right-occipitotransverse (R.O.T.).

FIG. 5-3. Right-occipito-anterior (R.O.A.).

FIG. 5-5. Right-occipitoposterior (R.O.P.).

means that the head is presenting with the occiput directed toward the left side of the mother and toward the front part of the pelvis. If the occiput were directed straight to the left with no deviation toward front or back of the pelvis, it would be termed left-occipitotransverse, or L.O.T. The occiput might also be directed toward the back or posterior quadrant of the pelvis, in which case the position would be left-occipitoposterior, or L.O.P. There are also three corresponding positions on the right side: R.O.A., R.O.T. and R.O.P.

The occipital positions are considered the most favorable for both mother and baby, and of these, the L.O.A. position is preferred. The same system of terminology is used for face, breech and shoulder presentations, as indicated in the following list of abbreviations (S indicating breech; M, chin or face; and A, shoulder).

Although it is customary to speak of all "trans- verse lies" of the fetus simply as shoulder presentations, the examples of terminology sometimes used to express position in the shoulder presentation are listed. Left-acromio-dorso-anterior (L.A.D.A.) means that the acromion is to the mother's left and the back is anterior.

POSITIONS—VERTEX PRESENTATION

L.O.A.—Left-occipito-anterior (Fig. 5-2)
L.O.T.—Left-occipitotransverse
L.O.P.—Left-occipitoposterior
R.O.A.—Right-occipito-anterior (Fig. 5-3)
R.O.T.—Right-occipitotransverse (Fig. 5-4)
R.O.P.—Right-occipitoposterior (Fig. 5-5)

POSITIONS—BREECH PRESENTATION

L.S.A.—Left-sacro-anterior
L.S.T.—Left-sacrotransverse

Fig. 5-6. Left-sacroposterior (L.S.P.).

Fig. 5-7. Left-mento-anterior (L.M.A.).

Fig. 5-8. Right-acromio-dorso-posterior (R.A.D.P.). This means that the *acromium* lies toward the *right* side of the mother and that the back (dorsum) of the infant lies toward the *posterior* part of the pelvis.

Fig. 5-9. Fetal head, showing transverse diameters.

L.S.P.—Left-sacroposterior (Fig. 5-6)
R.S.A.—Right-sacro-anterior
R.S.T.—Right-sacrotransverse
R.S.P.—Right-sacroposterior

POSITIONS—FACE PRESENTATION

L.M.A.—Left-mento-anterior (Fig. 5-7)
L.M.T.—Left-mentotransverse
L.M.P.—Left-mentoposterior
R.M.A.—Right-mento-anterior
R.M.T.—Right-mentotransverse
R.M.P.—Right-mentoposterior

POSITIONS—SHOULDER PRESENTATION

L.A.D.A.—Left-acromio-dorso-anterior
L.A.D.P.—Left-acromio-dorso-posterior
R.A.D.A.—Right-acromio-dorso-anterior
R.A.D.P.—Right-acromio-dorso-posterior
(Fig. 5-8)

Figures 5-9 and 10 show the principal measurements of the fetal skull. The most important transverse diameter is the biparietal; it is the distance between the biparietal protuberances and represents the greatest width of the head. It measures, on an average, 9.25 cm. There are three important anteroposterior diameters: the suboccipitobregmatic, which extends from the undersurface of the occiput to the center of the anterior fontanel and measures about 9.5 cm.; the occipitofrontal, which extends from the root of the nose to the occipital prominence and measures about 12.0 cm.; and the occipitomental, which extends from the chin to the posterior fontanel and averages about 13.5 cm.

In considering these three anteroposterior diameters of the fetal skull, it is important to note that with the head in complete flexion and the chin resting on the thorax, the smallest of these, the suboccipitobregmatic, enters the pelvis, whereas if the head is extended or bent back (with no flexion whatsoever), the greatest anteroposterior diameter presents itself to the pelvic inlet. Herein lies the great importance of flexion; the more the head is flexed, the smaller is the anteroposterior diameter which enters the pelvis. Figures 5-11 to 13 show this basic principle in diagrammatic form.

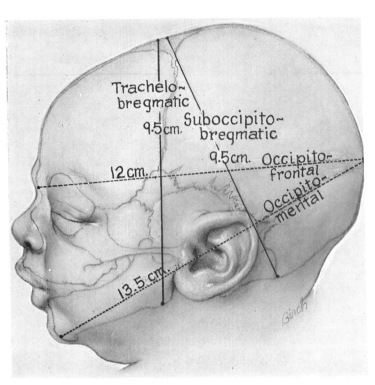

FIG. 5-10. Fetal head, showing anteroposterior diameters.

DIAGNOSIS OF FETAL POSITION

Diagnosis of fetal position is made in four ways: (1) abdominal palpation; (2) vaginal and rectal examination; (3) combined auscultation and examination; (4) in certain doubtful cases, the roentgenogram.

Inspection

Nurses thus should be able to determine whether a presentation is normal or otherwise, as work in rural, sparsely settled localities often may require of her knowledge not demanded in her hospital experience. Only under most unusual conditions would she be expected to ascertain this in any other way than by palpation.

Palpation

The nurse should familiarize herself thoroughly with this method. She will find it extremely helpful to palpate the abdomen before listening to the fetal heart tones. The region of the abdomen in which the fetal heart is heard most plainly varies according to the presentation and the extent to which the presenting part has descended. The location of the fetal heart sounds by itself does not give very important information as to the presentation and the position of the child, but it sometimes reinforces the results obtained by palpation. In order to obtain satisfactory information by abdominal palpation for the determination of fetal position, the examination should be made systematically by following the four maneuvers suggested by Leopold, often called the *Leopold maneuvers*.

The nurse should make certain that the patient has emptied her bladder before the procedure is begun. This will not only contribute to the patient's comfort but also will aid the nurse to gain more accurate results in the latter part of the examination. During the first three maneuvers the nurse stands at the side of the bed facing the patient; during the last one she faces the patient's feet. Although a diagnosis should not be made on the basis of inspection, actual observation of the patient's abdomen should precede palpation. For the examination the patient should lie flat on her back, with her knees flexed, to relax the abdominal muscles; the nurse should lay both hands gently, and at first, flat upon the abdomen. If done in any other manner than this, or if her hands are not warm, the stimulation of her fingers will cause the abdominal muscles to contract. She should accustom herself to palpate the uterus in a definite, methodical way, and it will be found

Fig. 5-11 (*Top*). Complete flexion allows smallest diameter of head to enter pelvis.

Fig. 5-12 (*Center*). Moderate extension causes larger diameter to enter pelvis.

Fig. 5-13 (*Bottom*). Marked extension forces largest diameter against pelvic brim, but it is too large to enter.

best to carry out successively the following four maneuvers.

First Maneuver. The nurse should ascertain, facing the patient, what is lying at the fundus of the uterus by feeling the upper abdomen with both hands; generally she will find there a mass, which is either the head or the buttocks (breech) of the fetus. She must decide which pole of the fetus this is by observing three points (Fig. 5-14):

1. Its relative consistency: the head is harder than the breech.

2. Its shape: if the head, it will be round and hard, and the transverse groove of the neck may be felt. The breech has no groove and usually feels more angular.

3. Mobility: the head will move independently of the trunk, but the breech moves only with the trunk. The ability of the head to be moved back and forth against the examining fingers is spoken of as ballottement.

Second Maneuver. Having determined whether the head or the breech is in the fundus, the next

FIG. 5-14. Palpation: (*top, left*) first maneuver; (*top, right*) second maneuver; (*bottom, left*) third maneuver; (*bottom, right*) fourth maneuver.

step is to locate the back of the fetus in relation to the right and the left sides of the mother. Still facing the patient, the nurse places the palmar surfaces of both hands on either side of the abdomen and makes gentle but deep pressure. If the hand on one side of the abdomen remains still to steady the uterus, a slightly circular motion with the flat surface of the fingers on the other hand can gradually palpate the opposite side from the top to the lower segment of the uterus to feel the fetal outline. Then, to palpate the other side, the functions of the hands are reversed (i.e., the hand which was used to palpate now remains

steady), and the other hand palpates the opposite side of the uterus. On one side is felt a smooth, hard, resistant plane, the back, while on the other, numerous angular nodulations are palpated, the small parts; these latter represent the knees and the elbows of the fetus.

Third Maneuver. This maneuver consists in an effort to find the head at the pelvic inlet and to determine its mobility. It should be conducted by gently grasping the lower portion of the abdomen, just above the symphysis pubis, between the thumb and the fingers of one hand and then pressing together. If the presenting part is not engaged, a movable body will be felt, which is usually the head.

Fourth Maneuver. In this maneuver the nurse faces the feet of the patient and places the tips of her first three fingers on both sides of the midline about 2 inches above Poupart's ligament. Pressure is now made downward and in the direction of the birth canal, the movable skin of the abdomen being carried downward along with the fingers. It will be found that the fingers of one hand meet no obstruction and can be carried downward well under Poupart's ligament; these fingers glide over the nape of the baby's neck. The other hand, however, usually meets an obstruction an inch or so above Poupart's ligament; this is the brow of the baby and is usually spoken of as the "cephalic prominence." This maneuver gives information of several kinds:

1. If the findings are as described above, it means that the baby's head is well flexed.

2. Confirmatory information is obtained about the location of the back, as naturally the back is on the opposite side from the brow of the baby, except in the uncommon cases of face presentation, in which the cephalic prominence and the back are on the same side.

3. If the cephalic prominence is very easily palpated, as if it were just under the skin, a posterior position of the occiput is suggested.

4. The location of the cephalic prominence tells how far the head has descended into the pelvis. This maneuver is of most value if the head has engaged and may yield no information with a floating, poorly flexed head.

Vaginal Examination

Vaginal examination is done by the physician and consists in identifying the fontanels and the suture lines of the fetal skull. During pregnancy the vaginal examination gives limited information concerning the position of the fetus because the cervix is closed. However, during labor, after more or less complete dilatation of the cervix, important information about the position of the baby and the degree of flexion of its head can be obtained.

Auscultation

The location of the fetal heart sounds, as heard through the stethoscope, yields helpful confirmatory information about fetal position but is not wholly dependable. Certainly, it never should be relied on as the sole means of diagnosing fetal position. Ordinarily, the heart sounds are transmitted through the convex portion of the fetus, which lies in intimate contact with the uterine wall, so that they are heard best through the infant's back in vertex and breech presentations, and through the thorax in face presentation. In cephalic presentations the fetal heart sounds are heard loudest midway between the umbilicus and the anterior superior spine of the ilium. In general, in L.O.A. and L.O.P. positions the fetal heart sounds are heard loudest in the left lower quadrant. A similar situation applies to the R.O.A. and R.O.P. positions. In posterior positions of the occiput (L.O.P. and R.O.P.) often the sounds are heard loudest well down in the flank toward the anterosuperior spine. In breech presentation the fetal heart sounds usually are heard loudest at the level of the umbilicus or above.

Roentgenograms

Roentgenograms are of particular value in diagnosis of fetal position in doubtful cases, particularly in obese women or in those with abdominal walls so rigid that abdominal palpation is difficult. In such situations the roentgenogram enables the physician to recognize the existence of conditions which might otherwise have escaped detection until late in labor. They give accurate information concerning position, presentation, flexion and descent of the fetal head (see Fig. 7-4).

SUGGESTED READING

Danforth, D. N.: Textbook of Obstetrics and Gynecology. New York, Hoeber Medical Division, Harper & Row, 1966.

Eastman, N. J. and Hellman, L. H.: Williams Obstetrics. ed. 13, New York, Appleton, 1966.

Greenhill, J. P.: Obstetrics. ed. 13, Philadelphia, W. B. Saunders, 1965.

Willson, J. R.: Obstetrics and Gynecology. ed. 3, St. Louis, C. V. Mosby, 1966.

CONFERENCE MATERIAL

1. What would be your responsibility to a friend who is pregnant and yet has not registered for delivery with either a doctor or a clinic?

2. How would you present the subject of human reproduction to a group of Girl Scouts or junior high school students?

3. What illustrative material and reference readings would you select for a group conference of young parents or those about to be married?

4. How would you go about looking up the costs of obstetric care in your community?

5. If a patient appealed to you to secure information about the best obstetric care available in a certain city in the United States, how would you get this information for her?

6. What authentic sources are available for obtaining maternal and infant mortality statistics?

7. What is the status of the midwife in this country? How does this situation compare with that in other countries?

8. What forces are in operation to improve the quality of maternity care?

9. How can you stimulate the interest of a lay group in the community which is willing to give time and some financial support to help with an educational program for the less fortunate?

SELF-EXAMINATION QUESTIONS FOR THE STUDENT

After each unit of this book some objectively scorable test questions are provided to aid you in making immediate *use* of the information and the knowledge that you have gained through studying each of these units. The questions are planned to enable you to see how some of the important facts function in the nursing care of patients, and how knowledge of the facts enables you to (1) recognize, analyze and interpret the nursing needs of maternity patients, (2) plan to meet these needs, (3) carry out the plan and (4) evaluate both the plan and the results.

These questions represent only a few sample instances in which information, facts and principles presented in the units function in nursing care. If you are successful in these samples, you may be in many more instances, but you should not assume that success here guarantees success in all. Likewise, failure on many of these items does not necessarily mean complete lack of understanding, but it is a rather good indication that you need to restudy the unit more carefully.

Use these tests as a study device. After you believe that you have mastered the important points in the unit, fill out the objectively scorable test questions at the end of the unit. Think through each question and response carefully. Complete the entire unit test and then (and not until then) turn to the key on page 000, where you will find the right answers. See how many you had correct. Look up the answers to those that you answered incorrectly.

You will observe that many of the questions demand that you use your previously acquired knowledge of anatomy and physiology, bacteriology, chemistry, pharmacology, psychology, nursing arts and nutrition, together with maternity nursing knowledge, for all nursing care demands the simultaneous functioning of facts and principles from many of these fields, along with those of the special clinical field.

In some judgments on debatable questions the answer given in the key may conflict with the current practice in your institution or locality. Ask your teacher how she thinks you should evaluate yourself on this knowledge.

Since the purpose of these self-scoring tests is to aid you in learning, you will be defeating that purpose and penalizing yourself if you misuse them. Carefully think through the question. *No one but you is interested in how well or how poorly you do on these tests.* When you have discovered how well or how poorly you have done, you will know better what you need to study again, and how much more study is necessary.

Your teacher's evaluation of your ability to use the material presented in each unit may sample some of these and many other points presented in the unit. Your best preparation for your teacher's appraisal in classroom and in the practice of nursing is your own evaluation of your attainment and study in light of your accomplishment. But, more important, your best preparation for giving skilled professional nursing care to maternity patients is to have a complete understanding of and ability to use the important principles that relate to that care, an understanding that is largely within your own power to obtain through your own efforts.

Study Questions

Unit One: Human Reproduction

Read through the entire question and place your answer on the line to the right.

1. Which of the following complications of pregnancy are responsible for the greatest toll in maternal mortality?
   A. Cardiac complications
   B. Toxemia
   C. Hemorrhage
   D. Infection
   E. Diabetes

   Select the number corresponding to the correct letters.
   1. A and B
   2. A, C and E
   3. B, C and D
   4. B, C and E   _____3_____

2. What improvement is believed to be the greatest single factor for decreasing maternal deaths during the past half century?
   A. Antepartal care
   B. Management of labor
   C. Analgesia during delivery
   D. Nursing care during delivery
   E. Care by the physician during delivery
   F. Care during the puerperium   _____A_____

3. A patient in the clinic, who was in the latter part of her pregnancy, reported to the nurse that she was suffering from backache and wanted to know the cause. What would be the most likely reason that the nurse could give her?
   A. The larger size of the fetus tires her more easily.
   B. Increased mobility of joints throws greater weight on surrounding muscles.
   C. She must have some abnormality in pelvic structures.
   D. The descent of the presenting part into the pelvic cavity prior to labor increases pressure against the sacrum.   _____B_____

4. In each of the following write the term or the phrase by which the pelvic measurement described is commonly called.
   A. Between the symphysis pubis and the depression below the 5th lumbar vertebra   A. Ext. conjugate
   B. From the lower margin of the symphysis pubis to the sacral promontory   B. Diagonal
   C. Between the lateral edges of the iliac crests   C. Intercristal
   D. The posterior portion of the symphysis pubis to the promontory of the sacrum   D. Conjugata vera
   E. From the inner aspects of the ischial tuberosities   E. Intertuberous diameter.

5. By using the letter or letters of the measurements described in Question 4 indicate:
   A. The one which must be estimated rather than measured directly   A. _____D_____
   B. The one which represents the most important diameter   B. _____D_____
   C. The one which represents the largest diameter   C. _____C_____

6. A patient's chart shows pelvic measurements of 11 cm. for the diagonal conjugate and 9.5 cm. for the true conjugate; therefore, the nurse caring for the patient in the labor room should anticipate that the patient might have:

A. An easy, rapid delivery
B. A delivery of reasonable duration
C. A protracted labor with difficult delivery   C

7. To give adequate care to the patient during and after delivery, the nurse should fully understand the structure of the uterus. Which of the following are true of the uterus?

A. Its muscular tissue is:
    1. Chiefly striated
    2. Chiefly nonstriated
    3. Entirely striated
    4. Entirely nonstriated   4

B. Its muscle fibers are arranged to run:
    1. Circularly
    2. Longitudinally
    3. In all directions
    4. In three layers, the inner and the outer circularly, the other longitudinally   3

C. Its blood is supplied directly from:
    1. Ovarian and uterine arteries.
    2. Abdominal aorta and uterine arteries.
    3. Internal iliac and ovarian arteries.
    4. Internal iliac and uterine arteries.   1

D. Normally, it is:
    1. Attached anteriorly to the bladder wall.
    2. Suspended freely movable in the pelvic cavity.
    3. Suspended between the bladder and the rectum.
    4. Attached posteriorly to the anterior wall of the sacrum.   3

8. The perineum lies between the vagina and the rectum. This structure has:

A. A single, strong elastic muscle
B. A strong elastic tendon
C. A tendon to which 5 muscles are attached
D. Two strong muscles, the anal and the transverse perineal   C

9. Every effort is made to prevent the tearing of the perineum during childbirth. The chief hazard to the patient from laceration of the perineum would likely be:

A. Incontinence
B. Postpartal hemorrhage
C. Perineal abscess
D. Prolapsed uterus   B

10. A patient with small breasts in her first pregnancy was worried about her ability to feed her baby.

A. The nurse could respond correctly to the patient by telling her that:
    1. She probably would be unable to feed her baby.
    2. The size of the breasts does not influence the amount of lactation possible.
    3. Mothers with small breasts usually have less difficulty feeding their babies.
    4. Her baby would be fed better by means of a formula.   2

B. Milk is produced by the process of:
   1. Dialysis
   2. Osmosis
   3. Secretion   _3_

C. The structures most directly involved in the production of milk are:
   1. Papillae
   2. Glands of Montgomery
   3. Acini cells
   4. Lactiferous sinuses
   5. Areola
   6. Lactiferous ducts   _3_

11. What are the ovarian hormones produced by the graafian follicle and the cells of the corpus luteum?
   A. Progesterone and gonadotropin
   B. Estrogen and progesterone
   C. Gonadotropin and FSH
   D. FSH and estrogen   _B_

12. A young mother-to-be told a nurse that she was sure that she would have a boy because her husband was such a strong, physically well-developed man. The nurse could respond correctly by saying:
   A. "It is the female cell which determines the sex of the child."
   B. "It is unlikely because there are more girls born than boys."
   C. "Physical strength does not influence the sex of the child."
   D. "You are probably right."   _C_

13. A patient expelled a fetus of 16 cm. prematurely. What would be the approximate age of the fetus?
   A. 2 months
   B. 3 months
   C. 4 months
   D. 5 months   _C_

14. Although the exact date of delivery cannot be predetermined, if a pregnant woman's last menstrual period began on September 10, the estimated due date would be nearest:
   A. May 6
   B. May 10
   C. June 10
   D. June 17   _D_

15. The only direct connection between the fetus and any other structure is through the umbilical cord. The umbilical cord contains which of these important structures?
   A. Umbilical artery
   B. Umbilical arteries
   C. Umbilical vein
   D. Umbilical veins
   E. Umbilical nerves
   F. Umbilical lymphatic duct
   G. Wharton's jelly

   Select the number corresponding to the correct letters.
   1. A, D and F
   2. B, C and G
   3. C, E and G
   4. All of them   _2_

16. After a protracted labor and a difficult delivery, the mother, upon seeing her baby, was shocked at the elongated appearance of the infant's head. The nurse could correctly reassure the patient by saying:

    A. "The baby's head is molded during delivery and will return to normal in a few days."
    B. "All newborn babies' heads are shaped this way."
    C. "The child's head shape was changed during delivery, and it will take six months for it to return to normal."
    D. "After the 'soft spot' closes, the head will return to normal."   _____A_____

17. Indicate the abbreviations that might be used on a patient's chart to represent each of the positions and the presentations described:

    A. Back of head directed straight to the left   A. _LOT_
    B. Back of head directed toward the left side and the front quadrant of the pelvis   B. _LOA_
    C. Back of head directed toward the right side and the back quadrant of the pelvis   C. _ROP_
    D. Breech presentation, buttocks at the left back quadrant   D. _SLSP_
    E. Face presentation, chin at the right front quadrant   E. _RmA_
    F. Transverse lie, shoulder is to the right of mother's pelvis, back is posterior F. _RADP_

    Note: The key to the correct answers to these questions is given on page 613.

UNIT TWO
Nursing in Pregnancy

Normal Pregnancy

Signs and Symptoms of Pregnancy

Antepartal Care

Social Factors in Maternal Care

Patient Teaching

Normal Pregnancy

INTRODUCTION

This chapter is concerned with the anatomic and the physiologic adaptations of the human organism to pregnancy. Knowledge of human reproduction, presented in the previous unit, is essential to the understanding of this phase of the reproductive process. From a biologic point of view, pregnancy and labor represent the primary function of the female reproductive system and should be considered as a normal process.

The length of human pregnancy varies greatly, but the average duration, if counted from the time of conception, is approximately 267 days or 38 weeks (see Chap. 3).

Many changes in maternal physiology occur during pregnancy. These adaptations to pregnancy, although most apparent in the reproductive organs, involve other body systems as well. Concomitant with these changes, the expectant mother usually has many emotional adjustments to make: sometimes fear, apprehension, worries (financial as well as physical) and family problems are present. The fact that delivery must be "faced," that there is no turning back or "changing the mind," can in itself sometimes create an overwhelming crisis (see Chaps. 8 and 10). However, these are all temporary alterations. Usually they regress after the birth of the baby (see Chap. 14).

PHYSIOLOGIC CHANGES OF PREGNANCY

The physiologic changes of pregnancy are those alterations, both local and general, which affect the maternal organism as the result of pregnancy, but subside at or before the end of the puerperium. Such changes are to be regarded as normal, inevitable and purely temporary. They are present in varying degrees in every instance, and in the case of a physically healthy woman there should be no significant traces of them after convalescence is complete. However, it must be remembered that after pregnancy the uterus does not return to its normal nulliparous size, though it does return to a normal nonpregnant state. The adult parous uterus is slightly larger and weighs more than that of a woman who has never borne children (Chap. 2).

LOCAL CHANGES

Uterus

The uterus increases in size to make room for the growing fetus. Naturally, the enlargement of the uterus is the most striking change in pregnancy. Moreover, it is directly responsible for other important alterations. The growth of this organ in gestation is phenomenal. It increases in size from approximately 6.5 cm. long, 4 cm. wide and 2.5 cm. deep to about 32 cm. long, 24 cm. wide and 22 cm. deep. Its weight increases from 50 to 1,000 Gm. The small, almost solid organ which has a capacity of about 2 cc. increases to become a thin-walled muscular sac capable of containing the fetus, the placenta and over 1000 cc of amniotic fluid. The tremendous growth is due partly to the formation of new muscle fibers during the early months of pregnancy, but principally to the enlargement of pre-existent muscle fibers which are 7 to 11 times longer and 2 to 7 times wider than those observed in the nonpregnant uterus (Fig. 6-1). Simultaneously, fibroelastic tissue develops between the muscle bands and forms a network about the various muscle bundles. This is of great importance in view of the function of the uterus in pregnancy and labor, because it strengthens the uterine walls. During early pregnancy the hypertrophy of the uterus is probably due to the stimulating action of estrogen on muscle fibers. The uterine wall thickens during the first few months of pregnancy from about 1 cm. to almost 2 cm., but thereafter it thins to about 0.5 cm. or less. By the end of pregnancy the uterus becomes a thin, soft-walled muscular sac which yields to the movements of the fetal extremities and permits the examiner to palpate the fetus easily.

The muscle fibers are arranged in three layers: the external hoodlike layer which arches over the fundus; the internal layer of circular fibers around the orifices of the fallopian tubes and the internal os; and the figure-8 fibers in the middle layer which make an interlacing network through which the blood vessels pass. This last group plays an important role in childbearing and will be referred to particularly in the care of the mother during labor and after delivery; for when these muscle fibers contract, they constrict the blood vessels.

Between the 3rd and the 4th months of pregnancy the growing uterus rises out of the pelvis and can be palpated above the symphysis pubis, rising progressively to reach the umbilicus about the 6th month and almost impinging on the xiphoid process at the 9th month (Figs. 6-2 to 5).

In the majority of pregnancies the uterus is rotated to the right as it rises out of the pelvis. This dextrorotation is probably caused by the presence of the rectosigmoid on the left.

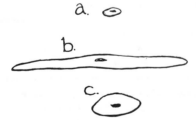

FIG. 6-1. Size of muscle cells. This illustrates the size of the muscle cells of the uterus (a) before pregnancy, (b) during pregnancy, showing the change in the size of these cells, and (c) in the puerperium. (After Stieve)

FIG. 6-2. Pregnancy should and usually does improve posture. The diagram illustrates the correct standing posture showing that a straight line may be drawn from the ear to the ankle. During pregnancy "walk tall, stand tall and sit tall."

As the uterus becomes larger, it comes in contact with the anterior abdominal wall and displaces the intestines to the sides of the abdomen. About 2 weeks before term, in most primigravidae the fetal head descends into the pelvic cavity. As a result, the uterus sinks to a lower level and at the same time falls forward. Since this relieves the upward pressure on the diaphragm and makes breathing easier, this phenomenon of the descent of the head has been called "lightening" (Fig. 6-6). These changes usually do not occur in multiparas until the onset of labor. By palpating the height of the fundus experienced examiners can determine the approximate length of gestation.

Since the full-term pregnant uterus and its contents weigh about 12 pounds, a gravid woman may be likened to a person carrying a heavy basket pressed against the abdomen. Such a person will instinctively lean backward to maintain equilibrium. This backward tilt of the torso is

FIG. 6-3. Changes in abdominal contour in pregnancy. Photographic study of actual patient.

20 weeks   24 weeks   28 weeks   32 weeks

36 weeks   40 weeks   7 days postpartum

characteristic of pregnancy. From a practical viewpoint it is important to note that this posture imposes increased strain on the muscles and the ligaments of the back and the thighs, and in this way is responsible for many of the skeleto-muscular aches and cramps so often experienced in late pregnancy.

An additional contributing factor is a relaxation of the ligaments which support the joints of the spinal column and pelvis. This feature is in-

creasingly prominent as pregnancy progresses. Relaxation of the sacroiliac joints and the pubic symphysis creates a certain amount of pelvic instability, producing additional strain on the back muscles and thighs. These changes account for the waddling gait observed in late pregnancy and in the early postpartal period.

The cervix undergoes certain remarkable changes during pregnancy. One of the first physical signs of pregnancy, softening of the cervix, may be

Fig. 6-4. Relative size of the growing uterus (front views), showing the fetus at 4 months, 6½ months and 9 months of gestation. The fundus reaches a height between the symphysis pubis and the umbilicus by the 4th month, is about the level of the umbilicus at 6½ months and almost impinges on the xiphoid process at about the 9th month of gestation.

Fig. 6-5. Relative size of the growing uterus (side views), showing the fetus at 4 months, 6½ months and 9 months of gestation. (See the last sentence of the caption for Fig. 6-4.)

apparent as early as a month after conception (see p. 122). The softening of the cervix in pregnancy is due to increased vascularity, edema and hyperplasia of the cervical glands. As shown in Figures 6-7 and 8, the glands of the cervical mucosa undergo marked proliferation and distend with mucus. As a result they form a structure resembling honeycomb and make up about one half of the entire structure of the cervix. This is the so-called "mucous plug" and is of practical importance for a number of reasons. First, it seals the uterus from contamination by bacteria in the vagina. Second, it is expelled at the onset of labor and along with it a small amount of blood; this gives rise to the discharge of a small amount of blood-stained mucus, which is known as "show." Frequently, the onset of labor is heralded by the appearance of show. While these changes in the uterus and the cervix are taking place, the vagina and the external genital organs are being prepared for the passage of the fetus at the time of labor. These parts become thick-

FIG. 6-6. The changes which take place in "lightening." (A) Pressure exerted on diaphragm before lightening. (B) Pressure relieved by falling forward of uterus. (C) Descent of head causes pressure on pelvic structures, particularly bladder.

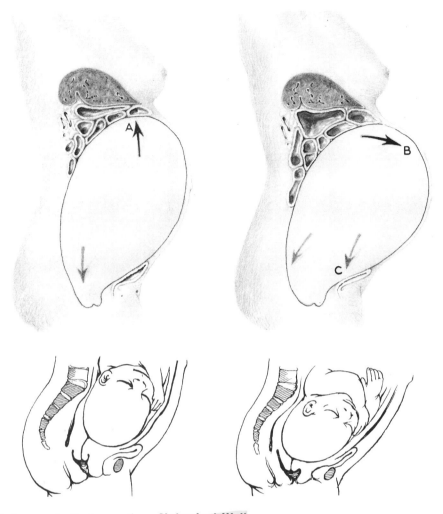

ened and softened, and their vascularity is greatly increased. This increase in the blood supply of the genital canal gives a dark violet hue to the tissues (Chadwick's sign), in contrast with the ordinary pink color of the parts, and is often described as a valuable sign of pregnancy. As the result of the succulence of the parts, the vaginal secretions may be considerably increased toward the end of gestation. The increased vascularity extends to the various structures in the vicinity (i.e., tissues in the perineal region, skin and muscle) and effects changes in preparation for labor.

As pregnancy advances, there is a marked change in the position of the ovaries. Ovulation ceases during pregnancy. New follicles do not ripen, and only the single large corpus luteum can be found on one of the ovaries. The large size of the corpus luteum of pregnancy is due mainly to the increased vascularity of the organ.

Abdominal Wall

The abdomen naturally enlarges to accommodate the increase in size of the uterus. The mechanical effect of this distention of the abdominal wall causes in the later months of pregnancy the formation of certain pink or slightly reddish streaks (or striations) in the skin covering the sides of the abdomen and the anterior and the outer aspects of the thighs. These streaks are known as *striae gravidarum* and are due to the stretching, the rupture and the atrophy of the deep connective tissue of the skin (Plate 3, *left, top and bottom*). They grow lighter after labor has taken place and finally take on the silvery whiteness of scar or cicatricial tissue. In subsequent pregnancies new pink or reddish lines may be found mingled with old silvery-white striae or striations. The number, the size and the distribution of striae gravidarum vary exceedingly in different women, and patients

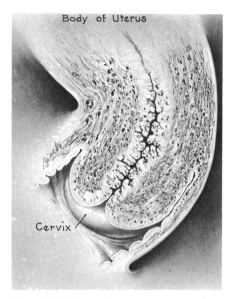

FIG. 6-7. Normal nonpregnant cervix.

FIG. 6-8. Cervix at full term, showing mucous plug.

occasionally are seen in whom there are no such markings whatever, even after repeated pregnancies. Striae are not peculiar to pregnancy but may be found in other conditions which cause great abdominal distention, such as the accumulation of fat in the abdominal wall or the development of large tumors of rapid growth.

Coincident with the uterine and the abdominal enlargement, the umbilicus is pushed outward until at about the 7th month its depression is completely obliterated, and it forms merely a darkened area in the smooth and tense abdominal wall. Later, it is raised above the surrounding integument and may project, becoming about the size of a hickory nut.

When the abdominal wall is unable to withstand the tension created by the enlarging uterus, the recti muscles become separated in the median line—so-called *diastasis recti*.

Breasts

Slight temporary enlargement of the breasts, causing sensations of weight and fullness, is noted by most women prior to their menstrual periods. The earliest breast changes of pregnancy are merely exaggerations of these changes. After the 2nd month the breasts begin to become larger, firmer and more tender; a sensation of stretching fullness, accompanied by tingling both in the

---

SOME IMPORTANT DEFINITIONS

Gravida: a pregnant woman.

Primigravida: a woman pregnant for the first time.

Primipara: a woman who has given birth to her first child. Usage is not uniform.

Multipara: a woman who has had two or more children.

Para I: a primipara.

Para II: a woman who has had two children (and so on up numerically, Para III, Para IV, etc.).

(The plural of these words is usually formed by adding "e," as "primigravidae.")

The term **gravida** refers to a pregnant woman, regardless of the duration of pregnancy. In reference it includes the present pregnancy. The term **para** refers to past pregnancies which have produced an infant which has been of viable age, whether or not the infant is dead or alive at birth. The terms **gravida** and **para** refer to pregnancies, not to fetuses.)

breasts and in the nipples, often develops, and in many instances a feeling of throbbing also is experienced. As time goes on, the nipple and the elevated, pigmented area immediately around it—the areola—become darker in color. The areola tends to become puffy, and its diameter, which in virgins rarely exceeds 1½ inches, gradually widens to reach 2 or 3 inches. Embedded in this areola lie tiny sebaceous glands which take on new growth with the advent of pregnancy and appear as little protuberances or follicles.

(Plate 3, *bottom, right*). In a few cases, patches of brownish discoloration appear on the normal skin immediately surrounding the areola. This is known as the secondary areola and is a sign of pregnancy, provided the woman never has nursed an infant previously (Plate 4, *center, right*). With the increasing growth and activity of the breasts, it is not surprising that a richer blood supply is needed; consequently, the blood vessels supplying the area enlarge. As a result the veins beneath the skin of the breast, which previously may have been scarcely visible, now become more prominent and occasionally exhibit intertwining patterns over the whole chest wall.

The alterations in the breasts during pregnancy are directed ultimately to the preparation for breast-feeding the baby. After the first few months a thin viscous yellowish fluid may be expressed by gentle massage, or appears spontaneously, from the nipples. This is a watery precursor of breast milk called colostrum.

METABOLIC CHANGES

Weight Gain

A desirable total weight gain in pregnancy for the average woman is about 20 pounds. During the first 3 months there may be a slight weight loss, or if weight is gained, it is perhaps only a small per cent. About one half of the increment is gained in the second trimester and a similar amount in the last trimester. However, there are wide individual variations observed, even in completely normal patients. The greater part of this 20-pound increment is quite understandable, as shown by the following figures:

Baby	7 pounds
Placenta	1 "
Amniotic fluid	1½ "
Increase in weight of uterus	2 "
Increase in blood volume	1 "
Increase in weight of breasts	1½ "
	14 pounds

The remaining 6 pounds gained by the pregnant woman represent, in part, general accumulation of fat and, in part, the increased amount of fluid that tissues tend to retain at this time. As pregnancy progresses, there is an increasing tendency toward salt retention. The salt holds water with it, and the net result is an accumulation of body fluid. This contributes to the total weight gain in pregnancy. A sudden increase in weight, especially in the last trimester of pregnancy, suggests excessive fluid retention. Recognition of this possibility is especially important, since abnormal water retention may presage the onset of toxemia (see Chap. 19). Normally, there is a diuresis, a rapid elimination of the accumulated salt and water, during the first 24 hours after delivery.

Gains between 15 and 20 pounds are natural and in keeping with good health; usually they are lost after the baby is born.

Carbohydrate Metabolism

Pregnancy has a decided influence on carbohydrate metabolism. In general, the levels of fasting blood sugar are lower, and the secretion of insulin by the pancreas is increased. The stress of pregnancy may actually bring to light sub-clinical diabetes (see Chap. 19). In fact, diabetes is often detected for the first time during the course of prenatal care.

CHANGES IN THE VARIOUS SYSTEMS
Blood

The total volume of blood in the body increases during pregnancy about 30 per cent. The minimal hematologic values for non-pregnant women apply to pregnant women, namely, 12 Gm. of hemoglobin, 3.75 million erythrocytes, 35 per cent hematocrit. If there are adequate iron reserves in the body, or if sufficient iron is supplied from the diet, the hemoglobin, the erythrocyte count and the hematocrit values remain within normal limits during pregnancy.

During pregnancy, there is an increased production of red blood cells by the bone marrow. At the same time, the maternal blood volume, the total amount of fluid circulating in the vessels, increases. Thus, under normal conditions, the actual concentration of red blood cells is relatively the same, and the normal values cited above apply.

The marked increase in production of red blood cells places an inordinate demand on bodily iron stores. Iron stores in the female are often marginal anyway because of the normal loss at menstruation. Iron deficiency anemia is often present prior to pregnancy, especially when there has been inadequate dietary intake of iron, frequently the case among patients in poor socio-economic circumstances. Iron deficiency is markedly aggravated by pregnancy because of the heavy demand for iron by the growing fetus, especially late in gestation. The increased demand for iron as a result of the changes associated with pregnancy should be kept in mind during the course of prenatal care, and the use of supplementary iron should be seriously considered.

Heart

An important aspect of this increase in blood volume relates to its effect on the heart. As a natural result of this change, the heart has more blood to pump through the aorta—about 50 per cent more blood per minute than it did prior to pregnancy. This augmented cardiac output attains a peak at the end of the second trimester, then declines to the non-pregnant level at the last weeks of gestation. Immediately following delivery there is a sharp rise again. In women with normal hearts this is of no particular concern. However, in women with heart disease this increase in the work that the heart has to do may add to the seriousness of the complication (see Chap. 19).

Palpitation of the heart is not uncommon; in the early months of pregnancy this is due to sympathetic nervous disturbance, and toward the end of gestation to the intra-abdominal pressure of the enlarged uterus.

Respiration

In the later months of pregnancy the lungs are subjected to pressure from the underlying uterus, and the diaphragm may be displaced upward as much as an inch. As a consequence, shortness of breath at that period is common. It might seem that this upward displacement of the diaphragm would decrease the capacity of the lungs, but a concomitant widening of the thoracic cage occurs which more than compensates for the other change. Actually, indeed, the pregnant woman breathes in much more air than the nonpregnant. This is necessary, since the mother is called upon to oxygenate not only her own blood but, by osmosis, that of her baby as well.

Digestion

The function of the digestive organs may be somewhat altered during pregnancy. During the early months the appetite may be diminished, particularly if nausea exists. Since the nutritional requirements to meet the needs of the mother's body and the growing fetus demand quality of the diet rather than an appreciable increase in the quantity of food ingested, this temporary manifestation should not produce injurious effects. As pregnancy advances, and the digestive apparatus seems to become accustomed to its new conditions, the appetite is increased and may be voracious. Heartburn and flatulence may occur at this time. Also, the pressure from the diaphragm and the diminished tone may delay the emptying time of the stomach. Constipation is exceedingly common in pregnancy; at least one half of all gravid women suffer from this disorder. This suggests that the entire gastrointestinal tract is limited by diminished tone and pressure of the growing uterus during gestation.

Skin

Striae gravidarum, which have already been discussed in relation to changes in the abdominal wall, often develop in the breasts, the buttocks and the thighs, presumably as the result of deposition of fat in those areas with consequent stretching of the skin. Certain pigmentary changes also are common, particularly the development of a black line running from the umbilicus to the mons veneris, the so-called *linea nigra* (Plate 3, *bottom, left*).

The external genitalia and any pigmented nevi also darken. In certain cases irregular spots or blotches of a muddy brown color appear on the face. This condition is known as *chloasma* or the "mask of pregnancy" (Plate 3, *top, right*). These facial deposits of pigment often cause the patient considerable mental distress, but her mind may be relieved by the assurance that they will often disappear after delivery. However, the increased pigmentation of the breasts and the abdomen never disappears entirely, although it usually becomes much less pronounced. All these pigmentary deposits vary exceedingly in size, shape and distribution and usually are more marked in brunettes than in blondes. Vascular spiders are minute, fiery-red blemishes in the skin with branching legs coming out from a central body. They develop more often in white women, however, they are of no clinical significance and will disappear. The skin changes may be associated with hypertrophy of the cortex of the adrenals.

In addition to the above skin changes, there is a great increase in the activity of the sebaceous and the sweat glands and of the hair follicles. The augmented activity of the sweat glands produces an increase in perspiration, an alteration which is helpful in the elimination of waste material.

Urinary System

The urine in pregnancy usually is increased in amount and has a lower specific gravity. Pregnant women show a tendency to excrete dextrose in the urine. Although a reduction in the renal threshold for sugar is often associated with pregnancy, the presence of any sugar in the urine should always be reported to the physician. Lactosuria may be observed at times, especially during the latter part of pregnancy and the puerperium. It is of no significance, being due to the presence of milk sugar which is supposed to be absorbed from the mammary glands.

The ureters become markedly dilated in pregnancy, particularly the right ureter. This change apparently is due in part to the pressure of the gravid uterus on the ureters as they cross the pelvic brim and in part to a certain softening which the ureteral walls undergo as the result of endocrine influences. These dilated ureters, the walls of which have now lost much of their muscular tone, are unable to propel the urine as satisfactorily as previously; consequently, stasis of urine is common. Following delivery, the ureters return to normal within 4 to 6 weeks. The stretching and the dilatation do not continue long enough to impair the ureter permanently unless infection has developed, or pregnancies are repeated so rapidly that a subsequent pregnancy begins before the ureters can return to normal.

The bladder functions efficiently during pregnancy. The urinary frequency experienced in the first few months of pregnancy is caused by pressure exerted on the bladder by the enlarging uterus. This is observed again when "lightening" occurs prior to the onset of labor.

EFFECTS ON THE PSYCHE

The effect of pregnancy on the psyche varies greatly. Although many women escape nervous manifestations entirely, some patients present more or less altered mental and emotional characteristics, varying all the way from cravings for unusual foods, fretfulness and peevishness to rare instances of true psychoses. In exceptional cases the change is to the opposite extreme, and a woman who is ordinarily of an irritable disposition becomes exceedingly amiable and agreeable. The more unstable emotionally the patient is, the more likely is her mental status to be affected by the strain of pregnancy.

ENDOCRINE CHANGES

Placenta

In Chapter 4 the placenta is considered simply as an organ designed to transmit nutritive substances from mother to fetus and waste products in the reverse direction. The placenta has another highly important function; it is one of the most important organs of internal secretion. The early chorionic villi of the implanted ovum secrete a gonad-stimulating substance, a hormone, *human chorionic gonadotropin,* which prolongs the life of the corpus luteum. The result is the continued production of estrogen and progesterone, which are so necessary for the maintenance of the endometrium. During pregnancy this hormone is excreted in the mother's urine and makes possible the standard tests for pregnancy (see p. 123).

In addition to its function in the formation of chorionic gonadotropin, the placenta takes over the production of estrogen and progesterone from the ovaries and after the first 2 months of gestation becomes the major source of these two hormones. The increase in these hormones in the maternal organism is thought to be responsible for many important changes that take place during pregnancy, such as the growth of the uterus and the development of the breasts. In the breasts, the development of the duct system is promoted by estrogen, and the development of the lobule-alveolar system by progesterone.

Pituitary Body

The pituitary gland enlarges somewhat during pregnancy, but, as such, is not essential for the maintenance of pregnancy. The *anterior lobe* of this small gland, located at the base of the brain, has already been referred to as the "master clock," which, under the influence of the hypothalamus, controls the menstrual cycle (see Chap. 3). In addition to gonadotropins, it secretes hormones which act on the thyroid and adrenal glands, and yet another hormone which influences the growth process. Production of these hormones continues during the course of pregnancy. Gonadotropins, on the other hand, are no longer released. The estrogen and progesterone produced by the placenta inhibit their release from the pituitary gland.

The *posterior lobe* of the pituitary secretes an oxytocic hormone, which has a very strong stimulating effect on the uterine muscle. That portion of extracts of the pituitary gland which contains this hormone, known as *oxytocin,* is widely employed in obstetrics to cause the uterus to contract after delivery, thereby diminishing postpartal hemorrhage. It is sometimes used also to initiate labor and to stimulate contractions during labor when they are of poor quality. Oxytocin also has an influence on the breasts. It causes "milk letdown," or ejection of milk from the nipples. This effect is of clinical usefulness in the care of the nursing mother. Oxytocin is marketed under the names Pitocin and Syntocinon, the latter a synthetic product, and is administered either parenterally or, for milk let-down, by a nasal spray.

Other Endocrine Glands

It is quite clear that the placenta is the major endocrine gland in pregnancy. Other endocrine glands display alterations during normal pregnancy. During the course of pregnancy, there is slight to moderate enlargement of the thyroid. It is now known that this hypertrophy of thyroid tissue is not associated with increased thyroid activity, although there is an elevation in the basal metabolic rate which increases throughout the course of pregnancy. This is merely a reflection of the increased oxygen consumption as a result of the metabolic activity of the products of conception. Other parameters for the measurement of thyroid function also display changes. The serum protein-bound iodine (PBI) and the butyl extractable iodine (BEI) levels increase, and the elevated levels are maintained until shortly after delivery. The increase is due not to increased thyroid activity as such but, rather, to an elevation in the level of thyroid-binding protein normally present in the blood. Thus, although there

is an increase in the amount of circulating thyroid hormones and, therefore, the total concentration of hormone is elevated, the actual amount of unbound or available hormone remains within normal limits. The triiodothyronine uptake test displays decreased values in pregnancy. This, again, is the result of an increase in the binding of circulating triiodothyronine. A similar increase in the level of thyroid-binding proteins is seen in the nonpregnant patient following the administration of estrogen, and it is likely that in pregnancy the increase is a reflection of the high level of circulating estrogen.

The *adrenal cortex* hypertrophies during pregnancy, and it is believed that its activity increases. The actual secretion of cortisol by the adrenals is unchanged, although there are alterations in the metabolism of cortisol as a result of the influence of estrogen. There is clearly an increase in the production by the adrenal glands of aldosterone the hormone responsible for the retention of sodium by the kidneys. This increase begins early in pregnancy and continues throughout. It is probably brought about under the influence of progesterone. The net result of the increase is a decreased ability of the kidneys to handle salt during pregnancy. In the absence of proper dietary control of salt intake, there is often fluid retention, and either occult or overt edema.

The *ovary,* except for the activity of the corpus luteum of pregnancy, remains relatively quiescent. Gonadotropin levels are low, inasmuch as their release is inhibited by the estrogen and progesterone produced by the placenta. Thus, follicular activity in the ovary remains in abeyance, and there is no further ovulation until after delivery.

SUGGESTED READING

Eastman, N. J., and Hellman, L. M.: Williams Obstetrics. ed. 13, New York, Appleton, 1966.

Eastman, N. J., and Russell, K. P.: Expectant Motherhood. ed. 5, Boston, Little, Brown, 1970.

Signs and Symptoms of Pregnancy

Classification of Signs and Symptoms • Presumptive Signs • Probable Signs • Positive Signs

CLASSIFICATION OF SIGNS AND SYMPTOMS

The first visit of the expectant mother to her physician is usually prompted by the query, "Am I really pregnant?" Oddly enough, this is the one question which the physician may answer equivocally, because even the most careful examination rarely will reveal clear-cut evidence of pregnancy until two menstrual periods have been missed, and occasionally the diagnosis may remain uncertain for a longer time. Some of the signs and symptoms of pregnancy can be recognized readily by the nurse, whereas others can be determined accurately only by one who has had a thorough medical or technical training.

Certain signs are absolutely indicative of pregnancy, but even these may be absent or lacking if the fetus has died in the uterus. Some so-called "positive" signs are not present until about the middle of gestation, and at that time the physician usually can make a diagnosis without them by the "circumstantial evidence" of a combination of earlier and less significant symptoms.

The signs of pregnancy are usually divided into three groups, as indicated in the following classification:

A. Presumptive signs

1. Menstrual suppression
2. Nausea, vomiting, "morning sickness"
3. Frequency of micturition
4. Tenderness and fullness of the breasts, pigmentation, etc.
5. "Quickening"
6. Dark blue discoloration of the vaginal mucous membrane (Chadwick's sign)
7. Pigmentation of the skin and abdominal striae
8. Fatigue

B. Probable signs

1. Enlargement of the abdomen
2. Fetal outline, distinguished by abdominal palpation
3. Changes in the uterus—size and shape and consistency (Hegar's sign)
4. Changes in the cervix
5. Braxton Hicks contractions
6. Positive pregnancy tests

C. Positive signs

1. Fetal heart sounds
2. Fetal movements felt by examiner
3. Roentgenogram—outline of fetal skeleton

PRESUMPTIVE SIGNS

Menstrual Suppression

In a healthy married woman who previously has menstruated regularly, cessation of menstruation strongly suggests that impregnation has occurred. However, not until the date of the expected period has been passed by 10 days or more can any reliance be put on this symptom. When the second period is also missed, the probability naturally becomes stronger.

Although cessation of menstruation is the earliest and one of the most important symptoms of pregnancy, it should be noted that pregnancy may occur without prior menstruation and that occasionally menstruations may continue after conception. An example of the former circumstance is noted in certain Oriental countries, where girls marry at a very early age; here pregnancy frequently occurs before the menstrual periods are established. Again, nursing mothers, who usually do not menstruate during the period of lactation, often conceive at this time; more rarely, women who think they have passed the menopause are startled to find themselves pregnant. Conversely, it is not uncommon for a woman to have 1 or 2 periods after conception; but almost without exception these are brief in duration and scant in amount. In such cases the first period ordinarily lasts 2 days instead of the usual 5, and the next only a few hours. Although there are instances in which women are said to have menstruated every month throughout pregnancy, these are of questionable authenticity and are probably ascribable to some abnormality of the reproductive organs. Indeed, vaginal bleeding at any time during pregnancy should be regarded as abnormal and reported to the physician at once.

Absence of menstruation may result from a number of conditions other than pregnancy. Probably one of the most common causes of delay in the onset of the period is psychic influence, particularly fear of pregnancy. Change of climate, exposure to cold, as well as certain chronic diseases such as anemia, likewise, may suppress the menstrual flow.

Nausea and Vomiting

About one half of pregnant women suffer no nausea whatsoever during the early part of pregnancy. About 50 per cent experience waves of nausea; of these perhaps one third experience some vomiting. "Morning sickness" usually occurs in the early part of the day and subsides in a few hours, although it may persist longer or may occur at other times. When this "morning sickness" occurs, it usually makes its appearance about 2 weeks after the first missed menstrual period and subsides spontaneously 6 or 8 weeks later. Since this symptom is present in many other conditions, such as ordinary indigestion, it is of no diagnostic value unless associated with other evidence of pregnancy. When the vomiting is excessive, when it lasts beyond the 4th month, when it begins in the later months, or when it affects the general health, it must be regarded as pathologic. Such

conditions are termed "hyperemesis gravidarum" or "pernicious vomiting" and will be discussed with complications of pregnancy in Chapter 19.

Frequent Micturition

Irritability of the bladder with resultant frequency of urination may be one of the earliest symptoms of pregnancy. It is attributed to the fact that the growing uterus stretches the base of the bladder, so that a sensation results identical with that felt when the bladder wall is stretched with urine. As pregnancy progresses, the uterus rises out of the pelvis, and the frequent desire to urinate subsides. Later on, however, the symptom is likely to return, for during the last weeks the head of the fetus may press against the bladder and give rise to a similar condition. Although frequency of urination may be somewhat bothersome, both at the beginning and at the end of pregnancy, it never should constitute a reason for reducing the quantity of fluid consumed, which should be not less than 6 or 8 glasses a day.

Breast Changes

The breast changes of pregnancy have already been described (p. 114). In primigravidae (women pregnant for the first time) these alterations are helpful adjuncts in the diagnosis of pregnancy, but in women who have already borne children, particularly if they have nursed an infant within the past year, they naturally are of much less significance.

"Quickening"

This is an old term derived from an idea prevalent many years ago that at some particular moment of pregnancy life is suddenly infused into the infant. At the time this notion was in vogue, the first tangible evidence of intra-uterine life lay in the mother's feeling the baby move, and the conclusion was only natural that the infant "became alive" at the moment these movements were first felt. As is reflected in the Biblical reference to "the quick and the dead," the word "quick" used to mean "alive," and the word "quickening" meant "becoming alive." Hence, our forebears were accustomed to say that when fetal movements were first felt, "quickening" or "coming to life" of the baby had occurred. We now know that the infant is a living organism from the moment of conception, but the old term "quickening" is still used in obstetric terminology, whereas among the laity "feeling life" is the common synonym. As used today, quickening refers only, of course, to the active movements of the fetus as first perceived by the mother.

Quickening is usually felt toward the end of the 5th month as a tremulous fluttering low in the abdomen. The first impulses caused by the stirring of the fetus may be so faint as to raise some doubt as to their cause; later on, however, they grow stronger and often become disturbingly active.

Many fetuses, although alive and healthy, seem to move about very little in the uterus, and, not infrequently, a day or so may pass without a movement being felt. Inability to feel the baby move does not mean that it is dead or in any way a weakling but, in all probability, that it has assumed a position in which its movements are not felt so readily by the mother. Should 3 or 4 days pass without movements, the physician should be asked to listen for the fetal heart sounds. If these are heard, it means beyond doubt that the fetus is alive and presumably in good condition. It might seem that the sensations produced by the baby's movements would be so characteristic as to make this a positive sign of pregnancy, but, oddly enough, women occasionally misinterpret movements of gas in the intestines as motions of a baby and on this basis imagine themselves to be pregnant. Therefore, the patient's statement that she feels the baby move cannot be regarded as absolute proof of pregnancy.

Vaginal Changes

On inspection of the vagina, the physician is able to observe discoloration of the vaginal mucous membrane due to the influence of pregnancy. The mucosa about the vaginal opening and the lower portion of the anterior wall frequently becomes thickened and of a dark bluish or purplish congested appearance instead of its customary pinkish tint in the nonpregnant state. This sign, known as *Chadwick's sign,* is of no special value in women who have borne children; and, as it may be due to any condition leading to the congestion of the pelvic organs, it can be considered only as a presumptive sign of pregnancy.

Skin Changes

The changes in the skin which may accompany pregnancy (i.e., striae gravidarum, linea nigra, chloasma, pigmentation of the breasts, etc.) have been referred to in the previous chapter. These manifestations often are observed in pregnant women but vary exceedingly in different persons, often being entirely absent. The pigmentation changes in particular are frequently absent in decided blondes and exceptionally well marked in pronounced brunettes. As already mentioned, this pigmentation may remain from former pregnancies and cannot be depended on as a diagnostic sign in women who have borne children previously.

Fatigue

During the early months of pregnancy the expectant mother becomes easily fatigued and experiences periods of lassitude and drowsiness. This condition frequently accompanies pregnancy and usually disappears after the first few months of gestation.

PROBABLE SIGNS

Abdominal Changes

The size of the abdomen in pregnancy corresponds to the gradual increase in the size of the uterus, which at the end of the 3rd month is at the level of the symphysis pubis. At the end of the 5th month it is at the level of the umbilicus, and toward the end of the 9th month, at the ensiform cartilage (Figs. 6-3 to 5). Mere abdominal enlargement may be due to a number of causes, such as accumulation of fat in the abdominal wall, edema, or uterine or ovarian tumors. However, if the uterus can be distinctly felt to have enlarged progressively in the proportions stated above, pregnancy may properly be suspected.

Fetal Outline

After the 6th month the outline of the fetus (head, back, knees, elbows, etc.) usually may be identified sufficiently well by abdominal palpation to justify a diagnosis of pregnancy. As pregnancy progresses, the outline of the fetus becomes more and more clearly defined. The ability to outline the fetus makes pregnancy extremely probable. In rare instances, however, tumors of the uterus may so mimic the fetal outline as to make this sign fallible.

Changes in the Uterus

Changes in shape, size and consistency of the uterus which take place during the first 3 months of pregnancy are very important indications.

These are noted in the bimanual examination which shows the uterus to be more anteflexed than normal, enlarged and of a soft, spongy consistency. About the 6th week the so-called Hegar's sign, so named for the man who first described it, is perceptible (Fig. 7-1). At this time the lower uterine segment, or lower part of the body of the uterus, becomes much softer than the cervix. So soft does it become that in its empty state (for it has not yet become encroached upon by the growing embryo) it can be compressed almost to the thinness of paper. This is one of the most valuable signs in early pregnancy. Another valuable sign found on vaginal examination is ballottement (from the French *balloter*, to toss up like a ball). During the 4th and the 5th months of pregnancy the fetus is small in relation to the amount of amniotic fluid present; a sudden tap on the presenting part makes it rise in the amniotic fluid and then rebound to its original position and, in turn,

tap the examining finger. When elicited by an experienced examiner, this response is the most certain of the probable signs.

Cervical Changes

Softening of the cervix usually occurs about the time of the 2nd missed menstrual period. In comparison with the usual firmness of the nonpregnant cervix (which has a consistency approximate to that of the cartilaginous tip of the nose), the pregnant cervix becomes softened, and on digital examination the external os feels like the lips or like the lobe of the ear (Goodell's sign) (see page 112).

BRAXTON HICKS CONTRACTIONS

Uterine contractions begin during the early weeks of pregnancy and occur at intervals of from 5 to 10 minutes throughout. These contractions are painless, and the patient may or may not be

FIG. 7-1. Hegar's sign.

conscious of them. They may be observed during the later months by placing the hand on the abdomen and during the bimanual examination. By means of these contractions the uterine muscles contract and relax, thereby enlarging in size to accommodate the growing fetus. These contractions are referred to as the Braxton Hicks sign, after a famous London obstetrician of the last century who first described them. They often account for false labor.

Pregnancy Tests

Since the very dawn of civilization efforts have been made to devise a satisfactory test for pregnancy. The priest-physicians of ancient Egypt, in the earliest writings handed down to us, tell of a test then in vogue based on the seeming ability of pregnancy urine to stimulate the growth of wheat and barley seeds. The itinerant physicians of classical Greece employed similar tests, and during the Middle Ages the omniscient physician merely gazed at the urine and claimed in this way to be able to diagnose not only pregnancy but also many other conditions.

Today, interestingly enough, as in the tests of old, urine is used in a large number of tests for pregnancy. The tests are based on the fact that the early chorionic villi of the implanted ovum secrete a hormone, chorionic gonadotropin, which is excreted in the maternal urine. The method of its detection is dependent on the fact that this hormone may be detected in urine by biologic or immunologic methods. Some of the biologic tests which were used extensively in the past include: (1) the Aschheim-Zondek test (immature female mouse), (2) the Friedman test (female rabbit), (3) the Hogben test (South African toad), (4) the American male frog test, (5) the Frenk-Berman test (immature female rat).

Recently, a number of systems for immunologic pregnancy testing have been devised. These have largely supplanted those which require the use of animals. Since chorionic gonadotropin is an antigen capable of producing specific antibodies when injected into an animal, such as the rabbit, the serum of the animal so injected will contain an antibody or antihormone specific for chorionic gonadotropin. This serum then can be used by reliable immunologic methods to establish the presence or absence of chorionic gonadotropin in pregnancy urine.

Kits for immunologic pregnancy testing are available and have been simplified so that with a little practice the test can be carried out within

minutes, by the physician or nurse. Immunologic tests have two main advantages over the older biologic ones: (1) They provide an answer within a few minutes rather than many hours; (2) they eliminate the need for maintaining an animal colony. These tests are at least as accurate as the older biologic methods.

The great value of the endocrine tests lies in the fact that they become positive very early in pregnancy, usually about 10 days after the 1st missed menstrual period, sometimes even a few days earlier than this. If any of the tests has been carried out properly, the results are accurate in more than 95 per cent of cases. They are not, therefore, absolutely positive signs of pregnancy, but very nearly so.

POSITIVE SIGNS

Although certain of the signs mentioned above —notably, the hormone tests, ballottement and palpating the fetal outline—are nearly positive evidences of pregnancy, they are not 100 per cent certain; errors in technique occasionally invalidate the hormone tests, and on rare occasions the other signs may be simulated by nonpregnant pathologic states. If the term "positive" is used in the strict sense, there are only 3 positive signs of pregnancy, namely, the fetal heart sounds heard, fetal movements felt by the examiner and the x-ray outline of the fetal skeleton.

Fetal Heart Sounds

When heard distinctly by an experienced examiner, the fetal heart sounds can leave no doubt about the existence of pregnancy. Ordinarily, they become audible at about the middle of pregnancy, or around the 20th week. If the abdominal wall is thin, and conditions are favorable, they may become audible as early as the 18th week, but obesity or an excessive quantity of amniotic

Fig. 7-2. Leff stethoscope for use with interchangeable bells (A). Weighted bell used for auscultation of fetal heart sounds (B). Small bell used to determine mother's blood pressure (C). (J. Sklar Manufacturing Co., Long Island City, N. Y.)

FIG. 7-3. Normal vertex position. (Bonner, K. P.: Radiography and Clinical Photography, Eastman Kodak Company, Rochester, N. Y.)

fluid may render them inaudible until a much later date. Although the usual rate of the fetal heart is about 140 per minute, it may vary under quite normal conditions between 120 and 160. The use of the ordinary bell stethoscope, steadied by rubber bands, is entirely satisfactory (Fig. 7-2), but in doubtful cases the head stethoscope is superior, since the listener receives bone conduction of sound through the headpiece in addition to that transmitted to the eardrum.

The nurse will find it advantageous to determine the fetal position by abdominal palpation before attempting to listen to the fetal heart tones, since ordinarily the heart sounds are best heard through the infant's back (see Chap. 5). Also, she will do well, while learning the characteristics of the fetal heart sounds, to accustom herself to place one hand on the maternal pulse and feel its rate at the same time that she hears the fetal heart tones through the stethoscope. Occasionally, the inexperienced attendant, particularly when listening high in the abdomen, may mistake the mother's heart sounds for those of the baby.

Since the two are not synchronous (fetal, 140; maternal, 80), the method suggested above will obviate this mistake; in other words, if the rate that comes to the ear through the stethoscope is the same as that of the maternal pulse, it is probably the mother's heart beat; on the other hand, if the rates are different, it is undoubtedly the sound of the fetal heart.

Two additional sounds may be heard in listening over the pregnant uterus: the funic souffle and the uterine souffle. Since the word "souffle" means a blowing murmur, or whizzing sound, the nature of these two sounds is similar, but their timing and causation are quite different. The word *funis* is Latin for umbilical cord, and, accordingly, the term "funic souffle" refers to a soft blowing murmur caused by blood rushing through the umbilical cord. Since this blood is propelled by the fetal heart, the rate of funic souffle is synchronous with that of the fetal heart. It is heard only occasionally, perhaps in 1 case out of every 6. The funic souffle is a positive sign of pregnancy, but it is not usually so listed,

FIG. 7-4. Normal breech position. (Bonner, K. P.: Radiography and Clinical Photography, Eastman Kodak Company, Rochester, N. Y.)

because almost always it is heard in close association with the fetal heart sounds. The uterine souffle is produced by blood rushing through the large vessels of the uterus. Since this is maternal blood, propelled by the maternal heart, it is synchronous with the rate of her heart beat. In other words, the rate of the funic souffle is ordinarily around 140 per minute (or the same as that of the fetal heart rate); the rate of the uterine souffle, near 80 (that of the maternal heart rate). The fetal heart may also be detected electronically or with ultrasound techniques described in detail in Chapter 21 (Fetal Diagnosis and Treatment).

Fetal Movements Felt by Examiner

As already noted, fetal movements supposedly felt by the patient may be very misleading in the diagnosis of pregnancy. However, when an experienced examiner feels the characteristic thrust or kick of the baby against his hand, this is positive evidence of pregnancy. Often this can be felt after the end of the 5th month.

Roentgenogram

A roentgenogram showing the outline of the fetal skeleton is, of course, undeniable proof of pregnancy. How early the fetal skeleton will show in the roentgenogram depends on the thickness of the abdominal wall, the x-ray equipment and other factors. It has been demonstrated as early as the 14th week and is quite easily demonstrated as a rule after the 20th week (Figs. 7-3, 4).

SUGGESTED READING

Eastman, N. J., and Hellman, L. M.: Williams Obstetrics. ed. 13, New York, Appleton, 1966.

Antepartal Care

8

INTRODUCTION

Within the last decade there has appeared a rising tide of comment about what constitutes "adequate antepartal care." In the literal sense antepartal* care refers to the medical supervision and the care given to pregnant women during the period between conception and the onset of labor. Opinions vary, but generally in current practice adequate antepartal care is that care which considers the physical, emotional and social needs of the woman and her unborn baby, her husband and their other children. It provides the best of medical science to protect the life and the health of the mother and the fetus, and it takes into consideration the social conditions under which the family lives (i.e., its economic status, educational level, housing, nutrition, etc. See Chap. 1), so that the mother may pass through pregnancy and labor and the puerperium with a maximum of mental and physical fitness. It also aims to increase the knowledge of the mother-to-be, so that she and her infant may be kept healthy and happy after the delivery. These aims are accomplished through the combined efforts of the expectant parents, the obstetrician, the nurse and the other members of the health team.

Antepartal care may be considered as the foundation for the normal development, the adequate growth, and the good health of the baby. During this formative period the teeth, the bones and the various systems of the body have their beginnings, as well as the foundations for his

---

* Derived from Latin, *partus* means birth and *ante*, before (i.e., before labor).

future health. Adequate antepartal care also aids in stabilizing the daily health of the mother. As pregnancy advances, the demands of the fetus increase. Since individuals react differently to pregnancy, this supervision is of the utmost importance in detecting these reactions; for it not only helps to relieve discomforts and to prevent accidents and complications, but also aids in ensuring a more rapid convalescence and continued good health.

THE IMPORTANCE OF PREVENTIVE CARE

Prior to the rise of present-day obstetrics, the physician usually had only one interview with his patient before he saw her in labor, and often at this interview he merely sought to compute the expected date of confinement. When he next saw her, she might be in the throes of an eclamptic convulsion or striving vainly to overcome the resistance offered by a contracted pelvis. It is in the prevention of such calamities as these that care and supervision of the pregnant mother have been found to be of such value. Indeed, antepartal care is an absolute necessity if a substantial number of women are to avoid disaster; and it is helpful to all.

From a biologic point of view, pregnancy and labor represent the highest function of the female reproductive system. As has been mentioned previously, this should be considered to be a normal process. But the numerous physiologic changes which occur in the mother's body during pregnancy (see Chap. 6) demonstrate that the borderline between health and illness is less distinctly marked during pregnancy than during the nonpregnant state. A slight variation in bodily function, which might be of little significance if the woman were not pregnant, may be a warning signal of a potential pathologic condition in pregnancy which could seriously threaten the health of the mother or the child or both. Examples of such symptoms might be a weight gain of several pounds during 1 week or a persistent headache. Health supervision and teaching begun early in pregnancy are often the means of avoiding complications of pregnancy; and in the event that symptoms do occur, their early detection and prompt treatment may avert serious problems.

The importance of early and continued medical supervision during pregnancy cannot be overemphasized. If it is possible, care should begin as early as the patient conceives or perhaps even earlier than that, not only at the very beginning of her pregnant period but ideally with her own mother's antepartal state, which likewise had everything to do with the patient's health. In recent years much has been accomplished through premarital and prepregnancy examinations to determine the patient's fitness for pregnancy. More and more physicians are offering this care and encouraging this plan toward positive health.

However, it must be noted that there are several forces in our society today that militate against the ultimate goal of high quality maternity care for all. These have been designated as the crisis* of quality, the crisis of logistics, the crisis of community agencies, and the crisis of medical economics.

The first of these, the crisis of quality, refers to the differential quality and delivery of medical services that often exist for the different socioeconomic groups in our society. Those in greatest need of good maternity care, who generally have the highest death and sickness rates, often lack confidence in the community facilities for their care. They believe that adequate health care is a right of citizenship; however, when they seek it, they often find that two kinds of care exist: one for those who can pay and another for those who cannot. Since so many people now feel that proper health care is a right of citizenship, the provision of adequate health services for all requires a restructuring of present national priorities and an escalation of the public's social consciousness. Most health professionals agree that any worthwhile program, in addition to providing

financial support, should also maintain the mother's dignity.

The second crisis is that of logistics and refers to the current anticipated problem of the shortage of maternity personnel at all levels: doctors, nurses, nurse-midwives, etc. While the number of births in the United States has fallen to the lowest point in 30 years, there is an expected increase in the near future as the babies of the post World War II baby boom begin to have their children. It is now recognized that maternity care in the future will be provided by a closely integrated team consisting of physicians, nurse-midwives, nurses, laboratory technicians, social workers, nutritionists, health educators and homemakers. None of these members are available in sufficient numbers today, and the quotas set by those planning high quality

Fig. 8-1. Clinic nurse weighing pregnant patient.

---

* The following discussion derives from the 50th Annual Report of the Maternity Center Association, 1969.

care will not be met in the foreseeable future, unless drastic recruitment for these team members ensues and more efficient use is made of existing personnel.

The third crisis arises in the community agencies. Agencies providing maternity care in this country are often competitive and repetitive in some communities, and entirely lacking in others. For example, there may be several public health nursing services in one area, such as the health department, the voluntary nursing agency and school nursing services. Many times they all serve one family, but hardly communicate with one another with respect to the total needs of the family. Similarly, some hospitals may be overcrowded, while others have empty beds. Nothing is done to relieve the shortage because the first hospital may be governed by economic considerations to the exclusion of considering the comfort and safety of its patients. There are ways to circumvent these problems with the use of innovation in building hospitals and planning patient care. Light unit-type buildings with interchangeable walls and rooms have been proposed. In some places, even motel type "half-way" houses staffed by nurse-midwives under medical supervision could provide adequate care. Unfortunately, many of these innovations are blocked due to long entrenched rules and regulations of local building codes, mortgage companies, etc. which require the massive stereotyped construction found in traditional hospitals. Thus, in many cases, we see vested interests of existing social and health agencies, professional and individual competition, politics, regulations, and false community pride standing in the way of services which can promote the health and life of future generations.

The final crisis is that of medical economics. The chief protection for the medical needs of most of America's young parents is voluntary and commercial prepayment insurance. Unfortunately, the maternity benefits traditionally have been distressingly low. Young people with low incomes are frequently saddled with a large medical and hospital bill at a time when they can least afford to pay. Many professionals feel that maternity care should be entirely covered, but the actuarians believe that the rates for this kind of coverage would be prohibitive. However, it might be noted that insurance companies have had this opinion about other forms of coverage and under public pressure have increased benefits. Many public health leaders feel that the resources of this country are so vast that full coverage is feasible if there is a public mandate to provide it. However, if this mandate does not come, these leaders foresee only increased costs to future parents.

While the above comments are perhaps unsettling, it is hoped that they give food for thought for tomorrow's nursing practitioners. Our society is undergoing a time of great social change and the commensurate stress that accompanies such change. The nurse, as she becomes better educated and increasingly knowledgeable regarding the forces in society that impinge on the health needs of her patients, is in an advantageous position to help her patients learn what forces and pressures they can bring to bear to help achieve their right of citizenship—adequate health care.

Mothers and Infants at Risk

In recent years the term "high risk" has been applied to groups of mothers and babies who have an actual or potentially higher incidence and prevalence of morbidity and mortality than the general population of mothers and infants. Unfortunately, there has developed a stereotype of these mothers as being chiefly unmarried, nonwhite, unemployed and from broken families. However, recent research indicates that this stereotype, as with most stereotypes, is not altogether useful in assessing whether or not the situation is truly "high risk." Many, if not most, of these mothers have children born in wedlock and are now members of intact families headed by a male, and in most cases, almost all the males have full time employment of some kind. However, the crucial factor is that the remuneration for this employment is often at a very low level—which makes the total economic picture precarious. Furthermore, many of these mothers do come from low economic status homes and hence, have experienced many deprivations during their formative years (see Chap. 9). While it is wise to beware of stereotyping these families, there are some commonalities that tend to appear. Many have inadequate pre- or postnatal care; some are teenagers and/or do not want their babies; the mothers may have metabolic or chronic diseases, take drugs, or have chronic cervical or vaginal infections or disease; finally the babies may sustain damage at birth or be one of a multiple birth. Early and continued prenatal care is a "must" for these patients to ensure both maternal and fetal salvage. However, case finding and motivating these patients to seek prenatal care present formidable problems.

Although maternity clinics across the country have been improved by federal funding, and satellite clinics have been opened·in many cities, many mothers, particularly those in the poverty group, are not seeking the care that is offered. Having been brought up in poverty and having known deprivation or medical indigence all their lives, they simply have never become accustomed to using medical care except in emergencies, and not surprisingly, they will not start when they become pregnant. These findings only reinforce the necessity of extending prenatal and preconceptual care back to childhood, through adolescence and adulthood. It must be remembered that this is not just a problem of prenatal care, but rather a problem of the ill-health and poverty of the total community. Similarly, it is not just a question of dietary supplements during pregnancy, but of life nutrition; nor is it just a problem of the organization of maternal and child health services, but a question of the organization of family health services. What is even more important is that it is not just a question of a considered referral to a prenatal clinic, but rather the way in which social agencies concern themselves with all the issues of health, and whether they encourage use of medical services preventively or curatively. Most expectant mothers who need motivation to seek prenatal care would go to the clinic if they could see some concrete benefits that accrue to them. Family planning services, for instance, are being found to more than double the attendance at postpartum clinics. In some programs, they also seem to exert a positive influence in attract-

FIG. 8-2. Clinic nurse taking blood pressure of pregnant patient.

ing women to prenatal clinics early, when they hear by word of mouth that family planning services are available.

Today's climate seems to call for innovation in thought and practice. It is likely that some form of national health insurance or prepayment scheme will be developed in the near future that will help cover some of the crises mentioned previously.

MEDICAL CARE

With today's emphasis on positive health, ideally every patient ought to be under the care of an obstetrician during the entire period of her pregnancy. This supervision aids greatly in determining the health status of those anticipating parenthood. The mother-to-be should be seen as early as possible and at least every 4 weeks thereafter until the 7th month. Then her visits can be made every 2 weeks until the last month of pregnancy, during which time it is most important that she be seen every week. The therapy of all patients should be individualized. In the case of an expectant mother who has some abnormal condition, the visits should be spaced according to the demands of the situation. Each physician has his own system. Some prefer to see their patients in groups in order to facilitate discussions of common concerns; some utilize nurse midwives, and some prefer to maintain a one-to-one relationship with their patients. Whatever the approach, at the first examination the history of the patient is taken, then a general medical examination is carried out, and finally the obstetric examination, which includes an examination *per vaginam,* is given. The examination may be carried out according to the following outline.

The History

The name and the address of the patient, her age and parity and the date of the latest menstrual period are recorded, and the date of delivery is estimated. Inquiries are made regarding the family history, with special reference to any condition likely to affect childbearing, such as hereditary disease, tuberculosis or multiple pregnancy. The personal history of the patient then is reviewed not only in regard to previous diseases and operations, but particularly in relation to any difficulties experienced in previous pregnancies and labors, such as miscarriages, prolonged labor, death of infant, hemorrhage and other complications. Inquiry is made into the history of the present pregnancy, especially in relation to nausea, edema of the feet or the face, headache, visual disturbance, vaginal bleeding, constipation, breathlessness, sleeplessness, cramps, heartburn, lower abdominal pain, vaginal discharge, varicose veins. Usually a suitable form for recording these particulars is employed. As a rule, obstetricians, hospital clinics and other community health agencies have their own forms for recording these details.

General Medical Examination

The general medical examination includes weighing the patient, taking the blood pressure, inspecting the teeth and the throat and making an examination by auscultation and percussion of the heart and the lungs. Opportunity is taken at this time to inspect the breasts and the nipples, particularly in relation to their suitability for subsequent nursing. From an obstetric viewpoint, one of the important details of the general medical examination is the measurement of the blood pressure (Fig. 8-2). This is usually carried out first and is also done when the patient is seen on subsequent visits. As will be explained subsequently, any substantial increase in blood pressure indicates one of the most serious complications in pregnancy—toxemia. A fact for the nurse to keep in mind is that any sudden or gradual rise in the systolic or the diastolic blood pressure is significant and may be alarming.

Obstetric Examination

The obstetric examination is comprised of three parts: (1) palpation and auscultation of the abdomen; (2) estimation of pelvic measurements; and (3) vaginal examination. Palpation and auscultation of the abdomen yield valuable information concerning the size and the position of the fetus and the rate of the fetal heart. The importance of careful pelvic measurements has already been emphasized, and the purpose of the vaginal examination (aside from its use in the diagnosis of pregnancy) is to rule out abnormalities of the birth canal (particularly those which might impede labor) and to take the diagonal conjugate measurement.

Laboratory Tests

The laboratory tests carried out in antepartal care are the urine examination, the blood test for syphilis, the estimation of the hemoglobin, tests for the Rh factor and blood type. At the first and subsequent examinations the urine is tested for albumin and sugar. The patient is instructed to collect a part of the first urine voided in the morning before breakfast. The reason for this is that glucose may spill into the urine of a normal pregnant woman due to a decreased kidney threshold for glucose. Hence, it is more likely to appear in the urine after a meal. The test for sugar is the same as that used to test a diabetic's urine; several simple tests are available today and may be completed quickly and accurately in a matter of minutes. Any positive reaction to sugar is reported to the physician so that the possibility of diabetes or a prediabetic condition can be ruled out.

The test for albumin also is simple. The principle involved here is the application of heat in chemical form, which solidifies any albumin present and causes a whitish precipitate. The presence of albumin in the urine is another symptom of possible toxemia and should be reported immediately. The sudden appearance of albuminuria is regarded as a symptom of preeclampsia.

FIG. 8-3. Clinic nurse explaining urinalysis to pregnant patient.

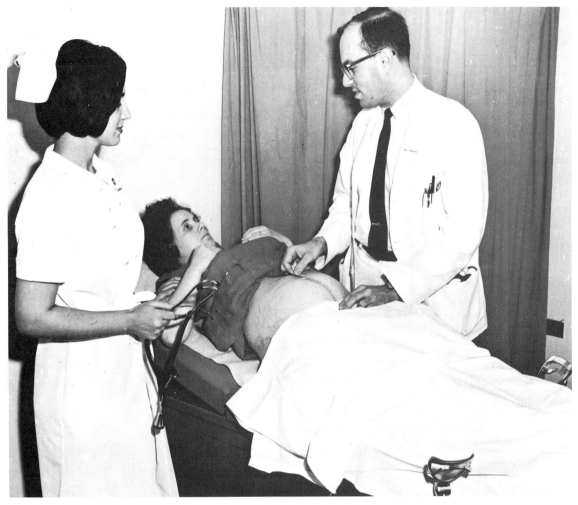

Fig. 8-4. Patient on examining table. Doctor is measuring the height of the fundus.

The blood for the Wassermann or other serologic test for syphilis is usually obtained by venipuncture. A sufficient quantity of blood is drawn at this time so that a portion may be employed for the Rh factor and hemoglobin estimation. Since many pregnant women develop anemia, the latter examination is highly important. A metabolism test is routine in the practice of some obstetricians.

If the test for the Rh factor shows the patient to be Rh negative, it may be necessary to check the husband. It is also a wise precaution for the doctor to have the husband's blood type (see Chap. 19).

In many antepartal and postpartal clinics the secretions in the cervix and the vagina are examined microscopically to ascertain whether the cells contained therein exhibit certain changes suggestive of incipient uterine cancer. A drop of the cervical or the vaginal fluid is placed on a glass slide, and after this has been spread out in a very thin layer, it is stained for microscopic study. This is called a Papanicolaou smear or Papanicolaou spread. According to the cellular picture seen, it is classified by number from Class 1 to Class 5. Smears in Classes 1 and 2 are characterized by the complete absence of malignant or "suspicious" cells. They are regarded as normal. Smears in Classes 3, 4 and 5 contain cells that either are suggestive of malignancy or actually malignant. These call for further investigation and, in some cases, intensive treatment. The rationale of this procedure is that it provides a method whereby incipient cervical cancer can

PLATE 3. (*Left, top*) Striae gravidarum.
(*Left, bottom*) Linea nigra and also striae gravidarum.
(*Right, top*) Mask of pregnancy (chloasma).
(*Right, bottom*) Montgomery's tubercles.

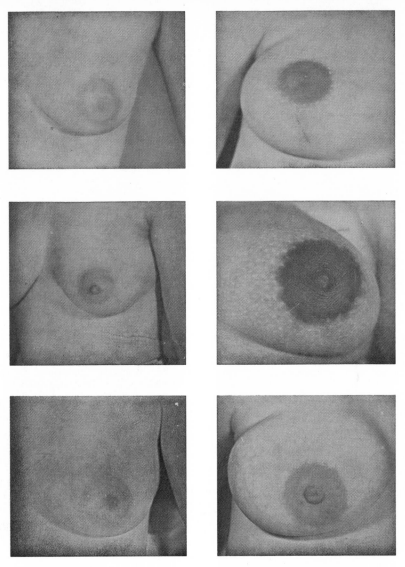

PLATE 4. (*Left, top*) Breast in nonpregnant blonde.
(*Right, top*) Breast in pregnant blonde, showing pigmentary changes.
(*Left, center*) Breast in nonpregnant brunette.
(*Right, center*) Breast in pregnant brunette, showing pigmentary changes
and marked secondary areola.
(*Left, bottom*) Breast in nonpregnant red-haired woman.
(*Right, bottom*) Breast in pregnant red-haired woman.

be detected in its earliest stages. Since the success of treatment in any form of cancer depends on early diagnosis and early treatment, the use of the Papanicolaou smear promises to prevent many fatalities from uterine cancer, one of the most common causes of death in women.

Weight

The routine estimation of weight at regular intervals during pregnancy is an important detail of antepartal care. Any *marked gain* or *loss* in weight will be discussed by the obstetrician. At first the average gain in weight of the fetus is 1 Gm. daily; nine tenths of the weight is gained after the 5th month, and one half of the weight of the fetus is acquired during the last 8 weeks. Most physicians agree that a weight gain of about 20 pounds is desirable for a woman who is average or "normal" in her prepregnant weight. However, there is increasing speculation and some evidence among some investigators that the weight gain for pregnancy needs to be individualized for every patient, particularly those of under and over average prepregnant weights. In the former case, a gain of 30 pounds or more has had no deleterious effects on the mother and has resulted in a healthy normal weight infant. In the case of the overweight prepregnant woman a large weight gain has resulted in overly large babies. Generally, in any excessive weight gain, or for a patient who is markedly overweight, one of the balanced low caloric diets may be prescribed in an effort to improve the nutritional state and control weight. For all patients the emphasis is becoming less centered on gain per se, but rather on a balanced nutritional status related to the patient's general physical condition.

Return Visits

At return visits careful inquiry is made into the general well-being of the patient, and questions are asked concerning any untoward signs and symptoms, such as edema of the fingers or the face, bleeding, constipation and headache. The patient then is weighed, her blood pressure is taken, and the urine is analyzed for albumin and sugar. An abdominal examination is usually carried out at this time. Abdominal, vaginal and rectal examinations should be done at regular intervals to determine that pregnancy is progressing at the expected rate and, following quickening, that the fetus is living. During these visits the patient should avail herself of the opportunity of asking the physician any questions that may be of concern to her.

Instructions to Patients

After the routine examination the doctor or the nurse may instruct the patient regarding diet, rest and sleep, daily intestinal elimination, proper exercise, fresh air and sunshine, bathing, clothing, recreation and dental care.

It is usually possible and always desirable to assure the patient that the findings on examination were normal, and that barring complications, she may anticipate an uneventful pregnancy followed by an uncomplicated delivery. However, at the same time, she is tactfully instructed regarding certain danger signals which demand immediate report to the physician. These symptoms are as follows:

1. *Vaginal bleeding, no matter how slight*
2. *Swelling of the face or the fingers*
3. *Severe continuous headache*
4. *Dimness or blurring of vision*
5. *Flashes of light or dots before the eyes*
6. *Pain in the abdomen*
7. *Persistent vomiting*
8. *Chills and fever*
9. *Sudden escape of fluid from the vagina*

In addition to this detailed supervision the patient needs an explanation of the changes that are taking place within her body. This point cannot be stressed enough. Intelligent exploration with the patient regarding her concerns about these changes and appropriate instruction will give her greater reassurance and self-confidence. An understanding and empathic attitude on the part of the doctor and the nurse will do much to buoy the patient's morale and to diminish unnecessary anxiety.

As the patient approaches full term, she should be instructed also about the signs and symptoms of oncoming labor, so that she may know when the process is beginning and when to notify the physician. At this time the physician will want to know the frequency of contractions and any other pertinent symptoms.

Most hospitals conduct routine tours of the maternity division for the registered maternity patients and their husbands. It is advisable to encourage the expectant parents to take advantage of this opportunity sometime during the pregnancy. Becoming familiar ahead of time with the surroundings where the mother-to-be will be delivered reduces the anxiety that may be experienced in going to a strange hospital for the first time after labor has begun. The details of the hospital admission routine should be explained, so that she is familiar with this procedure before being admitted for delivery.

NURSING CARE

Although adequate antepartal care is becoming more readily available throughout the nation, health workers find that because of one or several factors in the previously mentioned crises, many women who want this care often do not utilize available services, or they may discontinue their care at some point in the pregnancy. This is particularly true of those who attend clinics. There are several reasons that have been cited by patients as deterrents: (a) extremely long periods of waiting, (b) impersonal treatment by staff, (c) complicated procedures for clinic registration, (d) different doctors at each visit, (e) inadequate comfort facilities such as toilets and sitting room and (f) no evening or weekend clinic.

If those who provide care merely focus on a maintenance type of physical care and make no attempt to discover and help the expectant mother to satisfy her needs as she perceives them, the patient does not really receive good nursing care. Those who attend her must recognize that the pregnant woman is an individual involved in one of life's most important experiences. When the atmosphere of the hospital, the clinic or the doctor's office is such that a patient encounters regard for her human dignity and worth, and her concerns are listened to with interest and respect, she returns for care and profits by it. Therefore, one of the most important activities of the nurse who attends antepartal patients is to establish a relationship with the patient that conveys regard for her as a human being and permits free and frank discussion. This type of relationship not only will enable the nurse to instruct and counsel the mother more effectively about the various aspects of her pregnancy but also will allow the patient to express the more convert concerns and nuances of the pregnancy that are troublesome to her. The nurse then will be in a better position to deal with these herself or to refer them, as the occasion warrants, to the other members of the health team.

The nurse involved in antepartal care will find herself in one of three settings, a private doctor's office, a clinic or the community. Whatever the setting, the nurse should be skilled in communication techniques, since these are basic to establishing a productive nurse-patient relationship.

The nurse must be able to notice what goes on in the interaction between herself and the patient, to interpret what she observes, and to determine appropriate nursing intervention accordingly. In conferring with patients, the nurse needs not only to teach and give information, but also to be able to get it as well. Hence, she must be able *to listen* to what the patient is saying, to make non-judgmental responses, to question and to elicit significant information from the patient when it is appropriate, in order to increase her own understanding.

The nurse who *listens actively* to what the patient is saying will discern the covert as well as the overt cues. In conversation she can reflect the gist of the patient's remarks so that the patient, as well as the nurse, may gain insight into the topic under discussion. The skilled nurse can also probe gently but effectively to get at the crux of the problem or the concern. In helping the patient to separate fact from fiction in the situation and eventually to see what alternatives she has for action, the nurse helps the patient to confront her problems more realistically.

The nurse's understanding of human behavior will guide her in choosing the appropriate time and circumstances to help the patient in this way. The skillful nurse focuses her attention on the mother and listens, reflects and questions to learn more about the mother-to-be as an individual, her usual methods or ways of coping with problems, whether she needs help, and how she reacts to advice.

The Office and Clinic Settings

The Problem of Limited Time. The nurse who is accustomed to caring for patients on the inpatient hospital service, where she has rather continuous contacts with the same patient for days, or even weeks at a time, often finds the initial adjustment to an office or especially a clinic service difficult because of the limited time that the schedule usually permits for contacts with each patient. During the patient's brief appointment period in these last two settings, the nurse must evaluate the present and the continuing nursing needs of the individual and plan to meet these needs effectively. The nurse who recognizes and understands this problem of limited time will find the orientation period less frustrating, and as she becomes more skilled in communication and observation of nonverbal as well as verbal behavior, she will enjoy the satisfactions of giving patient care and guidance in these types of settings.

Fig. 8-5. Group counseling by the nurse in the clinic.

Teaching the Patient. In addition to assisting the physician with examinations and performing various procedures, the nurse in the office or the clinic can devote much of her nursing care to health teaching and anticipatory guidance (i.e., informing mothers about what to expect regarding their pregnancy, delivery, postpartal and child-rearing periods before they begin to worry or to make mistakes). Therefore, the nurse needs to have broad knowledge and understanding about the physiology of pregnancy and childbearing, general hygiene, nutrition, the emotional, psychological and sociologic-economic aspects of family living, and the part played by a family in the larger community. Her teachings are individualized for each patient, and should include instruction in ways of maintaining good health habits in daily living, interpretation of the reasons that these practices are important, and suggestions of ways in which undesirable habits may be changed or modified. It is important to remember that health teaching and anticipatory guidance in any setting involve motivating the patient—and consequently influencing the degree of her interest and her desire to change or to continue present patterns of behavior. To accomplish the desired end, the nurse first identifies the level of knowledge and understanding of the patient through exploration of what the patient knows and feels about the topic in question. Second, the nurse

clarifies any misinformation or misconceptions. Finally, she adds to the base of knowledge and understanding through reinterpretation, clarification, re-emphasis and reinforcement.

The problem of motivating patients is complex, and unfortunately no simple steps or methods exist to explain how to accomplish this. Generally, it seems that valid information about the subject, reference groups, and the patient's personal values are key "preconditions" to motivation. Another key "precondition" is the selection of a goal or "request" which the patient can reasonably achieve. If, for instance, a patient is well informed on a subject and can identify in some way with the group from which the request comes, and if the subject or the request is not at too much variance with the patient's values, he can comply without an enormous degree of change or effort; then the stage is set to "motivate."

THE INITIAL CONTACT with the patient is particularly important. By her pleasant greeting and professional manner the nurse can initiate a productive relationship that conveys her interest and concern for the patient. In making a patient comfortable who is waiting for her appointment with the physician, the nurse can utilize the opportunity to find out any questions, symptoms or problems that the mother may have and deal with them or report them to the proper person. This is an example of one way that the nurse can utilize limited contacts with the patient constructively.

REFERRALS. The problems that come to light are not always of a physical nature; emotional and social problems also may interfere with the patient's ability to derive full benefit from health services. It is the responsibility of the nurse to find out in what ways the patient needs help and to make appropriate referrals when they are indicated (e.g., to the nurse in the community, to allied community services or to other members of the extended health team). This is one of her most important nursing activities, since through the use of referrals she can keep lines of communication open between her particular health agency, the community and the members of the health team. Thus comprehensive care for the patient is assured.

VISUAL AIDS; TEACHING GROUPS. In hospitals and offices where the appointment system is used, the waiting time for the patient is minimized. In others the patient may have to wait longer periods. Waiting time in any setting may be utilized advantageously by providing reading material that will contribute to the patient's knowledge of her condition. Visual aids such as posters and charts may be both instructive and diverting. Flannelboard posters are excellent in this respect, since they can be changed frequently. These visual aids also provide an outlet for the creative ideas of the staff. Some offices and clinics use a group approach for discussion, teaching and guidance. These groups may be under the leadership of the nurse and provide a maximum amount of instruction and discussion for a large number of patients in a short period of time.

The Physical Examination. When the nurse assists the physician with the physical examination, she has an opportunity to learn more about the patient's condition. She should be alert to the cues and the events that transpire during this time, since she may be questioned afterward by the patient regarding her condition, or she may have to interpret the physician's instructions to make certain that they are understood. Often a patient is hesitant to discuss some matter with the physician, because she considers it too trivial, but she may feel comfortable in talking about it with the nurse. In turn, the nurse may consider this a problem of some importance, and on reporting it to the physician, she finds that it has a bearing on the course of treatment that he prescribes.

Another of the nurse's responsibilities is to prepare the patient for the physical examination. Since the initial examination is thorough, it is desirable that the patient disrobe completely and wear a gown that opens easily. In addition, the expectant mother should be covered with a small sheet to prevent unnecessary exposure and chilling. The nurse will want to instruct the mother to empty her bladder, since a full bladder is uncomfortable for the mother and may interfere with the physician's manipulations. A good footstool is imperative if the patient is to mount the table in safety and comfort. Many patients move somewhat awkwardly, especially as they near term, and the nurse can contribute a great deal to their safety and also help alleviate embarrassment by assisting the mother, as she changes her position, to move slowly but steadily. For the patient's physical and emotional comfort and for the doctor's protection, the nurse should be present during the entire examination.

THE PELVIC EXAMINATION. One aspect of the physical examination, the vaginal or pelvic examination, deserves special consideration, because often it is the most stressful part of the experience for the patient. This examination is carried out with the patient in the dorsal recumbent position. In this position the patient lies on her back with the lower limbs flexed and rotated outward. Her heels are supported in stirrups, which are level with the table, perhaps a foot in front of her buttocks. In this position the anxious patient, already under stress during the physical examination, is likely to tense her abdominal, pelvic and thigh muscles, attempting to adduct her thighs. Moreover, if the patient arches her back as her tension increases, her pelvis will be tilted downward, a position that makes the pelvic examination almost impossible to achieve.

The nurse can be most effective in assisting the patient to relax if she encourages her to keep breathing naturally, reminds her to breathe if she holds her breath, and helps her to let the small of her back press down on the table. Merely telling the anxious patient to relax is of no avail; thus the nurse needs to give the patient rather direct guidance, often step by step. For example, if the patient is clenching her fists, the nurse may say, "See, your wrists and hands are tense. Try to let them go limp—very limp—like a rag doll's. That's it—very limp." And a moment later, "Keep breathing naturally." Such short, explicit requests and instruction give the mother a simple task that she can do with guidance. This diverts her attention from the anticipated discomfort and promotes relaxation.

Since the doctor must see the cervix clearly, he will need a stool to sit on and a good light to focus into the vagina. Any equipment that he may need, such as vaginal speculum, swabs, cotton balls, slides, lubricating jelly, etc., should be close at hand, so that he can reach them readily.

The pelvic examination will begin with an examination of the external genitalia and will include the urethra, Skene's and Bartholin's glands. If any unusual discharge is present, a specimen may be obtained for culture or microscopic examination. Usually, the doctor will next insert a speculum into the vagina to distend the folds so that he may observe the cervix. If a Papanicolaou smear is to be taken, no lubricating jelly will be used; instead, the speculum may be rinsed under *tepid* running water to facilitate the ease of insertion. Occasionally, the dilatation of the vagina by the speculum may cause an unpleasant sensation of stretching. Unfortunately, the mother already may be tense from the effect of strange surroundings and experiences, and the intrusioin of this instrument may contribute to her discomfort, increasing her tenseness.

The fear, tension, pain syndrome in labor, described by Dr. Grantly Dick Read (see Suggested Reading), can affect the mother-to-be under these circumstances as well. Her fear of the examination increases her tenseness, which enhances the discomfort; hence a vicious circle is established. The nurse can do much to break this circle by encouraging the mother to breathe naturally while she is being examined. Allowing the patient to squeeze or to hold her hand is often very helpful, although the nurse should recognize that not all patients want or need this physical contact. It is wise to be readily available to the patient but to let her initiate the contact. In our culture it is important that people "conrol themselves"; this is difficult to do when one's privacy is invaded, as it is by these intrusive procedures. It becomes especially important, then, to help the patient to preserve a positive concept of herself in this obstetric situation, since these early encounters all help to form an integral part of the mosaic that determines her self-concept as a mother.

As the examination proceeds, the cervix is visualized, and the doctor will note its color and character. Normally, the cervix of the primi-gravida is pink or bluish and smooth, with a dimple for the os. The cervix of a multigravida may have an irregular os due to lacerations from previous deliveries. If erosions of the cervix are present, they may be treated with silver nitrate swabs. Any discharge, such as a purulent, a greenish or a frothy discharge, is considered to be abnormal, and a specimen may be secured for microscopic examination or culture.

After the cervix has been examined, the doctor will withdraw the speculum and proceed with the bimanual examination to evaluate the uterus and the adnexa. He will determine the size, the consistency and the contour of these organs as well as the relationship of the uterus to the pelvis. At this time he will take the internal measurements to determine the diameters of the pelvic inlet (see Chap. 2). The physician usually completes the pelvic examination with an examination of the rectum to ascertain the presence of hemorrhoids, polyps or other abnormalities.

At the completion of this examination, disposable tissues should be offered the patient so that she may wipe the perineum adequately. Optimally, further activity and demands should be kept at a minimum, so that the mother may recoup the energy which has been dissipated through trying to absorb all the new experiences and information. Further specific health teaching and counseling is better postponed until a subsequent visit, when the patient is not so overloaded with new stimuli and fatigue.

The Patient and Her Family. In a program which emphasizess family-centered service, the health problems of the individual patient and their relationship to other members of the family are of major importance. An example of a situation might be the case of Mrs. Brown, the wife of a laborer and the mother of a small toddler and a 4-year-old boy. Her physician has advised her that she needs more rest in the course of the day. Her husband is at work, and the older boy is in nursery school until noon. In order to get more rest, she needs help to make plans for the safety and the care of the children during these rest periods; otherwise the physical rest would not accomplish its purpose. Even the consideration of meeting the nutritional needs for this family with a limited income may require guidance. To give real help at this point requires some knowledge of nutrition and entails extra planning so that the meals supply the nutritional requirements for a pregnant woman, a father who performs hard physical labor and two small children. Wherever facilities and personnel permit, more clinics are utilizing the services of a "resident" nutritionist for guidance and counseling regarding nutritional aspects and planning. Depending on the clinic's procedure, the nurse may then have the responsibility of referring the patient to the nutritionist or arranging for the patient to join a group of mothers who meet with the nutritionist for planning. In the case where a nutritionist is not available, then the responsibility for this counseling falls to the nurse.

The nurse in the office or the clinic who is alert to such actual or potential health problems that affect both the patient and her family recognizes that a home visit by a public health nurse often is very helpful. If such a situation arises, she can tell the patient about available public health services and explain what a public health nurse might do while making a home visit and how such a visit could benefit the patient. With the doctor's knowledge and the patient's permission, she can institute a referral through the proper channels. Each institution or agency will have its particular method and procedure. Real value may be derived from a visit in which the nurse is able to see the patient in her usual surroundings. For instance, if the patient has the problem of excessive weight gain and is not responding to clinic therapy, the public health nurse, visiting the patient in her home, may gain some insight into the basis of the problem during her visit. In her report to the clinic or the office staff she would relate information that would contribute both to the medical and the nursing management of this pregnancy. In situations in which the clinic program is limited in educational opportunities, such as parents' classes and/or individual guidance, the public health nurse's visit to the home may be necessary to supplement the health care teaching and anticipatory guidance done in the clinic.

The Community Setting

The extensive adoption of early antepartal care by various institutions, both lay and medical, is doing much to improve obstetric standards; and, in connection with this movement, the public health nurse has proved to be an invaluable asset. During the period before antepartal care was fully accepted, a case-finding program was a part of the work done by some organizations (i.e., the nurse would canvass the district for pregnant mothers). In recent decades the demand for hospital deliveries has increased rapidly; thus the present trend is toward hospital care. This has resulted in an increased demand for hospital beds, and some hospitals, especially those in congested areas or those with limited facilities, have requested that patients register early in their pregnancy to be assured of adequate accommodations for their deliveries. This early registration has resulted in more mothers getting adequate antepartal supervision early in pregnancy. In some isolated rural areas the public health nurse does case finding in the course of her usual activities and can assist the local practitioner in the antepartal care of maternity patients in the community.

Ideal Role of the Public Health Nurse Serving in an Agency. The nurse in the community is "home-based" in either an official or a voluntary agency. The official health agency may have an antepartal clinic offering complete antepartal services for those families who are having financial crises that may or may not be a result of the pregnancy. Many agencies have recognized that the public health nurse is not being utilized to her fullest potential when she is responsible for the administrative aspects of the clinic. When the professional nurse is caught up in the mechanics of record work, room preparation, directing traffic and assisting with procedures, she can barely reinforce the physician's orders and perhaps clarify information relative to the obstetric condition. To utilize the time of the professional nurse more efficiently, so that she is free to counsel patients in depth in any matters relative to health, many agencies are employing registered nurses for clinic management who do not have the public health credential (i.e., formal preparation in public health and public health certification). In addition, to maximize patient care, various types of other auxiliary personnel may be utilized (e.g., lay volunteers, licensed vocational nurses, nursing aides, etc.). The clinic managers together with other nonprofessional personnel may be responsible for all of the clinic activities with the exception of patient counseling. Similarly, more hospital clinics throughout the nation are beginning to utilize a public health nurse for the health teaching and the anticipatory guidance aspects of patient care. As has been described already, most clinic schedules are very full, and the distribution of activities in such a manner results in more comprehensive patient care.

If the patient and/or her family has a problem that the public health nurse in the clinic thinks needs follow-up in th home (between clinic visits), she will contact her district counterpart and communicate the necessary information. In turn, the district public health nurse will inform the clinic personnel of any pertinent findings. If complete comprehensive care is to be given to patients, open lines of communication and an expeditious inter-agency referral system are basic to the best service of all members of the health team, whatever their level of responsibility.

Home Visits. The district public health nurse does not follow a stereotyped routine when she makes her home visits, since each visit involves an individual patient in her own home setting. She does not have the "captive audience" that the hospital nurse does; rather she is a guest in her patient's home, and this involves a somewhat different approach and orientation. In such a situation it is especially important to orient the visit to what the patient wants and needs to know. Repeated visits based on the *nurse's* needs (to impart certain information, instruction, etc.) may very well result in a firmly closed door and a consequent severing of the nurse-patient relationship. Astute assessment of the situation at each visit includes, first of all, finding out what the patient needs to know. Communication and observation skills (previously mentioned) are, of course, of paramount importance here. It is the wise nurse who takes her cues from the mother and handles each need as it arises without feeling compelled to "teach" a certain amount of material each visit. If the visits are managed in this way, topics may include basic information about pregnancy, hygiene and nutrition, specific preparations for the baby, how to handle sibling rivalry, and so on. These subjects may come up naturally in the course of the visits, or the nurse can guide conversation around to them as she explores with the mother certain areas of need. By the end of the antepartal supervision period all necessary counseling usually can be accomplished.

OPPORTUNITIES FOR FAMILY HEALTH SUPERVISION. During the course of antepartal care the nurse has many opportunities for family health supervision. In her observation of other children in the home, she may be the first person to notice a neglected orthopedic condition, to suspect a need for a chest roentgenogram or to observe a possible vision or hearing difficulty. In addition, observation of the mother's interaction with her children may give valuable clues to the patient's mothering patterns. This will aid the nurse in planning more effective anticipatory guidance and health teaching.

Comprehensive antepartal care, then, is a quality of patient care that is goal-directed toward the total health and the well-being of the pregnant woman. With this as the central objective, the combined efforts of several disciplines, in addition to those of medicine and nursing, may be required in the cooperative plan to achieve the ultimate goals. The practitioner-patient relationship is reciprocal, involving one giving and the other receiving care, and, to be meaningful, it must be a positive interaction. This type of interaction can be achieved only if the patient and her problems are understood and viewed with respect. The patient, in turn, must be helped to understand the goals of the health practitioners. A positive effort on the part of the health team becomes possible if each member has a clear understanding of his own role, appreciates and understands the contribution of the other professions represented on the team, knows something of the processes involved in the differing approaches, recognizes commonality of interest and skill, and has the intellectual and the emotional capacity to enter into a team relationship.

The Medical Social Worker

Although nursing care is the primary consideration in this section, one member of the extended health team will be mentioned specifically since she works so closely with the nurse in the care of the pregnant woman. Most hospitals today have a substantial Social Service Department; it is hoped that more public health agencies will be able to take advantage of this service as more funds and personnel make this possible.

The function of Social Service workers is to help people to meet and to cope with problems that interfere with social functioning. These problems may include the problems of unmarried parenthood, divorce, desertion, placing older children during the mother's hospital stay, arranging for a working housekeeper, planning convalescent care for the mother, or arranging financial or material assistance. In their professional role social workers are called on to evaluate these problems. Then, with the patient's cooperation they help her to mobilize her resources and assist her, when necessary, through referral and counseling to alleviate the condition. They

TABLE 8-1. RECOMMENDED DAILY DIETARY ALLOWANCES

Designed for the maintenance of good nutrition of practically all healthy people in the U.S.A.

	AGE[b] (years) From Up to	WEIGHT (kg)	WEIGHT (lbs)	HEIGHT (cm)	HEIGHT (in.)	kcal	PROTEIN (Gm)	VITAMIN A ACTIVITY (IU)	VITAMIN D (IU)	VITAMIN E ACTIVITY (IU)	ASCORBIC ACID (mg)	FOLACIN[c] (mg)	NIACIN (mg equiv)[d]	RIBOFLAVIN (mg)	THIAMIN (mg)	VITAMIN B6 (mg)	VITAMIN B12 (µg)	CALCIUM (g)	PHOSPHORUS (g)	IODINE (µg)	IRON (mg)	MAGNESIUM (mg)
Infants	0 - 1/6	4	9	55	22	kg × 120	kg × 2.2[e]	1,500	400	5	35	0.05	5	0.4	0.2	0.2	1.0	0.4	0.2	25	6	40
	1/6 - 1/2	7	15	63	25	kg × 110	kg × 2.0[e]	1,500	400	5	35	0.05	7	0.5	0.4	0.3	1.5	0.5	0.4	40	10	60
	1/2 - 1	9	20	72	28	kg × 100	kg × 1.8[e]	1,500	400	5	35	0.1	8	0.6	0.5	0.4	2.0	0.6	0.5	45	15	70
Children	1 - 2	12	26	81	32	1,100	25	2,000	400	10	40	0.1	8	0.6	0.6	0.5	2.0	0.7	0.7	55	15	100
	2 - 3	14	31	91	36	1,250	25	2,000	400	10	40	0.2	8	0.7	0.6	0.6	2.5	0.8	0.8	60	15	150
	3 - 4	16	35	100	39	1,400	30	2,500	400	10	40	0.2	9	0.8	0.7	0.7	3	0.8	0.8	70	10	200
	4 - 6	19	42	110	43	1,600	30	2,500	400	10	40	0.2	11	0.9	0.8	0.9	4	0.8	0.8	80	10	200
	6 - 8	23	51	121	48	2,000	35	3,500	400	15	40	0.2	13	1.1	1.0	1.0	4	0.9	0.9	100	10	250
	8 - 10	28	62	131	52	2,200	40	3,500	400	15	40	0.3	15	1.2	1.1	1.2	5	1.0	1.0	110	10	250
Males	10 - 12	35	77	140	55	2,500	45	4,500	400	20	40	0.4	17	1.3	1.3	1.4	5	1.2	1.2	125	10	300
	12 - 14	43	95	151	59	2,700	50	5,000	400	20	45	0.4	18	1.4	1.4	1.6	5	1.4	1.4	135	18	350
	14 - 18	59	130	170	67	3,000	60	5,000	400	25	55	0.4	20	1.5	1.5	1.8	5	1.4	1.4	150	18	400
	18 - 22	67	147	175	69	2,800	60	5,000	400	30	60	0.4	18	1.6	1.4	2.0	5	0.8	0.8	140	10	400
	22 - 35	70	154	175	69	2,800	65	5,000	—	30	60	0.4	18	1.7	1.4	2.0	5	0.8	0.8	140	10	350
	35 - 55	70	154	173	68	2,600	65	5,000	—	30	60	0.4	17	1.7	1.3	2.0	5	0.8	0.8	125	10	350
	55 - 75+	70	154	171	67	2,400	65	5,000	—	30	60	0.4	14	1.7	1.2	2.0	6	0.8	0.8	110	10	350
Females	10 - 12	35	77	142	56	2,250	50	1,500	100	20	40	0.4	15	1.3	1.1	1.4	5	1.2	1.2	110	18	300
	12 - 14	44	97	154	61	2,300	50	5,000	400	20	45	0.4	15	1.4	1.2	1.6	5	1.3	1.3	115	18	350
	14 - 16	52	114	157	62	2,400	55	5,000	400	25	50	0.4	16	1.4	1.2	1.8	5	1.3	1.3	120	18	350
	16 - 18	54	119	160	63	2,300	55	5,000	400	25	50	0.4	15	1.5	1.2	2.0	5	1.3	1.3	115	18	350
	18 - 22	58	128	163	64	2,000	55	5,000	400	25	55	0.4	13	1.5	1.0	2.0	5	0.8	0.8	100	18	350
	22 - 35	58	128	163	64	2,000	55	5,000	—	25	55	0.4	13	1.5	1.0	2.0	5	0.8	0.8	100	18	300
	35 - 55	58	128	160	63	1,850	55	5,000	—	25	55	0.4	13	1.5	1.0	2.0	5	0.8	0.8	90	18	300
	55 - 75+	58	128	157	62	1,700	55	5,000	—	25	55	0.4	13	1.5	1.0	2.0	6	0.8	0.8	80	10	300
Pregnancy						+200	65	6,000	400	30	60	0.8	15	1.8	+0.1	2.5	8	+0.4	+0.4	125	18	450
Lactation						+1,000	75	8,000	400	30	60	0.5	20	2.0	+0.5	2.5	6	+0.5	+0.5	150	18	450

* Recommended Daily Dietary Allowances (Revised 1968), Food and Nutrition Board, National Academy of Sciences—National Research Council, Washington, D.C.

[a] The allowance levels are intended to cover individual variations among most normal persons as they live in the United States under usual environmental stresses. The recommended allowances can be attained with a variety of common foods, providing other nutrients for which human requirements have been less well defined. See text for more-detailed discussion of allowances and of nutrients not tabulated.

[b] Entries on lines for age range 22-35 years represent the reference man and woman at age 22. All other entries represent allowances for the midpoint of the specified age range.

[c] The folacin allowances refer to dietary sources as determined by *Lactobacillus casei assay*. Pure forms of folacin may be effective in doses less than ¼ of the RDA.

[d] Niacin equivalents include dietary sources of the vitamin itself plus 1 mg equivalent for each 60 mg of dietary tryptophan.

[e] Assumes protein equivalent to human milk. For proteins not 100 percent utilized factors should be increased proportionately.

FIG. 8-6. Nutritional counseling by the dietitian in the clinic (with 2 patients).

may make home visits and interview the patient, and perhaps other family members, to aid them in diagnosing the extent of the problems. Social problems may seem overwhelming if the patient's physical condition is affected, and these concerns in turn may interfere with the benefit that the patient may derive from medical services. The social worker may act as an understanding counselor between the family and the patient during her hospital stay. In many hospitals the need for a social service referral is apparent when the patient is registered early in pregnancy. In that event the patient is interviewed after the initial medical examination, and from both the physical and the social findings plans are made with the patient to mobilize her resources.

By her observation, counseling and liaison work, the social worker combines her efforts with the other members of the health team to see the patient not only as an individual maternity patient but also as an important member of the family, and the family as an integral part of the community.

NUTRITION IN PREGNANCY

As previously mentioned, present day antepartal clinics are utilizing the services of nutritionists for dietary counseling and planning whenever possible. When nutritionists are available, the nurse will find that she can work in conjunction with them to provide adequate guidance. Her role in these cases may be to explore with the mother the extent of her need to have nutritional counseling and/or arrange for the mother to participate in some form of counseling under the auspices of the nutritionist. However, many areas do not have the services of a nutritionist and in these instances, a very important activity of the nurse is that of nutritional counseling. Attention has been focused on the diet of the pregnant mother in recent studies, and it has been demonstrated that the improved nutritional status of the mother promotes not only her well-being, but also her baby's. For instance, a significant relationship has been found between the protein intake of the mother and the physical condition of the infant. Moreover, some preliminary findings have indicated an association between inadequate protein intake during pregnancy and mental deficiency in the fetus, as well as low birth weight (see Suggested Reading). Thus, an appropriate diet promotes building materials for the growth and the development of her offspring. The student is advised to study the recommended dietary allowances so that she can compare necessary increases in pregnancy.

General Factors in Planning the Diet

Quality rather than quantity is the main consideration in planning the diet. During the first part of pregnancy the daily energy requirements for the average pregnant woman will be about the same as usual, in the neighborhood of 2,100 to 2,300 calories a day if she is moderately active, unless her weight needs to be regulated. It is important to consider the patient's activity in relation to her diet. In the latter part of pregnancy, if the patient maintains moderate activity, the daily caloric intake may be augmented because of the increased metabolic rate. If, however, activity slows down, as is often the case, and an inappropriate weight gain ensues, then caloric intake may be reduced. The physician will prescribe specifically for each mother to meet her individual needs, and the nurse or nutritionist then will follow through with counseling and planning as necessary. The Food and Nutrition Board of the National Research Council recommends daily allowances of specific nutrients for pregnancy and lactation, as shown in Table 8-1.

During the early months the appetite may be affected, and there may be phases of dislike for certain foods and beverages. Then later, there may be an increase in the desire for all food or certain types of food. The mother may need help to discipline her appetite in accord with the amount of food needed and the desirable weight gain. Thoughtful and cooperative meal planning with the patient, with specific and thorough direction as to quantity and quality of nutrients, do much to help the mother to maintain motivation and discipline during these difficult times.

One patient who had been told that she could eat "all the cottage cheese and tomatoes that she wanted" tearfully watched her weight climb each visit. When the matter finally was pursued, it was found that she had taken the words quite literally and was eating a pint of creamed cottage cheese and six medium-sized tomatoes for lunch each day. The quantity made up for the low calorie content of the food!

Also, it is well to counsel the mother early in her pregnancy to avoid sweets and high caloric desserts, as well as the habit of frequent nibbling, since these interfere with appetite for the more essential foods and only add additional weight. Early pregnancy is a good time to institute health teaching of this sort, since many mothers are motivated to attain good health for themselves and their impending child at this time and hence are very receptive to anything that will bring this about. Appetite tends to be diminished, and therefore appropriate choosing of the quantity of food may be easier; later, when the "newness" of the pregnancy has worn off, and [the] appetite is unleashed, self-discipline is much harder, especially without previous reinforcement. Occasional "cravings" for unusual articles of food may occur. These sometimes indicate the lack of a certain element in the diet that the body demands. Any desires of this nature may be granted with safety if they agree with the patient and are not exceptional in amount or content. If the diet supplies all the needs of the patient and the growing fetus, such cravings may not occur.

Salt Restriction. Another important point should be emphasized here, the importance of restricting excessive salt intake during pregnancy. First, the amount of salt consumed by the average person is far in excess of human requirements. Second, even if no salt were added to foods either in the kitchen or at the table, this mineral is distributed so widely in food materials that the likelihood of shortage would be exceedingly remote. Finally, there is a definite relationship between the amount of salt eaten and the amount of water retained by the body; that is, the greater the salt intake, the greater is the tendency of tissues to absorb water. The tissues of the pregnant woman manifest a particular avidity for water, as is evidenced by the tendency of the face and the fingers to become puffy, and if, superimposed on this tendency, there is an excess of salt in the diet, the tissues may become actually water-logged, with dire consequences.

Many physicians advise their patients early in pregnancy to watch their salt intake by avoiding salty foods, using salt judiciously in cooking, and avoiding the use of the saltshaker at the table. During the last trimester salt restriction is especially necessary, and it is important that the patient be so advised.

The Balanced Diet

The physician will regulate the patient's diet according to her condition, and the nurse will follow through, planning with the mother how best to implement his orders. If the patient's previous diet has been nourishing and well balanced, few changes will be necessary except to provide for the adjustment in protein, mineral and vitamin intake.

Counseling and Planning Sessions. To provide appropriate guidance for the mother and to better assess her level of understanding and knowledge about her diet, a brief diet history can be taken to find out her present eating patterns. The nurse may ask the mother to write down her usual daily and/or weekly meal pattern and any "extras" that she is likely to consume. These menus then are checked for an adequate intake of those foods that provide a substantial amount of the essential nutrients. As the nurse and the mother plan together, the patient's likes and dislikes are recognized, and those foods that provide the essential nutrients are encouraged. Suggestions may be given for the addition of certain foods or the modification of existing methods of selection and/or preparation. During these planning sessions it is important to remember that the mother is a member of a family, and although she plans the meals, many of her choices are dictated by the likes and dislikes of her family. The young teen-age bride who has just learned to fry cheeseburgers and french fries for her spouse may not be persuaded easily to broil and to bake instead; furthermore, she deserves recognition for accomplishing something as important as preparing a meal that is pleasing to her husband.

THE RELIGIOUS, RACIAL AND ETHNIC BACKGROUND of the patient and her family is another important consideration in counsel regarding nutrition, as well as in other aspects of care. Many families are fond of their regional or national diet and prefer it to the American "meat and potatoes" regimen. Whenever possible, the preferred diet should be considered and planned through the use of "exchanges" for food groups (see Suggested Reading). Many nutrition books give a "basic national" diet for the various countries, which provides a springboard for planning.

In considering the diet of persons of a different ethnicity, the nurse also should consider the degree of *acculturation* of the patient. This term refers to the acquisition by a group or an individual of the traits of another culture. For instance, in the case of a bilingual patient with the name of Munoz, it should not be assumed that beans and tortillas are staple in the diet. Mrs. Munoz may be a third-generation American and very familiar with and accepting of North American nutrition and eating patterns (i.e., she is acculturated).

PSYCHOLOGICAL ASPECTS OF NUTRITION. Other aspects to be considered are the stage of growth and development of the patient and the psychological factors involved in nutrition (e.g., the meaning that food has for the mother). We are aware, for instance, that foods enjoyed by adolescents are different from the foods enjoyed by older people; the hamburger-coke-french fry "typical" teen-age diet has received wide publicity. It seems to meet some need in much the same way as peanut butter sandwiches do for the preschooler. Many persons are marrying younger and becoming parents at an earlier age, and, of course, they carry their eating patterns into marriage with them. In addition, adolescence is a time for developing independence, and this is healthy. However, many foods are rejected (milk, vegetables, cereal, etc.), because they are associated with "home" and a dependency period. The desire to be free and to select the "forbidden" foods is very strong. Permitting assertion of independence is important if the overall developmental task is to be accomplished, and the patient is to make a healthy adjustment in roles from that of the child to that of the adult; yet limits often must be set if the health of the mother and the health of the baby are to be safeguarded. Therefore, incorporating the mother into the planning and allowing her choices whenever possible, helping her to increase her knowledge of nutrients, encouraging and reinforcing correct choices or willing adaptations, and giving firm guidance when indicated, all help the patient and the nurse to achieve their respective goals.

The psychological aspects of nutrition lend themselves less well to clear-cut analysis. It has been said that people can survive a state of celibacy, however uncomfortably, but no one has been able to survive without food. Food is a basic need, according to the survival criterion, more basic even than the need for sex. We know that hunger is the most fundamental of all sensations. Related to hunger, but of a very different origin, is appetite. Appetite is Nature's primary defense for the prevention of hunger. Based on the anticipation of eating, the impulse is determined by the person's previous experience. Only by coincidence and training does appetite become associated with health-giving foods. Factors affecting food-seeking behavior are the main determinants of eating (i.e., hunger, appetite and custom). The great deterrents to normal appetite are worry, fear, and preoccupation with troublesome or difficult problems—and these may be reflected in either an increase or a decrease of appetite. Some of the positive emotional stimulants include a situation of calm contentedness, a feeling of mild elation or a condition of ego-stimulation.

Present-day cuisine is a potpourri of heritage, superstition, custom, knowledge and opportunity. Subtle cravings are passed along from one generation to the next by the process of training and imitation. Unique methods of food preparation as well as food selection, combinations, and prejudices are embodied in this training. Congeniality and hospitality among normal people are enhanced by the serving of good food; and it has become the custom to serve food at practically all functions, business as well as social.

From infancy onward, food and closeness are associated with love and security. Food and eating, in and of themselves, are looked upon as symbolizing interpersonal acceptance, warmth and sociability. Throughout all societies this symbolic undertone is unmistakable; from the "breaking of bread" in antiquity to the modern banquet the serving of food is a vehicle for expressing honor, joy or mutual bonds. It is easy to see why food has become associated with the symbolism of motherliness. Feeding is not only kindly and warm in its emotional meaning to those who receive food, but it is also essential to growth and well-being; hence it has become bound up with the idea of the mother, the one who originally nurtured, loved and supported.

The pregnant woman makes a close identification with the concept of the mother, and selections and choices may be influenced profoundly by these symbolic meanings of food. She may respond to worry, frustration or anxiety by overeating—either by nibbling or gorging. Conversely, another patient may develop anorexia. Or she may crave certain foods and reject others, and not because of physiological factors. For instance, she may feel that certain foods will "mark" her baby or will give him strength. It is crucial that the meaning which food has for the patient be explored, and that her feelings and attitudes be respected. Care must be taken not to make her feel deprecated or deprived while she is helped to understand the dynamics involved in hunger and appetite.

In summary, if counseling is to be effective and the results lasting, the nurse should strive to elicit wholehearted cooperation from the patient through involving her in the planning; considering her and her family's needs, background, preferences and attitude; encouraging and reinforcing appropriate choices and preparation; providing gentle but firm limit-setting, when indicated, and careful, thorough explanation regarding the rationale behind the advice.

The following discussion might provide some guidelines in helping patients to plan their diet. Foods have been grouped according to four general classifications: dairy foods, meat group, vegetables and fruits, and breads and cereals.

Dairy Foods. The expectant mother should have a quart of milk in some form daily; milk is Nature's most nearly perfect food and is invaluable as a nutrient. It contains all the different kinds of mineral elements that are needed for fetal development. The high content of calcium and phosphorus in milk makes it almost indispensable for good growth of bone and teeth; it provides these minerals in the correct proportions and in a digestible form which permits optimum utilization by both mother and fetus. It is not only an excellent source of protein or tissue-building material but also the most readily digested and easily absorbed of all food proteins. Milk is also rich in energy-providing values, so that 1 quart a day alone furnishes almost one fourth of the total energy requirements. Finally, milk contains some of the most important vitamins, particularly vitamin A, which increases resistance to infection and safeguards the development of the fetus.

An effort should be made to have the mother drink 2 glasses of milk a day; the remainder may be taken in some other form, such as soups, custards, etc. If this is done, then total calories should be watched, since these other dishes involve additional nutrients. Evaporated milk and the instant dried milks are acceptable and may be substituted if fresh cow's milk is not available or desired.

For some patients, milk may be constipating,

or it may be distasteful. If it is found to be constipating, it is preferable to treat the constipation in some way other than by omitting the milk. If the milk is distasteful, it may be disguised in other foods, as has been mentioned. The instant nonfat and whole dry milks may be used in a quantity that provides an adequate intake. Approximately 5 tablespoons of dried skim milk will equal 1 pint of fluid milk. The milk may be used dry and worked into meatloaf, mashed potatoes, cereals, sandwich spreads, baked articles, etc. Reconstituted with less than the usual amount of water, it has a richer taste than the regular liquid skim milk. Certain condiments and flavorings (vanilla, nutmeg, instant coffee, cinnamon, etc.), when mixed with the milk, will enhance the flavor.

Some patients complain that milk is "fattening." In most instances the weight gain is due to the consumption of more food than is needed or an excess of such foods as bread, potatoes and desserts. These should be the articles that are restricted, and not the milk. Occasionally, however, it will be necessary to substitute skimmed milk or churned buttermilk for whole milk. This is acceptable and will reduce calories. Most dairies nowadays reinforce skim milk with vitamins A and D, which otherwise would be deficient. Many companies now have another variety of skim milk, one that is fortified by the addition of nonfat milk solids, 400 USP units of vitamin D and 4,000 USP units of vitamin A per quart. It has a standardized 2 per cent butter fat, so that the butter fat content in general is 1½ per cent less than that of whole milk.

American, Cheddar cheese and other dairy-made foods may be used occasionally as a substitute for a part or all of the milk allotment; 1 ounce of cheese contains approximately the same minerals and vitamins as a large glass of whole milk. However, the total protein and fat content of the diet then needs to be considered, since they may be altered.

If the mother can be helped to realize the importance of this one article of food in relation to the development of her baby, any sacrifices or modifications that may be involved can be made more willingly.

Meat Group. This is a rich source of one of the most essential nutrients, proteins. Two or more servings of beef, pork, lamb, veal, organ meats, fish, poultry, eggs or cheese are recommended daily. Legumes (dried beans, peas) or nuts may be used occasionally as alternates. In addition, these foods contain vitamins and valuable minerals, but their main value is in their amino acids or "building stones," as they sometimes are called. These are the elements that are needed not only by the mother but also by the fetus for the development of all the delicate and intricate systems of his body. Meat, eggs and fish contain complete proteins, with all the 10 amino acids that are necessary to maintain life and support growth. Oftentimes the family's budget restricts the quantity and the variety of these proteins, especially with respect to meat. The substitution of cheese, peanut butter, poultry, fish or legumes then may be suggested. The mother may also need advice regarding the preparation and the utilization of the organ meats that are so rich in protein, vitamins and minerals. Because some of these are relatively inexpensive, many women do not realize their nutritional worth and further avoid them because of the aesthetics that may be involved in the preparation—skinning, soaking, etc. Taste also is sometimes a factor. Nevertheless, with a little ingenuity and suggestions from a good nutrition and/or cook book, the nurse can do much to help the family to utilize this valuable and inexpensive source of protein. Liver, for instance, can be *lightly* broiled, ground and incorporated into a meatloaf or ground meat patties. The taste and looks are disguised, the nutritional value is retained, and the meat goes further.

Vegetables and Fruits. Four or more servings should be included from this group, especially the leaf, stem, green and yellow varieties of vegetables as well as the citrus fruits and tomatoes. It is desirable to serve at least one portion of each vegetable and fruit raw.

VEGETABLES, particularly, are rich sources of iron, calcium and several vitamins. At mealtimes there is no reasonable limit to the amount of lettuce, tomatoes, celery, string beans, carrots, beets and asparagus which may be eaten, provided that they are not heavily salted, sauced, buttered or served with a rich dressing. By increasing the quantity of such foods to several times the amount ordinarily taken, it is usually possible to satisfy the appetite without gaining abnormally in weight.

Fresh frozen vegetables are a good alternate. Canned vegetables may be used if fresh are not available. If a good brand is obtained, the vitamin content often is higher than that of vegetables cooked at home. Careful preparation and cooking of vegetables will help to retain the maximum vitamin and mineral content. Some vegetables contain several incomplete proteins which add to the total protein intake.

In addition to their value as nutrient agents, these vegetables deserve an important place in the diet as laxative agents, since their fibrous framework increases the bulk of the intestinal content and thereby stimulates the muscular, eliminative action of the intestines.

FRUITS. Citrus fruits—oranges, lemons and grapefruit—are the best sources of vitamin C. Most of these fruits also supply vitamins A and B. Tomatoes are also an excellent source of vitamin C; the amount, however, must be twice that of the citrus fruits to supply the same amount of vitamin. Other fruits, raw and cooked, such as prunes, raisins, apricots, contain important minerals (iron and copper) as well as vitamins. Fruits may stimulate a lagging appetite and counteract constipation. They may be used in many ways: as juices, combination of salads, additions to cereals or in-between meal refreshments and in desserts, such as gelatins and puddings. Fruits contain some incomplete proteins but only supplement the other proteins.

Bread and Cereals. Four or more servings should be included from this group. In the past it has been the practice to counsel patients to eliminate white bread and cereals and to substitute the darker and whole wheat varieties. This is no longer necessary, since almost all breads and cereals are enriched with vitamins, minerals and protein. A careful perusal of the label is usually all that is necessary. However, the darker varieties do provide a welcome change and, of course, are nutritious. When cereals are supplemented by milk, they become adequate for growth as well as for maintaining life. Bread that is buttered increases the vitamin A intake. The coarse cereals and the dark breads add roughage to the diet. Vitamin B and roughage both help to counteract constipation.

In addition to the four basic food groups, special attention should be given to the following:

Fluids. Fluids should be taken freely, averaging 6 to 8 glasses daily. Water aids in the circulation of the blood, body fluids, and the distribution of mineral salts, as well as in stimulating the digestion and the assimilation of foods. Fluids help to increase perspiration and to regulate elimination from intestines and kidneys. Tea and coffee may be included in the daily fluid quota if not found to be constipating or sleep-disturbing. Alcohol should be used sparingly, particularly if the mother must watch her weight, since beverages containing alcohol have a high caloric content. The use of alcohol by the pregnant woman has not shown a tendency to produce any pathologic changes in the mother or the fetus, and no effect on the course of pregnancy or labor has been demonstrated.

Vitamins. Vitamins are the *live* elements in food and are essential to life. The best sources are the natural foods. To retain the vitamin value in foods, they must be fresh, carefully prepared and not overcooked. During pregnancy and lactation the vitamin needs are increased, and so it is apparent that a well-balanced diet containing all the vitamins is of first importance. Some physicians add vitamin preparations to the diet to be sure that an adequate requirement has been met.

Vitamin A is essential in the diet for the maintenance of body resistance to infection. Foods which are good sources of this vitamin include whole milk, fortified skimmed milk, dairy products containing butter fat, eggs, green leafy and yellow vegetables and liver.

The vitamin B complex is essential to good nutrition. During pregnancy, thiamine (B₁) is necessary in increased amounts, as the fetus readily depletes the mother's reserve. Milk, eggs, lean meat and whole grain or enriched bread and cereal are good sources of thiamine. Riboflavin and nicotinic acid, absolute essentials in the diet, are found in such foods as meat, milk, eggs and green vegetables.

Vitamin C is necessary for the proper development of the fetus. Since an adequate reserve of this water-soluble vitamin is not stored in the body, an abundant supply of this vitamin is needed daily throughout pregnancy and lactation. Fresh citrus fruits, berries and green leafy vegetables (with the exception of lettuce) are foods which are a good source of vitamin C. These foods should be eaten raw as often as possible, since cooking destroys about half of their vitamin content.

Vitamin D is of great importance in safeguarding the mother and the fetus during pregnancy, since it bears some relationship to calcium and phosphorus metabolism. Liver, eggs, fortified sweet milk and fish (particularly Atlantic herring and mackerel) are food sources of vitamin D. The National Research Council recommends a daily intake of 400 I.U. for the pregnant and lactating woman. This amount, the Council says, will protect all normal growing individuals from deficiency with an adequate margin of safety. In evaluating vitamin D intake, all fortified foods in the diet should be taken into account, since large doses of either vitamin A or D may be toxic.

Minerals. Studies indicate that 13 or more mineral elements are essential for good nutrition. It is believed that if calcium, phosphorus, iron and iodine are provided in adequate amounts, the others also will be present in sufficient quantities.

CALCIUM. Although two thirds of the calcium in the fetus is deposited during the last month of pregnancy, the mother's daily requirement of calcium is increased during the entire course of pregnancy to prepare adequate storage for this demand. The principal foods from which calcium is obtained are cheese, eggs, oatmeal, vegetables and milk. A quart of milk alone supplies 1.2 Gm. of calcium.

PHOSPHORUS. This element is an essential constituent of all the cells and the tissues of the body. Milk provides an abundant source of phosphorus. Actually, since phosphorus is an almost invariable constituent of protein, a diet which includes sufficient protein-rich foods, such as eggs, meat, cheese, oatmeal and green vegetables, will provide also an adequate amount of phosphorus.

IRON. During the first two trimesters of pregnancy, iron is transferred to the fetus in moderate amounts, but during the last trimester, when the fetus builds up its reserve, the amount transferred is accelerated about 10 times. Therefore, the diet should be balanced and nutritious as well as rich in iron-containing foods. It is believed that certain amino acids, vitamin C and folic acid may be essential to normal iron absorption. If the daily diet contains egg yolk, lean meat (particularly liver), vegetables, fruit and whole grain cereals, the problem of anemia is less likely to occur. Recent studies indicate that expectant mothers who were in good health prior to pregnancy can maintain their hemoglobin concentration at known levels of health by eating a balanced diet (see Suggested Reading). However, many physicians prescribe additional iron in the form of such preparations as ferrous sulfate and ferrous gluconate. These preparations are administered 3 times a day, following meals, to allow for maximum absorption and to eliminate much of the intolerance for iron which would occur if the daily prescription for iron were administered in one dose.

IODINE. Only very small amounts of iodine are neeeded for the health of the mother and the fetus. This mineral is obtained very readily from seafoods; cod liver oil is another good source. In certain localities around the Great Lakes and in parts of the Northwest the water supply and the vegetables grown are poor in iodine. Hence, daily use of iodized salt ensures an adequate intake and prevents deficiency.

Following is a sample menu plan for a day*. Breakfast, midmorning, and bedtime patterns are approximately the same each day. Lunches and dinners are planned to provide other required food for the day. Wholegrain or enriched cereals and bread are to be used as well as butter or margarine.

BREAKFAST PATTERN

Citrus fruit—choose one: half grapefruit, medium orange, half cup canned grapefruit, 6 oz. fresh, frozen or canned orange, grapefruit or blended juice or tomato juice.†

Cereal—ready to eat or cooked cereal—½ to ¾ cup cooked cereal, or about one cup ready to eat cereal.

½ cup milk and 1 tsp; sugar (if desired).

2 slices bread or toast with 2 pats butter or margarine.

Note: Occasionally, the daily egg may replace one slice of toast, to provide extra variety.

MIDMORNING PATTERN

1 glass milk, warm or cold, or 1 cup cocoa made with milk. For variety, the milk may be flavored. An egg may be added on days when one is not used in other meals. Skim milk may be substituted.

SAMPLE LUNCH MENU #1

1 cup cream soup (homemade, canned, frozen made with milk)—potato, corn, tomato, pea, etc.,

4 crackers with soup,

Poached egg on toast with butter or margarine.

4 pieces fruit in syrup or ½ cup applesauce (homemade or canned) or a serving of fresh fruit,

1 glass milk.

SAMPLE LUNCH MENU #2

Egg-salad sandwich (2 slices bread, 1 tsp. butter or margarine, 1 hard cooked egg, chopped celery, dressing) peanut butter or lean meat may be used,

---

* Good Housekeeping Children's Center: Diet and exercise before and after the baby comes, New York, Hearst Corp., 1968.

† If you use tomato juice, use twice as much as you would orange or grapefruit juice, or include a citrus fruit at some other meal.

Raw carrot sticks, radishes, raw onions (if desired),

½ cup canned or frozen fruit or 1 serving fresh fruit,

2 graham crackers,

1 glass milk.

SAMPLE DINNER MENU #1

2 slices pot roast with gravy,

½ cup mashed potatoes,

½ cup buttered carrots or beans,

1 slice bread with butter or margarine,

Lettuce heart with french dressing or mixed green salad,

½ cup chocolate pudding (packaged or homemade) with 2 tblsp. light cream.

SAMPLE DINNER MENU #2

Broiled fish steak, shrimp, lobster or other lean meat,

½ cup scalloped potatoes,

½ baked acorn or ½ cup yellow squash,

Generous serving cole slaw,

1 slice bread with butter or margarine,

¾ cup fruited gelatin (homemade or package) with 1 tblsp. whipped cream.

Consult your doctor about the amount of tea and coffee he thinks you may have.

BEDTIME PATTERN

1 glass milk, warm or cold.

If the dinner hour is late, one may prefer to drink this glass of milk in the afternoon.

Other Information on Nutrition. When consultation with a nutritionist is advisable and one is not available on the clinic or hospital staff, one may be found in the area through the local public health department or a home economist's office. Publications and visual aids, charts, etc., may be secured from city, county and state health departments. The U. S. Government Printing Office is another invaluable source of publications. Certain professional organizations offer additional resources: Food and Nutrition Board, National Research Council, Council on Foods and Nutrition, American Medical Association, American Home Economics Association, American Public Health Association, etc. The above associations serve to illustrate only a few of the resources that the nurse and the physician have to assist their patients in planning for adequate nutrition.

Weight Control

An aspect of health closely associated with nutrition is weight control; this topic will be considered briefly before the other facets of counseling are outlined. During pregnancy a gain of 20 to 25 pounds is desirable and usually in keeping with good health. Given that the mother is of an average weight in her prepregnant state, a gain of about 20 pounds will generally result in an infant weighing from 6 to 8 pounds. Amniotic and other body fluids will account for about 2 to 3 pounds and the placenta from 1 to 1½ pounds; therefore, an increase in total pounds beyond the above amount for the average weight woman is undesirable for a number of reasons. First, they represent unnecessary poundage for the muscles of the legs and the back to carry about, and this suddenly imposed strain is a common cause of backache, pain in the legs and also easy fatigability. Second, certain serious complications of pregnancy, pre-eclampsia and eclampsia (see p. 449), are less common in patients whose weight increment is moderate. Third, excessive weight gain in pregnancy is likely to be a permanent acquisition, especially with successive pregnancies; thus, if the mother is interested in retaining her figure and health, she should be interested also in limiting weight gain at this time.

In the case of patients who are underweight and/or undernourished prior to becoming pregnant, the emphasis will be on providing balanced nutrition as well as a more generous caloric intake; thus, more than the usual 20 pounds may be permitted. With many of these patients, effort can be directed to teaching them economical ways of selecting and preparing foodstuffs since they are often poverty bound. However, with others, it is less a matter of economics than of knowledge and/or faulty eating habits; here the emphasis can be on instruction regarding the nutritional value of various foods together with mutual planning and reinforcement of appropriate choices by the nurse.

In general, obstetricians are emphasizing the importance of weight control in pregnancy and in particular they do so for the woman who is overweight in the prepregnant state. In these instances a gain of as little as 10 to 15 pounds is allowed. Some research has indicated that the obese patient can in fact lose weight during pregnancy with no adverse effects to herself or her infant. Infants of these mothers who lose weight are of normal birth weight and maturity and thrive just as infants of mothers who gain during pregnancy do.

In general then, if the patient's weight gain after the 3rd month is of the order of 3 pounds a month, it may be regarded as satisfactory; but if it exceeds 4 pounds a month, steps are usually taken to control it. Here a nurse can be of the utmost help in advising expectant mothers about certain simple steps that may be taken, particularly in regard to the curtailment of certain nonessential foods.

Some of the **specific suggestions** which may be made are as follows:

1. The patient can be acquainted with the amazing fattening potentialities of certain common *nonessential* foods—foods which, in many people's minds, scarcely deserve that term at all, because most of them are likely to be regarded as mere snacks without perceptible effects on total caloric intake. Actually, these little extras taken between meals or at bedtime constitute one of the most common causes for excessive weight gain in pregnancy and at other times. Even a glass of ginger ale or Coca-Cola averages 100 calories. A chocolate bar approximates more than 300 calories. A single cocktail or highball has 200 calories. A doughnut (without icing) plus a cup of cocoa yields 400 calories, and the average malted milk served at soda fountains contains some 500 calories. Pie àla mode approximates 600 calories. When it is recalled that 2,100 to 2,300 calories per day generally is recognized as a satisfactory (and generous) allowance for pregnancy, it is plain that these "little snacks" loom tremendously large in relation to the total caloric allotment. They simply must be eliminated if the patient is gaining excessively. If she is hungry between meals, she may take the glass of milk scheduled for dinner, omitting it from her evening meal. Raw vegetables and fruit also are helpful in assuaging hunger pangs.

2. The patient should be reminded that the way in which a food is prepared may affect its caloric or fattening value almost as much as the nature of the food itself. Failure to heed this fact has resulted in many women gaining weight on diets which should cause them, theoretically at least, to lose. Perhaps the simplest way to show how the preparation of a food affects its caloric value is to be found in fried foods. Although the caloric content of a poached or boiled egg is about 80 calories and is so calculated in dietary lists, once that egg is fried, its caloric value jumps to around 120 calories because of the fat absorbed by the egg in cooking. A level tablespoon of fat, let it be emphasized, yields approximately 120 calories. In regard to soups and desserts, it is common knowledge that those made with milk are of much less caloric content than those made with cream, and that those made with skimmed milk are still lower. When flour or cheese in addition to cream is used, as in escalloped or au gratin dishes, the calories soar to unbelievable heights; in general, for this group of foods, the smoother and the more delicious the taste, the higher is the caloric value.

The intrinsic caloric value of foods of the same type varies widely. Fruits show considerable variation according to their degree of sweetness. For instance, canned fruit can be very high in calories because of the sugar in the syrup. Therefore, the mother can be reminded to use fresh fruits regularly, and if for some important reason canned fruit must be served, the unsweetened varieties or those packed in light syrup are the only ones that should be taken. It might be added that these varieties are more economical than those packed in the rich heavy syrups. Likewise, meats vary greatly in their caloric contents; lean meats being low and those with much fat in their substance being high. As an example of the latter, an average serving of linked country sausage may exceed 600 calories. To summarize this aspect of weight control in pregnancy, the patient should be reminded that fried foods invariably possess a high caloric content and must be curtailed or eliminated altogether; that milk, preferably skimmed milk, should be substituted for cream in preparing soups and desserts; and that lean meat rather than fatty meat must be chosen, and fresh fruit rather than canned.

3. The next suggestion to make to the patient is to substitute skimmed milk for the whole milk included in the recommendation about diet in pregnancy. This reduces the caloric content of the diet by about 300 calories—no small sum. Fat-free or skimmed milk contains the same nutrients as whole milk, except for fat and vitamins A and D, but fortified fat-free milk contains much greater amounts of these two vitamins than does whole milk. However, be sure that the patient is taking this quart of milk every day. It provides more proteins, minerals and vitamins for less calories (and money) than any other food; and skimmed milk contains, of course, as much protein and minerals (including calcium) as does whole milk.

4. The next suggestion is an easy one to carry out, namely, to substitute saccharin for sugar, not only in coffee or tea but also for cereals, fruits

and cooking. Improvements in the manufacturing of this product have resulted in both liquid and solid forms, and most, if not all, of the former "bitter" and excessively "sweet" taste has been eliminated. Saccharin now can be used in cooking, and no difference in taste can be detected when it is used according to directions. In recent months there has been some controversy about the prolonged use of artificial sweeteners, especially the cyclamate variety. Some authorities are concerned about the utilization and excretion of these products. Therefore, it is wise that the doctor be consulted before recommending these sweeteners to determine his preference for his patient.

5. The salt ordinarily added to foods in the kitchen should be reduced drastically or eliminated altogether for the reasons mentioned previously (see p. 142). It is wise to counsel the mother-to-be to add no salt to the food at the table and in the kitchen to add a little less than she would like. In addition, she should be reminded to read carefully all labels on the foodstuffs that she buys to ascertain what salt and/or sodium content they have. For instance, frozen peas have salt added. Monosodium glutamate (MSG), a substance that brings out the natural flavor in foods, also should be avoided since it has a high sodium content.

As a substitute for flavor, herbs, spices, pepper, paprika, vinegar, lemon juice, vanilla or almond extract may be suggested. In the case of excessive weight gain in pregnancy, it is quite possible that a still further reduction in salt, as recommended above, will reduce superfluous body water and cause a substantial weight loss. At first, this salt-poor diet may seem so bland and tasteless as to constitute something of a hardship; with skillful use of herbs and with motivation and perseverance on the part of the patient, an adjustment can be made. However, it must be remembered that any modification of the meals has an impact on the family as well as the patient. They may need help in understanding and accepting the restrictions. If they cannot, then the patient is put in the position of having to prepare 6 meals a day instead of 3. This can be aggravating, to say the least, if not downright impossible; and certainly it will have implications for her own acceptance of the restrictions and her later follow-through. Thus, in these cases it is especially important to explore with the mother and the family their understanding, feelings and attitudes toward these new alterations rather than merely to issue dictums.

6. If the above recommendations do not serve to curtail weight gain, the patient should eliminate all rich desserts. Fresh fruits can be substituted, sweetened, if necessary, with saccharin.

7. It may be necessary to remind the patient to take servings of average size and only one serving.

Because of the importance of the subject, the nurse must understand that it will not suffice simply to tell the patients to reduce their food consumption or to eat less fattening foods. Directions, to be effective, must be specific as well as rather comprehensive and should be reviewed with the patients in an empathic and understanding way. Above all, it should be emphasized that no curtailment is to be made in food essentials—doubly essential in pregnancy—such as milk, green and yellow leafy vegetables, proteins, minerals and vitamins.

If the suggestions listed above, together with the other counseling mentioned, are not effective, the case is a special one, and the patient may require more meticulous medical supervision and/or the help of a nutritionist. The nurse is in the best position to keep the physician apprised of the dietary situation, and her follow-through is essential for proper referral.

GENERAL HYGIENE

The remainder of the counseling that the physician and nurse will want to give the mother falls under the heading of general hygiene. Pregnancy ought to be a normal, happy, healthy experience for a woman. During the months preceding labor, the physician and the nurse will advise her about her mode of life. She will be encouraged to continue her usual habits with very little change, unless, of course, it is found that she has been leading an existence not conducive to healthy living.

Rest, Relaxation and Sleep

Because rest and sleep are so essential to health, it is well to emphasize this detail in the nurse's teaching during the antepartal period. Pregnant women become tired more readily; therefore, the prevention of fatigue must be stressed very emphatically. The body is made up of various types of cells, each type with a specific function. Depletion of nerve-cell energy results in fatigue, and fatigue causes certain reactions in the body that are injurious. For all body processes, such as digestion, metabolism, working, playing and studying, nerve-cell energy is utilized. Nature has made provision for some reduction in normal energy without injury to health. Beyond this limit the symptoms of fatigue are evidenced in irritability, apprehension, a tendency to worry and restlessness. These symptoms are sometimes very subtle and misleading, but, in contrast, human beings are very conscious of tired muscles. It is more important to avoid fatigue than to have to recover from overfatigue. The pregnant woman should rest to prevent this fatigue. Rest and sleep replenish the cell energy. As Dr. Jastrow says of this code of rest and sleep, they "must be shaped according to the individual's nervous disposition, habits of life, age, and circumstances."

If patients cannot sleep, they can attempt to rest. Rest is the ability to relax. Patients often need to learn how to relax. There is no code so variable, so necessarily adapted to the individual, as that of rest and sleep. The final test is whether the day's work is done with zest and energy to spare. The expectant mother ought to get as much sleep as she feels she needs. Some people need more than others. In addition to a good night's sleep, it is advisable that the mother take a nap or at least rest for a half hour every morning and afternoon. If this is not possible, then shorter rest periods, preferably taken lying down (several times a day) are beneficial.

The nurse must recognize that all mothers are not able to follow the recommended rest periods to the letter. The woman who works throughout her pregnancy, the mother of several preschool children, all need special attention with respect to planning for adequate rest. Rigid recommendations are to be avoided, and the nurse can search with the mother for minutes in her busy day that can be utilized for rest; again, counseling the family may be necessary to maximize the mother's free moments. Although the nurse strives for flexibility, she also needs to emphasize the necessity of this aspect of general hygiene. It can be explained that rest means not only to lie down and perhaps to sleep, but also to lie down or to sit comfortably—to rest the body, the mind, the abdominal muscles, the legs and the back, and to stretch out whenever possible, and so make it easier for the heart to pump the blood to the extremities. During the last months of pregnancy a small pillow used for support of the abdomen, while the patient lies on her side, does much to relieve the discomfort common during this period and adds materially to the degree of rest that the patient gets in a given time.

Suggest to the patient that, instead of standing, she sit whenever possible, even while doing her housework. Sitting to rest for other brief periods during the course of the day can be beneficial if the feet and the legs are elevated.

Often the so-called minor discomforts of pregnancy can be overcome by rest. Rest and the right-angle position (see Fig. 8-11) are advised for swelling, edema and varicosities of the lower extremities. Rest and Sims's position (see Fig. 8-14) are advised for varicosities of the vulva and the rectum. Even for the more serious abnormalities, the simple aids included in "diet and rest" may help measurably until more specific orders from the obstetrician can be obtained. In such instances the nurse must be aware of the mother's interpretation of "rest," and, if indicated, she can provide the necessary guidance to help the mother to understand and to plan for it.

Exercise

Outdoor exercise during pregnancy is usually very beneficial, because it affords diversion in the sunshine and fresh air. However, for each patient the obstetrician usually decides whether the customary exercise should be increased or diminished. There are differences in the amount of exercise for the early and late periods of pregnancy. When pregnancy is advanced, exercise may be limited in comparison with the amount advised previously. Exercise usually means diversion, and, of course, this phase is most important. Exercise also steadies the nerves, quiets the mind, promotes sleep and stimulates the appetite, all of which are valuable aids to the pregnant mother.

Walking in the fresh air is quite generally preferred to every other form of exercise during pregnancy, because it stimulates the muscular activity of the entire body, strengthens some of the muscles used during labor and is available to all women. Exercise of any kind should not be fatiguing; to secure the most beneficial results, it should be combined with fresh air and sunlight, as well as periods of rest.

The woman who does her own housework needs little or no planned exercise from the physical viewpoint. However, she does need fresh air, sunshine and diversion. It is far better for the patient to be occupied than to sit idly, but standing for long periods of time should be avoided. Lifting heavy objects, moving furniture, reaching to hang curtains, any activity which might involve sudden jolts, sudden changes in balance which might result in a fall or the likelihood of physical trauma should be avoided. The more strenuous sports (i.e., horseback riding, skiing, hikes involving long climbs, rough water swimming) are subjects to be discussed with the obstetrician for his opinion and guidance. The pregnant woman who is accustomed to participating in certain sports and finds this participation an enjoyable form of recreation usually will be permitted to continue in moderation and at a mild pace, if it proves harmless.

Employment

The same attitude of moderation can be maintained whether for work or play. Ideally, no work or play should be continued to the extent of even moderate fatigue; however, it is not realistic to expect the mother to willingly discontinue her job because it is tiring, especially if it is essential to the family sustenance. If her employment is influencing her health adversely, then the matter needs conscientious exploration by the health team to see what realistic adjustments can be made. A referral to a social worker may be indicated, to better ascertain the economic situation of the family and/or the resources in the community that might be helpful. Different job opportunities can be discussed, and the patient's skills, satisfactions and preparation can be considered.

In general, jobs requiring moderate manual labor should be avoided if they must be continued over long hours, if they require delicate balance, or constant standing, or constant working on night shifts. Actually, the woman who has a "desk job" in an office often does less strenuous work than the average homemaker who does not go out to work. Nevertheless, positions which require the worker to sit constantly can be extremely tiring. Adequate rest periods should be provided for all pregnant women employed in such positions.

In some countries the time of discontinuing routine jobs has been regulated by law, and the limits, although arbitrary, are generally from 6 to 8 weeks prior to the expected date of confinement.

Many women are employed in industry, and the problem of pregnancy for the working mother in this type of employment is a most important one. To safeguard the interests of expectant mothers so engaged, the following Standards for Maternity Care and Employment of Mothers in Industry have been recommended by the Children's Bureau of the United States.

1. Facilities for adequate prenatal medical care should be readily available for all employed pregnant women; and arrangements should be made by those responsible for providing prenatal care, so that every woman would have access to such care. Local health departments should make available to industrial plants the services of prenatal clinics; and the personnel management or physicians and nurses within the plant should make available to employees information about the importance of such services and where they can be obtained.

2. Pregnant women should not be employed on a shift including the hours between 12 midnight and 6 A.M. Pregnant women should not be employed more than 8 hours a day nor more than 48 hours per week, and it is desirable that their hours of work be limited to not more than 40 hours per week.

3. Every woman, especially a pregnant woman, should have at least two 10-minute rest periods during her work shift, for which adequate facilities for resting and an opportunity for securing nourishing food should be provided.

4. It is not considered desirable for pregnant women to be employed in the following types of occupation, and they should, if possible, be transferred to lighter and more sedentary work:

a. Occupations that involve heavy lifting or other heavy work.

b. Occupations involving continuous standing and moving about.

5. Pregnant women should not be employed in the following types of work during any period of pregnancy, but should be transferred to less hazardous types of work.

a. Occupations that require a good sense of bodily balance, such as work performed on scaffolds or stepladders and occupations in which the accident risk is characterized by accidents causing severe injury, such as operation of punch presses, power-driven woodworking machines, or other machines having a point-of-operation hazard.

b. Occupations involving exposure to toxic substances considered to be extrahazardous during pregnancy, such as:

Aniline
Benzol and toluol
Carbon disulfide
Carbon monoxide
Chlorinated hydrocarbons
Lead and its compounds
Mercury and its compounds
Nitrobenzol and other nitro compounds of benzol and its homologs

Phosphorus
Radioactive substances and x-rays
Turpentine

Other toxic substances that exert an injurious effect upon the blood-forming organs, the liver, or the kidneys.

Because these substances may exert a harmful influence upon the course of pregnancy, may lead to its premature termination, or may injure the fetus, the maintenance of air concentrations within the so-called "maximum permissible limits" of State codes, is not, in itself, sufficient assurance of a safe working condition for the pregnant woman. Pregnant women should be transferred from workrooms in which any of these substances are used or produced in any significant quantity.

6. A minimum of 6 weeks' leave *before* delivery should be granted, on presentation of a medical certificate of the expected date of confinement.

7. At any time during pregnancy a woman should be granted a reasonable amount of additional leave on presentation of a certificate from the attending physician to the effect that complications of pregnancy have made continuing employment prejudicial to her health or to the health of the child.

To safeguard the mother's health she should be granted sufficient time off after delivery to return to normal and to regain her strength. The infant needs her care, especially during the first year of life. If it is essential that she return to work, the following recommendations are made:

a. All women should be granted an extension of at least 2 months' leave of absence after delivery.

b. Should complications of delivery or of the postpartum period develop, a woman should be granted a reasonable amount of additional leave beyond 2 months following delivery, on presentation of a certificate to this effect from the attending physician.

Diversion

Recreation is as necessary during pregnancy as it is at any other time in life. The patient is preparing for one of the most important role changes that she will undergo during life, and concomitant with any such change is the production of anxiety. It is to be expected that a certain amount of concern about the impending labor will be present; the additional responsibility of having a helpless new baby in the household, plus caring for and integrating him into the family unit, is also anxiety-provoking. The parents will have occasion to wonder whether they are equal to the enormous responsibility of rearing children, and whether or not they will be "good" parents. Therefore, activities which are diverting, healthful and relax-help the patient and the family to keep things in their proper perspective. Hence, it is beneficial to discuss with the mother some types of recreation that are most relaxing and pleasing for her and her family. Family group activities still can be enjoyed, even though the mother's energy and dexterity may be somewhat curtailed.

Consideration and understanding on the part of the husband, the family, the doctor and the nurse can do much to relieve any uncertainties or concerns that the mother may have. When the husband, in particular, understands more about the processes involved in the pregnancy (see Suggested Reading), his helpfulness can be increased. If a "blue" day comes, the husband can make it his particular responsibility to provide a means of counteracting it. On a home visit the nurse might discuss with the family ways in which they might help to diminish the strain in this period. This may necessitate changes in attitudes, understanding and habits; certainly it will mean increased tolerance and forbearance on the part of those involved; yet this is one of the ways that others can make their contribution to a successful pregnancy. The husband's gentleness and tenderness are especially appreciated and therapeutic at this time; the mother, for her part, can help him to maintain his supportive attitude and behavior by letting him know when his actions are helpful and gratifying. This type of "feedback" conveys her appreciation to the father and leads to reinforcement of his positive behavior. The husband is perhaps the key person in helping the mother to secure the kind of social relaxation that she enjoys most.

With respect to the activities themselves, books, radio, music, movies, sporting events, television, sewing clubs, church functions, visiting, drives, walks and entertaining friends are some of the means of providing relaxation and diversion. However, the mother should avoid crowds, chances of infection and all conditions likely to cause a sense of discomfort. Amusements, exercise, rest and recreation at proper intervals help to keep the pregnant mother well and happy in an environment conducive to her well-being and happy anticipation of the baby.

Traveling

This is perhaps a detail of antepartal care which most patients think very little about, unless they have a tendency to become nauseated or have had a previous miscarriage.

The restriction of travel to short trips had been a rule for maternity patients until World War II, when many women found it necessary to follow their husbands regardless of distance or modes of travel. It is now possible to apply the data compiled during that era to show that travel, almost regardless of distance and type of conveyance, has no deleterious effect on pregnancy.

Even though there is little restriction on travel from a medical point of view, this topic is to be discussed with the mother, so that any of her concerns or misinformation may come to light. The general information usually given to a pregnant woman is to avoid any trip which will cause undue fatigue, since she is prone to tire easily. For traveling long distances the railway or airplane is safer and provides greater comfort. If travel is by private automobile, rest periods of 10 to 15 minutes ought to be planned at least every 2 hours. This not only avoids fatigue, but the chance to stretch and walk about also benefits the general circulation.

Although traveling is not usually contraindicated during pregnancy, the expectant mother can consult her physician concerning the advisability of extensive travel at any time during the period of pregnancy.

Care of the Skin

The glands of skin may be more active during pregnancy, and there may be increased or decreased perspiration, resulting in irritation or dryness. Since the skin is one of the organs of elimination, bathing is obviously important, and baths should be taken daily, because they are stimulating, refreshing and relaxing. They not only act as a tonic and a general invigorator but also favor elimination through the skin as well. Elimination through the skin is thought to lessen the strain of elimination by the kidneys.

During pregnancy, showers or sponge baths may be taken at any time. The old idea that tub baths should be avoided because the wash water enters the vagina and thereby carries infection to the uterus now is believed to have little validity. There is only one objection to tub baths during the last trimester of pregnancy. At this period the heavy weight of the large abdomen may put pregnant women off balance and make climbing in and out of the tub awkward. Therefore, the likelihood of slipping or falling in the bathtub is increased. Chilling the body should be avoided; thus, cold baths, sponges or showers should be avoided if they produce this sensation.

Care of the Breasts

Special care of the breasts during pregnancy is one of the important preparations for breast feeding. During the antepartal period the breasts often have a feeling of fullness and weight and in fact do become larger, heavier and more pendulous. A well-fitted supporting brassière which holds the breasts up and in may relieve these discomforts. It may also help to prevent the subsequent tissue sagging so often noticeable after pregnancy due to the increased weight of the breasts during pregnancy and lactation.

There may be sufficient secretion of colostrum from the nipples to necessitate wearing a pad to protect the clothing. The daily care of the nipples and the reason for it, as well as the actual procedure, should be explained to the patient. Early in pregnancy the breasts begin to secrete, and this secretion often oozes out on the surface of the nipple and in drying forms fine imperceptible crusts. If these crusts are allowed to remain, the

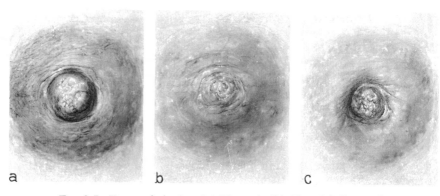

FIG. 8-7. Types of nipples. (a) Normal. (b) Flat. (c) Inverted.

skin underneath becomes tender; if left until the baby arrives and nurses, this tender skin area is likely to crack. With this condition there is always a possibility of infection. Nipples that are kept clean and dry do not have a tendency to become sore or cracked.

The breasts should be bathed daily; this may be done at the beginning of the bath, the shower or the sponge. The patient ought to use a clean washcloth and warm water. Some studies have demonstrated that the use of soap, alcohol and other such materials during the antepartal period and puerperium tends to be detrimental to the integrity of the nipple tissue, since they remove the protective skin oils and leave the nipple more prone to damage (see Suggested Reading). Therefore, the patient should discuss the use of these with the doctor. She should begin cleansing each breast by washing the nipple thoroughly with a circular motion, making sure that any dried material has been removed, then gradually continue working away from the nipple in this fashion until the entire breast is washed. Rinse the breast in this manner and dry with a clean towel. Rubbing the nipples with a rough towel during the last trimester of pregnancy may be helpful in attempting to toughen them. The physician may advise the use of Masse nipple cream, or some similar hydrous lanolin preparation, to prepare the nipples for nursing. This can be applied after the breasts are bathed. First, place a small quantity of cream on the thumb and the first finger, then grasp the nipple gently between the thumb and this finger and, with a kind of rolling motion, work the cream into the tiny creases found on the surface of the nipple. The position of the thumb and finger should be gradually shifted around the circumference of the nipple until a complete circuit has been made. This procedure should be limited to about 30 seconds on each breast.

A nipple which is flat or even slightly inverted in early pregnancy (Fig. 8-7) very probably will become protractile by delivery. If the nipples are inverted, some physicians prefer to start special care in the 5th or the 6th month of pregnancy or earlier. Dr. J. B. Hoffman[1] has suggested a treatment which has proved to be helpful. With the thumbs placed close to the inverted nipple, press firmly into the breast tissue and gradually push the thumbs away from the areola. The strokes should follow an imaginary cross drawn on the breast

(see Fig. 8-8) and be done 4 or 5 times in succession on awakening each morning. The nipple will assume an erect, projected position and then can be grasped as a unit and gently teased out a bit further. This is done daily, so that the nipples may be made more prominent for the baby to grasp. In extreme cases in which the nipples are badly inverted, the obstetrician will give instructions concerning the care needed.

Clothing

During pregnancy the clothes should be given the same or perhaps even a little more attention than at other times. The young mother who feels that she is dressed attractively and is well-groomed

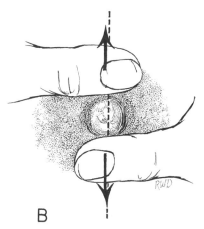

Fig. 8-8. A suggested treatment for inverted nipples. The thumbs are placed close to the inverted nipple, pressed firmly into the breast tissue, then gradually pushed away from the areola. The strokes should be directed horizontally (A) and vertically (B) and be done 4 or 5 times in succession.

---

[1] Hoffman, J. B.: A suggested treatment for inverted nipples. Am. J. Obstet. Gynec. 66:346, 1953.

will reflect this in her manner. Her clothing should be practical, attractive and nonconstricting. Most women are able to dress in the manner to which they are accustomed in the nonpregnant state until the enlargement of the abdomen becomes apparent. Maternity specialty shops and department stores have made maternity fashions available, which has settled the problem of suitable clothing during pregnancy. Today designers and stylists are giving consideration to the pregnant mother's clothing, so that she may dress attractively and feel self-confident about her appearance. The clothes are designed so that they are comfortable and "hang from the shoulders" to avoid any constriction; they are made in a variety of materials. The expectant mother can dress according to the climate and the temperature for her comfort.

Abdominal Support. Women who have been unaccustomed to wearing a girdle will scarcely feel the need of abdominal support, especially during the early months of pregnancy. Later, however, a properly fitted maternity girdle often gives the needed support to keep the mother from becoming fatigued. The natural softening of the pelvic joints which accompanies pregnancy and

Fig. 8-9. Maternity brassière for use during and after the nursing period. Special construction allows for sanitary gauze over the nipples and convenient opening for nursing. (Maiden Form Brassière Co., New York)

the increasing weight of the abdomen may encourage a change in posture to such a degree that severe backache results.

If the mother's abdomen is large, or if previous pregnancies have caused her abdomen to become lax or pendulous, a properly made and well-fitting maternity girdle will give support and comfort. The purpose of the garment is support, not constriction of the abdomen.

Breast Support. It is advisable that every pregnant woman wear a brassière that is well-fitted to support the breasts in a normal uplift position. Proper support of the breasts is conducive to good posture and thus helps to prevent backache (Fig. 8-9).

The selection of a brassière is determined by individual fitting and influenced by the size of the breasts and the need for support. It is important to see that the cup is large enough, and that the underarm is built high enough to cover all the breast tissue. Wide shoulder straps will afford more comfort for the woman who has large and pendulous breasts. The size of the brassière is, again, a matter to be determined according to the individual being fitted, but in most instances this is about two sizes larger than that usually worn. The mother who is planning to breastfeed will find it practical to purchase nursing brassières which can be worn during the latter months of pregnancy as well as during the postpartal period for as long as she is nursing her baby.

Garters. "Round garters" or any tight bands (rolled stockings, elastic tops on stockings) that encircle the leg tend to aggravate varicose veins and edema of the lower extremities and should be discarded in favor of suspender garters or some form of stocking supporters attached to an abdominal support. It will be remembered that arteries have muscular tissue in their walls, whereas veins have little or none, so that arteries are able to resist pressure. The external veins lie close to the surface, but the arteries are embedded deeper in the tissues. Hence, any constriction of any extremity affects the veins far more than the arteries. Blood which apparently meets no obstruction whatever in its flow down the extremity through an artery may on its return through the vein find at the point of constriction sufficient closure of the vessel to "dam it back" and so stretch the vein wall that a varicosity is formed. There is already a marked tendency toward this condition, because the enlarged and constantly enlarging uterus tends to impede the return circulation from the lower extremities by compression of the great abdominal vessels, and round garters definitely tend to aggravate the condition. Garters that encircle the leg never should be worn, even by growing children, for the tendency to varicosities always is present; and when once formed, they never entirely disappear and later may lead to great discomfort.

Shoes. A comfortable, well-fitting shoe is essential for the expectant mother. The postural changes which occur as the mother's abdomen enlarges may be aggravated by wearing high-heeled shoes, with resulting backache and fatigue. It is advisable that low-heeled shoes be worn during working hours and for busy daytime activities. For evening or more fashionable afternoon attire, a 2-inch heel is permissible if the patient does not develop backache from the increased lordosis induced by the heels, and if she can maintain adequate balance. However, the ingenious and attractive newer styles have taken much of the embarrassment out of wearing lower heels.

The nurse will want to remember that the height of the heel is but one consideration here, and that the support which the shoe gives the foot adds materially to the mother's comfort. Many of the flat-heeled and ballet-type shoes give little or no support to the feet and thus may be the cause of fatigue and aching legs and backs. A simple method to check the support of a shoe is to place the shoe flat on the floor, and then press the thumb down on the inner sole against the shank (the part that would come under the arch of the foot). If the shoe gives under this pressure, it indicates that it will give weak support to the foot.

Care of the Teeth

Good dental care is necessary, because the teeth are important in relation to adequate mastication of food. This care need be little different during pregnancy from what is considered to be good, general mouth hygiene in any person who is not pregnant. The teeth should be brushed carefully on arising, after each meal and before retiring at night. An alkaline mouthwash may be used, if desired. It is advisable for the expectant mother to visit her dentist at the very beginning of pregnancy and to follow his recommendations (Fig. 8-10). However, if he advises any extensive dental work to be done, the patient will want to consult her obstetrician.

The old saying, "For every child a tooth," based on a belief that the fetus takes calcium from the mother's teeth, has no real scientific basis. It should be carefully explained to the

FIG. 8-10. Dental care as part of obstetric health service. Because of the importance of good dental care, some hospitals have dental clinic facilities available as part of antepartal supervision. (School of Dentistry, Case Western Reserve University, Cleveland)

mother that an adequate diet during pregnancy will supply the baby with lime salts and other necessities in sufficient amounts to build his bones and teeth. Therefore, this old adage need not be true if proper attention is given to the care of the teeth and nutrition during pregnancy.

Bowel Habits

The pregnant woman who heretofore has adhered to regular habits of elimination usually experiences little or no change in the daily routine. Those who have a tendency toward constipation become noticeably more irregular during pregnancy due to (1) decreased physical exertion, (2) relaxation of the bowel in association with the relaxation of smooth-muscle systems all over the body, and (3) pressure of the enlarging uterus. Particularly during the latter part of pregnancy, the presenting part of the fetus exerts pressure on the lower bowel.

Personal habits of intelligent daily hygiene are the best resource that the expectant mother has to prevent constipation. The alleviation of this problem in modern society may be attributed to education, more reasonable bowel habits and greater latitude in physical exercise. During pregnancy the mother should pay close attention to bowel habits, drink sufficient quantities of fluid, eat fruits and other foods which add roughage to the diet and get reasonable amounts of daily exercise.

If these simple measures are not effective, the physician should be consulted about the problem. Harsh laxatives and enemas should be avoided unless the physician orders them specifically. He probably will prescribe some mild bulk-producing laxative and/or stool softener. If the mother has been taking a non-absorbable oil preparation, such as mineral oil, she should be advised to take the medication at bedtime, since it has the ability to dissolve and to excrete the oil-soluble vitamins if taken at mealtime, thus depriving her of the vitamins so necessary for good nutrition.

Constipation is conducive to the development of hemorrhoids and may be associated with the incidence of pyelitis. Aside from the discomfort associated with the passage of hard fecal material, this may injure the rectal mucosa and cause bleeding.

Douches

Vaginal douching, for so long considered by some women to be a requisite of feminine hygiene, should be kept at a reasonable minimum during pregnancy. If it is indicated because of excessive vaginal secretion or monilial or trichomonad infection, the physician will prescribe the kind of douche and the frequency with which it is to be taken. In the absence of excessive secretions or infection you might reassure the patient that a washcloth and soap and water are quite adequate for general cleanliness, with emphasis on washing anteriorly first, and the rectal area last. The use of the moist towelettes that are sold in foil packages is not contraindicated. The deodorant sprays are not contraindicated, but they can only be superficially effective because they do not reach the internal labial area. During pregnancy, the sebaceous glands in the genital area are quite active and there is a characteristic odor that some women find quite unpleasant. They will welcome any suggestions that you might volunteer for general cleanliness. They will find that the genital area is a little more sensitive to heat and cold and pressure during pregnancy, but reassure them that

there is nothing they can harm with the use of the above methods.

Specific instructions about douching are to be given, and the doctor usually gives this responsibility to the nurse. This instruction can be very time-consuming and, if she has permission, in either the clinic or private office situation she might consider writing out and having copies of instructions for douching that would agree with the philosophy of the office or clinic situation in which she is working. Women who avoid douching or douche infrequently have usually been instructed to do this in the bathtub, which is very awkward and time-consuming. Your instructions should also be clear enough for the patient who has never douched and knows nothing about it, and perhaps has never heard the word or seen it in print.

Your instructions should include the following points, making sure that the language and the vocabulary is understandable to the group of patients with whom you are working:

1. It is a four-minute procedure (after the initial few times).
2. It can be done while sitting on the toilet.
3. Use a gravity bag (never a hand bulb syringe).
4. During pregnancy the douche tip should not be inserted more than three inches.
5. The frequency and the solution are prescribed by the doctor.
6. The douche bag may be placed (hung or held) no higher than 2 feet above the level of the vagina.
7. The douche tip should be held at about the 3-inch length and inserted in the vagina, and the labial tissue in that area should be held around the douche tip with the same hand.
8. Allow the solution to run in until there is a slight feeling of fullness, then expel it (the douche bag will hold enough solution to do this four or five times).
9. The bag and the tube should be rinsed and hung to dry with a towel underneath.
10. The solution, for comfort, should only be barely warm to the hand. Holding the labial tissue around the douche tip allows the water to flow in without flowing out immediately, and this, along with rapid expelling, enables the solution to get into the folds of the wall of the vagina. In the non-pregnant woman there is no contraindication to inserting the entire douche tip or as much of it as the vagina will accommodate.

If douching is made a simple procedure, more women will use it both as a voluntary hygienic measure and, more important, as frequently as the doctor requests it for medicinal reasons. There is no need to get undressed and get into a bathtub (which many patients do not have) and spend a half an hour with a procedure that requires only 4 or 5 minutes.

Marital Relations

From the standpoint of both the physician and the nurse, the area of marital relations, because of its intimate nature, becomes one of the most difficult in which to give appropriate guidance. Many patients are reluctant to discuss the area of sex in general, especially when the patient-doctor-nurse relationship is new; and yet they are disturbed because of the changes which may be taking place in their feelings and emotions, with consequent influences on their marital relationship. Because of this reluctance, nurses (and doctors) often avoid exploring with the patient the possibility of any existing problem, and the counseling then consists mostly of prohibitions regarding the time and the frequency of intercourse. However, when there is a need, most patients will discuss the subject with a little help, especially when the doctor or the nurse conveys the idea that these are "expected" changes, and that there is nothing "shameful" or unique about them. Some patients prefer to speak only to the doctor regarding this matter, but some patients turn to the nurse at this time, because she is a woman and likely to experience similar feelings and concerns at some time or another. Since she may be utilized as a resource person, the nurse can prepare herself as she would for any other counseling activity. She should know about the anatomic, the physiologic and the psychological aspects involved; she can ascertain the physician's wishes regarding any general restrictions and limitations of the marital relationship during pregnancy, as well as any wishes involving the patient's relationship in particular. She should be aware that her approach here is extremely important and requires adroit use of communication skills, especially with respect to listening, reflecting and gentle probing. Finally, she can examine her own feelings and attitudes regarding sex, femininity, pregnancy and motherhood so that she can understand better and empathize with the patient's predicament.

Early pregnancy has an almost unpredictable effect on the sexual desire of the wife. Some women feel a sense of pleasant release from pregnancy fears, which enhances their desire; others find their ardor distinctly curbed. If this is a gross change from what is usual, concern may be generated in both wife and husband, especially if sexual activity is refused, and misunderstandings ensue. Sudden unexplained aversion to the husband also may occur, which is quite traumatic for both husband and wife. Fortunately, these idiosyncrasies are temporary, and desire and responsiveness soon return. It is important that the couple become aware of this fact before misunderstanding and hurt lead to the establishment of unhealthy and negative patterns of interaction. It is especially gratifying for the husband to realize that these apparent caprices of his wife's are only a temporary accompaniment of the new condition of pregnancy and do not signify any real change in her basic attitude or love for him. Some obstetricians advise that during the first trimester intercourse be avoided during the time of the regular menstrual periods because of the possible danger of abortion. If the patient has had previous abortions, coitus probably will be restricted until about 2 weeks after the third missed menstrual period. This restriction may prove to be burdensome especially for the husband, and since sexual excitement cannot be resolved in the usual way, it is wise to caution the couple to avoid arousing too much sexual interest. Usually the wish to have a happy, healthy pregnancy and a baby helps the parents to accept the restriction. In fact, there is rarely an indication to interdict intercourse or sex play during early pregnancy.

Abdominal protuberance does not in most cases interfere in any way with sexual activity until about the 5th month. At this time pressure on the abdomen may create discomfort or impede breathing. Positioning in this case becomes important. The side position for intercourse, placing pillows under the wife's hips and increased flexion of her thighs if she assumes the supine position enhance comfort for a time. By the 7th and the 8th months desire again may diminish, and most women find that they cannot participate very well in coitus in any position. The couple can be encouraged to experiment with positions that allow the wife to play a more passive role. Thus the husband can be satisfied and not feel deprived, and the wife can feel secure in the thought that she can still contribute to his gratification and happiness without exhausting herself in the process.

Some physicians advise abstinence from intercourse during the last weeks before term; others find no objection to intercourse through late pregnancy. Again, the same counseling as for any other period of restriction during the pregnancy is applicable here. Since relations should not be resumed until the doctor can determine that all has returned to normal, many couples feel a genuine deprivation. Recognition and acknowledgment of their sacrifice is one of the most effective ways of reinforcing positive behavior and helping to ease this final limitation on the marital relationship.

Smoking

The Surgeon General's report as well as other studies have indicated that cigarette smoking is a health hazard of sufficient importance in this country to warrant remedial action. Lung cancer and heart disease have been linked significantly with cigarette smoking. With respect to pregnancy, several studies have found a relationship between smoking and a lower birth rate, higher rates of prematurity and higher neonatal mortality. The mechanism is somewhat obscure, but it is thought that the nicotine in the cigarettes causes peripheral vasoconstriction, with subsequent changes in the heart rate, the blood pressure and the cardiac output that appear to have a detrimental effect on the development and the health of the fetus. Carbon monoxide also is found in higher concentrations in smokers, with a consequent decrease of oxygen; this apparently also affects the fetus.

The subject of smoking should be discussed thoroughly with the physician, and his recommendations followed. Several "smoking clinics" have been developed around the country, and books and articles have been published on the topic of "how to stop smoking." No one claims to have a sure answer. A combination of motivation, education in the destructive effects of smoking for both mother and infant and support seem to be the basic ingredients. The health team certainly can supply the last two and help the patient to achieve the first.

MINOR DISCOMFORTS

The so-called minor discomforts of pregnancy are the common complaints experienced by most expectant mothers, to some degree, in the course of a normal pregnancy. However, all mothers do not experience all of them, and, indeed, some mothers pass through the entire antepartal period without any of these discomforts. They are not serious in themselves, but their presence detracts from the mother's feeling of comfort and well-

being. In many instances they can be avoided by preventive measures, or entirely overcome by common sense in daily living, once they do occur.

Frequent Urination

One of the first signs the young woman may notice to make her suspect she might be pregnant is the frequent desire to empty her bladder. This is caused by the pressure of the growing uterus against the bladder and will subside about the 2nd or the 3rd month, when the uterus expands upward into the abdominal cavity. Later, during the last weeks of pregnancy the symptoms will reoccur (see p. 120).

Nausea

Nausea and vomiting of mild degree, the so-called "morning sickness," constitute the most common disorder of the first trimester of pregnancy. For many years it has been thought that this condition has an emotional basis. In all life's encounters, there are probably few experiences which are so anxiety provoking as the realization by a woman that she is pregnant. At first there is the anxious uncertainty before she can be sure of the diagnosis. Then, there are numerous adjustments that have to be made and responsibilities that may seem to be overwhelming. Emotionally, the implications of pregnancy extend far back into her childhood, long before she met her husband. It is understandable that women who cannot adjust themselves to all these new circumstances could have problems. However, the whole cause of nausea and vomiting should not be attributed to the neurotic factor. Symptoms may be caused by physiologic changes of normal gestation, such as slowing of peristalsis or changes in hormonal balance.

Symptoms usually appear about the end of the 4th or 6th week and last until about the 12th week. Nausea occurs in about 50 per cent of all pregnancies; of these, about one third experience some vomiting. Usually, it occurs in the morning only, but a small percentage of patients may have nausea and vomiting throughout the entire day.

The typical picture of morning sickness starts with the patient's experiencing a feeling of nausea on arising in the morning. The mother is unable to retain her breakfast, but by noon she has completely recovered and has no further episodes until the next morning. This does not always occur in the morning but may happen in the afternoon or in the evening. In a small percentage of patients the nausea and the vomiting may persist throughout the day and even be worse in the afternoon. With the majority of patients this problem lasts from 1 to 3 weeks and then suddenly ceases. There may be a slight loss of body weight but no other signs or symptoms.

Treatment. Often this condition can be controlled, and frequently it may be greatly relieved. Various "before breakfast" remedies often are used. If a half hour before rising the patient takes a dry piece of toast or a cracker, relief may be obtained. In some instances sips of hot water (plain or with lemon juice), hot tea, clear coffee or hot milk have been tried, with successful results. However, the dry carbohydrate foods seem to be more effective. After taking any one of these "before breakfast" remedies, the patient remains in bed for about a half hour; then she gets up and dresses slowly (meanwhile sitting as much of the time as possible). After this she is usually ready for her breakfast.

Greasy foods, and those known to disagree with the patient, should be avoided in the diet. Other suggested remedies include eating an increased amount of carbohydrate foods during this period of disturbance or eating simple and light food 5 or 6 times a day instead of the 3 regular full meals. Unsweetened popcorn during the morning is sometimes advised. The patient may be helped by drinking sweet lemonade, about half of a lemon to a pint of water sweetened with milk sugar. Usually, after vomiting, the patient is quite thirsty, and it is not difficult for her to drink lemonade. Small amounts of ginger ale or Coca-Cola also are often helpful.

Nausea and vomiting, if once established, are difficult to overcome; and so it is especially desirable to prevent the first attack, or at least to control this condition as soon as possible after it develops. It must be remembered that if the patient is unable to retain most of her food, her system is being depleted when daily health should be maintained. Pregnancies may differ, and what may help one person may not benefit another. The trial-and-error method often is necessary to obtain results. If persistent vomiting develops, as it does with a small number of these patients, the condition is no longer considered to be a minor discomfort but then may develop into a serious complication. (See Chap. 19, Complications of Pregnancy.)

Heartburn

This is a neuromuscular phenomenon which may occur any time throughout gestation. As a result of the diminished gastric motility which normally accompanies pregnancy, reverse peristaltic waves cause regurgitation of the stomach contents into the esophagus. It is this irritation of the esophageal mucosa which causes heartburn. It may be described as a burning discomfort diffusely localized behind the lower part of the sternum, often radiating upward along the course of the esophagus. Although referred to as heartburn, it really has nothing to do with the heart. Often it is associated with other gastrointestinal symptoms, of which acid regurgitation, belching, nausea and epigastric pressure are most troublesome. Nervous tension and emotional disturbances may be a precipitating cause. Worry, fatigue and improper diet may contribute to its intensity.

Very little fat should be included in the diet. Although fatty foods are especially aggravating in this disturbance, strangely enough, the taking of some form of fat, such as a pat of butter or a tablespoon of cream, a short time before meals acts as a preventive, because fat inhibits the secretion of acid in the stomach. However, this will not help if the heartburn is already present.

Home remedies are not to be used to relieve this condition. The physician usually will prescribe some alkaline preparation, because it gives the best results. However, *sodium bicarbonate is not to be used,* because the sodium ion tends to promote water retention. It is important to make sure that the patient undertstands this point. Equally effective medications are aluminum compounds, such as aluminum hydroxide gel, or this medication in tablet form with magnesium trisilicate.

Flatulence

This is a somewhat common and very disagreeable discomfort. Usually it is due to undesirable bacterial action in the intestines, which results in the formation of gas. Eating only small amounts of food which are well masticated may prevent this feeling of distress after eating. Regular daily elimination is of prime importance, as is the avoidance of foods that form gas. Such foods as beans, parsnips, corn, sweet desserts, fried foods, cake and candy ought to be avoided. If these measures fail to relieve the condition, the physician should be consulted.

Constipation

This is not unusual during pregnancy. It is due largely to impaired peristaltic motion of the intestine caused by pressure from the gravid uterus.

The patient should understand the importance of good bowel habits (see General Hygiene, p. 157), the influence of drinking adequate fluids and the appropriate diet in avoiding or alleviating this problem. Proper elimination cannot be emphasized too much, and daily regularity of habit aids in preventing constipation. In mild cases of constipation a diet of fruits, vegetables, dark breads and coarse foods, with several glasses of water daily, may relieve the condition.

Enemas, laxatives or cathartics are not to be used unless prescribed by the physician. Some obstetricians advise milk of magnesia or cascara for their patients. Cascara is easier to take in the pill form, but it seems to be less effective; when the fluid extract is given, the size of the dose and the frequency of its administration must be determined according to the individual patient's reactions. When the proper dosage has been determined, this drug is generally very satisfactory. The salines are usually reserved for the cases in which they are distinctly indicated, such as certain types of toxemia.

Simple measures, combined with a largely farinaceous diet, are ordinarily all that is necessary, and the obstetrician should be consulted before even these are used.

Backache

Most pregnant women experience some degree of backache. As pregnancy advances, the woman's posture changes to compensate for the weight of the growing uterus. The shoulders are thrown back as the enlarging abdomen protrudes, and, in order to maintain the body balance, the inward curve of the spine is exaggerated. The relaxation of the sacro-iliac joints, in addition to the postural change, causes varying degrees of backache following excessive strain, fatigue, bending or lifting. The mother can be advised early in pregnancy how to prevent such strain through measures such as good posture and body mechanics in everyday living and avoidance of fatigue. Appropriate shoes worn during periods of activity and a supporting girdle may be helpful (see Clothing, in General Hygiene).

A woman who has a pendulous abdomen, with a weak abdominal wall which allows the uterus to fall forward, will experience severe back pain, in addition to a "drawing sensation" in the abdomen and general discomfort in walking or standing. The physician will prescribe measures to be taken here or for any persistent complaint.

Dyspnea

Difficult breathing or shortness of breath occasionally results from pressure on the diaphragm by the enlarged uterus and may be sufficient in the last weeks of pregnancy to interfere considerably with the patient's sleep and general comfort. Usually it is not a serious condition, but unfortunately it cannot be wholly relieved until after "lightening" (p. 110) (the settling of the fetus into the pelvic cavity with relief of the upper abdominal pressure) or after the birth of the baby, when it will disappear spontaneously. It is most troublesome when the patient attempts to lie down, so that her comfort may be greatly enhanced by propping her well up in bed with pillows. In this semisitting posture she at least will sleep better and longer than with her head low. It is well for the nurse to demonstrate how these pillows may be arranged comfortably so that the patient's back is well supported.

In patients with known heart disease, shortness of breath, especially of rather sudden onset, may be a sign of oncoming heart failure and should be reported at once to the physician.

Varicose Veins

Varicose veins or varices may occur in the lower extremities and, at times, extend up as high as the external genitals or even into the pelvis itself. A varicosity is an enlargement in the diameter of a vein due to a thinning and stretching of its walls. Such distended areas may occur at short intervals along the course of the blood vessel; they give it a knotted appearance. Varicosities generally are associated with hereditary tendencies and are enhanced by advancing age, pregnancy and activities which require prolonged standing. During pregnancy the pressure in the pelvis due to the enlarged uterus, which presses on the great abdominal veins, interferes with the return of the

Fig. 8-11. Right-angle position for swelling, edema and varicosities of legs.

blood from the lower limbs. Added to this, any debilitated condition of the patient favors the formation of varicosities in the veins because of the general flabbiness and lack of tone in the tissues.

Naturally, the greater the pressure in the abdomen, the greater will be the tendency to varicose veins of the legs and the vulva. Therefore, any occupation which keeps a patient constantly on her feet, particularly in the latter part of pregnancy, causes an increase in abdominal pressure and so acts as an exciting factor.

Symptoms. The first symptom of the development of varices is a dull, aching pain in the legs due to distention of the deep vessels, and inspection will show a fine purple network of superficial veins covering the skin in a lacelike pattern. Later,

the true varicosities appear, usually first under the bend of the knee, in a tangled mass of bluish or purplish veins, often as large as a lead pencil. As the condition advances, the varicosities extend up and down the leg along the course of the vessels, and in severe cases they may affect the veins of the labia majora, the vagina and the uterus.

The treatment consists first and chiefly in the prompt abandonment, at the beginning of pregnancy, of round garters and all other articles of clothing that can cause pressure at any part of the body. If varicosities develop in spite of this precaution, the patient can be taught to take the right-angle position, that is, to lie on the bed with her legs extended straight into the air at right

Fig. 8-12. (*Top*) The method of applying the Ace bandage for varicosities or edema of the legs, which are sometimes treated by the application of Ace rubber-elastic bandage (Becton, Dickinson and Company) and Elastoplast bandage (Duke Laboratories).

Fig. 8-13 (*Bottom*) The Elastoplast bandage is applied firmly, adjusting the stretch to produce the amount of compression desired, each turn overlapping to avoid gaps.

angles to her body, her buttocks and heels resting against the wall (Fig. 8-11). At first this position is taken for 2 to 5 minutes several times a day, and that will soon demonstrate what can be accomplished. For some patients this position is very uncomfortable at first; but if it is explained, and the discomfort is therefore anticipated, the patient is less likely to discontinue the exercise. Late in pregnancy this position may be too difficult to assume because of pressure against the diaphragm.

In order to give support to the weak-walled veins, either an elastic stocking or elastic bandage often is recommended. The initial cost of elastic stockings is somewhat more than that of bandages, but they are easier to put on, more effective, have a neater appearance and a longer usefulness than bandages. A regular nylon stocking put on over the elastic hose further improves the appearance. Many hosiery companies are manufacturing "support" hose which do not have the strength of the elastic stockings but are very effective in giving a moderate amount of support. This type of stocking is useful in cases in which the varicosities are very mild or may not even be apparent peripherally, but may be suspected because of the ache they produce. Many women who must be on their feet a great deal, and do not have the opportunity to rest frequently, wear these stockings during working hours as a "prophylactic" measure. The nurse can be very helpful in apprising mothers of the varieties of hose now available and which will meet the needs of individual patients.

If bandages are used, they should be applied spirally with firm, even pressure, beginning at the foot and continuing up the leg above the varicosities (Figs. 8-12, 13). The nurse can demonstrate the technic of wrapping to the mother and let the patient practice in her presence; this will ensure that the mother understands and is able to wrap the bandages effectively. The patient also must be told that the stocking or the bandage should

FIG. 8-14. Sims's position for varicosities of vulva and rectum.

FIG. 8-15. The nurse helping the patient during a leg cramp, forcing the toes upward while making pressure on the knee to straighten the leg.

be removed at night for greater comfort and re-applied in the morning after the legs have been elevated so that the vessels will be less dilated. The longer stocking or bandage is more satisfactory when the varicosities are above the knee. Either the elastic stocking or bandage is washable; indeed, washing helps to maintain the original elasticity of these appliances. However, mild soap rather than detergent should be used.

Varicosities of the vulva may be relieved by placing a pillow under the buttocks and elevating the hips for frequent rest periods or by taking the elevated Sims's position for a few moments several times a day (Fig. 8-14). Patients suffering from this condition should not stand when they can sit, and they should not sit when they can lie down.

More important than the treatment of this condition is its prevention. Every pregnant woman should be advised to sit with her legs elevated whenever possible. And when the legs are elevated, care should be taken to see that there are no pressure points against the legs to interfere with the circulation, particularly in the popliteal space. Tight constricting garments, round garters, constipation, standing for long periods of time and an improper amount of rest, all tend to aggravate and excite this condition.

A varicose vein in the vagina may rupture during the antepartal or intrapartal period, but this is rare. The hemorrhage is venous and can be controlled readily by pressure. The foot of the bed can be markedly elevated.

Hemorrhoids

Hemorrhoids, varicosities of the veins about the lower end of the rectum and the anus, may develop during the antepartal period and may cause rectal bleeding. On the other hand, they may become thrombosed or protrude through the anus. The little bumps and nodules seen in a mass of hemorrhoids are the distended portions of the affected vessels. Like varicosities in other areas, they are due to pressure interfering with return venous circulation and are aggravated by constipation. They often cause great distress to the pregnant patient and, due to pressure at the time of delivery, may cause great distress during the postpartal period.

The first step is the prevention and the treatment of constipation. The guidance that the nurse gives the mother in this respect cannot be stressed enough. In addition, when internal hemorrhoids protrude through the rectum, the mother can be instructed to replace them carefully by pushing them gently back into the rectum. Usually the patient can manage this quite well, after a thorough explanation and/or demonstration. She lubricates her finger with petrolatum or mineral oil to aid ease of insertion and to avoid trauma to the veins. If the patient wishes, a finger cot can be used to cover her finger. Also taking either the knee-chest position (Fig. 14-22) or elevating her buttocks (Fig. 8-14) on a pillow facilitates replacement through gravity.

The application of an icebag, or cold compresses wet with witch hazel or Epsom salts solution, gives great relief. The physician may order tannic acid in suppositories, or compresses of witch hazel and glycerin. If the hemorrhoids are aggravated the first few days after labor, the same medications usually give relief. Surgery is seldom resorted to during pregnancy.

Cramps

Cramps are painful spasmodic muscular contractions in the legs. They may occur at any time during the pregnancy, but more generally during the later months due to pressure of the enlarged uterus on the nerves supplying the lower extremities. Other causes have been attributed to fatigue, chilling, tense body posture and insufficient calcium in the diet. They are commonly noted after the use of diuretics. A quart of milk in the daily diet has been generally recommended to meet the calcium needs during pregnancy. However, the studies of Page and Page can leave no doubt that large quantities of milk or dicalcium phosphate predispose to muscular tetany and leg cramps as the result of the excessive amount of phosphorus absorbed from these products (see Suggested Reading). Some authorities suggest that small quantities of aluminum hydroxide gel be taken with the quart of milk as it removes some of the dietary phosphorus from the intestinal tract. Immediate relief may be obtained by forcing the toes upward and by making pressure on the knee to straighten the leg (Fig. 8-15). Elevating the feet and keeping the extremities warm are preventives. Cramps, while not a serious condition, are excruciatingly painful for the duration of the seizure. If the husband has been taught the procedure for immediate relief, much pain will be prevented.

Edema

Swelling of the lower extremities is very common during pregnancy and is sometimes very uncomfortable. It is especially prone to occur in hot weather. Often it may be relieved by a proper abdominal support or by resting frequently during the day. Elevating the feet or taking the right-angle position often gives relief (Fig. 8-11). If the swelling is persistent, the patient may have to stay in bed, but ordinarily this condition proves to be no more than a discomfort. However, edema is one of the symptoms of toxemia, and it must never be overlooked.

When edema of the lower extremities is observed, careful investigation should be made to see if other parts are affected—the hands or the face, etc. The condition should be reported to the physician at once.

Vaginal Discharge

In pregnancy there is increased vaginal secretion so that a moderately profuse discharge at this time usually has no particular significance. However, it is wise to instruct the patient to call any copious and/or yellow or greenish foul-smelling or irritating discharge to the attention of the physician. For instance, a profuse yellow discharge may be regarded as a possible evidence of gonorrhea (see Chapter 20), especially when it is accompanied by such urinary manifestations as burning and frequency. A smear may be taken, and the microscopic result will indicate whether or not definite treatment is necessary. If any discharge becomes irritating, the patient may be advised to bathe the vulva with a solution of sodium bicarbonate or boric acid. The application of K.Y. jelly after bathing often relieves the condition entirely. Instructing a patient to wear a perineal pad is sometimes all the advice that is needed. A douche never should be taken unless the obstetrician orders it.

A particularly stubborn form of leukorrhea in pregnancy is caused by the parasitic protozoan known as the *Trichomonas vaginalis*. It is characterized not only by a profuse frothy discharge (white or yellowish in color), but also by irritation and itching of the vulva and the vagina. The diagnosis is easily made by the physician by taking a small quantity of the fresh secretion and putting it under the microscope in a hanging-drop. Here the spindle-shaped organisms, somewhat larger than leukocytes, with whiplike processes attached, can be seen in active motion.

One form of treatment used in this condition is the vinegar douche (3 tablespoons of vinegar in 2 quarts of water), followed by the insertion of an appropriate vaginal suppository into the fornix of the vagina. It is imperative that the expectant mother be given specific instructions about douching in pregnancy (see Douches, p. 158, General Hygiene). The husband of the woman who has trichomonas often becomes infected with this organism also; hence it is important that the husband be examined so that appropriate treatment may be instituted for him. Otherwise the mother-to-be will only become reinfected.

Moniliasis, a yeast infection caused by the *Candida albicans,* is another common cause of profuse vaginal discharge. The organism is frequently present in the vaginal canal without producing symptoms, but during pregnancy the physical changes in the vagina produce conditions that foster its development. It is characterized by white patches on the vaginal mucosa and a thick cottage-cheeselike discharge which is extremely irritating, so that burning or pruritus is present. Even the external genitalia often become inflamed, and occasionally extensive edema is observed. Bleeding may accompany the other symptoms if the patches on the mucosa are removed in any way.

It is not necessary to treat patients in whom *Monilia* are found if signs and symptoms are not present. Specific fungicidal suppositories are used to treat this condition. Although this treatment is effective, the infection is stubborn and likely to recur and require repeated treatment during the pregnancy. The *pruritus,* or itching of the skin, may be relieved to a marked degree if proper hygienic measures are employed to keep the area free of the irritating material being deposited on the skin surface. The mother who has a monilial infection may transmit it to her infant during the process of delivery. *Thrush* develops when the organisms attack the mucous membrane of the mouth.

PREPARATIONS FOR THE BABY

Layette

The baby's layette and equipment are of real interest to all parents—in fact, they are interesting to the majority of people. The cost of the layette should be in keeping with the individual economic circumstances. The entire layette can be purchased ready-made or can be made at home quite inexpensively. Much or little may be spent in its preparation, but nurses who are teaching parents should know why certain types of clothes and equipment are preferable. In the selection of clothing the following points should be considered: comfort, ease in laundering, ease in putting on and taking off, and that it be very light in weight. The new baby's skin is easily irritated by wool. Any clothing which comes in contact with the infant's skin should be made of soft cotton material. Knitted materials have the advantage of ease in laundering and sufficient stretch quality to allow for more freedom in dressing the baby. Garments that open down the full length and fasten with ties or grippers are easier to put on. Ties or grippers are not only less difficult to fasten than buttons but also are more desirable from the standpoint of safety. The geographic location and climate will greatly influence the selection of the infant's

clothing. Size 1 shirts and gowns are recommended, since the infant grows rapidly in the first 6 months and quickly outgrows his garments. It is well to remember that his clothing should not inhibit his normal activities. The complete outfit of clothes that the baby wears need not weigh more than 12 to 16 ounces.

The mother can be advised to prepare a very simple layette. As she sees how fast her baby grows, and what he will need, the additional items can be secured. The complete layettes which can be purchased often contain unnecessary items and are often costly. Also, many articles may be received as baby gifts. Therefore, it is wise to choose only those things which are necessary for immediate use.

FIG. 8-16. Family group at home. Baby clothes which have been stored away are being made ready for the new baby.

Layette necessities include:

5 or 6 shirts
3 to 4 dozen diapers (if diaper service is not used)
4 to 6 receiving blankets (These are very versatile items and can be used in various ways. For instance, they can be rolled firmly and used to support the infant's back when he is on his side; in emergencies, they can be used as bathtowels, diaper pads, sheets)
3 to 6 nightgowns, kiminos, or sacques
6 cotton covered waterproof diaper pads (11" x 16")
2 waterproof protectors for under diaper pads

2 afghans or blankets } (if climate is cold)
1 bunting
2 to 4 soft towels (40" x 40")
2 to 4 soft washcloths

Nursery equipment should consist of:

basket, bassinet or crib
mattress (firm, flat and smooth)
mattress protector (waterproof)
sheets or pillowcases for mattress
chest or separate drawer

FIG. 8-17. Family group at home, getting the bassinet ready.

cotton crib blankets
bathtub
diaper pail
toilet tray—equipped
absorbent cotton—or cotton balls
baby soap (bland, white, unscented)
rustproof safety pins
soap dish
bath apron (for mother)
table, for bath or dressing
chair (for mother)

Additional suggestions for layette and equipment are:

sweaters	footstool
crib spreads	diaper bag (for traveling)
bibs	disposable diapers
clothes drier	nursery light
chest of drawers	carriage
nursery stand	

Some further suggestions in relation to the selection of specific items are as follows:

Shirts, Gowns, etc. The sleeves should have roomy armholes, such as the raglan-type sleeve. If the pullover-type garments are used, the neck openings should be so constructed that they are large enough to be put on easily from over the feet or the head.

Diapers. Of the several varieties of diapers available, bird's-eye or gauze diapers are the most popular. The selection of diapers should be considered from the standpoint of their comfort (soft and light in weight), absorbency and washing and drying qualities. The mother who plans to use the services of a commercial diaper service may either use the company's diapers or her own. Disposable diapers are also available, but they are generally more expensive than cloth diapers or a diaper service, in the long run.

Receiving Blankets. These should be made of cotton flannelette 1 yard square. This square is used to fold loosely about the baby. If properly secured, the baby may lie and kick and at the same time keep covered and warm. In the early weeks these squares take the brunt of the service and in this way save the finer covers from becoming soiled so quickly.

Afghans or Blankets. These should be of very lightweight cotton or wool material. The temperature and the weather will determine the amount of covering needed.

Sheets. Crib sheets are usually 45″ x 72″ and are available in muslin, percale and knitted cotton materials. The knit sheets are practical for bottom sheets and do not need to be ironed. Pillowcases are very usable for the carriage or the basket mattress. Receiving blankets may be used for top sheets.

Waterproof Sheeting. *Various* waterproof materials are suitable to protect the mattress and to be used under the pads. Even though the mattress may have a protective covering, it is necessary to have a waterproof cover large enough to cover the mattress completely—something that can be removed and washed. (Waterproof material is not to be dried in the sun.)

Waterproof Pants. These offer protection for special occasions. If the plastic variety is used, they should not be tight at the leg or the waist. For general use, a square of protective material such as Sanisheeting or a cotton quilted pad can be used under the baby next to the diaper.

Bath Apron. This is a protection for both mother and baby and may be made of plastic material covered with terry cloth.

Nursery Equipment

In choosing the equipment, again the individual circumstances should be taken into consideration. Expense, space and future plans all influence the selection. Most nurseries are planned for the satisfaction of the parents. Eventually the baby's room becomes the child's room; and if economy must be considered, furniture should be selected that will appeal to the child as he grows and develops.

The Baby's Room. Preferably, the baby should have his own room. If this is not feasible, a quiet airy place, out of drafts, may be selected.

Bed. The baby should have his own bed. This may be a basket, a bassinet or a crib. The trimming on the basket or the bassinet should be such that it can be removed easily and laundered. A bed may be improvised from a box or a bureau drawer, placed securely on a sturdy table or on chairs which are held together with rope. Many parents may have a carriage that may be used as a bed. However, after about the first 2 months, the baby will need a crib. The crib should be constructed so that the bars are close enough together to prevent the baby's head from being caught between them. If it is painted, a paint "safe for babies" should be used.

Mattress. The mattress should be firm (not hard) and flat. All mattresses, including the waterproof-covered, should be protected by a waterproof sheeting to prevent the mattress from becoming stained and from absorbing odors. The

Fig. 8-18. Improvised toilet tray for baby. A household tray or baking pan and miscellaneous jars may be utilized. Comb has fine teeth with smooth rounded edges. Soap dish contains mild, white, unscented soap. (A) Jar for clean absorbent cotton. (B) Jar for safety pins.

waterproof sheet is easily washed and dries quickly.

Netting. This will be needed for the carriage, the basket or the crib during the insect season. If a Kiddie-Koop is used, it is screened to protect the baby from insects and animals.

Bathtub. The plastic tub is safe and easy to keep clean.

Bathtub Table. The table on which the tub is placed for the baby's bath should be of convenient height (Fig. 14-19). A kitchen table, or other sturdy table without wheels, may be used for this purpose.

Mother's Chair. The chair also should be a convenient height and comfortable for the individual mother.

Diaper Pail. It should be large enough for at least the day's supply of soiled diapers. It may be used also for boiling the diapers.

Toilet Tray. This tray can be prepared and ready for use immediately after the delivery of the baby (Fig. 8-18).

PLANS FOR AFTER-CARE OF MOTHER AND BABY

It is always a relief to the mother and her husband when the plans for delivery and the arrangements for the period following have been completed. The parents should make some provision for the mother to be free from other responsibilities until she has regained, in part at least, her physical strength, and until lactation has been established.

The nurse should make an effort to include the father when discussing the details of the mother's care. Often it is only with his help that his wife gets the full care she needs, care that the doctor and the nurse wish her to have (see Chap. 10).

Return to Employment

The expectant mother who is employed may desire to know how early she may return to work after the baby is born. Following delivery, 6 weeks are needed for the obstetrician to determine whether or not the reproductive organs are returning to their approximate normal size and position. Accordingly, no commitments should be made until the baby is from 6 to 8 weeks old. At the time of the postpartal examination, the obstetrician will discuss with the patient her future plans. It always must be kept in mind that the mother-child relationship during the first 6 years of a child's life is most important, and in making these future plans with the mother, this fact must not be ignored because of interest in re-employment. There are, of course, certain unavoidable circumstances within some family units which leave the mother no alternative but to return to work. In such a situation, the mother may require guidance not only from her physician but also from the nurse and the medical social worker to help her plan for this.

SUGGESTED READING

Apgar, V.: Drugs in pregnancy. Am. J. Nurs. 65: 104-106, March, 1965.

Auerback, A. B.: Meeting the needs of new mothers. Children 11:223, November-December, 1964.

Auerback, A. B., and Collier, G. B.: How do nurses take to the "new ways" in leading parent groups? Nurs. Outlook 6:674-677, December, 1958.

Barnes, A. C.: The clinical approach to the prevention of congenital anomalies. Am. J. Obstet. Gynec. 90: Part II: 1242, December 1, 1964.

Barnes, R. H.: Overemphasis in nutrition. New York State J. Med. 60:3126-3128, October 1, 1960.

Bing, E.: Six Practical Lessons for an easier Childbirth. New York, Grosset and Dunlap, 1967.

Bolton, J. H.: Dietary protein in pregnancy, its importance. The Australian and New Zealand J. of Obstet. Gynaec. 8:20-21, February, 1968.

Brandl, E.: Cigarette smoking and pregnancy. Nurs. Sci. 3:71-76, February, 1965.

Brandt, M. B.: Nutrition in pregnancy. Clinical Obstet. Gynec. 6:604-618, September, 1963.

Brook, M.: The use of artificial sweeteners in food products. Roy. Soc. Health J. 89:140-142, May/June, 1969.

Brown, E. L.: Newer Dimensions of Patient Care. Part 3, New York, Russell Sage Foundation, 1964.

Bruce, S. J.: Do prenatal educational programs really prepare for parenthood? Hosp. Topics 43:104, November, 1965.

Bruser, M.: Sporting activities during pregnancy. Obstet. Gynec. 32:721, November, 1968.

Buxton, C. L.: A Study of Psychophysical Methods for Relief of Childbirth Pain. Philadelphia, W. B. Saunders, 1962.

Caplan, G.: Psychological aspects of maternity care. Am. J. Public Health 47:25-31, January, 1957.

———: The mental hygiene role of the nurse in maternal child care. Nurs. Outlook 2:14-19, January, 1954.

Cashman, Rose: Trends in parent education. Health News 38:4-13, July, 1961.

Chaben, I.: Awake and Aware: Participating in Childbirth Through Psychoprophylaxis. New York, Dell, 1966.

Chow, B. F., et al.: Maternal nutrition and metabolism of the offspring: studies in rats and man. Am. J. Public Health 58:668-677, April, 1968.

Dalzell, Irene: Evaluation of a prenatal teaching program. Nurs. Res. 14:160-163, Spring, 1965.

Dansforth, D. N.: Pregnancy and labor—from the vantage point of the physical therapist. Am. J. Phys. Med. 46:653-658, February, 1967.

Davis, M. E., and Rubin, R.: DeLee's Obstetrics for Nurses. Philadelphia, W. B. Saunders, 1966.

de Watteville, P. H.: The use of obstetric analgesia at the Maternity Hospital of Geneva. Am. J. Obstet. Gynec. 73:473-491, March, 1957.

Eastman, N. J.: Williams Obstetrics. ed. 13, New York, Appleton, 1966.

Eastman, N. J., and Jackson, E.: Weight relationships in pregnancy. Obstet. Gynec. Survey 28: 1003-1025, November, 1968.

Editors: Behind the cigarette curtain. Trans-Action 2:3-8, January-February, 1965.

———: Iron and folic acid in pregnancy. Drug Ther. Bull. 5:21-23, March 17, 1967.

———: Moving Iron to the mother. J.A.M.A. 205: 33 and 36, September, 1968.

———: Obstet. Gynec. Survey 19:743, October, 1964.

Eichenlaub, J. E.: The Marriage Act. New York, Lyle-Stuart, 1961.

Estey, G. P.: Word from a mother. Am. J. Nurs. 69:1453-1454, July, 1969.

Fijalkowski, W.: New ways of psychophysical preparation for childbirth. Am. J. Obstet. Gynec. 92: 1018-1022, August, 1965.

Frazer, A.: Health Aspects of Artificial Sweeteners. Roy. Soc. Health J. 89:133-136, May/June, 1969.

Gage, M. A.: Educational aspects of prenatal care. Med. Serv. J. Canada 23:527-531, April, 1967.

Goldman, J. A., and Schechter, A.: Effect of cigarette smoking on glucose tolerance in pregnant women. Israel J. Med. Sci. 3:561-564, August, 1967.

Good Housekeeping Children's Center: Diet and Exercise Before and After the Baby Comes. New York, Hearst Corp., 1965.

Goodrich, F. W., Jr.: Natural Childbirth. New York, Prentice-Hall, 1950.

Hammel, F.: Nurses in private practice as monitrices. Am. J. Nurs. 69:1446-1450, July, 1969.

Haselkorn, F. (ed.): Mothers-at-risk. Perspectives in Social Work, Vol. 1, 1966.

Hendricks, C. H., and Brenner, W. E.: Patterns of increasing uterine activity in late pregnancy and the development of uterine responsiveness to oxytocin. Am. J. Obstet. Gynec. 90:485-492, October 15, 1964.

Highley, B.: Antepartal nursing intervention. Nurs. Forum 2:62-68, 1963.

Hillsman, G. M.: Genetics and the nurse. Nurs. Outlook 14:34-9, January, 1966.

Hoff, F. E.: How any nurse can help. Am. J. Nurs. 69:1451-1453, July, 1969.

Hulka, J. F., and Schase, J. T.: Obstetrics in adolescents. Obstet. Gynec. 23:678-685, May, 1964.

Hurvitz, N., and Berko, R. P.: Group counseling in private obstetric practice. Obstet. Gynec. 16:724-729, December, 1960.

Iyenger, L.: Effects of dietary supplements late in pregnancy on the expectant mother and her newborn. Indian J. Med. Res. 55:85-89, January, 1967.

Jache, M. C.: Nursing goals in working with families under multiple stress. Nurs. Clin. of N. Am. 4:69-75, March, 1969.

Jacobson, H. N., et al.: Effect of weight reduction in obese pregnant women on pregnancy, labor, and delivery, and on the condition of the infant at birth. Am. J. Obstet. Gynec. 83:1609-1616, June 15, 1962.

Johnston, R. A., et al.: Is prenatal care beneficial or necessary? Southern Med. J. 57:399-402, April, 1964.

Jonat, L. V.: Continuing maternal health care. Med. Serv. J. Canada, 23:531-534, April, 1967.

Keller, N. S.: Care without coordination: a true story. Nurs. Forum 6:280-323, 1967.

LaFever, John: The Lamaze method of natural childbirth—view from the side of the table. Am. J. Nurs. 63:67-69, June, 1963.

Lamaze, F.: Painless Childbirth. London, Burke, 1958.

LeMat, A. F.: The public health nurse in maternity service. Nurs. Outlook 12:58-61, October, 1964.

Lesser, M. S., and Keane, V. R.: Nurse-Patient Relationships in a Hospital Maternity Service. St. Louis, C. V. Mosby, 1956.

Madore, C. E., and Deutsch, Y. B.: Talking with parents. Am. J. Nurs. 62:108-111, November, 1962.

Mann, V. R.: Food practices of the Mexican-American in Los Angeles County. Los Angeles County Health Dept., 1963.

Manning, M. L.: The psychodynamics of dietetics. Nurs. Outlook 13:57-59, April, 1965.

Middleton, E., and Hugger, V.: Patients and their obstetricians. Psychosomatics 4:142-149, May-June, 1963.

National Institute of Child Health and Human Development: Optimal Health Care for Mothers and Children: A National Priority. Bethesda, Md., National Institutes of Health, 1967.

Newton, M., and Newton, N.: The normal course and management of lactation. Clin. Obstet. Gynec. 5:44-63, March, 1962.

Newton, M. E., et al.: Nutritional aspects of nursing care. Nurs. Res. 16:46-49, Winter, 1967.

Nikloayev, A.: Psychoprophylactic preparation of pregnant women for childbirth and painless parturition in the Soviet Union. J. of the International Federation of Gynec. and Obstet. 2:3-15, January, 1964.

O'Lane, J. M.: Some fetal effects of maternal cigaret smoking. Obstet. Gynec. 22:181-184, August, 1963.

Page, E. W., and Page, E. P.: Leg cramps in pregnancy. Obstet. Gynec. 1:94, 1953.

Pascatto, R. D., and Mead, B. J.: The use of posthypnotic suggestion in obstetrics. Am. J. Clin. Hypn. 9:267-268, April, 1967.

Peterson, W. F., et al.: Smoking and prematurity. Obstet. Gynec. 26:775-779, December, 1965.

Pike, R. L., et al.: Juxtaglomerular degranulation and zona glomerulosa exhaustion in pregnant rats induced by low sodium intakes and reversed by sodium load. Am. J. Obstet. Gynec. 95:604-614, July 1, 1966.

Pion, R. P., et al.: Prenatal care, a group psychotherapeutic aproach. Calif. Med. 97:281-285, November, 1962.

Psychophysical Preparation for Childbearing: Guidelines for Teaching. ed. 2, New York, Maternity Center Assoc., 1965.

Read, G. D.: Childbirth Without Fear. ed. 2, New York, Harpers, 1953.

Recommended Dietary Allowances, rev. ed., Publication No. 1146, Washington, D.C., National Academy of Sciences, National Research Council, 1963.

Reeder, S. R., and Reeder, L. G.: Some correlates of prenatal care among low income wed and unwed women. Am. J. Obstet. Gynec. 90:1304-1314, December 15, 1964.

Reeder, S. R., and Deck, E.: Nurses' participation in a group psychotherapeutic approach to antepartal management. Nurs. Forum 2:82-93, 1963.

Richie, J.: Using an interpreter effectively. Nurs. Outlook 12:27-29, December, 1964.

Ringrose, C. A. D.: Autohypnosis as an adjunct in obstetrics. Med. Trial Tech. Quart. 13:22-27, December, 1966.

Rose, P. A.: The high risk mother-infant dyad—a challenge for nursing. Nurs. Forum, 6:94-102, 1967.

Rosengren, W. R.: Social instability and attitudes toward pregnancy as a social role. Social Probl. 9: 371-378, Spring, 1962.

Rossi, J. P.: High risk babies: determining the problem. Conn. Health Bull., p. 267, November, 1964.

Rubin, R.: Behavioral definitions in nursing therapy, conference on Maternal and Child Nursing. Columbus, Ohio, Ross Laboratories, 1964.

———: Food and feeding: a matrix of relationships. Nurs. Forum 6:195-205, 1967.

Runnerstrom, L.: Expectant parent education. Nurs. Sci. 3:57-68, February, 1965.

———: Food iron intake and hemoglobin levels in pregnancy. Nurs. Sci. 1:187-197, August-September, 1963.

———: Food iron intake and hemoglobin levels in uncomplicated pregnancy: implications for nursing. Convention Clinical Sessions No. 11, Am. Nurses Assoc., 1964.

Semmens, J. P.: Fourteen thousand teen-age pregnancies. Am. J. Nurs. 66:308-311, February, 1966.

Specter, G. J.: An evaluation of the effect of health education methods on prenatal clinical attendance. Int. J. Health Ed. 9:183-187, October-December, 1966.

Sturges, S. H.: Opportunities and challenges of the premarital exam. Fertil. Steril. 13:209-219, May-June, 1962.

Taylor, E. S.: Four crises in maternity care. Obstet. Gynec. Survey 24:253, March, 1969.

Thoms, H.: A consideration of childbirth programs. New Eng. J. Med. 255:860-861, October 25, 1956.

Tokuhata, G. K.: Smoking in relation to infertility and fetal loss. Arch. Environ. Health 17:353-359, September, 1968.

Ulin, P. R.: Exhilarating moment of birth. Am. J. Nurs. 63:60-67, June, 1963.

———: Changing techniques in psychoprophylactic preparation for childbirth. Am. J. Nurs. 68:2586-2591, December, 1968.

———: The Lamaze method of natural childbirth—the exhilarating moment of birth. Am. J. Nurs. 63:60-67, June, 1963.

Vellay, Pierre: Childbirth Without Pain. New York, Dutton, 1960.

Watts, W.: Social class, ethnic background and patient care. Nurs. Forum 6:155-162, 1967.

Whiteside, M. G., et al.: Iron, folic acid and vitamin B_{12} levels in normal pregnancy, and their influence on birth-weight and the duration of pregnancy. The Med. J. Aust. 1:338-342, March 2, 1968.

Wohl, M., and Goodhart, R.: Modern Nutrition in Health and Disease. ed. 3, Philadelphia, Lea & Febiger, 1964.

Wright, E.: New Childbirth. New York, Hart, 1966.

Yahia, C., and Ulin, P. R.: Preliminary experience with a psychophysical program of preparation for childbirth. Am. J. Obstet. Gynec. 93:942-949, December, 1965.

Young, E. W.: Prepared childbirth: its impact on nursing. Canad. Nurse 64:39-43, January, 1968.

Younoszai, M. K., and Haworth, J. C.: Cigarette smoking during pregnancy: the effect upon the hematocrit and acid-base balance of the newborn infant. The Canad. Med. Assoc. J. 99:197-200, August 3, 1968.

Leo G. Reeder, Ph.D.
Professor of Public Health and Sociology
School of Public Health,
University of California at Los Angeles

Social Factors in Maternal Care

9

The Social and Cultural Meaning of Pregnancy
General Social Factors and Reproductive Performance
Social Factors Influencing the Outcome of Pregnancy • Sociocultural Patterns in Antenatal Care

INTRODUCTION

The concern with social, cultural and psychological forces as they impinge upon pregnancy outcome, although not of recent origin, is particularly manifested in modern health care. Stimulated by the efforts and interests of Sir Dugald Baird and other leaders in maternal care, modern social science research methods have been used to study a variety of problems associated with maternal health. In this chapter a number of issues related to maternal care will be discussed; these include the social and cultural meaning of pregnancy, the role of such factors as socioeconomic status, physique, age and parity, smoking, employment, illegitimacy and teen-age pregnancy in influencing the outcome of pregnancy, special problems of poverty, and sick role behavior. Given the scope of these topics, it will not be possible to consider each of them in depth; rather this chapter presents a survey of our current state of knowledge concerning social factors in relationship to maternal health.

Americans are accustomed to thinking of their health status as being the best and highest in the world. But despite many decades of experience with the complexity of health programs, the health care of the American people still is far short of its potential. The American Public Health Association recently noted that "while standard measures of health compare favorably with those of other advanced nations, large segments of the population are deprived of adequate medical care

and wide discrepancies persist in the quality of available services."[1] In fact, many of the recommendations made by experts in the field of maternal and child care (e.g., (1) increase the number of prenatal and postnatal clinics, (2) bring the antenatal and post-partum clinics to the population served, (3) establish special clinics for patients with special complications of pregnancy, etc.) have been implemented in recent years through programs of the Office of Economic Opportunity and the Children's Bureau as well as through units of the Public Health Service. Pilot programs have been initiated in urban and rural areas to develop neighborhood health centers in low-income areas and to bring maternal and infant care programs (MIC) closer to the populations most in need of such services. The critical issue concerns relative success of these programs in terms of the use made of them by the intended patient services. Unfortunately, these programs have not always fulfilled the high expectations and purposes toward which they were originally directed; they were only partial answers to old and familiar problems of maternity care in the United States.

How do we explain differential patterns of antenatal care? Why are some women at greater risk than others for complications of pregnancy or problematic pregnancy outcomes? Part of the

---

[1] Policy statement of the Executive Board of the American Public Health Association Social Policy and Medical Care, August, 1969.

answer to these questions is undoubtedly related to the way in which pregnancy is defined in different societies and within societies. In some societies, pregnancy is typically regarded as a "normal" life process, through which most women at some time pass. In other societies, pregnancy may be regarded as a kind of illness that must be overcome as quickly as possible. The expectations and the prescriptions for behavior surrounding pregnancy in Western Society are relatively ill-defined and in some situations they do not exist. Consequently women are oftentimes uncertain when and how often they ought to visit the doctor, whether they can continue in employment, and what is expected of them in relation to significant others. Part of the answer is related to the life styles of population sub-cultures and part of the answer lies in factors related to social structure (i.e., social class).

THE SOCIAL AND CULTURAL MEANING OF PREGNANCY

Childbearing Motivations

In order for nurses to function appropriately, to use their talents more creatively than in the past, the nurse must have an understanding of the social and cultural meaning of pregnancy. In the past fifteen years a large number of studies have appeared concerned with factors influencing the number of children desired by and born to married couples. Most of these studies have focused on the *number* of children desired rather than on the attitudes held by women regarding *why* they want children. A brief consideration of some of the social and psychological aspects motivating childbearing will be discussed.

No biological event has greater significance for society than reproduction and its outcome. Reproduction is important in family dynamics and population dynamics, and in turn, their impact weighs heavily on individual and national welfare. Women begin their preparation for childbearing early in life. In a sense, they begin it at the time of their own conception.

Society is primarily organized for the families with children and the argument for having children is very persuasive. Couples without children are generally made to feel "out of place," especially if they have been married very long. Many studies have demonstrated that the values of having children are generally accepted by the vast majority of Americans (R. O. Blood and D. M. Wolfe, 1960). In one study it was found that less than

1 per cent of the couples intended to have no children; that is, almost all people desire to have children of their own. In this context it is understandable that all levels of society should be organized in favor of children. Clearly, parenthood, at least in Western Society, is a highly valued phenomenon. As Rossi has noted, the cultural pressure to become parents is great enough that a couple may plan to bear children in spite of a latent desire to the contrary. For the female, the pressure to become a mother may be the equivalent of the cultural insistence that the male assume a productive occupational role.

The availability of acceptable means for preventing conception permits a portion of childbearing today to be a consequence of motivated human action rather than a mere biological result of sexual behavior. Regardless of when pregnancies occur or the presence or absence of deliberation, the number of children a couple has and the time at which they have them are partially a function of the nature of the couple's childbearing motivations (Mark Flapan, 1969).

There is a widespread belief in the United States that a higher amount of childlessness is present for white couples as compared with non-white couples. Actually, the extent of childlessness is generally not well known although various estimates have been made and these range from 6 to 15 per cent. The explanation of childlessness is complicated by the fact that two types of childlessness must be considered, voluntary and involuntary. Usually the literature fails to differentiate between these two types of childlessness. *Voluntary* childlessness includes those couples who make a decision that they will not have children. The assumption is made that these couples have technological knowledge to implement their decision to remain childless. *Involuntary* childlessness may be a consequence of many different factors (e.g., psychological or biological incapabilities). Unfortunately, data are not available to treat the two types separately. Many people today feel that nonwhite couples have a very *low* rate of childlessness, while white couples have a much higher rate of childlessness. This is a popular stereotype based on various myths involving white-nonwhite differences. On the other hand, demographers and students of fertility have long been cognizant of the opposite differential. In a recent reanalysis of census data, Kunz and Brinkerhoff demonstrated that, contrary to popular expectation, there were 8.9 per cent more nonwhite wives who were childless (Philip R. Kunz and

Merlin B. Brinkeroff, 1969). Although further study is necessary to determine the physical, social, and social psychological reasons for these differences, we can, at least, dismiss the generalized cultural myth that non-whites have lower childlessness and begin to analyze some of the broad differences and develop further knowledge from these.

Clearly, the childbearing motivations of women are complex and often interrelated. There is, for example, the social expectation to bear children, previously mentioned. A childless woman may wish to emulate her friends or relatives who already have children, or she may be supported in her desire to postpone childbearing by the fact that her friends are also childless. Some women are confident of their femininity and look forward to childbearing as a further confirmation of their feminine identity. On the other hand, a woman may doubt her femininity and require childbearing as a demonstration of her adequacy as a woman. A woman may desire motherhood as a substitute identity for unachieved career aspirations; or motherhood may be derogated as commonplace in comparison with her identity as a person or as a career woman and she may postpone childbearing indefinitely. There are various psychological factors related to feelings with regard to childhood memories and identifications, anticipation of expected relationships with children, that may be involved in childbearing motivations.

Finally, the woman's relationship with her husband, his interest in having children and her appraisal of his potential for fatherhood may also affect childbearing motivations. It's possible that a woman may consider her home incomplete without children. The child may serve as a symbol of the unity of the marriage or perhaps as an expression of her love for her husband. On the other hand, a woman may be reluctant to bear a child by a husband whom she neither loves nor respects. The husband's lack of interest in having children may undermine her childbearing motivations or support her own childbearing reluctance. These and many other factors are involved in the complex problem of childbearing motivations.

Transition to Parenthood: Problems of Adaption

The impact of the first-born child on each of the parents and on their marriage is a matter of concern to all in the field of maternity care. It is critical when counseling new parents to be alert to the problems that a new member of the family produces in the way of changes in attitudes and behavior. Although a number of "parenthood as a crisis" studies have been undertaken since the middle 1950s, little has been added to our basic understanding of the parenthood role. The major problem has been that most of the studies have been undertaken on samples that are small and nonrepresentative of the general population.

The research reported to date leaves no doubt that most parents find that the arrival of a child calls for major behavioral changes. The reports, however, are contradictory regarding the attitudes of new parents for these role changes. It would seem that future research needs to consider problems of sampling, to find standardized reliable and valid measuring instruments for determining gratifications and difficulties involved in the transition to parenthood and to determine a clear differentiation of the types of changes and adjustments required by parenthood and how these changes are perceived as affectively positive, neutral, or negative on the part of the parents (Arthur P. Jacoby, 1969 and Ann L. Clark, 1966).

GENERAL SOCIAL FACTORS AND REPRODUCTIVE PERFORMANCE

Socioeconomic and other social influences affect obstetric practice in at least two ways: "by their effect directly on the reproductive efficiency and habits of the mother herself and indirectly on the standard of obstetric care which is made available to her" (Sir Dugald Baird, 1965). The range and variety of possible social influences on childbirth or fetal health are very great, and this discussion can only be selective. Since socioeconomic status or social class has such a pervasive influence upon health and health care, it is well to describe briefly the usual procedure for measuring social class or socioeconomic status.

Social class, or socioeconomic status, is a complex concept referring to a theoretical formulation of relationships between subgroups in our society. It is a term frequently used by sociologists and epidemiologists in medical research as an effort to subdivide populations into a few descriptive categories which differ in a variety of social and economic characteristics, background, and behavior.

Membership in a specific social class or socioeconomic status group does not, per se, result in direct biological insult. Reference to socioeconomic status as a source of reproductive problems refers to behavior and conditions associated with a particular social class or socioeconomic status position and conditions which are linked to harmful physiological processes. For example, underlying early malnutrition or malnutrition during pregnancy may halt the growth of the fetus before it has reached the stage of viability. Thus, preventing perinatal deaths is very difficult or impossible. This is particularly true in the age group 15 to 19. It is difficult to prevent perinatal deaths in the 15 to 19 age group (which has the highest perinatal death rate together with the age group 35 plus) because such women tend to come from the lower socioeconomic group. They typically have the lowest standard of health and physique, the highest incidence of prenuptial conception and are the late-comers to the antenatal clinic.

Typically, in determining socioeconomic status, the usual procedure is to select as indicators of social differences one or several characteristics, each of which are closely related to: income, education, occupation, housing and place of residence, social values, and the general way of life of population subgroups. By far the most widely used indicator of socioeconomic status or social class is occupation. It is the best indicator of a person's income, education, standard of living, social values and a variety of other attributes. Thus, it has a practical property (ease of collection, accuracy, manageability) as well as social significance.

Not all social differences stem from occupational status. Dividing a population along one social dimension does not automatically provide categories which are socially meaningful in other respects. It can be demonstrated that such social variables as age, geographic region, height, parity, and socioeconomic status, each contribute independently to the total picture of social variation in pregnancy outcome. The same may be said of other more complex social influences.

Similarly, other social variables have limitations when studied out of context with other factors. For example, many studies have demonstrated, epidemiologically, that there is a relationship between customs, habits and general living conditions and a variety of medical disorders and health conditions. But such relationships are meaningful only in the sense that they indicate hypotheses for further study. They become meaningful to the clinician when it is possible to specify more clearly the nature of the linkage between these social background characteristics and biological consequences such as infant mortality and malnutrition.

SOCIAL FACTORS INFLUENCING THE OUTCOME OF PREGNANCY

It is not possible to speak of social influences independent of biological variables. There is a complex interplay between these social and biological factors. For example, the socioeconomic conditions which influence education, social values, opportunities and aspirations, also affect the material environment and nutritional experiences, which in turn influence intellectual functioning, growth patterns, etc. Thus, the social and cultural experiences and the physical environment tend to shape the physique and health of the individual, to influence emotional and intellectual growth and simultaneously develop certain sociocultural values and habits that influence behavior as an adult. The consequences of various social factors on biological variables are complex and often indirect. Nevertheless, a considerable amount of epidemiologic data exists on the interrelation of social and biological factors and pregnancy outcomes.

Perinatal and Infant Mortality

Perhaps the most traumatic and important of pregnancy outcomes concerns the viability of the fetus. The best available series of epidemiologic data are those for the experience in Great Britain. These data which have been systematically collected since 1911 indicated that there were socioeconomic differences in mortality, as between the social class groups (J. N. Morris and J. A. Heady, 1955). That is, mortality increased steadily with a decrease in socioeconomic status. For example, in the first month of life the death rates in the children of unskilled workers are approximately 50 per cent higher than those of professional workers. These differentials have persisted virtually unchanged since 1911, although the overall death rates in Great Britain have fallen dramatically and despite social and economic changes. The British data show that fetal loss, clinically defined, showed a social class gradient for each of eight separate cause groups distinguished with respect to stillbirths. The rate was higher for the lower social class groups than for the higher social class groups and this has been a consistent finding over the years. Data from other countries, although not as well documented, tend to confirm the evidence of a social class linkage to perinatal and infant mortality.

The geographic variations in perinatal and infant mortality are also worth observing. These geographic variations may be analyzed in terms of differences between countries, within regional areas of the same country, between urban and rural populations, and within residential sections of large metropolitan areas. There are voluminous data on the differences in national rates of infant mortality. The United States ranked 15th from the top in infant mortality rates in 1969. The mortality for nonwhites is double the overall national figure. Much less is known on complications of pregnancy, although such data that are available show that the Scandanavian countries regularly report low birth weights at 4 per cent and Britain and the United States at about 7 per cent for whites and 10 per cent for Negroes in the U.S. The so-called underdeveloped countries appear to have rates ranging from 18 to 35 per cent. It is not possible to make strict comparisons even with the so-called modern nations because of various factors that complicate the data (e.g., the underreporting of data such as early fetal deaths in the underdeveloped countries and the generally poor medical, environmental and other factors that make causal analysis rather impossible). A further complicating factor is that the differences within countries and between countries tend to change with regard to infant mortality at different stages of economic development. In general, however, there is an association between fetal loss and socioeconomic conditions.

The patterns of interaction between obstetrical variables and social class are very complex, and caution must be exercised in making inferences and interpretations. For example, one must not assume that for a specific complication the same social etiology applies at different times and places. The various components of social class tend to reflect the culture of the time and the place. Thus, one must be careful not to make misinterpretations of epidemiologic data.

As noted above, social class differentials in infant mortality have hardly changed in the modern nations although there have been great socioeconomic and medical changes over the past 50 years. One possible theory to explain these phenomena is that although great social and medical changes could be brought about rather quickly, the less changeable influences (e.g., customs, habits, utilization of available health facilities) would be much slower to change. Thus, it is argued that the better educated middle-classes might benefit the most from improved medical and socioenvironmental changes. This, in turn, would lead to wider class differences before there

would be any tendency toward equalization. The evidence with regard to public health campaigns in the field of early detection of cervical cancer lends weight to this argument (i.e., it is the middle class woman, who is at lower risk, who tends to obtain early and regular checkups for cervical cancer).

Illsley has postulated another type of explanation (1955). His study indicates that a process of upward social mobility of women from the lower socioeconomic groups to higher socioeconomic groups by marriage may be a factor in the results that are obtained on pregnancy outcome and social class. Illsley postulates a continuous process of social mobility which tends to concentrate healthy and taller women in the upper social groups and the least healthy and shorter in the lower social groups. This process would keep class mortality rates apart as long as there were differences in social equality. His study* showed that women from lower socioeconomic groups who married up the social ladder tended to be taller and of better physique than those who remained in the lower social classes at marriage. These women also gave birth to heavier babies and they had fewer perinatal deaths. On the other hand, women who were downwardly socially mobile at marriage tended to have high prematurity and perinatal death rates. Concurrently, if the size of the lower social class groups is decreasing, and if there is selective upward social mobility, this would tend to increase the concentration of less healthy mothers in these groups and would tend to counteract any movement toward improvement in their mortality rates.

Stature and physique are examples of biological factors that have a specific social composition and the significance of these biological categories is considered below together with other biological variables such as age and parity.

Physique and Maternal Health

In a series of pioneering studies, Baird demonstrated that women with poor physique had rates of caesarean section, prematurity, and perinatal death at least twice as high as those with very good health and physique. These studies showed a strong association between poor physique and short stature and both occurred more frequently in the lower socioeconomic status groups. It is well known that stature or adult height is strongly influenced by nutritional and socioenvironmental

---

* The study was conducted in Great Britain.

experiences from early childhood onward. More recent evidence tend to confirm these findings. In the United States, Kaltreider (1963) in a study of patients in Maryland found that short women had more pre-eclampsia, more caesarean sections, and higher prematurity and perinatal loss rates. These relationships of maternal height with various aspects of reproductive performance are well documented and accepted today. Clearly, the relationship between maternal stature and reproductive performance indicate the impact of certain health status characteristics in the lifetime of the patient prior to her pregnancy. It is important to recognize that height is not determined solely by genetic factors. The social correlates of height must also be considered. Thus, in Western Society short stature tends to be associated with lower levels of education, early marriage, prematurity, illegitimacy, high parity, low nutritional status, poor housing and lack of use of medical services.

These findings may be summarized as indicating that children reared in different societies, socioeconomic groups, cultural groups, and geographic areas, receive varying nutritional diets and live in physical environments that may influence development and growth. These experiences in childhood allow those groups in the more favored environment to attain their genetic potential of stature in contrast to the less favored, poorer groups with a resultant of better reproductive performance.

Age and Parity

Age and parity are two additional biological categories that have specific social significance. Perinatal mortality rises steadily with age in all pregnancies. Stillbirths are affected much more than the deaths that occur in the first week by increasing age. In discussing the interrelationships of age and parity it should be noted that there are substantial social class differences in the age at first pregnancy. As indicated above, primigravidae in the lower social classes are much younger than those in the upper social classes. It is generally recognized that reproductive efficiency of lactation is at its peak at about eighteen years of age in primigravidae and decreases afterwards. Thus, best results in a first pregnancy are obtained by tall women age eighteen or nineteen who have been reared in a good social environment. Unfortunately, primigravidae of eighteen or nineteen are not usually tall and healthy; those who are, tend to be over twenty-

five years of age, by which time reproductive efficiency is declining.

Smoking in Pregnancy and Pregnancy Outcome

Since the interesting paper by Campbell (1936), smoking in pregnancy has received spasmodic but increasing attention. A few workers have presented evidence to suggest that smoking may prevent a successful outcome to the pregnancy (Frazier, Davis, Goldsten, and Goldberg, 1961; Zabriskie, 1963; Butler, 1965; Russell, Taylor, and Maddison, 1966; Steele and Langworth, 1966). Most of these have not been able to show any relationship between smoking and pregnancy outcome. In 1957, Simpson reported a higher incidence of premature births (by weight) among smokers and since then an increasing number of workers have been able to show that when smokers and nonsmokers are compared, the smokers have the smaller babies (Russell, Taylor and Law, 1968). Despite the large number of studies that have demonstrated this relationship in recent years, a number of questions still remain to be answered. There is no longer any reasonable doubt that comparative studies of smokers and nonsmokers indicate that the former have smaller babies but there are differences of opinion as to the meaning of these results. Most workers subscribe to the view that the smaller babies born to smokers are smaller because of a direct effect of the smoking.

Recent evidence, based on a prospective study in England, has shown that fetal size and growth were related to the maternal smoking pattern and to various associated matters particularly maternal blood pressure (Russell, et. al., 1968). The result indicated that highly significant differences in maternal blood pressure and smoking were obtained. Their data showed that the percentage of unsuccessful pregnancy (abortion, stillbirth or neonatal death) was considerably higher for smokers than for nonsmokers, even when controlled on blood pressure. Smoking was also associated with the social class of the father, maternal age, and parity. Russell and his colleagues also examined the relationship of fetal weight and maternal smoking and found that the effect of smoking was clearly distinguishable as a separate effect. Thus, maternal smoking appears to be associated with lower fetal weight and this association seems to be independent of maternal age, parity, height, educational level, attitude to pregnancy or work in pregnancy, father's social class, partner's social class, and sex of the child or premature delivery.

Russell and his co-workers make the unequivocal statement that smoking per se, rather than associated factors, is implicated with the birth of smaller babies "without any reasonable shadow of doubt." Thus, the implications for prevention are clear. Counseling and health education directions for young women are clearly implied by the results of these studies.

Maternal Employment During Pregnancy

There are a number of reasons for interest in the proportion of women who are employed during their pregnancy. First is the medical aspect. A number of studies have indicated that the chance of a successful pregnancy is significantly lowered if the woman worked during her pregnancy. Some evidence indicates that women who were employed had a higher rate of prematurity than women who did only housework. Secondly, the proportion of women in the labor force has been increasing in recent years, and the increase has been particularly rapid for married women with children. Another reason is the effect that a woman's birth experience may have on the number and the spacing of her children.

Most of the studies on employment and pregnancy outcomes have been done in Great Britain. There is, according to these studies, an association between maternal employment, particularly heavy and prolonged manual work, and low birth weight. It should be noted that most of the British studies show that the duration of work in pregnancy is also associated with socioeconomic status, maternal height and age, prenuptial conception, and other sociomedical conditions.

In the United States one third of the women are employed outside the home at some time during pregnancy. This is particularly true for first mothers. Almost half of the wives who work are still employed during the third trimester of pregnancy. Of particular interest is the fact that employment rates during pregnancy increased as the woman's level of education increased according to the available data. Furthermore, employment rates also increased as family income increased.[2] Thus, in the United States, employment during pregnancy tends to be associated with the higher socioeconomic status women, who are, of course, at lower risk for problematic pregnancy outcomes.

Finally, there is no evidence that employment, per se, results in poor pregnancy outcomes.

Maternal Nutrition

Recent studies have shown that deficiencies in the diet of a pregnant woman can have profound effects on a number of pregnancy outcomes. For example, it has been shown that nutritional and genetic factors may interact during prenatal development, "with consequent irreversible results which endure for the lifetime of the individual. Specifically, the interaction of the trace element manganese in a specific gene has been studied. The most striking effect of maternal dietary deficiency of manganese during pregnancy is an irreversible congenital ataxia characterized by abnormal body-righting reflexes" (Lucille S. Hurley, 1969). Although Hurley's study was done with mice, it is worth noting its implications. Her research is an example of how a diet during pregnancy, high in manganese, can prevent what was previously thought to be a "predetermined" unchangeable congenital defect carried by an abnormal gene. The diet change did not change the genetic composition of the mice but it did overcome one of the biochemical effects of its inherited pallid gene. It is an example of how both heredity and environment are important in individual development. Hurley states:

> these studies of genetic-nutritional interactions during development may have significance for abnormal conditions in man . . . the studies of both manganese-deficient and *pallid* animals exemplify the notion that congenital abnormalities, even structural malformations, may exist at birth without becoming apparent until a later stage in the developmental life of the individual. That this relationship is of importance for human patients is seen by recent statistics which show higher incidences of congenital defects in the same group of children after one year than were seen at birth. One cannot help but wonder how many of the disorders that beset mankind may have developmental origins, possibly connected with nutritional factors in interaction with genes and *other* components of the environment.[3]

Deficiencies in the diet of pregnant women can have profound effects on the development of her baby's brain and this is one of the most important recent discoveries in the field of mental retardation. It is estimated that one-tenth of the children born today are seriously affected as a con-

[2] National Center for Health Statistics: Employment during pregnancy, legitimate live births, United States, 1963, Vital and Health Statistics, Series 22, Number 7, Washington, D.C.: US Department of Health, Education and Welfare, Public Health Service, September, 1968.

[3] Hurley, L. S.: Nutrients and genes: interactions and development, Nutr. Rev. 27:5, 1969.

sequence of malnutrition. Recent work at the National Institutes of Health suggest that there is a correlation between the level of the amino acids in the blood of a pregnant woman and the subsequent intelligence of her baby.

The effects of nutritional deficiencies on other outcomes of pregnancy are not so clear. Extremely low birth weights have been reported among poorly fed groups in Asia and Africa. The relationship between low birth weight and malnourished populations may be more complex than a simple nutritional explanation. Rather than dietary deficiency in pregnancy as the major factor, the small size of the baby may reflect long-term maternal under-nutrition dating back to the early childhood of the woman. Conceivably, malnutrition over many generations in the underdeveloped societies may have favored the emergence of genetically different kinds of women with lower dietary requirements. This, however, is highly speculative and needs much carefully designed research to confirm such a possibility.

Recent evidence on the geographic distribution of eclampsia has led Theobald to the "inescapable conclusion that the pregnancy toxemias were inextricably bound up with nutrition. Indeed, no adequate alternative explanation has been advanced" (G. W. Theobald, 1969). Eclampsia has largely been a condition associated with the very poor and particularly those in towns or urban places rather than rural places. However, this latter situation may be a result of differential diagnosis and the availability and the use of services in urban and rural areas among poverty level populations. As a matter of fact, epidemiological studies of the toxemias of pregnancy are problematical because of differential definition and diagnosis.

The effect of socioenvironmental influences was dramatically illustrated in the Second World War in Great Britain. During this period the mortality from the pregnancy toxemias fell dramatically (Fig. 9-1). The underlying reason for the drop in mortality resulting from this condition, in England and Wales, was that large numbers of women were evacuated from their homes in the cities into the country. The antenatal clinics were understaffed and improvisational. The major advantage brought about by this change of social environment was that the rationing system benefited expectant and nursing mothers, and children. For the first time, women of the lower socioeconomic groups were fed as well as other population groups and better than previously. Suffice

to say that eclampsia as a syndrome is most commonly seen in poor and badly-nourished populations and that there is some evidence that the incidence has been profoundly modified by environmental changes either situational or behavioral.

Undernutrition has been identified as one of the causes of low birth weight in infants born to poor urban mothers. In a study based on consecutive autopsies of stillborn and newborn infants, and which excluded fetal or maternal disorders that may have effected fetal growth, the study population was divided into poor and non-poor, living in the same area within New York City and of similar racial distribution. Both the poor and the non-poor constituted high-risk groups (Naeye, et al., 1969). These investigators found, upon examination of mean organ and body weights, that undernutrition appears responsible for the prenatal gross retardation in infants from poor families. Their findings were similar to what has been observed in both human beings and animals who have experienced chronic alimentary undernutrition, as well as what has been often observed in a variety of placental and uterine disorders in which the flow of nutrients to the growing fetus was restricted. Since these investigators excluded all multiple births and cases with a known uterine or placental disorder from their study, they concluded that maternal malnutrition during gestation contributed to the fetal undergrowth. Obviously, there is a complex interaction between undernutrition, poverty and other environmental or genetic factors.

FIG. 9-1. This figure shows the mortality rates per 100,000 live births for eclampsia, pre-eclampsia and nephritis. This dramatic fall occurred during the greatest war in history. (G. W. Theobald: The pregnancy toxemias seen in perspective. J. Reproductive Med. 3:79, August, 1969)

Clearly, malnutrition or undernutrition in pregnancy is associated with a complex of other socio-environmental factors, notably poverty. In the so-called underdeveloped areas of the world malnutrition may be *situational,* in the sense that there are nutrients lacking in the soils and in the environment. In addition, it may be *behavioral,* in the sense that individuals and groups may, by their beliefs and customs, maintain an undernourished diet. Similarly, in the well-developed nations, *situational* factors over many generations where there is interaction of social and biological factors, result in certain groups being at greater pathologic risk. These groups generally are in the lower socioeconomic status categories of the population. On a behavioral level, these groups are the ones who fail to maintain good antenatal care practices, including nutrition.

SOCIOCULTURAL PATTERNS IN ANTENATAL CARE

It is generally accepted that adequate medical care during pregnancy, particularly in the early stages of pregnancy, reduces the incidence of neonatal mortality, congenital malformations or other birth defects, maternal mortality, prematurity, etc. The relationship between low socioeconomic status and failure to receive adequate antenatal care, has been well documented. The data appear to be similar in the United States, Great Britain and in various other Western nations. Not only do the lower social class women typically comprise the highest proportion of those who have not received antenatal care, they are also the women, as a group, who contribute to the highest proportion of underutilizers of antenatal care (John B. McKinlay, 1970).

According to the latest sources of data for the United States, the average American woman made 11.5 visits for medical care during the year before her child was born. On the average, white mothers made 12.2 visits in a twelve month period and nonwhite mothers 7.7. Thus, the average white mother had 60 per cent more visits than the average nonwhite mother. This is undoubtedly related to other findings concerning the influence of socioeconomic status and antenatal care. According to these data, as family income in-

TABLE 9-1. CUMULATIVE PERCENT DISTRIBUTION OF MOTHERS[1] ACCORDING TO TIME OF FIRST VISIT, BY GEOGRAPHIC REGION AND COLOR: UNITED STATES, 1963 BIRTHS*

GEOGRAPHIC REGION AND COLOR	3 MONTHS BEFORE CONCEPTION	TRIMESTER OF PREGNANCY			NO MEDICAL CARE
		FIRST	SECOND	THIRD	
	PERCENT DISTRIBUTION				
United States	22	58	78	98	2
White	23	62	81	99	1
Nonwhite	15	35	60	94	6
Northeast	20	58	79	99	1
White	21	61	81	99	1
Nonwhite	14	33	63	98	2
North Central	25	64	82	99	1
White	25	65	83	98	1
Nonwhite	24	46	66	98	3
South	20	52	73	96	4
White	24	60	79	97	3
Nonwhite	11	31	56	92	8
West	22	59	78	98	1
White	22	61	80	99	1
Nonwhite	23	46	70	98	3

[1] Excludes mothers whose date of first visit is unknown.

* U.S. Department of Health, Education, and Welfare, Public Health Service: Vital and Health Statistics, Series 22, Number 4, Table E, Washington, D.C., U.S. Government Printing Office, 1968.

TABLE 9-2. NUMBER AND PERCENT DISTRIBUTION OF MOTHERS, BY TIME OF FIRST MEDICAL VISIT DURING THE 12 MONTHS PRIOR TO BIRTH ACCORDING TO METROPOLITAN STATUS AND 1962 FAMILY INCOME: UNITED STATES, 1963 BIRTHS*

METROPOLITAN STATUS AND 1962 FAMILY INCOME	NUMBER OF MOTHERS IN THOUSANDS	3 MONTHS BEFORE CONCEPTION	TIME OF FIRST MEDICAL VISIT				
			TRIMESTER OF PREGNANCY			NO MEDICAL CARE	UNKNOWN
			FIRST	SECOND	THIRD		
ALL AREAS			PERCENT DISTRIBUTION				
All incomes	4,097	21.3	35.1	19.1	19.6	2.0	3.0
Under $3,000	820	15.9	26.6	25.9	26.2	4.4	1.0
$3,000-$4,999	1,030	20.8	33.8	22.6	20.2	2.1	0.6
$5,000-$6,999	920	24.0	42.9	16.4	15.2	1.3	0.2
$7,000-$9,999	667	27.7	44.9	13.6	12.3	1.1	0.5
$10,000 and over	307	28.3	48.0	11.5	10.9	1.0	0.3
Illegitimate and unknown	352	10.7	8.1	17.4	35.3	..	28.6
METROPOLITAN AREAS							
All incomes	2,656	21.4	36.7	18.5	19.4	1.5	2.6
Under $3,000	429	15.1	27.2	26.0	27.8	3.0	1.0
$3,000-$4,999	612	20.5	33.2	22.5	21.0	2.0	0.8
$5,000-$6,999	625	23.2	44.0	16.5	15.2	1.0	0.2
$7,000-$9,999	506	27.3	45.6	13.3	12.1	1.2	0.4
$10,000 and over	249	27.2	51.5	11.8	8.7	0.5	0.4
Illegitimate and unknown	236	11.3	8.7	17.7	38.5	..	23.8
NONMETROPOLITAN AREAS							
All incomes	1,440	21.2	32.1	20.4	19.8	2.9	3.6
Under $3,000	391	16.7	26.0	25.9	24.4	6.0	1.0
$3,000-$4,999	419	21.1	34.6	22.8	19.0	2.1	0.2
$5,000-$6,999	294	25.6	40.7	16.1	15.2	2.1	0.3
$7,000-$9,999	161	28.7	42.7	14.5	12.8	0.6	0.6
$10,000 and over	59	32.9	33.4	10.2	20.2	3.2	..
Illegitimate and unknown	117	9.4	6.8	16.8	28.6	..	38.3

* U.S. Department of Health, Education, and Welfare, Public Health Service: Vital and Health Statistics, Series 22, Number 4, Table 12, Washington, D.C., U.S. Government Printing Office, 1968.

creased, the number of visits for medical care also increased. Women living in families below the poverty level made, on the average, 9.3 visits for medical care; women from middle income families averaged 13.7 visits. Most of the women in the lowest income group visited medical facilities (clinics, hospitals) for their care as contrasted to the women in the highest income group where the majority visited physicians for medical care.

Income appears to be a major factor in the number of visits for antenatal care. There is a large jump in number of visits when the income goes above the poverty line (i.e., $5,000 and over). As would be expected, the average number of visits for medical care was also higher

for women had completed more years of school. Primiparous women made more visits than multiparous women. According to the National Natality Study only 2 per cent made no visits at all during the 12 months before childbirth. On the other hand, almost 20 per cent of the women made no visits either to a physician or to a medical facility until the third trimester of pregnancy.

The evidence we have to date indicates that white mothers receive care earlier in pregnancy than nonwhite mothers. There is a consistent difference between white and nonwhite mothers and the receipt of medical care during each of the trimesters of pregnancy (see Table 9-1). There is evidence (Table 9-2) that women living in metropolitan areas receive care earlier than those outside metropolitan areas; this held true for both white and nonwhite women. Furthermore, more of the nonwhite women in metropolitan areas are known to have received care than nonwhite women residing outside metropolitan areas. It is worth noting, though, that for any given income or educational group the differences between metropolitan and non-metropolitan areas are insignificant with regard to the time when mothers first receive medical care.

Several factors are worth mentioning with regard to differences in antenatal care patterns. As noted, the lower socioeconomic status groups tend to come later in their pregnancy for prenatal care than do the middle and upper socioeconomic status groups. Furthermore, there is a differential by age and parity; the women in the younger age group tend to come later than women in the other age groups. This is probably due to the fact that the highest rates of illegitimacy are in the youngest age groups. Women in the lower socioeconomic status groups tend to receive their antenatal care in clinics and other medical facilities; women in the middle and upper socioeconomic status groups tend to receive their prenatal care from private physicians. Similarly, those in the lower socioeconomic status groups tend to have higher rates of illegitimacy and, given the stigma attached to this status, they are not likely to be seen by private practitioners but rather in the clinics. The stigma of illegitimacy would probably be a major factor contributing to underutilization of antenatal services by the young primigravidae.

There are crucial differences in the delivery of health services to clinic populations and to private patients. A number of sociomedical factors influence the availability and use of obstetric services. Not only are there variations in the services available but there are variations also in the quality of antenatal care for obstetric management. Secondly, there are differential resources available to the low socioeconomic status groups as contrasted to the higher socioeconomic status groups. That is to say, there are relatively fewer maternal care facilities as well as general medical facilities available to ghetto residents and other socioeconomic status groups than to other sociocultural groups.

The differential distribution of maternity care services is influenced by a complex interaction of many factors. These include population mobility, concentration of services in highly urbanized areas, and the problems of attracting sufficient and qualified professional staff to isolated rural or poor communities. But even where the best facilities exist, there is continued underutilization by the lower socioeconomic groups as demonstrated by the experience in the United States, Great Britain under the National Health Service, as well as in other European countries that have national or prepaid health schemes such as Yugoslavia. Thus, the processes that lead individuals or groups to make use of antenatal services and the social attitudes toward care and toward medical institutions, needs considerably more study. Similarly, more research is needed on the different levels of care provided by different units of the same medical service and the degree to which population groups of varying socioeconomic status receive unequal care from the same institution.

Teenage Pregnancy, Illegitimacy and Maternal Care

In the United States and certain other countries, such as England and Wales, the number of maternities to teenage women has been increasing in recent years. In part, this is due to increased births to unmarried girls; in part, it is a result of a trend toward early marriage. However, the major factor is derived from other social changes occurring in society. As noted earlier in this chapter, young women are known to have comparatively high rates of perinatal death and low birth weights. The increased risks associated with illegitimate pregnancy have been recognized for many years, but there is a complex web of interaction between social and biological factors that make interpretation of data rather difficult. For example, mothers in the age group under 20, both legitimate and illegitimate, are drawn primarily from the lower socioeconomic status groups with their attendant characteristics high risk of pregnancy outcomes. Problems associated with pregnancy are particularly acute in the very young mothers age 12 to 15. Physical immaturity, like maternal stature and physique, represent hazards to successful pregnancy outcomes.

Before proceeding much further, it is important to note that statistics on illegitimate births are universally poor. In the United States, national data on illegitimacy are based on reports from 34 states and the District of Columbia. The estimate of illegitimacy in the United States is made on the assumption that those states not reporting tend to have the same experience as reporting states in the same region of the country. These statistics are influenced by unevenness in the methods and inaccuracy of reporting among the 34 states that ask about legitimacy on their birth certificates, as well as by lack of information by nonreporting states. The available data indicate that about 40 per cent of unwed mothers are under 20 among white women as compared to 49 per cent in this age group among Negro women. For most, but not all, of the teenage unwed mothers, their first child is usually illegitimate.

Studies made in the United States, Scandinavia, and the United Kingdom all tend to show that premarital pregnancy is rather common among married white couples as well as nonwhite couples, particularly in the younger age groups. Studies also show that premarital pregnancy is more likely to result in marriage before birth of the child for a white teenage girl than for a Negro teenage girl. The problems of illegitimacy may be most acute in the age group under 20 but it is worth noting that women age 20 to 24 account for as many illegitimate births as do women under age 20. In fact, those in their 20's showed the highest rate of illegitimate births.

The illegitimate birth rate for the country as a whole has risen fairly steadily since 1940, though in recent years it has remained approximately the same (A. A. Campbell and James D. Cowhig, 1967). Although less information is available about illegitimate than about total births, we may assume that concealment of illegitimacy is more frequent for white women than for Negro women. But differences of concealment are not likely to account for the very great differences in illegitimate birth rates that appear in the data that are available. White women are not only more likely to conceal an illegitimate birth, they are also more likely to use contraception in the first place. Furthermore, if conception does occur, white women are more likely either to marry before the baby is born or to have an abortion. Thus, the illegitimacy figures presented here, though they have many limitations, can be considered to reflect a real situation. These statistics are important primarily because of the fact that they demonstrate the importance and significance of the problem of illegitimacy. Illegitimacy is a problem of all social and cultural groups, although some groups have a greater or more widespread problem than others.

Viewed from a sociological perspective, the great disparity of illegitimacy rates between white and nonwhite mothers can be analyzed in terms of incentive for marriage, sanctions and norma-tive orientations regarding marriage. From the perspective of incentives, or the advantages and disadvantages of marriage, most Negro women, married or unmarried, can expect less than white women from marriage on all of the usual expectations or rights. The Negro woman may be making a rational decision if she does not marry, even if she is thereby forced to care for her own child (for Negroes adoption is not usually considered and less often possible). The Negro woman often cannot expect her husband to solve her problems and, in fact, he may create some additional ones. Companionship and related aspects of marriage, supposedly highly prized by the middle-class, are not very salient for the low-income population, white or black. Typically, this population desires such things in a marriage as: support, emotional as well as economic; respect; and responsible conduct from their spouse. Much of what is taken for granted by the advantaged population groups, is only a dream for the disadvantaged. In short, the rewards of marriage, normally taken for granted in the middle-class culture, may be absent for the lower-class woman. Furthermore, the Negro, less often than the white unwed mother, will be encouraged to marry by significant others and this is borne out by data on premarital pregnancy. She may expect fewer sanctions from people around her and hence is less likely to keep her pregnancy a secret (Hallowell Pope, 1969).

Illegitimate children are not only stigmatized socially by their legal status but they also suffer handicaps with respect to their physical development at birth and their subsequent health. This can be shown in two health-related characteristics that are reported uniformly on the birth certificates of all states: the birth weight of the child and the attendant at birth and place of delivery (J. Pakter, 1961). Unmarried mothers receive less prenatal care and have more complications of pregnancy than married mothers. The number of visits (7.1) for prenatal care is the lowest for mothers of illegitimate children. There is a higher rate of prematurity among the illegitimate children than among legitimate births and their risk of death is considerably higher.

Various studies have shown that unmarried pregnant women tend to receive poor prenatal care compared to married pregnant women. That is, even when the unmarried pregnant woman shows up for antenatal care, the quality of care received is not as high as that of the married woman. Most of their visits are to clinics, hospitals, and other medical facilities where care is likely to be provided by residents, part-time physicians or foreign trained physicians. This tends to be reflected in the birth weight of their offspring. The median weight of legitimate infants born in 1964 was 3310 grams; it was only 3110 grams for illegitimate infants. The percentage of babies born weighing less than 2501 grams (i.e., those defined as immature) is a good index of future health because of the morbidity and mortality in this low birth weight group. By this criterion, 14.6 per cent of the illegitimate infants born in 1964 were immature as compared with 7.7 per cent of the legitimate babies.[4] The differences by color are striking: more nonwhite legitimate babies (13.0%) were immature than were white illegitimate ones (11.3%), but the gap between legitimate and illegitimate births was wider for white infants. In other words, nonwhite infants had a high rate of immaturity regardless of their legitimacy status, whereas legitimacy made a substantial difference for white infants (6.8 per cent of legitimate babies and 11.3 per cent of illegitimate babies were immature). These results were particularly true for first-order births. This difference may reflect a difference in socioeconomic environment and medical care between mothers of first illegitimate births and mothers who have second and higher order illegitimate births.

Thus, it is clear that illegitimate children begin life with more precarious health than do other children. In addition, of course, illegitimate babies have social handicaps and very little is known about the conditions under which children with these disadvantages grow to maturity. The role of the nurse in coping with teenage pregnancies and mothers of illegitimate children is particularly important. As has been pointed out elsewhere, punitive attitudes of nursing and medical personnel do little more than increase the guilt associated with an illegitimate pregnancy. The nurse has a crucial role to play in emotional support, education with regard to future antenatal care practices, use of contraception, and guidance with regard to disposition of the baby, for pregnant teenagers and mothers of illegitimate children.

Poverty: its Relationships to Maternal Care

Earlier in this chapter, the concept of socioeconomic status or social class, was briefly dis-

cussed. Unlike that concept, the concept "poor" is very ancient, dating back to biblical times (i.e., "The poor always ye have with you,"—John 12:8). This concept, like socioeconomic status or social class, also expresses social differences between men and has gained general acceptance. It has been used to describe rural tenant farmers, mountain folk in Appalachia, and ethnic and other groups in urban ghettos. The importance of a discussion of poverty and health with particular reference to maternity care, is obvious from the foregoing discussion in this chapter which has indicated a close relationship between low socioeconomic status and maternal health care.

Before discussing how the characteristics of lower-income persons influence their behavior in connection with the issues of health, illness, and the utilization of medical services, it is appropriate to briefly discuss some aspects of medical organization and medical care for lower-income groups.[5] The national commitment for equality of medical care for all citizens has led to a variety of important legislative acts. Many of these are now having their impact at the local level through the Department of Health, Education and Welfare and the Office of Economic Opportunity. The emphasis is on extending and improving the system of medical organization so that medical care can be offered more rapidly, more effectively, and more efficiently to the poor as well as those more economically advantaged. For example, the maternal and infant care projects (MIC) supported by the US Children's Bureau has had an important impact on maternity care throughout the United States. These projects are supposed to help reduce the incidence of mental retardation and other handicapping conditions caused by complications associated with childbearing and to help reduce infant and maternal mortality. These projects are concentrated in low-income areas of large and small cities. The emphasis is on early, comprehensive prenatal care for all patients in the geographic area served. A variety of allied health personnel has been recruited to provide and extend a range of services. According to a recent report (Warren H. Pearse, 1970), the number of antepartum visits per patient has risen markedly; postpartum return visits have quadrupled; perinatal mortality, stillbirths and neonatal mortality have declined sharply. As with many of these new programs, there are many problems that have yet to be resolved before they can be called truly successful.

---

[4] National Center for Health Statistics: Trends in illegitimacy, United States, 1940-1965, Vital and Health Statistics, Series 21, Number 15, Washington, D.C., US Department of Health, Education and Welfare, Public Health Service, February, 1968.

[5] The sick poor. Am. J. Nurs. 69:2424-2454, November, 1969.

The Maternity and Infant Care Program is probably one of the more successful programs of outreach to lower-income groups because of its unusual methods of communicating with the poor. On the other hand, there is a serious question as to whether the inequities in the medical care system can be overcome unless changes are made reflecting greater understanding of lower-income life styles. It is well known that when medical facilities are set up in convenient proximity to lower-income housing, they do not automatically draw clientele. No doubt, medical facilities located near the homes of lower-income people are more likely to draw and keep patients, but their mere presence does not solve the problem of delivering effective care to most people in the nearby locale.

There are two factors which contribute to inequities of medical care. The first of these relates to the way in which medical organization facilities are structured; the second factor is concerned with the characteristic life styles of lower-income groups. Both factors are obstacles to the delivery and receipt of quality medical care.

What are the features of medical care organization that tend to blunt the effectiveness of medical care for lower-income patients (Anselm L. Strauss, 1969)? These negative features of medical organization include the following: first, there is the massiveness of medical organization itself. Most of the lower-income women, as noted earlier in this chapter, tend to visit medical facilities such as hospitals and clinics. These are often large and complex organizations. They are characterized not only by great specialization of function and specialized clinics but by a fair degree of impersonality which is felt even by midde-class patients (who register this as one of their chief complaints about hospital care). Lower-class patients are ill-equipped by lack of education and experience to cope with complex bureaucratic organization. Little explanation is provided to the patient for the reasons for diagnostic tests, the necessity of visiting a variety of clinics, etc.

A second feature of medical organization that tends to decrease the quality of care for lower-income patients is the professionalization of health workers. This greater specialization with its resultant characteristic set of goals, its perspectives toward work and patients, results in a gap between the patients and the professionals. Lower-income people are less skilled in interviewing matters to get at information that the professionals have but are not yielding. They tend to be less aggressive in demanding explanations. On the

other hand, higher-income patients have greater aggressive and interactional skills and can cope more effectively with the professionals' failure to communicate. There are other, more subtle, disadvantages stemming from professional stances, which lower-income patients suffer. These have been discussed by a number of investigators with regard to the field of mental disorders. That is, middle-class patients are preferred by most treatment agents, and are seen as more treatable. In other words, there may be a distinct bias expressed against the lower-income patient, based honestly on professional conceptions. Many regimens are impossible for low-income patients to carry out. Even the simple order that medication is to be taken "with each meal" may not recognize that many lower-income families eat irregularly and may not have three meals a day.

Another characteristic of medical organization that influences the quality of medical care is the middle-class bias of most professional health workers. The staff members, typically, do not understand the perspective, attitudes, customs and life-styles of the patients. They simply take for granted that the patients have the same attitudes regarding health as they do. Hence, they tend to issue orders that are not understood or cannot be easily followed by lower-income patients. Furthermore, there is a tendency to think of lower-income people in stereotyped terms, "they cannot keep appointments, they have little sense of time or responsibility, they are shiftless, irresponsible, they have children out of wedlock, they are dirty." Lower-income patients may perceive these class biases and this may affect not only the quality of medical care which the patients receive, but also the underutilization of medical services.

The many hours of waiting, the impersonal routines of institutional care in large hospitals or clinics, particularly in the municipal and county hospitals, and in the larger cities these tend to be massive, complex, crowded and busy, the real or imagined perceptions of racial and class bias, tend to maximize dissatisfactions of lower-income patients and reduce the possibility of utilization of health facilities. Furthermore, the distances that patients must travel to the medical facilities and the cost of transportation are realistic matters. Customarily, poor people organize their lives so as not to go far for the necessities of living. This is one of the factors in the relative success of the MIC program (i.e., it has reached out into the lower-income communities and brought the clinic facilities into the neighborhood). Similarly, OEO neighborhood health centers have been relatively successful for this reason.

Finally, it is important to briefly take into account the characteristic life-styles of the poor. The lower-income person's experience of himself and his world is highly distinctive in our country. It is also distinctive for its problems and crisis-dominated character. As S. M. Miller has commented about these people, their "life is a crisis-life constantly trying to make do with string where rope is needed." In other words, health concerns are minor to those who feel they confront much more pressing troubles. Health problems are just one crisis among many that they must try to cope with, control, or just live with.

Another problem is that many lower-income households are often much more under-staffed than those of higher income. This under-staffing of households means that each individual's health receives relatively little attention as far as preventive measures are concerned, and when someone is sick it is more difficult to care for him at home. When the main family member is sick, he or she will be in a disadvantaged position in caring properly for himself or herself. There is a necessity for poor people to learn to live with illness rather than to use their limited financial and psychological resources to do something about illness. The pressing problems of daily existence tend to minimize the problem of illness so that symptoms that do not incapacitate are often ignored.

Furthermore, self education is much less advanced among lower-income groups than among people of higher income. Lower-income people do not conform to the expectations of how "good" and "considerate" patients should behave in medical settings. Their behavior is often frustrating and annoying to medical and nursing personnel for a variety of reasons. Finally, lower-income persons do not respond well to the "impersonality" of the professional role; they tend to seek personal rather than professional relationships with staff, as they do in behavior outside of medical settings. As a result there may be considerable anxiety when the lower-income patient is in the medical setting of large hospitals. This pervasive anxiety has been described in Rosengren's study of obstetric patients (W. R. Rosengren, 1964). Her lack of experience maneuvering within organizational structures makes this a problematic situation, even when she is a paying patient.

In this section an effort has been made to depict some of the problems associated with the delivery of services to the poor even when resources, equipment and finances are made available, by focusing upon some of the disparities between the assumptions made about lower-income patients by professional staff and the realities of lower-income life, attitude and behavior. Yet, such knowledge concerning the poor has not been adequately built into either the training of health professionals nor has it affected the organization of medical care in hospitals, clinics, and other medical facilities. It is important, therefore, that greater understanding and awareness of the characteristic life-styles of the poor gain greater currency among health professionals, if we are indeed, to meet the national commitment of good health care for *all* American citizens.

The Sick Role, Illness, and Pregnancy

How a society or groups within a society define pregnancy and cope with pregnancy tends to vary considerably. In some societies, pregnancy is regarded as a "normal" situation—a kind of status passage through which most women, at some time or other, will pass. In other societies, pregnancy may be regarded as an illness and is reacted to as other illnesses are. As previously noted in this chapter there is considerable variation even within societies, in the way health and illness are perceived by different social classes, ethnic groups, and age categories.

The sick role has been developed as a concept by sociologists to study the role behavior of persons who are considered sick or as having an illness (T. Parsons, 1964). In brief, the sick role concept refers to the process by which every society ensures that an adequate level of health and normative conformity exists among the majority of its members, most of the time. Society has various mechanisms for accomplishing this purpose. Illness as a form of deviance, is one method by which society accommodates individuals or groups who are ill and hence deviating from expected behavior, by placing them in a special position or status. The term "social role" refers to both the regular way of acting expected of persons occupying a given position and the social position itself. Typically there are certain rights or privileges, as well as expectations, associated with given social positions. Parsons has presented an insightful and systematic analysis of the expectations associated with occupancy of the sick role. There are two main rights:

a. The sick person is allowed exemption from the performance of normal social role obligations

b. The sick person is allowed exemption from responsibility for his own state.

In addition there are two main obligations:

c. The sick person must be motivated to get well as soon as possible.
d. The sick person should seek technically competent help and cooperate with medical experts.

The sick role is generally conceptualized by sociologists as an ideal type for the purposes of understanding the processes contributing to and the various conditions to be fulfilled in the legitimation of illness conditions. There is an attempt to detect and account for certain uniformities in the behavior of ill persons. Since this is a theoretical model, the concept permits a study of the effects of legitimation on both the individual and on his social milieu. In reality, the concept is not universally applicable to all who claim to be ill; it varies depending on the unique background of the person, the particular illness involved, and the social context within which legitimation is sought.

Sociologists have made a number of criticisms of the sick role including the fact that Parsons has left open the problem of the chronically ill as well as some illness that is not considered serious enough to warrant more than a slight reduction in normal activities. Furthermore, much illness never reaches the stage of formal consultation with a qualified doctor. Individuals who are ill may receive what they consider to be competent help from others than professional medical personnel. Furthermore, Parsons has suggested that his sick role formulation is especially applicable to psychiatric or emotional illnesses. Finally, Parsons' formulation may not be relevant to all societies, and various studies have demonstrated that there are both intercultural and intracultural variations in the definitions of the conditions to which the sick role is thought to be applicable.

The state of pregnancy in its modal or normal situation, where there are no resultant obstetric or delivery complications, must be considered in the discussion of the applicability of the sick role concept. If a woman is experiencing complications of pregnancy, then certainly this would make her eligible for the sick role as discussed above. The question that arises is whether pregnancy is in fact a "normal" state.

One may conceivably take the position that illness, or sickness, is statistically normal in most of the population, at some point in their life; similarly, pregnancy can likewise be considered statistically normal in that most of the population of possible conceivers at some time are in this state. Pregnancy can also be considered "normal" in the sense that it is a necessary biological function for the species. In deed, it can even be considered a desirable state of affairs. In this latter sense, it is not similar to illness at all. In a recent paper, McKinlay has noted that pregnancy differs from illness by "calling forth in both the woman and her significant others a set of responses which are in many ways different from those elicited with the onset of an illness" (John B. McKinlay, 1970). Considering whether the four sick role expectations noted above apply to pregnancy, McKinlay suggests that for a variety of reasons, the state of pregnancy is in some ways different from illness and cannot be analyzed in terms of any of the four expectations associated with the sick role.

There is a tendency in the more advanced societies to consider at least some point during pregnancy as illness and to treat it in a manner similar to that in which illness is handled. For example, women are discouraged from home deliveries and are increasingly hospitalized for delivery. Blood pressure, height, weight, etc. are usually taken at several points during the pregnancy. Treating women "as if" they are ill may perhaps encourage the adoption of certain roles because the women perceive this type of treatment as being similar to that for an illness. In sum, the state of pregnancy and the expectations covering it differ from routine illness behavior and the situation is relatively unstructured. This relatively unstructured situation may produce a sense of role ambiguity or strain in pregnant women. Women may take matters into their own hands and reduce such strain or ambiguity by structuring the situation in particular ways.

On the other hand, in the situation where women cannot maintain their homeostatic mechanisms under the physiological strain of pregnancy, there is a meaningful situation where the sick role becomes an important role behavior. For women who are at greater risk, either latent or manifest, and who react excessively or unfavorably under the strain of pregnancy, the sick role becomes meaningful and relevant.

Thus, in the "normal" circumstances of pregnancy and under pathologic conditions, the sick role is an important feature of maternal care.

SUGGESTED READING

Baird, Sir Dugald: The social aspect of obstetric practice. Obstet. Gynec. Survey 20:410-430, June, 1965.

Blood, R. O., and Wolfe, D. M.: Husbands and Wives. Glencoe, Ill., The Free Press, 1960.

Butler, N. R.: The problems of low birthweight and early delivery. J. Obstet. Gynaec. 72:1001-1003, 1965.

Campbell, A. A., and Cowhig, J. D.: The incidence of illegitimacy in the United States. Welfare in Review 5:1-6, May, 1967.

Campbell, A. M.: The effect of excessive cigaret smoking on maternal health. Am. J. Obstet. Gynec. 31:502-508, 1936.

Clark, A. L.: The adaption problems and patterns of an expanding family: the neonatal period, Nurs. Forum 5:93-108, 1966.

Flapan, M.: A paradigm for the analysis of child-bearing motivations of married women prior to birth of the first child. Am. J. Orthopsychiat. 39:402-417, April, 1969.

Frazier, T. M., Davis, G. H., Goldstein, H., and Goldbert, I. D.: Cigarette smoking and prematurity: a prospective study. Am. J. Obstet. Gynec. 81:988-996, 1961.

Hurley, L. S.: Nutrients and genes: interactions and development. Nutr. Rev. 27:3-6, January, 1969.

Illsley, R.: Social class selection and class differences in relation to stillbirths and infant deaths. Brit. Med. J. 2:1520-1524, 1955.

————: The sociological study of reproduction and its outcome, in Richardson, S. A., and Guttmacher, A. F.: Childbearing: Its Social and Psychological Aspects, Baltimore, The Williams & Wilkins Co., 1967. Jacoby, A. P.: Transition to parenthood: a reassessment, J. Marr. Fam. 31:720-727, November, 1969.

Kaltreider, D. F.: Effects of Height and Weight on Pregnancy and the Newborn, Springfield, Ill., Charles C Thomas, 1963.

Kunz, P. R., and Brinkerhoff, M. B.: Differential childlessness by color: the destruction of a cultural belief. J. Marr. Fam. 31:713-719, November, 1969.

McKinlay, J. B.: The new latecomers for antenatal care. Brit. J. Prev. Soc. Med. 24:52, February, 1970.

————: The sick role, illness and pregnancy in McEwan, P. J. M. (ed.): Problems in Medical Care. London, Travistock, 1971.

Morris, J. N., and Heady, J. A.: Social and biological factors in infant mortality: I. Objects and methods. Lancet 1:343-349, 1955.

Naeye, R. L., Diener, M. M., Dellinger, W. S., and Blanc, W. A.: Urban poverty: effects on prenatal nutrition, Science 166:1026, November 21, 1969.

National Center for Health Statistics: Employment during pregnancy, legitimate live births. United States, 1963, Vital and Health Statistics, Series 22, Number 7, Washington, D.C., US Department of Health, Education and Welfare, Public Health Service, September, 1968.

————: Natality statistics analysis. United States, 1965-1967, Vital and Health Statistics, Series 21, Number 19, Washington, D.C.: US Department of Health, Education and Welfare, Public Health Service, May, 1970.

————: Trends in illegitimacy. United States, 1940-1965, Vital and Health Statistics, Series 21, Number 15, Washington, D.C., US Department of Health, Education and Welfare, Public Health Service, February, 1968.

Pakter, J., et al.: Out-of-wedlock births in New York City :I—Sociologic aspects. Am. J. Public Health 51:683-696, May, 1961.

Pakter, J., et al.: Out-of-wedlock births in New York City: I—Sociologic aspects. Am. J. Public Health 51:846-865, June, 1961.

Parsons, T.: Definitions of health and illness in the light of American values and social structure, Social Structure and Personality, pp. 257-291, 436-437, Glencoe, Ill., The Free Press, 1964.

Pearse, W. H.: The maternity and infant care program. Obstet. Gynec. 35:114-119, January, 1970.

Pope, H.: Negro-White differences and decisions regarding illegitimate children. J. Marr. Fam. 31: 756-764, November, 1969.

Rosengren, W. R.: Social class in becoming "ill" in Shostak, A. B., and Donberg, W., (eds.): Blue Collar World. Englewood Cliffs, N.J., Prentice-Hall, 1964.

Rossi, A.: Transition to parenthood. J. Marr. Fam. 30:33, February, 1968.

Russell, C. S., Taylor, R., and Law, C. E.: Smoking in pregnancy, maternal blood pressure, pregnancy outcome, baby weight and growth, and other related factors. Brit. J. Prev. Soc. Med. 22:119-126, 1968.

Russell, C. S., Taylor, R., and Maddison, R. N.: Some effects of smoking in pregnancy. J. Obstet. Gynaec. 73:742-746, 1966.

The sick poor. Am. J. Nurs. 69:2424-2454, November, 1969.

Simpson, W. J.: A preliminary report on cigarette smoking and the incidence of prematurity. Amer. J. Obstet. Gynec. 73:808-815, 1957.

Steele, R., and Langworth, J. T.: The relationship of antenatal and postnatal factors to sudden unexpected death in infancy. Canad. Med. Ass. J. 94:1165-1171, 1966.

Strauss, A. L.: Medical organization, medical care in lower-income groups. Soc. Sci. Med. 3:143-177, 1969.

Theobald, G. W.: The pregnancy toxemias seen in perspective. J. Reproductive Med. 3:76-91, August, 1969.

Zabriskie, J. R.: Effect of cigaret smoking during pregnancy: study of 2,000 cases. Obstet. Gynec. 21:405-411, April, 1963.

Patient Teaching

10

Teaching and Learning • Group Discussion Programs • Preparation for Childbearing

INTRODUCTION

Childbirth in modern society reflects the progress brought about by cultural influences, social change, technologic advances and, above all, the progress of nursing and medical science.

Preparation for parenthood actually begins with the mother's own birth or earlier (as was stated in the last chapter), and its development is influenced by an accumulation of her experiences through infancy, childhood, adolescence and maturity. The father's feelings and attitudes are influenced in a like manner by his previous experiences. The addition of courses in sex education and marriage and family living to the high school and the college curricula has had a positive effect on the attitudes of young people. Much has also been accomplished through premarital and prepregnancy examinations and counseling.

In Manchester, England, during the 18th century, Dr. Charles White wrote a book on instructions for the supervision of mothers during pregnancy, and how to help them in labor and make them comfortable; so we know the idea of teaching patients is not an entirely new approach in patient care. In our own country, within the last 3 or 4 decades, the emphasis placed on the education of parents for childbirth has stimulated them to attend antepartal classes, which, in part, have helped further to dispel misunderstandings or lack of knowledge and to increase the understanding of childbirth as a normal physiologic body process. In addition, classes have been developed for mothers following delivery, as a part of postpartal nursing, in the majority of hospitals which have maternity units.

The concept of family-centered care which prevails in all health services today could have no more appropriate application than to the beginning of a new life in the family unit. Having children is no longer the mother's responsibility alone; it is a joint undertaking of both parents. From the moment of conception, when the baby begins his existence, the husband is encouraged to attend antepartal classes with his wife and begin to assume his role as father. A helpful, understanding and sympathetic husband can do much to make the pregnancy an experience that will contribute to the foundation of a more enriched family life.

The authors realize that the gigantic task required to present the subject matter for patient teaching in maternity nursing would consume an entire book. In this chapter some concepts of the teaching-learning process will be introduced. The student is encouraged to read more widely on the subject in the current literature in psychology and education. A number of excellent references are included in the Suggested Reading.

The focus in patient education here will be directed to groups of patients, though the principles would be applicable in teaching individuals. Parent education is a term used to cover a wide range of educational programs geared to help parents increase their competence as parents and develop effective methods of child care. The first phase of parent education is preparation for childbearing, which is our focus here in maternity nursing.

TEACHING AND LEARNING

"Teaching is an interactive process between a teacher and one or more learners."[1] The teaching-learning process is a complex entity and composed of various interrelated parts. These parts might

---

[1] Redman, B. K.: The Process of Patient Teaching in Nursing, p. 11, St. Louis, C. V. Mosby, 1968.

be summarized as: (1) identifying the need or needs of the learner, (2) determining the motivation of the learner, (3) establishing the objectives of learning, and (4) evaluation in terms of desired learning. Learning may be defined as a (desired) change in behavior.

Health teaching has long been considered an integral part of professional nursing care. Teaching in maternity nursing begins with making an assessment of what the expectant mother, or mother with her newborn, needs to learn. In planning for teaching, the motivation of the mother for learning must be considered in the nurse's plan for the learning experience.

The mother may not be highly motivated to learn about her new baby and his care the first day or so following delivery. One should consider the physiological and psychological changes which occur in the immediate puerperium as an important influence in determining the mother's readiness for attending even small group classes. Rubin speaks of the process of regeneration, the "taking-in" period in the puerperium which lasts for the first 2 or 3 days.[2] During this restorative period the mother has a great need for sleep, may indeed have "sleep-hunger" for several days. Among other normal reactions associated with this taking-in phase is the mother's passive and dependent behavior. However, when the "taking-hold" phase follows, the mother is physically and psychologically more ready to participate in such activities as group classes for postpartal mothers in the hospital. Once her dependency needs have been met in the taking-in phase, she needs to move forward toward independence.

In the context of education in general, Alfred Gorman says

Teachers are beginning slowly to understand that any group setting is packed with human relations needs that have to be met before people can get on with the learning of subject matter. Large numbers of students find the traditional classroom actively harmful to their self-images day after day. Many withdraw physically and become dropout statistics; much larger numbers stay physically while withdrawing psychologically. Still others do not withdraw, but learn to play the highly sophisticated game of teachers and students much in the same way that they role-played cops and robbers at earlier ages. Their real world

of personal meaning, where they can authentically play themselves, usually exists *outside* the classroom.[3]

Teaching is accomplished only when the learner (in this case the mother) learns, when she retains what she learns, and is able to use it now and later after discharge from the hospital. Thus, nurses should understand about the learner as well as learning.

The following list is illustrative rather than exhaustive. The student is encouraged to read more deeply in the field and to develop his own basic set of concepts to guide his teaching.

1. Learners (and teachers) bring with them to the classroom a cluster of understandings, skills, appreciations, attitudes, and feelings that have personal meaning to them and are in effect the sum of their reactions to previous stimuli.

2. Learners (and teachers) are individually different in many ways even when ability grouped.

3. Learners (and teachers) have developed concepts of self, which directly affect their behavior.

4. Learning may be defined as a change in behavior.

5. Learning requires activity on the part of the learner. He should not be passive.

6. Learners ultimately learn what *they* actively desire to learn; they do not learn what they do not accept or come to accept.

7. Learning is enhanced when learners accept responsibility for their own learning.

8. Learning is directly influenced by physical and social environment.

9. Learning occurs on successively deeper levels.

10. Learning is deepened when the learning situation provides opportunity for applying learnings in as realistic a situation as is feasible.

11. Learners are motivated when they understand and accept the purposes of the learning situation.

12. Learners are motivated by success experiences.

13. Learners are motivated by teacher acceptance.

14. Learners are motivated when they can associate new learnings with previous learnings.

[2] Rubin, R.: Puerperal change. Nurs. Outlook 9:754, December, 1961.

[3] Gorman, A. H.: Teachers and Learners in the Interactive Process of Education, p. 12, Boston, Allyn and Bacon, Inc., 1969. Reprinted by permission of the publisher.

15. Learners are motivated when they can see the usefulness of the learning in their own personal terms.[4]

Classes

Today there are definite courses offered for mothers and fathers in preparation for childbearing. These classes are included as a part of the programs of private "public health" agencies such as the Visiting Nurse Association, official public health agencies such as the local and state Departments of Health, private organizations such as Maternity Center Association in New York City, and many hospitals throughout the states. There is a growing trend in the United States for maternity hospitals or general hospitals with an active obstetric department to provide these classes for expectant parents, as well as classes for mothers in the hospital after the new baby has arrived. Some of these classes are given for expectant mothers or fathers alone; in others the parents attend classes together. In the latter group the classes aid the parents in their mutual appreciation of the value of antepartal preparation and tend to promote the idea of sharing parenthood. The goals set for the parents in any of these classes are similar, namely, to gain increased knowledge about childbearing and increased understanding of ways to promote and to maintain optimum health through the practice of good health habits in daily living.

Several disciplines may be represented in teaching any one group of classes, so that those who teach may be nurses, obstetricians, pediatricians, nutritionists, health educators and, in some courses which include exercise classes, physical therapists. Material related to the physiology of pregnancy and labor, general hygiene and the care of the mother during pregnancy, labor and the puerperium is included, as well as that related to the baby. All of the class content is approved by a medical council or advisory board, but the details of the classes usually are worked out by nurses to suit the conditions under which the courses are conducted.

The classes are attended by individuals from various social, cultural and economic groups, each with his or her own needs and desires. Those who teach must be realistic about their teaching and never forget that although they have set up

---

4 Ibid., pp. 13-14.

objectives for the students (in this case, the parents), they must help them to attain the goals that they have set up for themselves. For instance, a mother who has the satisfaction of appetite as her goal for family nutrition considers that if her family is not hungry, they are well fed. This goal may astound the nutritionist or the nurse who sees the importance of planning well-balanced meals. In this instance the job of health teaching requires the application of sound educational principles in order not to destroy the mother's goal with one fell swoop. The nurse's teaching can be most effective if she first identifies their common goals, and then, gradually, as she teaches, begins to change the mother's objective without undermining her security.

These educational programs can enhance, strengthen, and broaden the care and services provided by the physician or clinical staff members. Programs in parent education should be related segments in the total constellation of services provided to families. In order to make these sessions truly a preparation for parenthood and family-centered nursing, special attention has to be given to timing and availability of these courses. Sometimes hospitals and institutions arrange classes at times which are not feasible for the parents attending, especially for the father and often for the mother (e.g., in the middle of a busy day). Therefore, attendance is sparce and limited to mothers who are late in their pregnancies and who have a narrow focus of trying to accomplish a partial goal (e.g., management of pain in labor). Many valuable aims of the programs are thus thwarted.

Conventional Type of Program

This is the most widely used program in this country. It is planned to serve everyone in the community and places its emphasis on a general type of "education for childbirth." The course usually includes the physiology of childbearing, general hygiene, including nutrition during pregnancy and lactation, preparations for the baby, and the care of the mother and her baby after the delivery. In this type of program a multidisciplinary approach may be used in the teaching, or the nurse may be responsible for teaching all of the content.

In general, the material is usually covered in a lecture-type format with time allowed for questions and discussion. At times a semi-structured approach may be used, with certain topics being

Fig. 10-1. The Mothers' Round Table, a form of group teaching planned for small groups of postpartal patients through guided group discussions in the hospital. (MacDonald House, University Hospitals of Cleveland, Cleveland)

suggested by the participants and additional relevant information introduced by the nurse-discussion leader as it seems appropriate.

GROUP DISCUSSION PROGRAMS

In this type of class format no structured curriculum is set in advance. Group discussion is developed from the contributions of the class members. The leader is responsible for guiding the discussion and for opening essential areas not probed by the group members. The various areas described in the conventional type programs (i.e., physiology of childbearing, general hygiene, etc.) are covered as the nurse-leader introduces these topics as they fit with the areas brought up by the participants. The group situation demands that the nurse develop a new concept of herself as a leader and that she acquire new skills. She must have a knowledge and an understanding of what material is relevant so that she can draw on it as the group needs it. Hence, she must be totally prepared each time that the group meets since the discussion may range from nutrition in the first trimester of pregnancy to the physiology of labor. In addition, she must be skilled in communication techniques with the ability to listen, to probe, and to reflect so that she can help the group elaborate on germaine comments and statements. She must recognize the importance and the implication of "iceberg questions" or, as some-times spoken of, "the question behind the question," knowing that such questions may indicate an underlying concern of the questioner. For example, an expectant mother in the last trimester of pregnancy asks "how common is going crazy after having a baby?" In such instances the professional nurse should be able to explore and to sift alternatives until the real question can be asked and appropriate action may be taken. In this instance the patient really was not concerned with how often people became psychotic after childbirth but rather she wanted to know whether she was likely to experience this malady. Because of a history of mental illness in her family and her own extreme emotional lability during this pregnancy she was afraid that she might become psychotic after delivery. For a more thorough discussion of the group approach to antepartal management see Suggested Reading.

Since training group leaders is a costly and time consuming business (and it is essential that those who manage parents in this way must be trained in the techniques) group education is not a commitment to be undertaken lightly by either the participating nurses or the sponsoring agencies. Unfortunately, many of these agencies rate the success of a program by the numbers attending; and in the group situation, by definition, only *small groups* can be served at one time. However, it has been amply demonstrated that the actual behavior change,[5] to say nothing of satisfaction with the program, has resulted with this type of management (see Suggested Reading). Moreover, group education has the advantage of not limiting the discussion to certain topics usually discussed by particular class groups, and it can focus upon any of the aspects of pregnancy or childbearing which are of interest to the group.

Whatever the approach, the nurse who participates in parent classes is in a favorable position to help the patients and families to develop a better understanding of their immediate situations, together with a balanced view of the sociology of pregnancy and parturition, growth and development, and the psychological and emotional aspects of family life.

Natural Childbirth

Childbirth as a normal or natural process has received increasing emphasis during the past

[5] Hair, A. P.: Interpersonal Relations in the Small Group, in Faris, R. E. (ed.): Handbook of Modern Sociology, pp. 225-226. Chicago, Rand McNally, 1964.

decade. The reader will develop more understanding of this broad concept of maternity care from the writings of Read, Thoms and Goodrich (see Suggested Reading).

The interpretation of "labor" as "pain" has been held by women from time immemorial, with the result that today many women still approach childbirth in dread of an ordeal. Much of the misunderstanding, fear and apprehension can be overcome by understanding gained from education. This is no simple way to a painless or easy childbirth, but a means to enable a woman to gain more self-understanding, to help herself in labor and to increase her self-confidence.

Increasing emphasis has been placed on the fact that there is an "emotional labor" which is as definite and important as its physical counterpart. There can be no doubt that the attitude of a woman toward her confinement has a considerable influence on the ease of her labor. This fact was stressed for many years by the British obstetrician, the late Dr. Grantly Dick Read, and has been endorsed by various groups in this country, notably the Maternity Center Association of New York and by Drs. Thoms and Goodrich of New Haven and others. Dr. Read emphasized certain psychological aspects of labor—that "fear is in some way the chief pain-producing agent in otherwise normal labor." The neuromuscular mechanism by which fear exerts a deleterious effect on labor is obscure, but the general validity of Read's contention is in keeping with common clinical knowledge. The mother builds up a state of tensions because she is frightened, and these tensions create an antagonistic effect on the muscular activity of normal labor, with resulting pain. The pain causes more fear, which further increases the tensions, and so on, until a vicious circle is established.

Rather unfortunately, certain overzealous people have inferred that a spontaneous delivery, to be psychologically rewarding, *must* be accomplished entirely without medication of any kind. Furthermore, they have implied that if medication was either requested or required, the parturient somehow had "failed" to accomplish delivery by the natural childbirth method. Thus, the connotation of "painless childbirth" also was injected here, an interpretation that is not accurate.

The family-centered approach to maternity care, which is a fundamental part of the natural-childbirth program, is not basically different from that practiced when deliveries were conducted at home with the father present. But changes are apparent.

The current trend to have babies born in the hospital has the advantage of increased safety provided by improved medical techniques and modern obstetric practice. For so long women approached childbearing without any real understanding of what to expect or, for that matter, without much knowledge of the anatomy and the physiology of their reproductive organs. The majority of husbands were included insofar as they were present in the household, but they were not actually made to feel that they were really participating in the event. The natural-childbirth program provides an opportunity to help both parents gain more knowledge and the satisfaction of mutual participation.

The program of education during pregnancy is designed to eliminate fear. Facts which concern the anatomy and the physiology of childbearing and the appropriate care of the mother are taught. The mother not only learns how labor progresses but also is helped to gain an understanding of the sensations likely to accompany labor and methods of working cooperatively with them. The exercises which are included are designed for the muscles which will be used in labor, as well as those which will promote the general well-being of the body. In the performance of any skill the individual is more efficient if the muscles involved are in the best condition. The exercises are not strenuous and, for the most part, are ones that will contribute to improved posture, body balance, agility and increased strength and endurance. The mother learns breathing techniques that will aid her ability to relax in the first stage of labor, and techniques that will help her to work effectively with muscles used in the delivery. To enable the parents to meet better the needs of their baby after he is born, information about his growth and development also is included in these classes.

An important consideration throughout the program is "to help the mother help herself," so that her pregnancy will be a healthy, happy experience, and at the time of labor she will be better able to participate actively in having her baby. In former days when mothers often were given heavy sedation, they were unable to have this satisfying experience.

The encouragement and the support of those about her are particularly important to the expectant mother, especially during labor. Every modern obstetric aid for the mother's safety and comfort is at her disposal. It should be emphasized that the proponents of natural childbirth have never claimed that labor should be conducted without anesthetic aids, or that it can be made devoid of pain (Thoms). The response to pain is individual, and if the mother and/or the physician decides that some assistance in the form of medication is necessary, it is readily available. It would be rather incongruous to suggest that any program would reject medical advances which have made such important contributions to obstetrics. However, many mothers who are "prepared" for natural childbirth often are reluctant to accept any form of medication, feeling that it is rather a personal blow to their integrity. In such a case the mother needs help to understand that this will not detract from her experience, but rather will enhance it. She may need help to remember that the physician is the one person capable of making the final decision as to what is best for her and her baby. The use of medication should not be a criterion in the consideration of "how well the mother did" during labor and delivery. The real measure of success can be determined only by the satisfactions which the mother derives from being able to cooperate with the natural processes of labor to the best of her ability. The new infant is really the important entity and, after he is born, should be the mother's chief concern, not an elaboration of her physical feats.

In summary, satisfactory results in connection with natural childbirth are aided by such factors as attaining good physical health and emotional stability; learning about the baby's development during the antepartal period; understanding the muscular processes that take place during labor and delivery; preparing for labor by attending classes where supervised exercises are practiced and perfected; having empathic understanding and "support" during labor; planning for the postpartal period, the physical and the emotional adjustment of the mother, and the care of the new baby; and the integration of the father into the events of pregnancy and parturition.

Psychoprophylactic Childbirth

Psychoprophylactic preparation for childbirth is a somewhat less permissive version of natural childbirth. It was first propounded by two Russian doctors, Nicolaiev and Velvovskiy. The rationale of the program was based on Pavlov's concept of pain perception and his theory of conditioned reflexes (i.e., the substitution of favorable conditioned reflexes for unfavorable ones).

The Lamaze method often is cited as an ex-

ample of this technique. The theory intrigued a Paris obstetrician, Fernand Lamaze, who studied Russian trained mothers-to-be in a Leningrad clinic. Lamaze returned to France and began to prepare his patients in "psychoprophylaxis" or "mental prevention" of pain in childbirth. He gradually introduced certain adaptations, the most important of which was the rapid shallow breathing which came to characterize the Lamaze method. As the technique spread throughout Europe and Latin America the "Lamaze Method" and "psychoprophylaxis" became synonomous. The late Marjorie Karmel was perhaps the most responsible for introducing this technique to America. There are now programs in psychoprophylaxis throughout this country. Many are under the auspices of the American Society for Prophylaxis in Obstetrics (ASPO) which was founded through joint efforts of Mrs. Karmel and a physical therapist, Elizabeth Bing, and others. In general, the teaching in the program consists of combating the fears associated with pregnancy and childbirth by instructing the pregnant woman in the anatomy and the neuromuscular activity of the reproductive system and the mechanism of labor. The underlying theory of these programs remains firmly based on the neurophysiology of cortical excitation and conditioned response. That is, the mother is taught to replace responses of restlessness, fear and the loss of control with more useful activity. Its usefulness lies in the fact that a high level of activity can excite the cerebral cortex efficiently to inhibit other stimuli, in this case, the pain usually associated with labor. In some programs nutrition and general hygiene are included. Exercises which strengthen the abdominal muscles and relax the perineum are taught, and breathing techniques to help the process of labor are practiced. Thus, the mother is conditioned to respond with respiratory activity and dissociation (or relaxation) of the uninvolved muscles. She then controls her perception of the stimuli associated with labor and learns to work more effectively with the obstetric team. Heretofore, the breathing techniques differed from those used in other methods of prepared childbirth in that the original Lamaze technique emphasized slow deep intercostal breathing at the beginning of each contraction in early labor. Then, as labor progressed, the mother's concentration-effort intensified until, toward the end of the first stage, she changed to rapid, superficial panting which reached a peak of intensity at the height of each contraction and diminished as the contraction subsided. The degree of muscle relaxation some mothers achieved was impressive; however, for those inadequately trained or untrained mothers attempting this type of breathing, undue fatigue and hyperventilation with subsequent carpopedal spasm resulted. Maternal respiratory alkalosis and a paradoxical acidosis in the fetus are also possibilities if hyperventilation is prolonged. It has been reported that a comparative physiological study carried out with four groups of mothers in labor demonstrated that under certain circumstances hyperventilation did occur. Each group of mothers in the study had different preparation during pregnancy: (1) no antepartal training, (2) training in psychoprophylaxis, (3) trained in psychophysical technique, (4) autohypnosis. Breathing patterns, alveolar gas samples and acid-base balance of maternal and umbilical cord blood were compared for the four groups of mothers. Hyperventilation was observed in all four groups of women, but the mothers prepared by the psychophysical method were more relaxed and overbreathed less than any other group.[6] Perhaps because of these minor difficulties, and in the natural course of the evolution of treatment, changes have taken place in various countries (see Suggested Reading) which include the introduction of a polysaccharide in the ninth month of pregnancy to enhance rapid dilatation of the cervix (Vellay in France). In America, the greatest change has come about with respect to breathing techniques. Many practitioners of psychoprophylaxis in the United States have deleted the rapid, shallow breathing from their teaching and now subscribe to a more moderate pattern which can be accelerated to follow the rhythm of the contraction and provide oxygen in sufficient quantity to prevent hyperventilation. The technique of Erna Wright of Great Britain has been incorporated in the many breathing patterns by the United States "prophylaxis" practitioners. The highest level of breathing is normal respiration while the patient silently but emphatically mouths the words to a song while simultaneously tapping the rhythm with her fingers. In her antepartal preparation she has chosen the song and practiced the mouth and tapping repeatedly. Today in these programs there is less emphasis on "one way" of breathing. Dr. Vellay, for instance, while advocating his particular breathing pattern, stresses that individual need, not formal rules, ought to govern the respiratory activity. After all, it is but part of the total scheme of conditioning.

The psychoprophylactic method and that of natural childbirth as introduced by Read and practiced by Thoms and others have, in fact, several points in common even though they derive from different theories (prophylaxis from the cortical-stimulation-conditioning response and natural childbirth from the fear-tension-pain syndrome). Both methods believe that (1) fear enhances the perception of pain but may diminish or disappear when the parturient knows about the physiology of labor, (2) psychic tension enhances the perception of pain but the parturient may relax more easily if childbirth takes place in a calm and agreeable atmosphere, and if good human contacts have been established between her and the personnel attending her, (3) muscular relaxation and a specific type of breathing diminish or abolish the pains of labor.[7]

Hypnosis

This technique is an induced state of extreme suggestibility in which the patient is insensible to outside impressions, except the suggestions of her attendant. There is no particular "program" associated with the use of this technique, rather training in achieving an hypnotic state or autohypnosis is usually given by an obstetrician who himself is especially trained in this area. While there is no general regimen for learning this technique the conditioning required is usually presented in several individual sessions at the time of the prenatal visits, usually in the latter half of pregnancy. The "modus operandi" of hypnotically induced relaxation has been explained by suggesting that whenever all the voluntary muscles are completely relaxed during labor, the uterus has a monopoly on available energy and hence can work more efficiently. In addition, it is likely that when fears are abolished or diminished efficient uterine action is promoted. The utilization of comfort measures, such as low back massage, has also been suggested as enhancing the hypnotic state. The major drawback to this technique lies in the difficulty in securing adequately prepared physicians.

[6] Buxton, R. St. J.: Maternal Respiration in Labor. The Obstetric Association of Chartered Physiotherapists, St. Albans, Herefordshire, England, 1969.

[7] de Watteville, P. H.: The use of obstetrical analgesia in the maternity hospital of Geneva. Am. J. Obstet. Gynec. 73:473, 1957.

PREPARATION FOR CHILDBEARING*

The Maternity Center Association has instituted a comprehensive program of parent education which has played an important part in making the events of pregnancy, labor, and the postpartal period more satisfying for families. The preparation aims at helping a mother to manage her body well in activity and rest, to use her natural resources effectively during labor, and to achieve optimal postpartal restoration. In addition, in this series of classes mothers and fathers discuss maternity care, general parental adjustment and infant needs, all of course, under the direction of a professional instructor. The exercises utilized to prepare the mother for labor emphasize an approach based on the principles of relaxation and are correlated with the total program of expectant parent education and antepartal care. It is important to remember that this method, as well as others, is not a substitute for pharmaceutical analgesics. However, it often lessens the need for chemical pain relief and sedation during labor and reinforces their effects. Whenever indicated, medication should be given and accepted early enough to enable the mother to stay in control of herself and to achieve her goal of conscious participation in her labor. The predominant consideration at all times is the health and well-being of the mother and infant.

Maternity Center Association emphasizes an approach to exercises which are utilized to prepare the mother for labor based on the principles of relaxation. Although there are other approaches the Association has found that the techniques described in their booklet enable mothers to achieve their objectives simply, without fatigue, and without imposing unnecessary strains or pressures.[8] Some of the exercises will enable the expectant mother to improve her muscle tone and carry out activities of daily living more easily. Others embody techniques more directly related to preparation for labor (i.e., for increasing muscle control and coordination) to facilitate the mother's response to the guidance of her professional attendants during labor. The third category of exercises here involve the return of the mother's body to the prepregnant state (postpartal restoration).

Comfort in pregnancy. The majority of women can maintain their usual work and play activities. However, changes do occur in weight and weight distribution. Comfort in pregnancy can be significantly improved by good posture and body mechanics in everyday activities. It is often possible to reduce or overcome discomfort by correct positions, body movements and exercises. Since the major postural changes begin in the second trimester of pregnancy, this is the logical time for learning. Correct posture for standing, sitting, and stair climbing, and good body mechanics for carrying packages or lifting objects should be reinforced. The spinal muscles and joints should be protected from undue strain, thus the mother needs to know how the feet can be used efficiently for balance and for movement.

Certain principles are applicable to activities in everyday living. For instance, activities should be varied (e.g., walking, standing, sitting, and they may need to be of shorter duration. Walking back and forth is preferable to standing still. When the mother does housework which requires standing (e.g., using equipment such as a mop), she should stand with one leg forward to enable her to shift her weight easily and efficiently from foot to foot and turn her body comfortably.

As she walks, she should keep her head erect, back upright and chin up and forward.

When the mother climbs stairs she should place her entire foot on the stair and use leg muscles to lift herself up each step, without leaning forward.

Whenever possible, the expectant mother should avoid stooping and lifting. When it becomes necessary to stoop, she should squat down in front of an object she wants to reach or lift. She should then squat down keeping her feet wide apart and her back straight. A good axiom to remember is "use the legs to spare the back." As an alternate method of squatting, have the mother place one foot in front and to the side of the other, as when taking a step forward, then she is ready to squat. In carrying bulky packages such as groceries, the load should be divided and carried in two hands if it seems heavy. Better still, the mother should let someone else do the lifting for her. Whenever possible a cart that rolls easily should be employed to carry heavy loads.

---

* Preparation for Childbearing is the title of a publication produced by the Maternity Center Association, 48 East 92nd Street, in New York. The illustrative material and much of the information in this section were provided through the courtesy of Maternity Center Association.

[8] Maternity Center Association: Preparation for Childbearing. Ed. 2, New York, 1969. Material on this subject as presented on pages 198 to 204 is either a condensation or direct quotation from this source. (Also see Table 13-2.)

A word should be mentioned about the height of the work surfaces in the home. These should be adjusted for the individual mother to minimize stooping and stretching. A footstool is often an invaluable aid for the mother when she is sitting.

For rest and comfort during pregnancy, the mother should learn the position for lying on her side, on her back, in the side relaxation position, and equally important, how to get up and out of bed without strain.

Backache is one of the most common complaints and *pelvic rocking* performed daily will help to relieve abdominal pressure and low back pain during pregnancy and early labor. This exercise is useful also to firm the abdominal muscles following the birth of the baby.

Other exercises to promote comfort and give relief from some of the common discomforts of pregnancy include *rib cage lifting, shoulder circling, leg elevating, hip elevating, and calf stretching* (see below and Maternity Center booklet "Preparation for Parenthood[9]").

Muscle Control

Two muscle groups undergo great changes during pregnancy, the abdominals and the muscles of the pelvic floor. The abdominal muscles stretch from the pressure of the enlarged uterus, the pelvic floor muscles soften to prepare for the vaginal delivery. Loss of muscle tone can be minimized during pregnancy and can be regained after delivery through proper exercise.

Abdominal contraction is an exercise which increases muscle tone and thus helps to strengthen the abdominal wall during pregnancy and the postpartal period. The mother should assume any comfortable position, even standing or walking, and tighten her abdominal muscles as much as she can, hold them for a few seconds, then relax. This should be repeated frequently throughout the day, and may be performed simultaneously with *pelvic floor contraction*. The latter exercise reduces congestion and general discomfort in the pelvic region and increases ability to control the muscles surrounding the orifice of the vagina, bowel, and bladder. It also improves muscle tone, thereby providing better support for the pelvic organs. Whenever exercises are taught to the patient with instructions to "repeat frequently throughout the day," the patient should understand about muscle fatigue and its consequences which may result from overdoing.

[9] Op. cit., pp. 4-23.

Relief of Common Discomforts that May Occur During Pregnancy

Discomfort	Exercise or Position
Leaking urine when coughing, laughing	Pelvic floor contraction
Abdominal pain when coughing	Abdominal contraction
Heaviness in pelvis	Knee-chest; pelvic floor contraction
Hemorrhoids and swelling around vagina	Knee-chest; resting with hips elevated; pelvic floor contraction
Low back pain—one side	Knee-chest
Cramps in thighs, buttocks	Knee-chest
Cramps in legs	Leg elevating; calf stretching
Tired legs	Leg elevating; calf stretching
Varicose veins in legs	Leg elevating; calf stretching
Shortness of breath	Good posture; good body mechanics; rib cage lifting
Low backache	Pelvic rocking; good posture; pushing posture; squatting
Middle backache	Pushing position
Upper backache	Shoulder circling; good posture
Numbness in arms and fingers	Shoulder circling; lying on side
Abdominal muscle spasm (stitch)	Squatting; pushing posture

Conscious Relaxation

Relaxation is one of the most natural activities known to man. However, human beings living in a civilized society, unlike their feline pets, seem to have forgotten how to relax naturally.

Relaxation enables a person to obtain maximum benefit from any rest period, it relieves bodily tensions that cramp muscles, producing fatigue, and promotes a feeling of physical and mental well-being.

Physical relaxation may reduce the pain of labor and equally important, can put the mother in a calm frame of mind which permits her to cope more effectively with the demands of her situation.

The key to relaxation may be found in two principles—**correct posture** and **proper breathing.** Correct posture minimizes muscular stress, and coupled with this, controlled breathing makes it easier to relax.

Once the mother has developed the art of relaxing by using the following techniques, she is advised to practice regularly and at other times when she is under pressure or excited. The mother may need to be reminded that her ultimate purpose in this preparation is to be able to relax during labor, when feelings of excitement and tension are apt to run high.

Complete Breath and Breath Control—Technique 1

A complete breath is one in which the chest wall epands and the diaphragm descends to its maximum extent. The breath is let out slowly under pressure so that a more complete exchange of oxygen and carbon dioxide can take place. It is used periodically during relaxation and should be followed by slow, quiet, easy respiration (see Fig. 10-2).

1. Breathe in once as deeply as possible.
2. Hiss or blow the air out slowly, letting your whole body go limp.
3. Continue breathing quietly, easily and rhythmically.
4. Let yourself go completely loose.
5. Soon your body will begin to feel very heavy and any exertion will be difficult. You can test this out:
   a. Gradually bend an elbow bringing your hand toward your chin. Notice how much effort this requires.
   b. Slowly lower your arm to its resting position. Again you will find yourself actually working to prevent its falling too quickly.

Breath Control in the First Stage of Labor

Application of Complete Breathing to Labor

1. Pretend that you are having a contraction lasting 30 to 45 seconds.
2. At the beginning of each contraction take a complete breath and hiss or blow it out.
3. Breathe deeply, slowly and rhythmically (see throughout the remainder of the contraction).

Fig. 10-2. Complete breath and breath control. (Maternity Center Asssociation: Preparation for Childbearing, ed. 2, p. 27, Fig. 22, New York, 1969)

4. When the contraction has ended, take another complete breath and hiss or blow it out slowly.
5. Return to normal breathing between contractions.
6. During labor, you will continue to use this pattern of breathing with contractions as long as it continues to be helpful (Fig. 10-3).

Modified Complete Breathing

As labor advances and contractions increase in strength, there is often a desire on the mother's part to keep the diaphragm as still as possible. Yet, the uterus continues to need a good supply of oxygen. For this reason the mother should breathe deeply as the contraction begins and ends, and modify her breathing so that it is quiet and shallow at the peak of each contraction. To practice this:

1. Pretend that you are having stronger contractions, lasting almost a minute.
2. Breathe in deeply as the contraction starts. Then slowly hiss or blow out, letting yourself go completely limp.
3. Make each of the next four or five breaths a little shallower than the previous one. Soon you will notice that you are breathing very lightly.
4. Light breathing is quiet and effortless, almost like a throat breath. Experiment to find your own comfortable rate and continue for 15 to 45 seconds. If you become dizzy or lightheaded, your breathing is too vigorous. If you have trouble getting enough air or difficulty maintaining the rhythm, try taking a quick, deep breath, and return to light breathing.
5. Make each of the next four or five breaths a little deeper than the previous one.
6. End the breath pattern with one complete breath (see Fig. 10-4).

Fig. 10-3. Application of complete breathing to labor. (Maternity Center Association: Preparation for Childbearing, ed. 2, p. 30, Fig. 23, New York, 1969)

Fig. 10-4. Modified complete breathing. Maternity Center Association: (Preparation for Childbearing, ed. 2, p. 30, Fig. 24, New York, 1969)

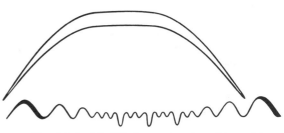

Fig. 10-5. Modified complete breathing with adaptation for transition. (New York Maternity Center: Preparation for Childbearing, ed. 2, p. 31, Fig. 25, New York, 1969)

Further Adaptation for Transition

(For the latter part of the first stage of labor, if you feel a tendency to hold your breath or to push during strong contractions) do the modified complete breath, but with one important change: *During light breathing, puff out gently as you exhale on every third or fourth breath* (see Fig. 10-5).

Pushing Position with Pushing Breath for Second Stage

During the second stage of labor, the mother pushes, actively helping in the delivery of her baby. Contractions at this time last 60 to 65 seconds and generally are accompanied by a strong urge to push. To practice for this (see Fig. 10-6):

1. Lie on your back with head and shoulders elevated. Pillows may be used for practice at home. In the labor room the head of the bed may be elevated.
2. Bend your knees and separate your legs.
3. Take a deep breath and hiss or blow out.

4. Breathe in as quickly and deeply as you can; then hold your breath. (In labor, this "held" breath will help to fix your diaphragm so that your abdominal wall will make more effective downward pressure on the uterus and baby, aiding the baby's birth.)
5. Draw up your legs against your abdomen, in a squatting position, holding your legs or feet with your hands. (On the delivery table your feet and legs will be supported in stirrups so that you won't have to hold them, and there will be handle on which to pull.) Raise head.
6. During practice, do *not* actually push. You will be able to do so in labor.
7. Take *catch breaths* as needed. A catch breath is a short breath that may be taken whenever you can no longer hold your breath comfortably. Try to take no more than two or three catch breaths in each 60 to 65 second breath pattern.
   a. Maintain the pushing position.

b. Exhale, moving your head back.
   c. Take in a quick, deep breath.
   d. Tilt your head forward again and hold your breath.
8. When the contraction is over, relax completely, take a deep breath and sigh it out.

Note: *You may wish to practice breath holding and catch breaths without assuming the pushing position. You may do this while sitting in a chair by following the instructions relating to breathing described above.*

Practice Position for the Delivery Table

On the delivery table the mother's legs and feet are supported in stirrups, adjusted to the mother's comfort. It is important that the inner thigh and pelvic floor muscles be relaxed so that they offer no resistance to the baby's oncoming head (see Fig. 9-7). Practice relaxation of these muscles as follows:

FIG. 10-6. Pushing position. (Maternity Center Association: Preparation for Childbearing, ed. 2, p. 32, Fig. 26, New York, 1969)

Fig. 10-7. Practice position for the delivery table. (Maternity Center Association: Preparation for Childbearing, ed. 2, p. 33, Fig. 27, New York, 1969)

1. Lie flat on your back.
2. Draw up your knees and place your feet flat on the bed.
3. Tense your inner thigh and pelvic floor muscles.
4. Relax these muscles, allowing your knees to drop apart gradually.
5. Have your husband apply gentle pressure to your knees and outer thighs so that he is supporting them in a widely separated position and you do not experience a pulling sensation.
6. Remain in this relaxed position for a few minutes.

Panting

Your doctor may tell you to pant or to stop pushing in the middle of a contraction. If so, begin panting immediately. This will make your diaphragm move up and down. Although this will not decrease the desire to push, it will physically prevent you from doing so. To practice panting:

1. Start doing the exercise described on pages 201-202 (Pushing Position with Pushing Breath).
2. All at once, drop your head and shoulders, allowing your arms and hands to relax.

3. Breathe in and out very quickly, keeping your mouth open—like a panting dog.
4. Continue breathing this way until contraction ends (see Fig. 10-8).

Postpartum

During the puerperium, the 6 weeks following childbirth, the body undergoes major changes. The organs that had adjusted during pregnancy to make room for the growing baby gradually return to their original positions in the mother's body.

Fig. 10-8. Diagrammatic breath pattern for panting. (Maternity Center Association: Preparation for Childbearing, ed. 2, p. 34, Fig. 28, New York, 1969)

Fig. 10-9. Prone position for rest and relaxation postpartally. (Maternity Center Association: Preparation for Childbearing, ed. 2, p. 35, Fig. 29, New York, 1969)

The uterus, cervix, and vagina slowly return to the non-pregnant state. Important hormonal changes also occur. In effect, a bodily transformation that took 9 months to complete is being reversed in the course of a few weeks.

Good nutrition and adequate rest are essential during this period. A new mother needs at least one rest period each day. Lying on the abdomen may help her uterus to return to good position (see Fig. 10-9). A pillow under the hips when lying this way prevents back strain.

Knee-chest Position. Such exercises as the knee-chest position are advised and regulated by the obstetrician, according to the individual mother's condition. If the mother has had an abnormal delivery or any extensive perineal repair, exercises may not be advisable. Any exercises prescribed for the mother should not be strenuous or tiring when used in moderation. They should be practiced slowly and rhythmically, only a few times at first and gradually increased from day to day (see Chap. 8).

The knee-chest position may be advised by some physicians to encourage the uterus to return to its normal position, particularly if the organ is retroverted. When this exercise is employed, the physician usually instructs the patient to start the exercise about the 3rd postpartal week, beginning with 2-minute periods each morning and evening and gradually increasing the time to 5 minutes twice daily. Patients should never be put in the knee-chest position *without specific orders from the physician.* Because of the anatomic relationship of the bladder to the uterus, the patient should empty her bladder first. The advantage to be gained from this exercise depends on the position of the pelvis. In order to attain the correct attitude of the pelvis, the patient's thighs should remain erect (perpendicular to the floor) while her back is carefully positioned so that it does not sag (Fig. 15-22). Care must be taken to see that the external genitalia are not drawn open to allow air to enter the vagina. The danger of a fatal air embolism occurring in such situations has been reported (see Suggested Reading). To avoid this tragic complication, postpartal knee-chest exercises should be withheld until the first 4 weeks post delivery.

SUGGESTED READING

Teaching and Learning Process:

Cantor, N.: The Dynamics of Learning. ed. 2, Buffalo, New York, Foster and Stewart, 1950.

————: The Teaching-Learning Process. Buffalo, New York, Dryden Press, 1953.

Gorman, A. H.: Teachers and Learners: The Interactive Process in Education. Boston, Allyn and Bacon, 1969.

Redman, B. K.: The Process of Patient Teaching in Nursing. St. Louis, C. V. Mosby, 1968.

Teaching Expectant Parent Groups:

Auerbach, A. B.: Parents Learn Through Discussion: Principles and Practices of Parent Group Education. New York, John Wiley & Sons, 1968.

————: Training for leadership in parent group education. Nurs. Outlook 14:38-40, April, 1966.

Bing, E.: Six Practical Lessons for an Easier Childbirth. New York, Grosset and Dunlap, 1967.

Brim, O. G.: Education for Child Rearing. New York, The Free Press, 1965.

Buxton, C. L.: A Study of Psychophysical Methods for Relief of Childbirth Pain. Philadelphia, W. B. Saunders, 1962.

Dalzell, I.: Evaluation of a prenatal teaching program. Nurs. Res. 14:160-163, Spring, 1965.

Fielding, W., and Benjamin, L.: The Childbirth Challenge: Common Sense Versus "Natural" Methods. New York, Viking Press, 1962.

Fyalkowski, W.: New ways of psychophysical preparation for childbirth. Am. J. Obstet. Gynec. 92: 1018-1022, August 1, 1965.

Gardiner, S. H.: Expectant Parent and Sex Education. Proceedings from American Medical Association National Conference on Infant Mortality, August 12-13, 1966.

Genne, W. H.: Husbands and Pregnancy. New York, Association Press, 1956.

Goodrich, F. W., Jr.: Preparing for Childbirth. Englewood Cliffs, Prentice-Hall, 1966.

Karmel, M.: Thank You, Dr. Lamaze. Philadelphia, J. B. Lippincott Co., 1959.

Leppert, P., and Williams, B.: Birth films may miscarry. Am. J. Nurs. 68:2181-2183, October, 1968.

Maternity Center Association: Preparation for Childbearing. ed. 2, New York, The Association, 1969.

McCaffery, M. S.: An approach to parent education. Nurs. Forum 6:77-93, 1967.

Perchard, S.: Hypnosis and the pregnant woman. Nurs. Mirror 124:i-v, April 7, 1967.

Read, G. D.: Childbirth Without Fear, Rev. ed., New York, Harper Brothers, 1953.

Ulin, P.: Changing Techniques in psychoprophylactic preparation for childbirth. Am. J. Nurs. 68:2586-2591, December, 1968.

———: The exhilarating moment of birth. Am. J. Nurs. 63:60-67, June, 1963.

Yahia, C., and Ulin, P.: Preliminary experience with a psychophysical program of preparation for childbirth. Am. J. Obstet. Gynec. 93:942-949, December 1, 1965.

Study Questions

Unit Two: Nursing in Pregnancy

Read through the entire question and place your answer on the line to the right.

1. Below are some signs, symptoms and conditions commonly associated with pregnancy. Those which the patient might notice and describe in the first trimester of pregnancy are:
   A. Amenorrhea
   B. Enlargement and tenderness of breasts
   C. Enlargement of uterus
   D. Frequent micturition
   E. Goodell's sign

   Select the number corresponding to the correct letters.
   1. A and C
   2. A, B and D
   3. B, D and E
   4. All of them   _2_

2. A. In pregnancy, morning sickness is most common during which of the following periods?
      1. First month
      2. First 6 weeks
      3. Sixth to 12th week
      4. First 4 months
      5. Eighth to 16th week   _3_

   B. A patient complains of morning sickness. Which of the following measures should the nurse suggest as a possible means of overcoming this discomfort?
      1. Keep the stomach empty when nausea is present.
      2. Drink plenty of water upon arising.
      3. Eat 6 small meals instead of 3 per day.
      4. Increase daily intake of whole milk.   _3_

3. A pregnant woman seen for the first time in the antepartal clinic has a hemoglobin of 70 percent. The nurse should understand that this condition is:
   A. A true anemia
   B. Caused by increased blood volume
   C. Dangerous to baby's development
   D. Predisposing to postpartal hemorrhage   _B_

4. The nurse in the obstetrician's office should instruct the patient regarding the collection of the specimen for the Aschheim-Zondek test by telling the patient to:
   A. Save the first voided specimen in the morning.
   B. Withhold fluid intake during the night and collect the first voided specimen in the morning.
   C. Report to the laboratory in the morning for a blood specimen.
   D. Take a warm voided specimen to the laboratory.   _B_

5. Though the pregnant woman is usually advised to include a quart of milk in her diet daily, which of the following, if any, would justify the omission of milk?
   A. Milk makes her constipated.

B. She is gaining weight too rapidly.
C. She is not gaining fast enough and needs more concentrated foods.
D. Milk causes a feeling of fullness, decreasing her appetite for other foods.
E. Milk causes heartburn.
F. None of the above; milk should not be omitted.   _F_

6. The most essential foods in a 2,300-calorie diet for a pregnant woman are:
A. High in carbohydrate, low in protein
B. High in protein, low in carbohydrate
C. High in protein, low in fat
D. High in fat, low in protein   _C_

7. The nurse in the antepartal clinic will encourage the pregnant woman to see her dentist at the earliest convenience because:
A. Each baby causes the mother to lose one tooth.
B. Bone development of the baby requires calcium.
C. Foci of infection should be removed early in pregnancy.
D. The increased carbohydrate needed in pregnancy is detrimental to sound teeth.   _C_

8. What instruction should the clinic patient be given concerning the care of her breasts during pregnancy?
A. A brassière should:
  1. Not be worn
  2. Be worn snugly enough to support and lift up the breasts
  3. Be worn snugly enough to press the breasts flat against the chest wall
  4. Be worn snugly enough to apply constant firm pressure toward the midline   _2_

B. Special care of the nipples should begin:
  1. As early as pregnancy is confirmed
  2. Between the 3rd and 4th months
  3. Between the 6th and 7th months
  4. At the beginning of the 9th month   _3_

9. "Preparation for Childbearing" is a term applied to a maternity center's program in antepartal education.
A. The program includes certain "exercises" as one aspect of preparation. Which of the following are these "exercises" intended to accomplish?
  1. Promote control of muscle tension for coordination and economy of effort in all the mother's activities
  2. Develop intra-abdominal space for uterine enlargement
  3. Obviate the need for pharmaceutical analgesics   _1_

B. The program prepares the pregnant patient for some of the experiences of labor. In addition to muscular control, which of the following measures will be most helpful to her during labor?
  1. Sympathetic care
  2. Moderately heavy sedation
  3. Understanding the progress of labor   _3_

C. Which of the following best explains the purpose of conscious control of respiration during the first stage of labor?
  1. Gives mechanical relief of pressure by depression of the diaphragm to expand the abdominal wall
  2. Limits the downward movement of the diaphragm through restriction of breathing to the upper chest
  3. Gives the patient a calming rhythmic activity upon which to concentrate   _3_

10. A. If the pregnant woman complained of painful, swollen veins in the legs, the nurse would understand that the condition would be likely to be due to:
   1. Infection of the blood-vessel wall
   2. Toxins accumulating in the blood
   3. Pressure against the veins in the pelvis
   4. Pressure directly against the walls of the arteries
   5. Force of gravity   ___3___

   B. To remedy this condition, the nurse would expect that the patient would be advised that she should:
   1. Refrain from wearing restricting clothing around the legs or the abdomen
   2. Refrain from wearing a girdle
   3. Lie down each day for an hour's rest
   4. Apply an Ace bandage, starting above the source of obstruction   ___1___

11. The nurse teaching parents' classes should stress the importance of which one of the following?
   A. Husbands doing the housework for their wives during the period of pregnancy
   B. The idea of sharing responsibility in parenthood
   C. The causes of invalidism during pregnancy
   D. The moral responsibility of being parents   ___B___

12. If a woman 6 months pregnant asked if she should or should not wear a girdle, in your opinion the patient should be advised:
   A. To avoid wearing any girdle
   B. To adjust her regular girdle loosely
   C. To wear a girdle that will keep the uterus from rising too high in the abdomen
   D. To wear a girdle that will firmly support the lower portion of the abdomen and the back
   E. To wear a girdle that will not disclose her condition   ___D___

13. The reason that pregnant women are warned against wearing high-heeled shoes from the 7th to the 9th months is:
   A. To avoid additional backstrain
   B. To increase venous pressure in the legs
   C. To allow freer movement in taking daily exercises
   D. To dress themselves according to current styles   ___A___

14. The expectant mother who is employed as a stenographer should be advised that:
   A. Rest periods are unnecessary if the job requires only "desk work."
   B. Part-time employment should be requested after the 4th month of pregnancy.
   C. A position which requires moderate manual labor would be more advantageous because it affords physical exercise.
   D. Employment should be discontinued if the work causes moderate fatigue.   ___D___

15. The clinic nurse would expect the pregnant patient to be advised to get in touch with her doctor *immediately* as soon as she observed which of the following?
   A. Abdominal pain
   B. Bleeding with bright blood
   C. Blood-streaked mucus
   D. Chills and fever
   E. Constipation

                            Select the number corresponding to the correct letters.
                            1. A, B and D
                            2. B, C and E
                            3. C, D and E
                            4. All of them

16. In teaching the pregnant woman how to take a vaginal douche prescribed by the physician, the following should be emphasized:
    A. A hand-bulb syringe is satisfactory if the mother is accustomed to using it.
    B. The medicated solution must be prepared according to the physician's instructions.
    C. The external genitalia should be cleansed with soap and water before taking a douche.
    D. The douche may be aken while sitting on the toilet if the douche bag is placed no higher than 2 feet above the level of the hips.
    E. The douche nozzle should be inserted gently into the vagina as far as it will go.

    Select the number corresponding to the correct letters.
    1. A and B
    2. B and C
    3. B, D and E
    4. All of them   2

17. During her first visit to the clinic the mother confides to the nurse that she is afraid to have a baby. The most appropriate response of the nurse might be:
    A. "Modern obstetrics makes having a baby so safe that you have absolutely nothing to fear."
    B. "Perhaps if you discussed this with a psychiatrist he would help you to overcome this feeling."
    C. "Many women feel this way, so I wouldn't be concerned about it if I were you."
    D. "I can understand that you might feel this way. What is it in particular that you are worried about?"   D

    Note: The key to the correct answers to these questions is given on page 613.

Study Questions

Unit Two: Nursing in Pregnancy

Read through the entire question and place your answer on the line to the right.

1. Below are some signs, symptoms and conditions commonly associated with pregnancy. Those which the patient might notice and describe in the first trimester of pregnancy are:
   A. Amenorrhea
   B. Enlargement and tenderness of breasts
   C. Enlargement of uterus
   D. Frequent micturition
   E. Goodell's sign

   Select the number corresponding to the correct letters.
   1. A and C
   2. A, B and D
   3. B, D and E
   4. All of them   _____

2. A. In pregnancy, morning sickness is most common during which of the following periods?
   1. First month
   2. First 6 weeks
   3. Sixth to 12th week
   4. First 4 months
   5. Eighth to 16th week   _____

   B. A patient complains of morning sickness. Which of the following measures should the nurse suggest as a possible means of overcoming this discomfort?
   1. Keep the stomach empty when nausea is present.
   2. Drink plenty of water upon arising.
   3. Eat 6 small meals instead of 3 per day.
   4. Increase daily intake of whole milk.   _____

3. A pregnant woman seen for the first time in the antepartal clinic has a hemoglobin of 70 percent. The nurse should understand that this condition is:
   A. A true anemia
   B. Caused by increased blood volume
   C. Dangerous to baby's development
   D. Predisposing to postpartal hemorrhage   _____

4. The nurse in the obstetrician's office should instruct the patient regarding the collection of the specimen for the Aschheim-Zondek test by telling the patient to:
   A. Save the first voided specimen in the morning.
   B. Withhold fluid intake during the night and collect the first voided specimen in the morning.
   C. Report to the laboratory in the morning for a blood specimen.
   D. Take a warm voided specimen to the laboratory.   _____

5. Though the pregnant woman is usually advised to include a quart of milk in her diet daily, which of the following, if any, would justify the omission of milk?
   A. Milk makes her constipated.

UNIT THREE
Nursing During Labor and Delivery

Phenomena of Labor
Analgesia and Anesthesia for Labor
Conduct of Normal Labor

Phenomena of Labor

11

Labor refers to the series of processes by which the products of conception are expelled from the mother's body (Fig. 11-1). The terms "childbirth," "travail," "accouchement" and "confinement" have all been used at one time or another to refer to labor. The word "delivery" refers, as a rule, to the actual delivery of the baby.

PREMONITORY SIGNS OF LABOR

During the last few weeks of pregnancy a number of changes indicate that the time of labor is approaching. Particularly in primigravidas, "lightening" occurs about 10 to 14 days before delivery. This alteration is brought about by a settling of the fetal head into the pelvis (Fig. 11-2). This may occur at any time during the last 4 weeks, but occasionally does not occur until labor actually has begun. Lightening may take place suddenly, so that the expectant mother arises one morning entirely relieved of the abdominal tightness and diaphragmatic pressure that she had experienced previously (Fig. 6-6). But the relief in one direction often is followed by signs of greater pressure below, such as shooting pains down the legs from pressure on the sciatic nerves, an increase in the amount of vaginal discharge and greater frequency of urination due to pressure on the bladder. In mothers who have had previous children, lightening is more likely to occur after labor begins.

For a varying period before the establishment of true labor, the patients often will suffer from so-called "false labor." The nurse should be able to distinguish between this and effective uterine contractions. True labor contractions will produce a demonstrable degree of dilatation of the cervix in the course of a few hours. On the other hand, false labor contractions do not affect the cervix. The crux of the matter, then, between true and false labor is whether or not the uterine contractions effect cervical effacement and dilatation.

False contractions may begin as early as 3 or 4 weeks before the termination of pregnancy. They are merely an exaggeration of the intermittent uterine contractions which have occurred throughout the entire period of gestation but are now accompanied by discomfort. They are confined chiefly to the lower part of the abdomen and the groin and do not increase in intensity, frequency and duration. The discomfort is rarely intensified if the mother walks about and may even be relieved if she is on her feet. Examination will reveal no changes in the cervix. The signs that accompany true labor contractions present a contrasting picture. True labor contractions usually are felt in the lower back and extend in girdlelike fashion from the back to the front of the abdomen. They have a definite rhythm and gradually increase in frequency, intensity and duration. In the course of a few hours of true labor contractions a progressive effacement and dilatation of the cervix is apparent.

Another sign of impending labor is pink "show." After the discharge of the mucous plug that has filled the cervical canal during pregnancy, the pressure of the descending presenting part of the fetus causes the minute capillaries in the cervix to rupture. This blood is mixed with mucus and therefore has the pink tinge. The nurse should understand that pink show is simply the appearance of a small amount of blood-tinged mucus. Any substantial discharge of blood should be reported to the physician.

FIG. 11-1. "The Birth Relief." This distinguished sculptured relief depicts the 9 stages of birth with vertex presentation from before labor through the delivery of the placenta. (Dickinson-Belskie models, Cleveland Health Museum, Cleveland)

Fig. 11-2. Before labor, showing the uterus relaxed with the cervix closed and thick pelvic floor. (Dickinson-Belskie models, Cleveland Health Museum, Cleveland)

Occasionally, rupture of the membranes is the first indication of approaching labor. It used to be thought that this was a grave sign, heralding a long and difficult dry labor, but present-day statistics show that this is not true. Nevertheless, the physician should be notified at once; under these circumstances, he may advise the patient to enter the hospital immediately. After the rupture of the membranes there is always the possibility of a prolapsed cord if the presenting part does not adequately fill the pelvic inlet. This is more likely if the infant presents as a footling breech, or by the shoulder, or in the vertex presentation when the fetal head has not de-scended far enough into the true pelvis prior to the rupture of the membranes (see Fig. 20-6).

CAUSE OF ONSET OF LABOR

Regardless of species, whether the fetus weighs 2 Gm. at the end of a 21 day pregnancy, as in the mouse, or whether it weighs 200 pounds at the end of a 640-day pregnancy, as in the elephant, labor usually begins at the right time for that particular species, namely, when the fetus is mature enough to cope with extra-uterine conditions but not yet large enough to cause mechanical difficulties in labor. The process responsible for this beautifully synchronized and salutary

Fig. 11-3. First stage of labor. The rhythmic contractions of the uterus aid the progressive effacement and dilatation of the cervix, as well as the descent of the infant. (Dickinson-Belskie models,
Cleveland Health Museum, Cleveland)

achievement is obscure. A number of theories
have been advanced to explain the phenomenon.
Some of them are increased sensitivity of the
myometrium to oxytocin, decreased local sub-
placental progesterone level, and increased uterine
irritability as a result of stretching from expanding contents.

UTERINE CONTRACTIONS

In all languages the word for the uterine contractions of labor has been interpreted the same,
namely, "pain." The degree of discomfort during
labor varies considerably from patient to patient.
The patient who anticipates a painful experience
will have more pain than the patient who is

properly prepared for what can be a good experience. In order to allay preexisting fear, one
should refer to uterine contractions as "contractions," not "pains." The duration of these contractions ranges from 45 to 90 seconds, averaging
about 1 minute. Each contraction presents three
phases: a period during which the intensity of
the contraction increases (increment), a period
during which the contraction is at its height
(acme), and a period of diminishing intensity
(decrement). The increment, or crescendo phase,
is longer than the other two combined. The
contractions of the uterus during labor are intermittent, with periods of relaxation between, resembling, in this respect, the systole and the

diastole of the heart. The interval between contractions diminishes gradually from about 10 minutes early in labor to about 2 or 3 minutes in the second stage. These periods of relaxation not only provide rest for the uterine muscles and for the mother, but also are essential to the welfare of the fetus, since unremitting contractions may so interfere with placental functions that the resulting lack of oxygen produces fetal distress. Another characteristic of labor contractions is that they are quite involuntary, their action being not only independent of the mother's will, but also of extra-uterine nervous control.

During labor, the uterus is soon differentiated into two identifiable portions—the upper and lower uterine segments. The upper segment is the active, contractile portion of the uterus. Its function is to expel the uterine contents. It displays a decreasing gradient of intensity of contractions from the fundus downward. As labor progresses, a passive lower segment is developed. With each contraction, the muscle fibers of the upper segment retract, becoming shorter as the fetus descends. The upper segment, therefore, becomes thicker. Fibers of the lower segment stretch and, consequently, it becomes thinner. The distinct boundary between the upper and lower uterine segments is referred to as a physiologic retraction ring.

DURATION OF LABOR

Although there is usually some degree of variation in all labors, an estimate of the average length of labor can be based on studies of records of some several thousand primigravidas and multiparas.

The average duration of first labors is about 14 hours, approximately 12½ hours in the first stage, 1 hour and 20 minutes in the second stage, and 10 minutes in the third stage.

The average duration of multiparous labors is approximately 6 hours shorter than for first labors; for example, 7 hours and 20 minutes in the first stage, a half hour in the second stage, and 10 minutes in the third stage.

During the first stage of labor full dilatation

MEAN LABOR CURVE

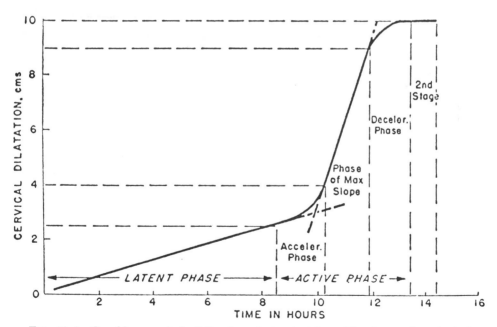

FIG. 11-4. Graphic appraisal of the time factor in labor. The *latent phase* includes that portion of the first stage between the onset of labor contractions and acceleration in the rate of cervical dilatation. The upswing in the curve denotes the onset of the *active phase* of the first stage of labor, which includes the accelerated phase, the phase of maximum slope and the deceleration phase. (Friedman, E. A.: Graphic appraisal of labor. A study of 500 primigravidas, Bull. Sloane Hosp. Wom. 1:42, 1955)

of the cervix (10 cm.) is accomplished, but for the greater part of this time the progress of cervical dilatation is slow. This has been clearly demonstrated in Friedman's study of 500 labors of primigravidous women (Fig. 11-4). From his study labor is divided into the latent phase and the active phase. The *latent phase,* from the onset of uterine contractions, takes many hours and accomplishes little cervical dilatation. But with the beginning of the *active phase,* cervical dilatation proceeds at an accelerated rate and then reaches a deceleration phase shortly before the second stage of labor.

The first 4 cm. of cervical dilatation occurs during the slow, latent phase. The remainder of cervical dilatation is accomplished much more rapidly in the active phase. Hence, 5 cm. of dilatation has taken the patient well past the halfway point in labor, even though 10 cm. represents full dilatation. In fact, at that point the average labor is more than two thirds over.

THE THREE STAGES OF LABOR

The process of labor is divided, for convenience of description, into three distinct stages.

The first stage of labor, *or the dilating stage, begins with the first true labor contraction and ends with the complete dilatation of the cervix.*

This stage may be further subdivided into the latent phase and the active phase.

The second stage of labor, *or the stage of expulsion, begins with the complete dilatation of the cervix and ends with the delivery of the baby.*

The third stage of labor, *or the placental stage, begins with the delivery of the baby and terminates with the birth of the placenta.*

The First Stage of Labor

In the beginning of the first stage the contractions are short, slight, or 10 or 15 minutes or more apart and may not cause the patient any particular discomfort. She may be walking about and is generally quite comfortable between contractions. Early in the first stage the sensation is usually located in the small of the back, but, as time goes on, it sweeps around, girdlelike, to the anterior part of the abdomen. The contractions recur at shortening intervals, every 3 to 5 minutes, and become stronger and last longer. Indeed, the contractions which immediately precede full dilatation are often of increased intensity. At this time, there is usually a marked increase in the amount of show due to rupture of capillary vessels in the cervix and the lower uterine segment.

As the result of the uterine contractions, two important changes occur in the cervix during the

Fig. 11-5. Cervix in primigravida. (*Top, left*) At beginning of labor; no effacement or dilatation. (*Top, right*) About one half effaced, but no dilatation. (*Bottom, left*) Completely effaced, but no dilatation. (*Bottom, right*) Complete dilatation. (Bumm)

Fig. 11-6. Full dilatation: cervix high, head deep in birth canal, membranes intact. (Dickinson-Belskie models, Cleveland Health Museum, Cleveland)

first stage of labor—*effacement and dilatation* (Fig. 11-3).

Effacement is the shortening of the cervical canal from a structure 1 or 2 cm. in length to one in which no canal at all exists, but merely a circular orifice with almost paper-thin edges. As may be seen in Figure 11-5, the edges of the internal os are drawn several centimeters upward, so that the former cervical mucosa becomes part of the lower uterine segment. In primigravidas, effacement is usually complete before dilatation begins, but in multiparas it is rarely complete, dilatation proceeding, as a rule, with rather thick cervical edges. Synonymous with effacement are the terms "obliteration" and "taking up" of the cervix.

Dilatation of the Cervix. This means the enlargement of the cervical os from an orifice a few millimeters in size to an aperture large enough to permit the passage of the fetus—that is, to a diameter of about 10 cm. When the cervix can no longer be felt, dilatation is said to be complete. Although the forces concerned in dilatation are not well understood, several factors appear to be involved. The muscle fibers about the cervix are so arranged that they pull upon its edges and tend to draw it open. The uterine contractions make pressure on the amniotic sac and this, in turn, burrows into the cervix in pouchlike fashion exerting a dilating action (Fig. 11-6). In the absence of the membranes, the pressure of the presenting part against the cervix and the lower uterine segment has a similar effect.

Dilatation of the cervix in the first stage of labor is solely the result of uterine contractions which are involuntary. In other words, there is nothing that the mother can do, such as bearing down, which will help the slightest in expediting this period of labor. Indeed, bearing-down efforts at this stage serve only to exhaust the mother and cause the cervix to become edematous.

The Second Stage of Labor

The contractions are now strong and long, lasting 50 to 70 seconds and occurring at intervals of 2 or 3 minutes. Rupture of the membranes usually occurs during the early part of this stage of labor, with a gush of amniotic fluid from the vagina. Sometimes, however, membranes rupture during the first stage and occasionally before labor begins. In rare cases the baby is born in a "caul," which is a piece of the amnion that sometimes envelops the baby's head. Superstitious parents consider this to be a good omen.

During this stage, as if by reflex action, the muscles of the abdomen are brought into play; and when the contractions are in progress the patient will strain, or "bear down," with all her strength so that her face becomes flushed, and the large vessels in her neck are distended. As a result of this exertion she may perspire profusely.

Fig. 11-7. Extreme bulging of perineum showing patulous and everted anus.

During this stage the mother directs all her energy toward expelling the contents of the uterus. There is a marked pressure in the area of the perineum and rectum, and the urge to bear down is usually beyond the control of the patient.

Toward the end of the second stage, when the head is well down in the vagina, its pressure causes the anus to become patulous and everted (Fig. 11-7), and often small particles of fecal material may be expelled from the rectum with each contraction. This should receive careful attention to avoid contamination. As the head descends still further, the perineal region begins to bulge, and the skin over it becomes tense and glistening. At this time the scalp of the fetus may be detected through a slitlike vulvar opening (Fig. 11-8). With each subsequent contraction the perineum bulges more and more, and the vulva becomes more dilated and distended by the head, so that the opening is gradually converted into an ovoid and at last into a circle. With the cessation of each contraction the opening becomes smaller, and the head recedes from it until it advances again with the next contraction.

The contractions now occur very rapidly, with scarcely any interval between. As the head becomes increasingly visible, the vulva is stretched further and finally encircles the largest diameter of the baby's head. This encirclement of the largest diameter of the baby's head by the vulvar ring is known as "crowning." The physician usually does an episiotomy at this time, supports the tissues surrounding the perineum and delivers the head. One or two more contractions are normally enough to effect the birth of the baby.

Whereas in the first stage of labor the forces are limited to uterine action, during the second stage two forces are essential, namely, uterine contractions and intra-abdominal pressure, the latter being brought about by the bearing-down efforts of the mother. (The force exerted by the mother's bearing down can be likened to that used in forcing an evacuation of the bowels.) Both forces are essential to the successful spontaneous outcome of the second stage of labor, for uterine contractions without bearing-down efforts are of little avail in expelling the infant, while, conversely, bearing-down efforts in the absence of uterine contractions are futile. As explained in Chapter 13, Conduct of Normal Labor, these facts have most important practical implications.

The Mechanism of Labor. In its passage

Fig. 11-8. Second stage of labor. "Caput," or top of infant's head, begins to appear through the vulvar opening. (Dickinson-Belskie models, Cleveland Health Museum, Cleveland)

through the birth canal, the presenting part of the fetus undergoes certain positional changes which constitute the mechanism of labor. These movements are designed to present the smallest possible diameters of the presenting part to the irregular shape of the pelvic canal, so that it will encounter as little resistance as possible. The mechanism of labor consists of a combination of movements, several of which may be going on at the same time. As they occur, the uterine contractions bring about important modifications in the attitude or habitus of the fetus, especially after the head has descended into the pelvis. This adaptation of the baby to the birth canal, as descent takes place, involves four processes, flexion, internal rotation, extension and external rotation (Fig. 11-9).

For purposes of instruction, the various movements will be described as if they occurred independently.

Descent. The first requisite for the birth of the infant is descent. When the fetal head has descended such that its greatest biparietal diameter

is at, or has passed, the pelvic inlet, the head is said to be *engaged*. This provides a clear indication that the pelvic inlet is large enough to accommodate the widest portion of the fetal head and is, therefore, of adequate size. For the average fetal head, the linear distance between the occiput and the plane of the biparietal diameter is less than the distance between the pelvic inlet and the ischial spines. Thus, when the occiput is at the level of the spines, its biparietal diameter has usually passed the pelvic inlet, and the vertex is therefore engaged. However, one cannot assume that engagement has occurred simply because the vertex is at the spines. When the fetal head has been molded markedly, with consequent increase in the distance between the occiput and the biparietal diameter, the vertex may be felt at the spines, but its longest diameter may still be above the pelvic inlet.

The ischial spines are used as a landmark to describe the relative position of the fetal head in the pelvis. When the vertex is at the level of the spines, it is at 0 station. If 1 cm. below, it is a

Fig. 11-9. L.O.A. Positional changes of head in passing through birth canal.

+1 station; 2 cm. below, +2 station; 3 cm. below, +3 station. When the vertex is 1 cm. above the spines, it is a −1 station; 2 cm. above, −2 station; 3 cm. above, −3 station. This relationship is evaluated during the course of each pelvic examination and recorded, along with the assessment of cervical dilatation and effacement.

In primigravidas, engagement often precedes the onset of labor. This is the process of "lightening." Because the vertex is frequently deep in the pelvis at the onset of labor, further descent does not necessarily begin until the second stage of labor. In multiparas, on the other hand, descent often begins with engagement. Once having been inaugurated, descent is inevitably associated with the various movements of the mechanism of labor.

Flexion. Very early in the process of descent the head becomes so flexed that the chin is in contact with the sternum, and, as a consequence, the very smallest anteroposterior diameter (the suboccipitobregmatic plane) is presented to the pelvis.

Internal Rotation. As seen in Chapter 2, the head enters the pelvis in the transverse or diag-onal position. When it reaches the pelvic floor, the occiput is rotated and comes to lie beneath the symphysis pubis. In other words, the sagittal suture is now in the anteroposterior diameter of the outlet (Fig. 2-7). Although the occiput usually rotates to the front, on occasion it may turn toward the hollow of the sacrum. If anterior rotation does not take place at all, the occiput usually rotates to the direct occiput posterior position, a condition known as persistent occiput posterior. Since this represents a deviation from the normal mechanism of labor, it will be considered in Chapter 20, under Abnormal Fetal Positions.

Extension. After the occiput emerges from the pelvis, the nape of the neck becomes arrested beneath the pubic arch and acts as a pivotal point for the rest of the head. Extension of the head now ensues, and with it the frontal portion of the head, the face and the chin are born (Fig. 11-11).

External Rotation. After the birth of the head, it remains in the anteroposterior position only a very short time and shortly will be seen to turn

FIG. 11-10. Successive stages of extrusion of placenta: (*left*) by Schultze's mechanism; (*right*) by Duncan's mechanism.

to one or another side of its own accord—*restitution*. When the occiput originally has been directed toward the left of the mother's pelvis, it then rotates toward the left, and to the right when it originally has been toward the right. This is known as external rotation and is due to the fact that the shoulders of the baby, having entered the pelvis in the transverse position, undergo internal rotation to the anteroposterior position, as did the head; this brings about a corresponding rotation of the head, which is now on the outside. The shoulders are born in a manner somewhat similar to that of the head. Almost immediately after the occurrence of external rotation, the anterior shoulder appears under the symphysis pubis and becomes arrested temporarily beneath the pubic arch, to act as a pivotal point for the other

shoulder (Fig. 11-12). As the anterior margin of the perineum becomes distended, the posterior shoulder is born, assisted by an upward lateral flexion of the infant's body. Once the shoulders are delivered, the infant's body is quickly extruded (expulsion).

The Third Stage of Labor

The third stage of labor is made up of two phases, namely, *the phase of placental separation* and *the phase of placenta expulsion*.

Immediately following the birth of the infant, the remainder of the amniotic fluid escapes, after which there is usually a slight flow of blood. The uterus can be felt as a firm globular mass just below the level of the umbilicus. Shortly thereafter, the uterus relaxes and assumes a discoid

FIG. 11-11. Head extends upward: pelvic floor retreats. (Dickinson-Belskie models, Cleveland Health Museum, Cleveland)

FIG. 11-12. Birth of shoulders: rotating to accommodate to birth passage. (Dickinson-Belskie models, Cleveland Health Museum, Cleveland)

FIG. 11-13. Separation of placenta. (Dickinson-Belskie models, Cleveland Health Museum, Cleveland)

shape. With each subsequent contraction or relaxation the uterus changes from globular to discoid shape until the placenta has separated, after which time the globular shape persists.

Placental Separation. As the uterus contracts down at regular intervals on its diminishing content, the area of placental attachment is greatly reduced. The great disproportion between the reduced size of the placental site and that of the placenta brings about a folding or festooning of the maternal surface of the placenta (Fig. 11-13); with this process separation takes place. Meanwhile, bleeding takes place within these placental folds, and this expedites separation of the organ. The placenta now sinks into the lower uterine segment or upper vagina as an unattached body.

The signs which suggest that the placenta has separated are: (1) the uterus becomes globular in shape and, as a rule, firmer; (2) it rises upward in the abdomen; (3) the umbilical cord descends 3 or more inches farther out of the vagina; and (4) a sudden gush of blood often occurs. These signs usually occur within 5 minutes after the delivery of the infant.

Placental Expulsion. Actual expulsion of the placenta may be brought about by bearing-down efforts on the part of the mother if she is not anesthetized. If this cannot be accomplished, it is usually effected through gentle pressure on the uterine fundus by the physician after he has first made certain that the uterus is hard. Excessive pressure should be avoided to obviate the rare possibility of "inversion" of the uterus (see Chap. 20).

The extrusion of the placenta may take place by one of two mechanisms. First, it may become turned inside-out within the vagina and be born like an inverted umbrella with the glistening fetal surfaces presenting. This is known as Schultze's mechanism and occurs in about 80 per cent of

SUMMARY OF MECHANISM OF LABOR

First Stage—Dilating Stage

Definition. Period from first true labor contraction to complete dilatation of cervix.

What Is Accomplished? Effacement and dilatation of cervix.

Forces Involved. Uterine contractions.

Second Stage—Expulsive Stage

Definition. Period from complete dilatation of cervix to birth of baby.

What Is Accomplished? Expulsion of baby from birth canal—facilitated by certain positional changes of fetus: descent, flexion, internal rotation, extension, external rotation and expulsion.

Forces Involved. Uterine contractions plus intra-abdominal pressure.

Third Stage—Placental Stage

Definition. Period from birth of baby through birth of placenta.

What Is Accomplished? (A) Separation of placenta; (B) expulsion of placenta.

Forces Involved. (A) Uterine contractions; (B) intra-abdominal pressure.

cases. Second, it may become somewhat rolled up in the vagina, with the maternal surface outermost, and be born edgewise. The latter is known as Duncan's mechanism and is seen in about 20 per cent of deliveries (Fig. 11-10). It is believed that the Schultze's mechanism signifies that the placenta has become detached first at its center, and usually a collection of blood and clots is found in the sac of membranes. The Duncan mechanism, on the other hand, suggests that the placenta has separated first at its edges, and it is in this type that bleeding usually occurs at the time of separation.

The contraction of the uterus following delivery serves not only to produce placental separation but also to control uterine hemorrhage. As the result of this contraction of the uterine muscle fibers, the countless blood vessels within their interstices are clamped shut. Even then, a certain amount of blood loss in the third stage is unavoidable, the average being about 250 to 300 cc. It is one of the aims of the conduct of labor to reduce this bleeding to a very minimum.

SUGGESTED READING

Eastman, N. J., and Hellman, L. M.: Williams Obstetrics, ed. 13, New York, Appleton, 1966.

Quilligan, E. J. (ed.): Symposium on physiology of labor. Clin. Obstet. Gynec. 11:13-191, 1968.

Analgesia and Anesthesia for Labor

12

General Principles • *Methods* • *Special Obstetric Anesthesia Problems*

The discomfort endured by women in childbirth has been related in the historical records since the time of early civilizations. It was not until the middle of the 19th century that medical science introduced anesthesia to relieve this discomfort. Two important pioneers who made important contributions in the use of anesthesia in obstetrics were Sir James Y. Simpson, of Edinburgh, and his contemporary in this country, Dr. Walter Channing, of Boston. A knowledge of the historical development of relief for obstetrical discomfort will assist the nurse to gain an increased understanding of modern practices utilized in this approach to providing the mother with more comfort during labor. In addition, she will find that this study provides fascinating reading material. Space will not permit an adequate discussion here; thus the student is advised to pursue it in appropriate texts. (See Suggested Reading and Chapter 26, History of Obstetrics.)

GENERAL PRINCIPLES

In spite of the fact that delivery may be several months away when the pregnant woman makes her initial visit to the obstetrician, she is often anxious to know about labor and delivery and anesthesia and analgesia. She may have some rather definite ideas as the result of previous experience, the experience and advice of friends and relatives, or her own research into the matter. Others have no particular opinions but are nonetheless anxious to hear those of the obstetrician. It is well for the physician to advise the patient, at this time, of the several methods which exist, briefly describing each and suggesting reading material, if applicable. Generally, it is well to leave the matter open, especially if the obstetrician has not had an opportunity to get to know the patient. The patient should also be advised that, although she may help to decide upon the type of analgesia or anesthesia for a normal labor and delivery, complications may dictate a change in plans. Having had an initial discussion with the patient, it is well to rediscuss the subject as the time of delivery approaches. The physician and the nurse should help the patient avoid preoccupation with the type of anesthesia and direct her thoughts to the birth of a healthy baby.

Every woman experiences a degree of discomfort during labor, unless there has been an interruption of the nerve supply to the uterus, as would be the case in a paraplegic. This discomfort is the result of several factors, including the stimulation of pressure-sensitive nerve endings in the cervix and ischemia of the uterine muscle during contractions. The amount of pain recognized by the woman in labor is modified by numerous factors, including previous experiences, prenatal education, emotional stability, parity, fetal size and position, pelvic capacity, and the emotional support of those attending her labor. In addition, there are a variety of analgesic and anesthetic methods which can be used by the obstetrician in conjunction with the anesthesiologist. In every method which will be described, a balance must be struck between the comfort of the patient and possible adverse effects upon the fetus. Any method selected must be clearly outlined to the patient and to her husband, if he is participating. Departures from the plan, if dictated by the obstetric situation, should also be explained to the patient, if time permits.

METHODS

Natural Childbirth

This term applies to a rather broad and general philosophy of labor management. Such methods are based upon the principle that, with careful prenatal education, the support of obstetrician, nurses and husband, and the application of controlled breathing and voluntary muscle relaxation, the need for anesthesia and analgesia can be minimized, if not eliminated. The effectiveness of these methods is not based primarily on the physical techniques employed, but rather on the total involvement and acquired knowledge of the patient and her husband, and the interest of the people supporting her.

The methods outlined by the British obstetrician, Grantley Dick Read, have more recently been replaced in popularity by the Lamaze method or psychoprophylaxis, an approach involving controlled breathing and active participation by the husband. Instructions in the use of such an approach are available in most areas through private tutors, or an organization known as the Childbirth Education Association. If such instruc-

Fig. 12-1. Pudendal block done transvaginally with the examiner's finger guiding the needle to the ischial spine and pudendal nerve.

tion is not available, there are a number of books which the obstetrician and his patient may use. Such an approach is not applicable to all patients, and the key to a successful application of the technique is motivation. Those interested only because of intellectual curiosity, or those talked into the idea, generally do poorly. Patients who select this approach should understand that, even though they may fail to get through their entire labor without anesthesia, they have still accomplished something and should not feel guilty. When used successfully, this approach can be a very rewarding experience for all concerned.

Hypnosis

This technique is infrequently used but has some of the same advantages as the natural childbirth approaches, namely, the absence of agents which might depress the fetus. However, the use of hypnosis, requires special training for the obstetrician, a patient who is a good subject, and often a considerable amount of prenatal training of the patient.

Narcotics

Narcotics are the most common form of analgesia used in this country. The most common narcotic used is the synthetic compound meperidine hydrochloride (Demerol). Demerol resembles morphine as an analgesic, although many feel it is less depressant to respiration. The drug may be given intravenously or intramuscularly in doses of 50 to 100 mg. The dose is smaller and the duration of action less when the intravenous route is used. As a general principle, narcotics are withheld until labor is in the active phase. This avoids prolongation of the latent phase. It is also well to avoid a dose of Demerol late in labor. This would produce a high blood level of Demerol in the baby at birth. Although it is often said that an average dose of narcotic will not depress a healthy fullterm fetus in an uncomplicated labor, the number of qualifying conditions is such that unnecessary chances are not justified.

Tranquilizers

These drugs, in the form of phenothiazines and other agents (e.g., Phenergan, Largon, Vistaril, Sparine), have become very popular in recent years. These agents are used in combination with narcotics whose action they potentiate, thus reducing the dose of narcotic to be used. In addition to this action, these drugs are also effective anti-nauseants and reduce anxiety.

Barbiturates

These are hypnotics and are effective in reducing the tension and fear of the patient in labor. These agents are not analgesics, and they produce excitement rather than sedation if administered alone in the presence of pain. Barbiturates are not well handled by the newborn and should generally be avoided in advanced labor. Thus, these agents are most useful in the patient in early labor whose major problem is apprehension, rather than pain. The more common barbiturates in use are Nembutal (pentobarbital sodium), Seconal Sodium, and Amytal Sodium. They may be used orally, intramuscularly, or intravenously in doses of 100 to 300 mg.

Scopolamine

This belladonna alkaloid depresses the parasympathetic nervous system and is used in labor because it is also capable of producing amnesia. The latter effect is desired by some patients, although this approach is less popular now than it was several years ago. In the presence of pain, if adequate analgesia is not provided along with the scopolamine, excitement, and even hallucinations and delirium, may result. This is a most unpleasant situation, and when it occurs the patient may even sustain injuries as a result of the uncontrolled activity. When the patient is in labor under the influence of this drug, she may respond to the discomfort of contractions by crying out

Fig. 12-2. Paracervical blocking, using the "Iowa Trumpet" to guide the needle into the paracervical area.

or grimacing but remembers nothing of it when it is over, unless specifically reminded. Every precaution should be taken to protect the patient from injury (this includes side rails on the labor bed) including constant observation.

FIG. 12-3. Sagittal section of sacral canal, with caudal needle properly placed in the caudal space.

Regional Anesthesia and Analgesia

This designation refers to all those techniques which produce anesthesia in the anatomical area supplied by the nerve or nerves blocked. These techniques have the common advantage of reducing discomfort in the mother without significant effect on the fetus. All of these techniques are of course risky if the patient is allergic to one or more of the "caine" drugs, or if the amount used and consequently absorbed into the circulation is too great. In questioning a patient regarding reaction to these agents, it is important to ask about previous dental procedures for which they are commonly used.

Local Infiltration can be used for performing and repairing episiotomies, as well as for the repair of lacerations. Procaine and Xylocaine are the commonly used agents, in 0.5 to 1.0 per cent solution.

Pudendal Block produces more extensive perineal anesthesia, as well as relaxation of the superficial perineal muscles. Although this injection can be made through the perineal skin, it is more comfortable and more successful when the injection is made through the vaginal mucosa directly over the ischial spines (Fig. 12-1). The block is done on both sides just prior to delivery; it does not have any effect on the discomfort of uterine contractions.

FIG. 12-4. Continuous caudal analgesia: catheter method. The patient is in modified Sims's position, with legs properly placed as necessary for "laying" the caudal catheter. The Pitkin's syringe for continuous technique is shown attached to the caudal catheter in place in the caudal canal. Note method of taping the catheter in place.

A Paracervical Block is the transvaginal injection of an anesthetic solution on each side of the cervix (Fig. 12-2). This can relieve the pain of uterine contractions for 45 to 60 minutes. The technique is relatively simple to master, is effective in a high percentage of patients, and is especially useful in the multiparous patient whose labor is progressing rapidly. The need for repeated injections when a longer period of analgesia is required makes the technique somewhat cumbersome, although, recently, several types of indwelling paracervical catheters are being tested. Transient fetal bradycardia occurs occasionally following the injection, probably because of rapid absorption of the anesthesia from the very vascular paracervical area. To avoid this, the total dose and concentration of the anesthetic should be reduced.

Caudal Anesthesia is a form of analgesia and anesthesia achieved by "blocking" the nerves in the peridural space. The anesthetic agent is introduced into the peridural space via the sacral hiatus. This opening leads to a space within the sacrum known as the caudal canal or the caudal space (Fig. 12-3). The space is really the lowest extent of the bony spinal canal. Through it a rich network of sacral nerves passes downward after the nerves have emerged from the dural sac a few inches above. The dural sac separates the caudal canal below from the spinal cord and its surrounding spinal fluid above.

When the patient is in active phase labor, with the presenting part well down in the pelvis, caudal analgesia may be started. By the addition of anesthetic solution through the indwelling caudal catheter at appropriate intervals, the desired effect can be maintained throughout labor and provide anesthesia for delivery as well.

To insert the catheter, the obstetric patient is placed on her side in a modified Sims's position, with the upper leg well flexed at the hip and knee joints and the lower leg extended (Fig. 12-4). The sacral and coccygeal area is cleansed with an antiseptic solution. The area is surrounded with sterile towels or a sterile drape. The physician wears sterile gloves for the procedure, since it requires aseptic technique. After the pliable needle or fine plastic catheter has been inserted into the caudal space, a test dose of 8 cc. of the local anesthetic solution, such as Metycaine 1.5 per cent, Pontocaine 0.15 per cent, Xylocaine 1 per cent or Nesacaine 3 per cent, is injected. When 5 minutes have elapsed, the following test for spinal anesthesia is made to be assured that the drug has not been injected into the sub-

arachnoid space. If the 8 cc. dose has been accidentally placed in the subarachnoid space, spinal rather than caudal anesthesia will result, and within 5 minutes the patient will experience difficulty in moving her legs and will also have a sensory block above the pubic symphysis. At this time the physician also will check the anal sphincter for loss of tone and examine the lower extremities for increasing skin temperature. If these two observations prove to be positive (i.e., the anal sphincter is relaxed, and the patient's feet are be-

FIG. 12-5. Cutaneous dermatomes to illustrate sensory anesthetic levels.

coming warmer and dry), they are an indication that the caudal catheter is placed properly in the caudal space. Only after this is certain is the patient given the obstetric dose of 20 to 30 cc. of medication. This will block the afferent sensory nerve supply from the uterus and usually will provide anesthesia to the 10th thoracic dermatome. This level (Fig. 12-5) is at the umbilicus and is required to eliminate the discomfort of uterine contractions. The large volume (20 to 30 ml.) of anesthetic solution in the peridural space is necessary to achieve this level.

At first the patient experiences a sense of fullness along the distribution of the sciatic nerve in one or both legs, which may cause temporary discomfort. About 15 minutes after the injection, relief is obtained from the abdominal discomfort of uterine contractions, and in about 20 minutes the analgesia should be complete. One observes the lower extremities for pronounced vasodilatation and cessation of sweating as one of the first effective signs. The great toe and the ball of the foot are the first parts to develop vasomotor block; thus this area is the first to become pink, warm and dry. The heel will be the last to show these signs. The effect may be unilateral at first, and some minutes may elapse before it affects the other side, or the physician may have the patient lie on the unaffected side to encourage diffusion of the anesthetic agent. The nurse should remember that the physician should be consulted before changing the patient's position to one side or the other during this early stage of analgesia. After anesthesia has been well established, there is usually no contraindication to changing the patient's position so long as the pliable needle or plastic catheter is protected. If the procedure is successful, the patient experiences no pain whatsoever in labor and is not conscious of either uterine contractions or of perineal distention, except for some minor degree of pressure.

Provided that the maternal systolic blood pressure does not fall below 100 mm. Hg, with resulting fetal hypoxia, a continuous caudal has the advantage of exerting the least possible effect on the infant, because it does not cross the placental barrier in significant pharmacologic doses. This factor is an advantage to the premature infant particularly, as well as the fact that caudal analgesia tends to retard rapid and forceful labor and enables the physician to perform an easy, controlled delivery. It also lessens the strain of labor for mothers handicapped with heart disease, pul-

monary tuberculosis, acute respiratory infections or diabetes.

POSSIBLE COMPLICATIONS. One of the commonest complications of conduction analgesia for labor is *maternal hypotension*; thus it is important for the nurse or the physician in attendance to keep a constant check on the patient's blood pressure. Hypotension can be controlled by alertness and prompt action on the part of the attendant. One of the first clues that may alert the nurse that the patient's blood pressure has dropped abruptly is a sudden episode of rather severe nausea, accompanied promptly by the other signs of sudden hypotension. When the mother in labor becomes hypotensive, immediate action should be taken to restore the blood volume to the central circulation. The most expedient measure in this instance is to elevate the patient's legs, either by raising the foot of the bed or merely elevating her legs. The patient may require oxygen at this time. If her blood pressure does not return to normal, she should be turned on her left side (with the foot of the bed elevated) and continue to breathe oxygen. Lying on the left side relieves the uterine pressure exerted on iliac veins and the inferior vena cava, and thus facilitates venous return from the lower extremities. Patients receiving caudal anesthesia should have an infusion of 5 per cent dextrose in water, started before the block is administered. If hypotension occurs, increasing the rate of this infusion will often correct the situation. If the above measures are not successful, the physician may decide to administer small divided doses of a vasopressor drug.

In addition to the tendency to produce hypotension, *other disadvantages* of continuous caudal are (1) it increases the frequency of forceps deliveries, (2) it may prolong labor, especially if started too early in labor, and (3) if the anesthesia reaches a high level, uterine atony may result. Caudal anesthesia would be contraindicated in the case of shock or hemorrhage because of its vasodilator tendencies and, for the same reason, it should be used cautiously in toxemia. Any infection of the skin over the sacral area would also be a contraindication for its use. A final disadvantage of the technique is that careful supervision is necessary, placing heavy demands on personnel. If adequate personnel are not available, the technique should not be used.

Lumbar Epidural is another form of peridural anesthesia in which the space is approached from the lumbar rather than the caudal area. The advantages of this technique as opposed to caudal

FIG. 12-6. Circle filter anesthesia apparatus. With this type of machine any combination or mixture of gases can be administered to the patient. Heidbrink Division, Ohio Chemical & Surgical Equipment Co., Madison, Wis.)

are technical; the end result for the patient is essentially the same. The anesthetic agents used are the same as those used for caudal, the only difference being that a smaller volume is necessary when injected at the higher lumbar site. Although the anatomy of the lumbar spine is more consistent than that of the caudal area, thus making the injection simpler in some ways, the risk of penetrating the dura and thus obtaining an inadvertent spinal anesthetic is greater. As with caudal anesthesia, skill is required and careful supervision is most important, as long as anesthesia is maintained.

Spinal Anesthesia is a popular form of obstetric anesthesia in the United States and has the advantage of other forms of regional anesthesia (i.e., good pain relief with little or no effect on the fetus). The term saddle block has been applied to the use of a low-dose hyperbaric (drug heavier than spinal fluid) spinal anesthetic. This technique is used for terminal anesthesia in delivery, generally with a sensory level from T-9 to T-11. This provides a pain-free delivery and does not interfere with uterine contractions. As with most spinal anesthetics, the drug is usually introduced at the L-3—L-4 level. Although the level of anesthesia obtained is to some extent the result of the dose and volume of anesthetic solution used, and to a lesser extent the level of injection, the most important factor is the position of the

patient after the injection. To obtain the lower levels in saddle block for vaginal delivery, the injection is made with the patient sitting up, and she remains sitting for 30 to 120 seconds, permitting the hyperbaric solution to fall. Higher dose spinal anesthesia is generally reserved for cesarean sections. Levels of anesthesia from T-6 to T-8 are required. This is achieved by using a larger dose than for saddle block (6 to 8 mg. instead of 4 mg.), and by positioning the patient after the injection. For cesarean section, the injection is usually made with the patient in a lateral rather than a sitting position. Continuous catheter spinal anesthesia has virtually no place in modern obstetric practice.

The major problems with spinal anesthesia are hypotension and headaches. The hypotension is, as it is in peridural anesthesia, the result of sympathetic block and to a great extent is related to the level of anesthesia obtained. Post-spinal headache is probably the result of leakage of spinal fluid at the puncture site, with consequent reduction in spinal fluid pressure. This problem occurs more often in the pregnant than the non-pregnant patient, probably because of the natural diuresis which occurs postpartum and may also involve pressures during uterine contractions. The typical spinal headache, although self-limited (5 to 10 days), may be incapacitating until it resolves. The treatment includes: Increase of fluid intake, antihistamines, such as benadryl and dramamine, tight abdominal binders, caffeine sodium benzoate, and in resistant cases the injection of dextrose or saline solution into the peridural space.

General Anesthesia

This implies the use of an agent, either by inhalation or injection, which will provide analgesia and render varying levels of unconsciousness. As a group, these agents have several problems in common. The first of these problems is that the anesthetic action of the agents is related directly to the blood concentration, and such blood levels are reflected quickly in the fetal circulation. Fetal narcosis and respiratory depression at birth is then a major concern. A second and really serious problem is vomiting and aspiration. The obstetric patient is not the well-prepared patient one anesthetizes for elective surgery. When labor begins, intestinal motility and gastric emptying virtually cease. Thus, even though delivery may occur many hours after the last meal, the stomach may still be full and vomiting may occur during induction of anesthesia. This is less likely to occur with agents such as nitrous oxide in analgesic concentration, because in this concentration the cough reflex is maintained. When vomiting does occur, great skill is required on the part of the anesthetic to avoid aspiration. If aspiration occurs, the immediate and most ominous consequence may be respiratory failure and cardiac arrest. Unfortunately, this is one of the leading causes of maternal deaths in the United States. Aspiration pneumonia is a delayed complication of considerable gravity. The remaining problems with the general anesthetics are related to the specific agents and are discussed individually.

Nitrous Oxide in combination with varying concentrations of oxygen is probably the most common anesthetic agent used for obstetrics in this country. This gas is not capable of producing total surgical anesthesia but does afford excellent analgesia. Since the level of anesthesia is not profound and consciousness is not lost, especially if the agent is used intermittently with contractions, nitrous oxide poses less risk of vomiting and aspiration. The concentration of nitrous oxide should never exceed 80 per cent (with 20 per cent oxygen) and preferably should be lower to avoid fetal hypoxia. It is necessary to use either local infiltration or pudendal block for the episiotomy and repair to provide complete anesthesia for that area and obviate the need for prolonged continuous administration of the gas.

Trichlorethylene (Trilene) is a volatile analgesic agent which is usually self-administered, using an inhalator strapped to the patient's wrist. There is a safety factor with the trilene mask; the patient will drop the mask as soon as she is sufficiently depressed. Profound surgical anesthesia cannot be obtained in this fashion. If the agent is used in an anesthesia machine with a carbon dioxide absorber, one must be cautious, because an increase in heat may cause the formation of a toxic gas, phosgene. The same precaution applies to patients who have been using Trilene for analgesia and subsequently require surgical anesthesia. Delivery room personnel should not hold the Trilene mask on patient's face, and its use is contraindicated in patients with heart disease because of a tendency to produce cardiac arrhythmias.

Choloroform is another volatile anesthetic which is now of greater historic than practical interest, having been administered to Queen Victoria in 1853. Since its toxic level is only slightly above that required for anesthesia, its use has been discontinued in American hospitals. The toxicity is cardiac in nature, and arrhythmias are common if epinephrine or oxytocin is used in conjunction with the agent. Advantages include the fact that choloform is pleasant and rapid and, if necessary, can produce excellent uterine relaxation.

Ether for many years was the mainstay of obstetrical anesthesia. The reasons for the popularity of ether included its safety, because of its slow action, and the fact that distinct stages of anesthesia could be observed. The agent can be administered either by an open drop technique or with a standard semiclosed anesthesia machine. Disadvantages of ether include those of all inhalation agents (i.e., the dangers of vomiting and aspiration); also, ether is irritating to breathe, often causing coughing and a prolonged induction of anesthesia. In addition, ether produces profound uterine relaxation, which is helpful if one is doing a version and extraction or manual removal of a placenta, but it is a distinct disadvantage in a normal delivery. Since ether is cleared very slowly from the lungs, the uterine relaxation is prolonged, thereby increasing the postpartum blood loss. Induction with ether takes considerable time, so it is not the agent of choice when deep anesthesia is needed quickly.

Cyclopropane is an anesthetic gas which has the major advantage of being able to produce profound surgical anesthesia very quickly (within a few minutes). It can be administered in relatively low concentrations, thereby maintaining a high oxygen concentration and can, if the level of anesthesia is deep enough, produce uterine relaxation. This gas should never be used unless complete precautions have been taken to avoid an explosion, including conductive shoes or shoe covers. Cyclopropane is usually administered in a closed system machine, and, although very helpful in many obstetric emergencies, it is probably "more anesthesia" than is necessary for a normal vaginal delivery.

Halothane (Fluothane) is a rapid-acting volatile anesthetic agent which produces excellent uterine relaxation very quickly and, for this reason, is probably the agent of choice when such is needed. Fluothane should not be used in patients with liver disease and, like cyclopropane, is probably excessive anesthesia for normal obstetrics.

Methoxyflurane (Pentharne) is another halogenated ether which has found use in obstetrics. It does not produce uterine relaxation like halothane and can be used in analgesic concentrations for a normal delivery. As with halothane, a history of liver disease contraindicates its use.

Thiopental Sodium (Pentothal Sodium), the only intravenous agent in use in obstetric anesthesia, is used for vaginal deliveries, as well as cesarean sections. Because pentothal reaches the same concentration in the fetal circulation as in the maternal very rapidly (within 5 minutes), it is not a popular agent for normal deliveries. Blood levels of barbiturates in the newborn are not usually cleared quickly, and neonatal depression is a problem. Laryngospasm in the mother is also a serious problem which can produce fetal as well as maternal hypoxia, and a skilled anesthetist is essential. Thus, although pentothal is easy to administer, its potential problems are so significant that most obstetricians avoid its use.

SPECIAL OBSTETRIC ANESTHESIA PROBLEMS

Breech

This presentation poses a particular anesthesia problem. Most obstetricians prefer to have a cooperative patient who can bear down during the second stage, but they also need adequate anesthesia available, if there is difficulty in delivery of the shoulders, or the after-coming head. Caudal, epidural and spinal anesthesia have the problem of impairing the ability of the patient to push. This increases the frequency of breech extrac-

tions, with their inherent risk. It is preferable to use local anesthesia or a pudendal block, along with intermittent nitrous oxide analgesia, which permits the patient to bear down, and to have an anesthetist present who is prepared to add a more profound agent such as cyclopropane or halothane, if difficulty occurs with the shoulders, or after-coming head.

Cesarean Section

Since more complete anesthesia is required before the operation may be started, and since the time required to deliver the baby may be longer than for a normal delivery, there is greater risk of neonatal depression. Several techniques are in common use for cesarean section. Spinal anesthesia has been favored by many because it provides adequate anesthesia without fetal depression. The major problem with spinal anesthesia is the frequent hypotension resulting from the sympathetic block and the uterus compressing the vena cava. Cyclopropane anesthesia with a rapid induction can provide adequate anesthesia but forces the surgeon to proceed rapidly, in an effort to deliver the baby before the gas equilibrates across the placenta. A third technique involves a small dose of pentothal, just sufficient to induce sleep, followed by nitrous oxide and oxygen along with a muscle relaxant such a succinylcholine. This affords adequate oxygenation with minimal fetal depression. In some circumstances, the anesthesia of choice is local infiltration of the abdominal wall. Cesarean section can be accomplished with this approach if the operator is skilled in the use of local anesthesia and avoids undue peritoneal traction. Of course, as with any surgical situation, circumstances will dictate the choice of approach (e.g., one would avoid spinal anesthesia in a patient with bleeding, who would be prone to hypotension. On the other hand, one might select spinal anesthesia in a patient who has recently eaten).

Uterine Relaxation

Several obstetrical procedures—internal version, breech extraction, manual removal of the placenta, intrauterine examination, and cervical cerclage operations—require uterine relaxation. Although ether, chloroform, cyclopropane and halothane all can produce such relaxation, halothane does it more quickly and efficiently and is, therefore, the agent of choice.

SUGGESTED READING

Bonica, J. J.: Principles and Practice of Obstetric Analgesia and Anesthesia. Philadelphia, F. A. Davis, 1967.

Buxton, C. L.: A study of Psychophysical Methods for Relief of Childbirth Pain. Philadelphia, W. B. Saunders, 1962.

Crawford, J. S.: Principles and Practice of Obstetric Anesthesia. ed. 2, Philadelphia, F. A. Davis, 1965.

Flowers, C. E., Jr.: Obstetric Analgesia and Anesthesia. New York, Hoeber, 1967.

Greenhill, J. P.: Analgesia and Anesthesia in Obstetrics. Springfield, Charles C Thomas, 1962.

Greiss, F. C., and Grandell, D. L.: Therapy for hypotension induced by spinal anesthesia during pregnancy. J.A.M.A. 191:793.

Hingson, R. A., and Hellman, L.: Anesthesia for Obstetrics. Philadelphia, J. B. Lippincott, 1956.

Lucas, W., Kirschbaum, T., and Assali, N. S.: Spinal shock and fetal oxygenation. Am. J. Obstet. Gynec. 93:583, 1965.

Marx, G. F., and Orkin, J. R.: Physiology of Obstetric Anesthesia. Springfield, Charles C Thomas, 1969.

Maternity Center Association: Psychophysical Preparation for Childbirth: Guidelines for Teaching. ed. 2, New York Maternity Center Association, 1965.

Moore, D. C.: Anesthetic Techniques for Obstetrical Anesthesia and Analgesia. Springfield, Charles C Thomas, 1965.

Moya, F., and Smith, B.: Spinal anesthesia for cesarean section. J.A.M.A. 179:609, 1962.

Read, G. D.: Childbirth Without Fear. New York, Harper, 1962.

Shnider, S. M., and Moya, F.: Effects of meperidine on the newborn infant. Am. J. Obstet. Gynec. 89:1009, 1964.

Stoelting, V. K.: Fluothane in obstetric anesthesia. Anesth. Analg. 43:243, 1964.

Van Praagh, I. G. L., and Povey, W. G.: Paracervical block anesthesia in labour. Canad. Med. Ass. J. 94:282, 1966.

Vellay, P.: Childbirth Without Pain. New York, Dutton, 1960.

Conduct of Normal Labor

DIMENSIONS OF EFFECTIVE NURSING CARE

Perhaps at no other time during the maternity cycle is the nurse in such an advantageous position to give nursing care as she is during the time of parturition. It is a unique and humbling experience, this miracle of giving birth, not only for the mother and the father, the main participants, but also for the physician and the nurse who share this experience, and upon whom so much depends. From the parents' point of view, labor looms as a critical period in the process of childbearing; often it is considered by them, and especially by the mother, as the end of a long-drawn-out process rather than the beginning of new life. Hence they attribute enormous significance to events and people who are necessary and helpful to them at this time. They indicate repeatedly that they consider the nurse in particular to be one of those necessary, helpful people. Indeed, she can be if she utilizes the opportunity.

Effective nursing care during labor provides for maximum well-being and comfort for both mother and infant and at the same time allows the father to participate in the process, insofar as he is able, and to derive a sense of satisfaction from that participation. The nursing intervention is purposeful but flexible, based always on the needs of each individual patient, infant and husband. To execute such care, the nurse must have knowledge and understanding of the course of normal labor, ability to recognize deviations from the normal, and judgment and ability to cope with stressful and emergency conditions. In addition, she should have a mastery of certain skills, both technical and communicative, which she can apply appropriately to meet the exigencies of the situation. The importance of teamwork between doctor and nurse should not be overlooked, and it is especially important to keep the physician informed through accurate reporting and recording of the progress of the mother in labor.

However, knowledge and technical ability are not sufficient in themselves, for the nurse must also be able to convey warmth and empathy if she is to be really effective. The empathic nurse is able to enter into the feelings of her patient and at the same time to retain her separateness. Thus, objectivity is maintained, which contributes to more effective care. Yet the worth and the individuality of each mother always are recognized. In addition, the nurse ought to be accepting and non-judgmental regarding the behavior of the mother or the father, realizing that this is a stressful period, and that their usual behavior may be drastically different. She strives to sustain her patient and to reinforce her confidence whenever necessary, thus helping the mother to attain the greatest amount of comfort and satisfaction from the labor experience. By assisting the patient and her husband to mobilize their resources and strengths, she is able to work with them in a positive way and to reinforce their concept of themselves as adequate people.

The mind and body of the nurse boggle a bit when she is faced with this considerable responsibility; certainly the young student has some trepidation when she is called upon to assume these duties. Yet with competent guidance and instruction she learns to function efficiently in this role. In order to help the student and/or young graduate prepare for her responsibility, the authors in this chapter have focused on both the patient and the nurse as they move through the successive stages of labor. Although it is the mother who truly delivers her infant, the other important people in this event—the husband, the doctor and ancillary personnel—are not to be forgotten, for they also play important roles.

The Process of Clinical Judgment

Implicit in the idea of effective nursing care is the ability to make effective clinical judgments. Clinical judgments and the acts associated with them represent, in fact, nursing practice. Various terms have arisen in the literature: nursing diagnosis, clinical judgments, clinical nursing, to name a few. All of these constitute in some way the anatomy of nursing care. Certainly the ability to make nursing diagnoses and appropriate clinical judgments is utilized not only in attending the labor patient, but throughout all nursing. However, the process is introduced and specified at this point because the nature of nursing care during labor and the exigencies under which it is given require a great facility with this process. There is much that is unpredictable in the delivery area. Patients may be admitted with great rapidity; labors may progress in a similar manner. Unforeseen emergencies may occur no matter how well organized and efficient the personnel, and when they do occur, they may be serious. Hence the nurse may be called upon to exercise a great deal of judgment "on her feet" so to speak, without specific direction or the luxury of thinking through the problem. In the midst of crises where human lives are at stake, calm fact finding and judicial deliberations become increasingly difficult. Some of our most crucial problems arise from conflicts between principle and expediency. Hence, we need to have a method so internalized as to be second nature so we can operate without conscious step by step proceedings. Thus, we can arrive quickly at appropriate decisions and conclusions regarding our patients.

The "components" will help the student understand how nursing practice (and hence the process) can be made operational. While the various components have been categorized under arbitrary headings, one is not to assume that these categories are mutually exclusive or stand alone. Many authors, for instance, would consider data collection and implementation as part of the nursing diagnosis; some would consider what we have termed "the process of clinical judgment" as a nursing diagnosis (see Suggested Readings). One could also think of the process in terms of (nursing) diagnosis, therapy and prognosis. Thus, dif-

COMPONENTS OF THE PROCESS OF CLINICAL JUDGMENT[1]

Information gathering or data collection	1. Examine the patient and his environment.
	2. Identify findings having implications for stability or instability in the patient's behavior (i.e., determine the nature of the patient problem).
	3. Determine the nature of the intervention needed. a. Does the patient need assistance? b. What assistance is needed; what is the nurse's responsibility?
Nursing Diagnosis	4. Examine alternatives for action considering resources, obstacles and anticipated consequences for the patient.
	5. Decide a course of action. a. What action and by whom. b. How is it to be implemented and in what sequence.
Implementation	6. Initiate the course of action.
	7. Consider the need for modification of the course of action. a. Modify as indicated. b. Reassess the situation.
Prognosis	8. Examine the consequences of the implemented course of action. a. Was the goal accomplished? Were there other outcomes? b. How could the nursing plan be altered in terms of consequences (evaluation). c. Attempt to classify this information. (These classifications aid future study and care and give direction to necessary research).

[1] These components were developed through the joint efforts of the UCLA School of Nursing Undergraduate Faculty (1964-1967) who taught the Senior Clinical Nursing courses.

ferent terminology has been used to describe nursing decision making and care giving.

We are using the term "clinical" in reference to health-illness study and practice based on actual observation and treatment of patients (as apart from experimental or laboratory study). By "judgment" we mean the ability to come to a decision based on understanding and good sense. We have incorporated the word "process" into the phrase to underline the notion of fluidity. That is, the process is constantly changing, subject to reassessment based on new information, and changing conditions. It includes the implementation, modification, evolution and predictions regarding the care that is planned and given. We can consider a patient problem to exist if the behavioral stability or integrated behavior which is functional for the patient is threatened or disrupted, either by disease processes, stressful events (i.e., pregnancy, labor), changes in role or other conditions of a health-illness nature which the patient may experience.

As we review the process, it can be seen that components 1 and 2 constitute a reconnoitering stage in which information is gathered and the diagnosis begun. Resources such as the chart, the family, the patient himself, members of the health team and elements in the environment can be utilized. The nurse also may utilize her ability to "role take" to speed up the data collection. (For a detailed definition and explanation of the concept of "role taking" and its application in maternity nursing, see the Turner and Reeder articles in the Suggested Readings.) This term refers to the ability of the nurse to put herself in the place (position) of the patient in order to imaginatively construct the role of the patient, so as to provide herself with appropriate cues for predicting and understanding the meaning of the patient's behavior, and thus, for determining appropriate behavior for herself. The process by which the role of each particular patient is inferred stems from basic knowledge about the patient role in general, prior experience with the individual or others like him, and/or a specific bit of behavior that is being manifested. As the student gains more experience with various individuals involved in the patient role who are confronted with different kinds of health-illness conditions (including maternity patients) she will find her role-taking ability facilitated. As we acquire our data, we become able to decide the existence and extent of a problem. We can say in the most general terms, that a problem does exist when

there is a health goal to be obtained but the individual (patient) sees no well defined, well established means of attaining it. For instance, she may be too ill or weak to help herself. Again, the goal may be so vaguely defined or unclear that the patient cannot determine relevant means of achieving it. Thus, the patient may not understand or know how to accept conditions and instruction regarding achieving the goal of health.

A decision about the existence and extent of the problem initiates the diagnosis. As previously stated, there are many definitions of this term. For our purposes we shall regard a nursing diagnosis as a conclusion based on a systematic and scientific appraisal of an individual's health-illness problems, resulting from critical analysis of his behavior (alone and with others), the nature of his illness and the numerous other factors, environmental, social, psychological, that may affect his condition. This conclusion serves as a guide for our nursing care. It is well to remember also that the statement of the diagnosis may be several words, and more descriptive than etiological. As we find out additional information about our patients we may move from descriptive to more etiological statements. Moreover, there may be several diagnoses relating to a constellation of interrelated problems the patient has; for instance, if the nurse were to write the diagnosis regarding a labor patient the diagnosis might be: "anxiety regarding process of labor;" "elevated temperature;" "inefficient but painful contractions." Finally, one can have the same nursing diagnosis but have different pathological conditions which give rise to it. In the case of a newly delivered infant, for instance, the diagnosis might be "inadequate oxygenation"; the cause for one infant might be a congenital heart defect; for another infant, immature lungs associated with prematurity. Thus, the total interrelationship of all the influencing factors is to be considered as it gives direction to our care plan. As we do this we progress through components 3 to 5.

Components 6 and 7 are concerned with the actual implementation of knowledgeable intervention in the form of nursing activities (which can include everything from comfort measures to counseling). These activities are directed toward moving the patient toward increased positive adaptation to his environment. Again it is important to remember that the implementation also is fluid since it is based upon the diagnosis (or diagnoses) which is constantly being reassessed. Moreover, as we administer care, the patient's condition will be expected to change, which will necessitate a new diagnosis and hence a modification of care. Therefore, there is a continuous spiral process.

Component 8 includes both evaluation and prediction facets. A worthwhile evaluation should include an estimation of the results of our past nursing care activities to help us predict the validity of our care for the future. Any statement of the effectiveness and reliability of our actions is best made with qualifications indicating the degree or amount of effectiveness and reliability claimed. *Were all symptoms relieved? What was the extent of the results? On what evidence (observation of self, others, verbal response, cessation of symptoms)? Who was involved (nurse, patient, others)? In what contexts (what else was happening when the action was performed)?* If these points are established, then we can begin to build categories of nursing action that are effective under certain circumstances for certain patients given certain conditions. As we ascertain the extent of our effectiveness we are then in a better position to predict the patient's potential for change toward stability and/or a wellness condition. Thus, we arrive at his nursing prognosis.

The student is encouraged to utilize the Suggested Readings for the articles regarding nursing diagnosis and clinical judgment for a thorough and varied treatment of the subject. Let us continue with some of the events that the mother will be experiencing.

PRELUDE TO LABOR

The prodromal signs heralding the onset of labor begin several weeks before true labor commences (see Chap. 11). Lightening may occur any time during the last 4 weeks of pregnancy; in primigravidas it usually occurs about 10 days to 2 weeks prior to labor. This phenomenon causes a sensation of decreased abdominal distention produced by the descent of the presenting part of the baby into the pelvis. In multigravida this may not occur until the labor has begun. The painless Braxton Hicks contractions which have occurred intermittently throughout the latter part of pregnancy may increase so much that they become annoying. They may cause the mother many restless or sleepless nights that contribute to her gradually increasing tension and fatigue. Since the rise in the anxiety level contributes to heightened awareness, the mother becomes more sensitive to various stimuli: if the baby is generally less active, she may worry; if he moves more than usual, she may worry. She wonders about the 2- to 3-lb. weight loss that may occur 3 to 4 days before the onset of labor. Ordinarily this would be an occasion of great rejoicing, but now it may give her some concern. Even the increased vaginal mucous discharge may have an ominous significance for her. The spurt of energy that may occur 1 to 2 days before labor begins often leads her into activities that are overfatiguing, and she will need anticipatory guidance from the nurse and the physician to help her to set limits on activity.

This is the time to finish packing her suitcase and to simplify her housekeeping duties. She may want to complete meal preparations for the family's use when she is in the hospital; if this is done daily little by little, then it should not become bothersome. Last-minute details for the care of the other children or the functioning of the household can be taken care of at this time. Short walks in the fresh air are a good way to release extra tension without overfatigue. The mother should be encouraged to achieve a happy balance between activity and rest.

During the latter part of pregnancy the mother will have been instructed about what to do when she thinks labor has begun. As term approaches, it is wise for the nurse to explore with the mother her preparations for coming to the hospital. The patient and her husband should know ap-

TABLE 13-1. DIFFERENTIAL FACTORS IN TRUE AND FALSE LABOR

TRUE LABOR	FALSE LABOR
Contractions:	*Contractions:*
Occur at regular intervals	Occur at irregular intervals
Intervals gradually shorten	Intervals remain long
Intensity gradually increases	Intensity remains the same
Located chiefly in back	Located chiefly in abdomen
Intensified by walking	Walking has no effect; often gives relief
Show:	*Show:*
Usually present	None
Cervix:	*Cervix:*
Becomes effaced and dilated (this can be determined by digital examination)	Usually uneffaced and closed

proximately how long it will take them to reach the hospital and what alternate means of transportation are available if the husband may not be able to take his wife. What entrance to the hospital they should use and what admission procedures they must go through also are important. A tour of the ward for the parents can be arranged during the antepartal period so that they can become more familiar with the surroundings.

THE ONSET OF LABOR

Most physicians instruct their patients to notify them if the labor contractions become rhythmic and regular and/or the bag of water breaks. To prepare the patient adequately for what to expect, and to instruct her on an appropriate course of action, it is necessary that the nurse have an understanding of the physiology of labor as well as other factors (p. 133). Since the nurse will be with the patient more constantly than the doctor after the patient is admitted to the hospital, the nurse will be expected also to report on the general character of the labor contractions as well as the other symptoms of labor. First, it must be determined whether the patient is actually in labor. Although this is occasionally a difficult problem to settle, usually a decision can be reached on the basis of the differential points between true and false labor (Table 13-1). It is important that the patient be aware of the difference, too, since it will save herself and the doctor innumerable telephone calls and concern if she does not think every contraction is indicative of true labor.

ADMISSION TO THE HOSPITAL

As previously stated, the mother who has been given adequate antepartal care will have received instruction from the physician or the nurse on what to anticipate when she comes to the hospital to have her baby. If this is the mother's first hospital experience, it will be much easier for her if she has been told about the necessary preliminary procedures, such as vulvar and perineal preparation, the methods of examination employed to ascertain the progress of labor, and the usual routines exercised for her care in the course of labor. It is important for the mother to understand that she should come to the hospital at the onset of labor; for as labor progresses, these activities are more difficult to carry out and are much more distressing to the patient. If the mother has not had adequate prenatal care to

prepare her, then her labor may be rather advanced upon admission and she may not know what to expect. It will then fall to the nurse to reassure this mother and orient her as quickly as possible to the process of labor and the physical environment. In these instances, the nurse will find her ability to make decisive clinical judgments, especially with regard to establishing priorities of care, extremely helpful and necessary.

The preparation for delivery will of necessity vary in different hospitals, since every hospital has its own admission procedure. The nurse should be aware that many details may be accomplished in a number of ways. Very few institutions employ precisely the same technique in preparing a mother for delivery. Actually, the differences are in details only, for the principles are the same everywhere—namely, asepsis and antisepsis, together with careful observation of the mother for any deviations from the normal.

ESTABLISHMENT OF THE NURSE-PATIENT RELATIONSHIP

For many a young mother in labor, admission to the maternity unit may mark her first aquaintance with hospitals as a patient. Her immediate reaction may be one of strangeness, loneliness and homesickness, particularly if the husband is not permitted to stay with her in the labor room. Regardless of the amount of preparation for this event, whether she is happy or unhappy, whether she wants the baby or not, every mother enters labor with a certain amount of normal tension and anxiety (see p. 240). Moreover, not infrequently mothers are thoroughly afraid of the whole process. This may be attributed in part to the fact that the mother's preparation for childbearing has been limited, or she may have been reared in an environment fraught with mysteries and old wives' tales about childbirth. If she has had previous children, she may have had unfortunate and fear-producing experiences. All these factors make her fear understandable.

In addition, the nurse's contact with the patient during the labor and delivery process is very short term. Thus, the nurse is faced with the problem of providing high quality care in a short space of time. The key to the problem appears to lie in her ability to utilize whatever time she has available, whether it be 5 minutes or an hour, to provide an atmosphere of receptivity to her patients' needs. Her ability to determine needs lies in her ability in the collection and diagnosis portion of the process of clinical judgment. When she im-

TABLE 13-2. GUIDELINES TO MOTHERS PARTICIPATION IN LABOR*

WHAT IS HAPPENING	HELPING YOURSELF	BREATHING PATTERN IN CONTRACTION	OTHER HELPS
PRELUDE TO LABOR Lightening (2-4 weeks before 1st baby comes). Braxton-Hicks contractions may increase. Increase vaginal mucous discharge. Weight loss of 2-3 lbs. (3-4 days before labor). Baby less active. Spurt of energy (1-2 days before labor).	Have hospital suitcase packed. Simplify housekeeping. Conserve energy.		
ONSET OF LABOR You may notice any one or a combination of: Regular contractions (felt as backache, pelvic pressure, gas, menstrual cramp, etc.). Show. Rupture of membranes.	Check signs; time contractions. Call doctor and report. If daytime, continue usual light activity. If night, rest.		Husband or other chosen companion offers diversion and relieves possible tension-producing situations in home.
EARLY FIRST STAGE Cervix effacing, dilatation beginning. Contractions become strong enough so that you feel need to do something. Dilatation continuing; contractions becoming somewhat closer and stronger. If contractions are causing backache.	When contractions start, breathe out and relax. Continue slow deep breathing through contraction. Try sitting positions. In between contractions rest, read, watch TV, etc. Go to hospital as doctor directs. Relax as much as possible in sitting or lying positions during travel and admitting procedures. Lie on side, breathe deeply and slowly while rocking pelvis very gently throughout contraction.		Admitting procedures, including questions, examinations, checking baby's heart, perineal shave, enema; medication as indicated. Firm pressure against lower back or slow deep massage during contractions.

LATE FIRST STAGE

Dilatation continuing; contractions becoming markedly closer, stronger, and of longer duration.

Try lying on back.

Breathe regularly but more shallowly during contraction.

When further need felt, change to accelerated breathing, shallow at height of contraction.

Relax during contraction.

Direction in control of relaxation and of breathing rhythm and depth.

Face sponged with cool cloth; lips moistened.

No distracting conversation.

Medication as indicated.

TRANSITION:

10 to 20 strong, long contractions, close together but may be somewhat irregular. These contractions complete dilatation.

Rectal pressure may cause desire to bear down.

There may be tremors, nausea, perspiration, hiccups.

During contraction continue to try to relax.

Concentrate on breathing control.

As contraction starts, begin breathing fairly deeply. Puff out occasionally if there is urge to push. Don't hold breath! Don't push.

Reassurance about normality of sensations and probable limitation of their duration.

Understanding acceptance of possible expressions of irritability.

SECOND STAGE

Baby moves gradually through birth canal.

Contractions change in character, remaining very strong but slightly further apart.

Continuing strong contractions pushing baby down against pelvic floor and causing stretching, perhaps burning sensation.

Baby's head seen at vaginal opening.

As doctor slowly delivers head, there may be strong desire to push.

Shoulders are born one at a time. Relief is experienced as birth of baby is completed.

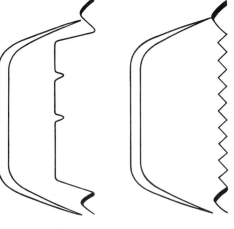

During contractions use position shown in Fig. 10-6.

Push toward vaginal opening as directed, relaxing pelvic floor and steadily reinforcing work of uterus.

Between contractions relax completely.

While being moved to delivery room, pant deeply through contractions.

When settled on delivery table, push as directed through contractions, remembering to relax pelvic floor and thighs.

Rest completely between contractions.

Pant deeply to control pushing urge; relax thighs.

If requested to push, push very gently.

Pillows arranged to support mother in comfortable position for pushing.

Direction of pushing effort and encouragement of complete relaxation between contractions.

Transfer to delivery room. (Anesthesia as indicated). (Episiotomy as indicated).

Direction for controlled pushing and panting.

THIRD STAGE

Rhythmical contractions, less intense.

Abdomen sensitive.

Placenta delivered.

Push as directed.

Lie back and enjoy baby!

* Maternity Center Association: Preparation for Childbearing. ed. 2, pp. 40-41, New York, 1969.

plements effective care, her facility with therapeutic communication, plus technical understanding and skill are key issues.

There has been a good deal of time and effort spent in nursing research to determine the needs of patients (see Suggested Readings), especially the needs above and beyond those related directly to the physiological and/or pathological conditions of the patient. These needs have generally been classified as "emotional" or "psychosocial." Whatever their label, they are especially important for consideration in the maternity patient. A recent study[2] has indicated that when questioned, patients expressed a preponderance of needs that were emotional in origin. These fell into the following general areas: the need to have one's *identity* recognized and maintained in the face of disability, the need to have some *control* over events relating to oneself, and needs deriving from *fear, anxiety* and *loneliness* which become translated into concern for *safety* and *comfort*.

Encouragement. Accordingly, one of the first responsibilities of the nurse is to recognize that, in addition to the physical manifestations, there are these psychosocial factors that influence each mother's pregnancy and have a bearing on her individual needs for care (see Chaps. 8 and 10). Therefore, every mother deserves encouragement that tends to inspire assurance during her labor. Her discomfort never should be minimized, and an effort should be made to help her to keep in control when her labor is painful. Attention should be directed to the fact that progress is being made, and that her efforts to work cooperatively with her labor are helpful and necessary.

Awareness of Physical and Behavioral Signs. In addition, the nurse must be constantly alert to the physical and behavioral signs associated with the progress of normal labor. She can be extremely helpful by giving the couple anticipatory guidance in this respect so that they will know what to expect during this experience. At the same time, she must watch vigilantly for any sign that may point to abnormal developments. For instance, an increase in pulse rate, a rise in temperature, excessive bleeding, changes in the character of uterine contractions, passage of meconium with a vertex presentation, or alterations in the fetal heart sounds are changes which

may have profound implications for the mother's welfare.

Rapport. The nurse who is cordial, empathic and interested in the welfare of her patients establishes good rapport with relative ease and, with astute interviewing, secures the necessary information that will enable her to gain greater insight into the mother's nursing needs. The establishing of rapport is essential in giving effective supportive care. Rapport may be thought of as a relationship consisting of interrelated thoughts and feelings that include empathy, compassion, sympathy, interest and respect for each individual as a unique human being. One of the crucial components of this type of relationship is empathy; that is, the ability to enter into the feeling or spirit of another person, with a consequent sense of being similar to or nearly identical with him. In a therapeutic nurse-patient relationship the feelings thus engendered are subjected by the nurse to critical scrutiny for the purpose of making more astute nursing diagnoses and hence, planning effective care. Empathy also enters into the nurse's ability to "role-take" as we have previously stated. Perhaps the most important quality necessary for the nurse to begin to empathize with the patient is the ability to identify with the patient. (For an interesting discussion of why student nurses often identify more quickly with certain patients see the Yeaworth article in the Suggested Readings.) Identification has been described as the mechanism which enables a person to take up any attitude toward another's mental life. Certain changes take place in the ego structure when this mechanism is employed resulting in an expansion of ego boundaries to include the attitude once observed in the other and now made a part of one's self. This type of identification is seen in children as they learn their various social roles, for instance. However, in the therapeutic relationship, the altered ego structure is only a temporary experience and remains "ego segregated" but available for reality testing and further thought. Certainly to be able to identify and share with another and then revert to one's own identity requires flexibility of the ego boundaries, and this flexibility can become enhanced with repeated use of the mechanism. After the nurse has attempted to experience the patient's feelings, she must be able to step back, that is, to narrow her ego boundaries back to reality. She then uses her intellectual processes to review what has occurred from three perspectives: (1) what is known about the patient, (2) what is known about herself, (3)

[2] Newman, M. A.: Identifying and meeting patients' needs in short-span nurse-patient relationships. Nurs. Forum, 5: pp. 76-86, 1966.

what is known from theory. Thus, subjectivity is converted into objectivity and permits valid assessment of needs and problems. In order for effective nursing therapy to be instituted, empathy must operate within a sound conceptual framework, backed by theoretical knowledge and clinical experience. It is a valuable aid in designing and implementing care, but is not to be considered a substitute for careful planning and rational evaluation. Unfortunately, we do not know if and how empathy can be taught or learned. We do know the ability to utilize the identification mechanism has something very vital to do with the empathy process. It is to the identification-empathy-rapport linkage that more research needs to be directed.

In addition to the notion of empathy, the concept of rapport also involves positive communication that contributes to mutual understanding and acceptance. While no "method" or "rules" have yet been determined to establish this positive, therapeutic communication, the student may find the following general behavioral principles useful when attempting to institute an effective relationship. (1) The nurse's verbalization regarding an aspect of the patient's behavior or appearance confronts the patient with the nurse's perception of the immediate situation. This tends to elicit the patient's agreement or disagreement and any subsequent explanation, especially when non-directive probes are used. Here the nurse indicates her attention and concern and the patient has the option of responding. (2) By being alert to the patient's cues regarding her various social roles (mother, wife, possible breadwinner, career women) and by demonstrating a genuine interest in her roles, the nurse can collect more data upon which an evaluation of her immediate and future needs can be based. This allows the patient to keep her identity and gives her some feeling of control in the situation. (3) Communication can be facilitated when the nurse acknowledges to the mother that she does not understand what she is saying and asks for further clarification. (4) All members of the health team (and family also if appropriate) ought to be informed of any needs of the patient that cannot be handled by the nurse alone; moreover subsequent actions by personnel (and family) are to be communicated to the patient so that she may recognize that communication lines are open and her needs and problems are recognized and attended to as they arise. This retards feelings of helplessness and loss of control. (5) Therapeutic communication is more likely to be initiated and facilitated if the nurse assumes a relaxed and/or sitting position, *close* to the patient if possible. Standing at the foot of the bed or in the doorway is not conducive to satisfying conversation. In the hustle and bustle of the labor and delivery suite, the nurse often falls into the habit of "popping in and out" with the result that the mother may never have a chance of more than a rhetorical answer to "How are you coming along?" This of course demolishes any attempts at positive communication, and promotes the feelings that many mothers have of the delivery staff as being "too busy to care."

The nurse who establishes rapport with her patient will, then, demonstrate understanding and acceptance of the mother. The mother, in turn, is able to trust the nurse, and an effective nurse-patient relationship is facilitated.[3]

First Impressions. The kind of greeting that the patient receives as she enters the delivery suite is extremely important and sets the tone for future interaction with the health team. Some institutions permit the father to accompany his wife to the area; others prefer to admit the mother first and then let the husband and the wife remain together; still others do not allow the husband to be with his wife at all during labor. If the husband is present, the nurse should be mindful that he is to be considered and welcomed in an appropriate way, as is his wife.

The mother should be made to feel welcome, expected and necessary (remember that it is she who delivers the baby). Thus she and her husband, if he is present, should be called by name and shown personally by the nurse to the labor room that the mother will occupy. Once there, the patient can be helped, if necessary, to undress and to get into bed.

Orientation. The mother and the father will need to know some of what will be expected of them, and what they in turn can expect as participants in this new situation. Hence, the nurse can begin an orientation to the process of labor as well as to the general environment. It is to be remembered that there is no set form or content for this orientation and no set time for the introduction and the continuation of this process; rather the nurse must first explore what the parents do know about the environment and the

---

[3] A more thorough discussion of the various concepts involved in rapport and their implementation has been described in the writings of Travelbee, Kachelski, and Jourard (see Suggested Reading).

labor process, so that she can judge what needs to be introduced, reinforced, etc., and when the most appropriate time to do this would be. An easy conversational manner may be employed rather than a rapid fire explanation of dos and don'ts.

The rationale for any procedures and/or restrictions always should be given. The patient should not be overloaded with too much stimuli at one time and should be allowed to absorb any new information and explanation before additional material is presented. The nurse can structure the situation to allow the patient to "feedback" information, so that she knows how much the mother really understands.

Generally, the mother and her husband will need to know what procedures and activities will be performed and the reason for them. In addition, the couple should know the limits of the mother's activity, and what restrictions of food and fluids there will be. What the patient and her husband can expect regarding the progress of labor should be included also (i.e., what will be happening physically, how the mother will be feeling, and how she and her husband can participate in the labor experience. See Table 13-1, Guidelines to Mother's Participation in Labor, and Chap. 11. The father, if present, can be included in any explanations, etc., since he may be participating in the care of his wife. As implied, this orientation will continue throughout the entire course of labor and possibly delivery. The nurse will determine when and how each phase will be instituted, according to the cues given by the mother and the husband.

CONTINUING CARE

After making the mother comfortable in the labor room, the nurse will need to find out some rather specific information regarding the mother's general condition (i.e., the frequency, the duration and the intensity of her contractions, the amount and the character of show, and whether the membranes have ruptured or are intact). At this point it is expedient to learn when the first signs of labor became apparent to the mother and the nature and timing of the uterine contractions from that time. Since the mother's emotional status often has bearing on her physical labor, it is wise to be continuously alert to her behavior—whether she seems *unduly* apprehensive, or whether she is relatively relaxed or calm. Restlessness, excessive conversation, rapid, darting eye movements, arm and body rigidity, and plucking at the bedclothes are all signs of the former. The nurse reports all findings to the physician as soon as possible.

Although the nurse will want to avoid any outward display of rush or hurry, she should proceed with the admission as quickly as possible. It must be remembered that the mother's labor usually will become progressively stronger; hence the more procedures, orientation, etc., that can be accomplished early in labor, while she is able to be more responsive with relative ease, will enhance the patient's comfort and well-being. Also, there generally will be several other people concerned with the care of the mother—the doctor, intern, laboratory technician—and they often cannot carry out their activities until the patient is fully admitted. Finally, an expeditious completion of the admission procedures leaves more time for the mother and her husband to be together before the actual delivery.

Prior to the physician's examination the nurse will take the mother's temperature, pulse, respiration and blood pressure and listen to the fetal heart tones. A voided urine specimen will be obtained for the admission specimen and will facilitate the physician's vaginal examination. If the patient is allowed to use the bathroom, a receptacle should be placed under the toilet seat since the physician will want to have available for examination whatever material may be passed per vagina, as well as the urine specimen. If the patient is in labor, the doctor probably will order such procedures as shaving and cleansing of the vulva.

Enema. Unless labor is progressing too rapidly, a cleansing enema may be ordered. The nurse will use the same principles in giving the enema as for any other patient; however, she may find it more difficult to insert the tube because of the pressure of the presenting part of the fetus or of hemorrhoids that the mother may have. Hemorrhoids and/or the strength of the contractions may make the enema discomforting for the patient. It is essential that the nurse let the mother know that she is aware of the possible discomfort, and that she will do all she can to give the enema carefully and comfortably. Giving a step-by-step explanation of the procedure as well as telling the mother specifically what she can do to help to allay the discomfort will go far to alleviate the discomfort. Helpful remarks are: "Let me know when you're having a contraction, and I'll clamp the tubing. Relax your buttocks when you begin to feel the tube being inserted. I'll give this very slowly, so as not to increase cramping. Let me know if it's too uncomfortable, and I can stop the flow for a little while."

An admission bath is rarely a routine procedure. Most patients have sufficient warning at the onset of labor to enable them to bathe prior to coming to the hospital. When a bath is deemed desirable, the type used will depend to some extent on the facilities of the hospital. The types usually given are the shower and the sponge bath. The hand spray may be used as an improvised shower when the shower stall is not available.

Vulvar and Perineal Preparation. The aim in shaving and washing the vulva is to cleanse and disinfect the immediate area about the vagina and to prevent anything contaminated from entering the birth canal. During labor, pathogenic bacteria ascend the birth canal more readily, and every effort should be made to protect the mother from intrapartal infection. In some hospitals a sterile gauze sponge or a folded towel is placed against the introitus to prevent contaminated matter, such as hair or soapy fluid, from entering the vagina during the preparation procedure. In addition, the nurse should be aware that infection from the nasopharynx is possible, and she should avoid unnecessary coughing or talking which might contaminate the vulva from this source.

Some physicians do not require that the mons pubis be shaved because of its distance from the episiotomy area and because of the discomfort that the regrowth of the hair causes; clipping the hair in this area often suffices. Some do not even wish the perineum shaved although episiotomy repair is certainly facilitated in the absence of perineal hair. However, most physicians still require the traditional pubic and perineal shave. When this is done, the pubic and the vulvar hair are lathered prior to shaving to facilitate the procedure and make it more comfortable for the mother. An ordinary safety razor is used, and, beginning at the mons veneris, with the direction of the stroke being from above downward, the area of the vulva and the perineal body is shaved. The nurse can stretch the skin above each downward stroke and permit the razor to move smoothly over the skin without undue pressure. When the entire area anterior to an imaginary line drawn through the base of the perineal body has been shaved, the patient can be turned to her side to enable the nurse to complete the shaving of the anal area. With the upper leg well flexed, the anal area is lathered and shaved, again with a front-to-back stroke. It must always be remem-

bered that anything which has passed over the anal region must not be returned near the vulvar orifice.

The solutions as well as the techniques used in cleansing the genitals will vary in different hospitals, but warm water with soap is probably the most commonly employed. More recently, pHisoHex has come into popular usage. A little of this antibacterial liquid cream, used with water and applied to the area with friction, creates a lather and cleanses the skin. On repeated use it develops cumulative bacteriocidal and bacteriostatic properties. Some patients do get a local mucosal reaction manifested by edema and tenderness when pHisoHex is used full-strength. In these cases the pHisoHex should be discontinued and a non-irritating soap substituted. The reaction disappears spontaneously in several hours, and no specific treatment is required other than to remove the solution thoroughly with water.

In washing the genitals, the nurse cleanses thoroughly first the surrounding areas, using sterile sponges or disposable washcloths for each area and gradually works in toward the vestibule. The strokes must be from above downward and away from the introitus. Special attention should be paid to separating the vulvar folds in order to remove the smegma which may have accumulated in the folds of the labia minora and/or at the base of the clitoris. Finally, the region around the anus is cleansed. It should be emphasized here again that a sponge which has passed over the anal area must not be returned near the vulvar orifice but should be discarded immediately. The patient is instructed not to touch the genitals lest she infect herself.

EXAMINATIONS IN LABOR

General. The pulse, respiration and temperature are taken, as previously stated, and are repeated every 4 hours. In cases in which there is fever, or in which labor has lasted more than 24 hours, it is desirable to repeat these observations every 2 hours. The blood pressure is recorded by either the physician or the nurse and is repeated every hour; in cases of toxemia of pregnancy, this may be done more frequently, according to the physician's instructions. As soon as possible after admission, a complete examination of the heart and the lungs is carried out by the physician to make certain that there are no conditions present which might contraindicate the type of analgesia or anesthesia to be used.

Fig. 13-1. Rectal examination, showing flexion of thumb of the gloved hand to prevent contamination of the vulva.

Abdominal. The abdominal examination is similar to that carried out in the antepartal period, comprising estimation of fetal size and position and listening to the fetal heart sounds.

Rectal. The majority of the examinations during labor are abdominal and rectal; vaginal examinations may be performed for special reasons. It was previously thought that rectal examinations were much safer than vaginal examinations, since they reduced the risk of carrying pathogenic bacteria from the introitus and the lower vagina to the region of the cervix and the lower uterine segment. Studies and general experience show that this supposed advantage of rectal examinations over vaginal examinations has been greatly exaggerated. Nevertheless, rectal examinations do have the advantage of not requiring preliminary disinfection on the part of the physician or the patient.

For either rectal or vaginal examination the patient lies on her back with her knees flexed. The nurse should drape the patient so that she is well protected, but with the perineal region exposed. In making a rectal examination the index finger is used, the hand being covered by a clean but not necessarily sterile rubber glove. As shown in Figure 13-1, the thumb should be fixed into the palm of the hand, because otherwise it may enter the vagina and introduce infection. The finger is anointed liberally with a lubri-

cating jelly and introduced slowly into the rectum. The cervical opening usually can be felt as a depression surrounded by a circular ridge (Fig. 13-2). The degree of dilatation and the amount of effacement are noted. Very often the membranes can be felt bulging into the cervix, particularly during a contraction. The level of the fetal head is now ascertained and correlated with the level of the ischial spines as being a certain number of centimeters above or below the ischial spines. After the completion of the examination the patient's perineum is wiped, and the examiner's hands are washed. The rectal glove is cleansed and sterilized if it is to be reused; otherwise, it is discarded.

The frequency with which rectal examinations are required during labor depends on the individual case; often one or two such examinations are sufficient, while in some instances more are required. The nurse who stays with the mother constantly will find that she becomes increasingly skillful in her ability to follow the progress of labor to a great extent by careful evaluation of subjective and objective symptoms of the mother (i.e., the character of the uterine contractions and the show, the progressive descent of the area on the abdomen where fetal heart sounds are heard, the mother's over-all response to her physical labor, etc.).

FIG. 13-2. Rectal examination, showing how the examining finger palpates the cervix and the infant's head through the rectovaginal septum.

Vaginal. If the mother is to have a vaginal examination, she may be prepared by cleansing the vulvar and the perineal region in a manner similar to that used in preparation for delivery. The physician scrubs his hands as for an operation and dons sterile gloves. Before introducing his fingers into the vagina, he takes care to separate the labia widely in order to minimize possible contamination of his examining fingers if they should come in contact with the inner surfaces of the labia and the margins of the hymen. Then the index and the second fingers of the examining hand are gently introduced into the vagina (Fig. 13-3). Vaginal examination is more reliable than rectal, since the cervix, the fontanels, etc., can be palpated directly with no intervening rectovaginal septum to interfere with the tactile sense. Some authorities feel that the danger of introducing infection into the birth canal is increased with repeated vaginal examinations and thus attempt to limit the number of times the examination is repeated, using it only as necessary.

CONDUCT OF THE FIRST STAGE

The first stage of labor (dilating stage) begins with the first symptoms of true labor and ends with the complete dilatation of the cervix. The physician examines the patient early in labor and sees her from time to time throughout the first stage but may not be in constant attendance at this time. In normal labor his examinations (fetal heart, rectal, etc.) will show that the baby is in

good condition and that steady progress is being made. Furthermore, the rate of progress often will give some indication as to when delivery is to be expected. Since the physician is usually unable to be with the mother constantly during

FIG. 13-3. Vaginal examination.

Fig. 13-4. Expectant parents share experience of labor together. (MacDonald House, University Hospitals of Cleveland)

this stage, he must rely on the nurse not only to safeguard the welfare of mother and fetus but also to notify him concerning the progress of labor.

Support During Labor

As already emphasized, it is as important for the nurse to have an empathic supportive attitude toward the mother, so she can interpret the progress of labor and perform certain technical procedures skillfully. It should be pointed out that "supportive care" includes not only aspects of emotional support but also aspects of physical care which in the total context of care contribute to the well-being and the comfort of the mother and hence to her emotional equilibrium. Thus, a sponge bath, oral hygiene, a backrub, an explanation before a procedure, etc., all enhance her comfort and help the mother to feel that she is a special, worthwhile person. Many

of the physical care activities that nurses perform consist, in part at least, of "laying on of hands," which is known to be necessary and helpful to patients in maintaining or reachieving good health. These activities, then, can be valuable entrées in establishing and maintaining rapport and hence an effective relationship. Even the intrusive procedures which are so often painful or distasteful, if done with gentleness and skill, show the patient that her dignity and integrity are respected.

Related to this "laying on of hands" aspect is the effectiveness of the use of touch. Although this has not been explored to any great degree scientifically, its importance was recognized as far back as the mid-19th century.[4] More recently, research indicates that the patient's ability to work

[4] Mauriceau, A. M.: The Married Women's Private Medical Companion. New York [publisher unknown], 1859.

effectively with her labor contractions increased when extensive physical contact was introduced and then decreased when physical contact was withdrawn (see Suggested Reading). This contact can take the form of a backrub, allowing the patient to grasp the nurse's hand, stroking the patient's brow, etc. However, touch should not be used indiscriminately, as excessive and/or inappropriate touching is offensive to many people. The need will vary from patient to patient, and the mother will indicate which type of touch is helpful and who will be the most appropriate person to give it. The nurse must use her professional judgment regarding its use, and her rapport with the patient will help her to make a correct decision. This type of communication can be a way of demonstrating the nurse's concern and empathy, especially when verbal communication is difficult or impossible. It is also an effective means of incorporating the husband into the care and the support of his wife.

The more cheerful, flexible environment of the modern labor room undoubtedly is conducive to putting the patient and her husband more at ease, but this in itself is not enough. Once labor is well established, the mother should not be left alone. The morale of women in labor is sometimes hopelessly shattered, regardless of whether or not they have been prepared for labor during pregnancy, when they are left by themselves over long periods of time. During labor the mother is more sensitive to the behavior of those about her, particularly in relation to her perception of how much concern the personnel about her show for safety and well-being. As labor progresses, there is a normal narrowing of the phenomenal field, an "inward turning," which results in easy distortion of stimuli and perception. For instance, careless remarks dropped in conversation often are misinterpreted as indicative of negligence or unfeelingness. It is well to remember that comments and laughter overheard in the corridor outside the patient's room may contribute to her uneasiness. Therefore, the nurse must be on guard against unfortunate happenings of this kind.

The nurse should be aware that her own anxieties in the situation may be communicated to the patient. The process of labor and the forthcoming delivery will produce normal anxieties which are no more than a healthy anticipation of the events to come (in both patient and nurse). Thus, most patients tolerate their labor much better if they are told the kind of progress that is being made and assured that they are doing a good job working with their contractions. This is part and parcel of the continuing orientation to the labor process that was mentioned earlier (see p. 245).

Another point that is apropos here is the usefulness and the effectiveness of suggestion for the mother in labor. It has been shown that the pregnant woman is extremely passive and vulnerable; this increases her sensitivity and makes her receptive to both positive and negative suggestion from virtually total strangers. The nurse can utilize this suggestibility to great advantage in her supportive care, since the mother responds very readily to suggestions, especially in early labor. The groundwork can be laid at this time for the more complicated instructions that may be necessary later in labor concerning relaxation, breathing technics and the management of pain.

The mother who has attended antepartal classes that have included exercise and relaxation techniques is usually better prepared for labor, but nevertheless she needs to be coached in utilizing the technics which will enable her to cooperate with the natural forces of labor. During early labor the patient usually prefers to move about the room and frequently is more at ease sitting in a comfortable chair. She can be permitted and encouraged to do this and whatever else seems to be most relaxing and pleasant to her. If hospital policy permits the husband to be in the labor room, his presence can be a valuable asset because of the support that it gives his wife. Several studies have documented the presence of the husband during labor as a major source of support for the mother (see Suggested Reading). This not only benefits the mother but also helps the father to feel that he has a more vital role in participating with his wife in the birth of their child (Fig. 13-4).

Progression of Active Phase of Labor. When the mother begins to mind her labor, she may need help to get into a comfortable position and to relax. During the contractions she can be coached as necessary in the application of the slow deep-breathing technique described in Chapter 8. Regardless of how diligently the mother has practiced the various breathing and relaxing techniques during pregnancy, or the level of her understanding about the physiology of labor, the situation is changed somewhat for her by active labor. Each mother may react in a slightly different way, for each is an individual. Some analgesic medication may be required for the mother's comfort after good labor is established (see p. 228). The nurse

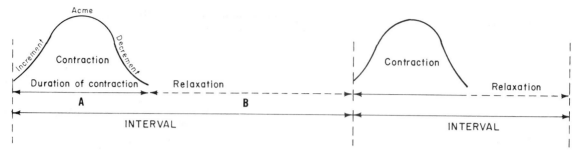

FIG. 13-5. The interval and the duration of uterine contractions. The frequency of contractions is the interval timed from the beginning of one contraction to the beginning of the next contraction. The interval consists of two parts: (A) the duration of the contraction and (B) the period of relaxation. The broken line indicates an indeterminate period, since this time (B) is usually of longer duration than the actual contraction of (A).

may observe in time that as the active phase progresses (i.e., the 7 to 10 cm. dilation) slow deep breathing becomes difficult for the patient. The mother herself is aware that "her diaphragm won't cooperate." Rapid, shallow breathing (accelerated breathing) with the contractions is usually easier and more effective.

Uterine Contractions

The term "pains" has been associated with uterine contractions of childbirth since time immemorial. One finds this term still in common usage, so that even today many young women approach childbirth with fear of pain. It is no easy task to dispel this age-old fear, but throughout the childbirth experience a conscious effort must be made to instill a wholesome point of view in the mother. The nurse should avoid the use of the word "pain" whenever possible because of the very connotation of the word, and it is hoped that she will not use it in reference to uterine contractions. It is important to remember, however, that as labor progresses, the contractions often become painful. This is not just a figment of the patient's imagination. Therefore, it is the nurse's responsibility to help the mother to distinguish between the *fear and anticipation* of pain and the *actual* pain she may be experiencing, and to help her to cope effectively.

Studies of pain have demonstrated that the anticipation of pain raises the anxiety level significantly to cause the pain reaction threshold to lower. Thus, the patient reacts sooner to even minimal pain stimuli. The pain is subjectively intensified and even a slight amount of pain seems to be much greater. Furthermore, other sensations are misinterpreted as pain (e.g., pressure, stretching, etc.), which explains why the digital

examinations and even the pressure of the nurse's fingers on the abdomen as she times contractions "hurts." Therefore, "everything" is painful, and the heightening of the anticipation of pain in turn increases the response to pain, and soon a vicious cycle is established. The nurse can help to break this cycle or to prevent it from becoming established by intervening at the anticipation-anxiety junction. She does this by reminding the patient when a contraction is over (and the pain is gone), that another contraction is not expected for several minutes: thus, this is the time for the mother to rest and to relax. The anxiety related to the anticipation of pain then is lowered or eliminated (the mother knows now she is free from pain for several minutes and can rest), and the subjective intensification is diminished. It is obvious that the nurse or some other reliable person must be in continuous attendance in order to do this. Moreover cultural (and sub-cultural) factors play an important part in the meaning and interpretation of pain for patients. While pain is basically a physiological phenomenon, the meaning pain has and the kinds of responses to pain that are deemed appropriate are matters of cultural prescription. Cultural orientations, social conditioning, and sociocultural sanctioning play a large part in molding patterns of response to painful experiences which are modal (i.e., occur most frequently) in a group, and these modal patterns are meaningful in terms of the values and beliefs of a particular group. Therefore, a culture or subculture from which a person comes conditions the formation of his particular reaction patterns to pain, and a knowledge of a group's attitudes toward pain is extremely important to the understanding of the reaction of a particular member of that group. (For a more thorough discussion of the responses and interpretation of pain by various cultural and sub-cultural groups see Suggested Readings.)

The frequency, the duration and the intensity of the contractions should be watched closely and recorded. The frequency of contractions is timed from the beginning of one contraction until the beginning of the next. The duration of a contraction is timed from the moment the uterus first begins to tighten until it relaxes again (Fig. 13-5). The intensity of a contraction may be mild, moderate or strong at its acme. Since this is a relative factor, it is difficult to interpret unless one is at the mother's bedside. For the sake of description, one might say that during a mild contraction the uterine muscle becomes somewhat tense; during a moderate contraction the uterus becomes moderately firm; during a strong contraction the uterus becomes so firm that it has the feel of woody hardness, and at the height of the contraction the uterus cannot be indented by pressure of the examiner's fingers.

When the mother first becomes aware of the contractions, they may be 15 to 20 minutes apart and lasting perhaps 20 to 25 seconds. Since these are of mild intensity, she usually can continue with whatever she is doing, except that she is alert to time the subsequent contractions (to have specific information to give the physician when she calls him). If this is her first pregnancy, he may advise her to wait until the contractions are 5 to 10 minutes apart before coming to the hospital (depending on the other signs of labor). However, if she is a multipara, she will more than likely be told to come to the hospital as soon as a regular pattern of contractions is established (again, depending on other criteria).

As labor progresses, the character of the contractions will change (see Chap. 11). They will become stronger in intensity, last longer (a dura-

Fig. 13-6. Mother in active first-stage labor (cervix 8 cm. dilated) being assisted by husband and nurse to accomplish conscious relaxation. (MacDonald House, University Hospitals of Cleveland)

tion of 45 to 60 seconds) and come closer together (at a frequency of every 2 to 3 minutes). The only effective method the nurse can employ to time contractions is to keep her fingers lightly on the fundus. The fingers are recommended because they usually are more sensitive than the more calloused palm. However, for some people the whole hand is helpful. It should be emphasized that enough of the fingers should be used to ensure adequate contact with the abdomen; too slight a contact does not enable the nurse to ascertain the contractions accurately.

As the nurse times in this manner, she is able to detect the contraction, as it begins, by the gradual tensing and rising forward of the fundus, and to feel the contraction through its 3 phases until the uterus relaxes again. The inexperienced nurse can get some idea of how a contraction will feel under her fingertips if she feels her own biceps contract. First, the forearm should be extended and the fingertips of the hand on the opposite side placed on the biceps. Then, the arm is gradually flexed until the muscle becomes very hard, held a few seconds, and gradually extended. This should take about 30 seconds to simulate a uterine contraction. It is not reliable to ask the mother to let you know when contractions begin, because often she is unaware of it for perhaps 5 or 10 seconds, sometimes even until the contraction reaches its acme. It is important for the nurse to observe the rhythm of the contractions and to be assured that the uterine muscle relaxes completely after each contraction. As the labor approaches the transition, the contractions will be very strong, last for about 60 seconds and occur at 2 to 3 minute intervals. If any contraction lasts longer than 70 seconds and is not followed by a rest interval with complete relaxation of the uterine muscle, this should be reported to the physician immediately because of its implications for both the mother and her infant (see Chap. 20, Complications of Labor).

Particularly during the late active phase the need for human contact—someone to hold on to—during the severe contractions will be seen. The mother responds less well to other physical contact, stroking, sponging, etc.; she may even say, "Leave me alone," meaning, of course, "Don't disturb me." However, it is helpful for her, to have someone's hand to hold, and she should be allowed to do this if she indicates the need.

Since during the first stage of labor the uterine contractions are involuntary and uncontrolled by the patient, it is futile for her to "bear down" with her abdominal muscles, because this only leads to exhaustion. The mother who has been prepared for "natural childbirth" has been schooled in breathing techniques, such as diaphragmatic breathing or rapid shallow costal breathing, and with coaching from her husband or her nurse is usually able to accomplish conscious relaxation.

With the "unprepared" mother a different situation exists. These mothers can best be helped to relax by encouraging and coaching them to keep breathing slowly and evenly during the early contractions and then more rapidly and shallowly during the late active phase. They should be reminded not to hold their breath during the contractions. One cannot expect perfection in the breathing techniques with these patients; however, this activity gives the inexperienced mother a point of concentration, and her feeling that she is actually participating and "controlling" her labor to some degree is helpful to her. Most mothers in labor, whether they are "prepared" or not, want to cooperate, and the calm, kind, firm guidance of an interested nurse can do much to help the mother utilize her contractions effectively.

Show

This mucoid discharge from the cervix is present after the discharge of the mucous plug. As progressive effacement and dilatation of the cervix occur, the show becomes blood-tinged due to the rupture of superficial capillaries. The presence of an increased amount of bloody show (blood-stained mucus, not actual bleeding!) suggests that rather rapid progress may be taking place and should be reported immediately, particularly if associated with frequent severe contractions.

A perineal pad is not to be worn during labor because of the nature of the vaginal discharge. The tenacious mucoid discharge frequently comes in contact with the anus and could easily be smeared about the external genitalia and vaginal orifice when the patient moves about the bed or adjusts the pads. A quilted pad placed under the mother's buttocks serves very well to absorb material discharged from the vagina. This pad should be changed frequently and the perineum cleansed as necessary to keep the mother clean and dry.

Fetal Heart Tones

The behavior of the fetal heart beat in labor is of great importance. When taking the fetal heart sounds, one should listen and count for 1 full minute in order that any irregularity or slowing may be detected. As already explained, the fetal heart rate normally is between 120 to 160 beats per minute, except during and immediately after a uterine contraction, when it may fall to as low as 70 to 110. Hon[5] found that in multigravidas the fetal heart rate might fall from 140 to 110-120 beats per minute at the acme of a contraction. In primigravidas the drop is greater, at times reaching 60 to 70 beats per minute (Fig. 13-7). This physiologic bradycardia begins after the onset of a contraction and ends 10 to 15 seconds prior to its end. It is believed to result from compression of the fetal skull by the partially dilated cervix rather than from fetal hypoxia. It appears to occur most commonly between 4 and 8 cm. of cervical dilatation.

It may be difficult to hear the sounds during a contraction, because the uterine wall is tense, and, in addition, it is more difficult for the mother to lie still during this period. But it is particularly important to listen at this time, since these observations inform the listener how the fetus reacts to the contraction. From a clinical standpoint any prolonged slowing should be reported to the obstetrician. Should the slowing be below 100 beats per minute, and should it last more than 30 seconds after the termination of a contraction, then it is no longer considered to be

5 Hon, E. H.: Electronic evaluation of fetal heart rates. Am. J. Obstet. Gynec. 83:333-358, February 1, 1962.

physiologic and is taken as a sign of fetal distress. Occasionally, this prolonged slow rate is accompanied by the passage of meconium, another sign indicative of fetal distress if it occurs in a vertex presentation. It must be remembered that, unless the membranes have ruptured, the meconium will not be apparent. Any unusual observations must be reported to the physician promptly so that measures can be instituted before permanent damage is done to the infant.

Repeated auscultation of the fetal heart sounds constitutes one of the most important responsibilities in the conduct of the first and the second stages of labor (see Chap. 6, Normal Pregnancy). During the early period of the first stage of labor the nurse should record the fetal heart rate every hour, and once good labor is established, every half hour, or even more often if indicated. During the second stage of labor it should be done every 5 minutes and recorded.

The fetal heart tones should be checked immediately following the rupture of membranes, regardless of whether they rupture spontaneously or are artificially ruptured by the physician. With the gush of water that ensues, there is a possibility that the cord may be prolapsed, and any indication of fetal distress from pressure on the umbilical cord can thereby be detected.

Electronic Monitoring

In the past decade, a good deal of work has gone into the electronic measuring of uterine

FIG. 13-7. Electronic evaluation of fetal heart rates, showing normal slowing of the fetal heart rate during uterine contraction. (Hon, E. H.: Observations on "pathologic" fetal bradycardia, Am. J. Obstet. Gynec. 77:1084, 1959)

forces in labor (tokodynamometry, electrohy-stereography) and fetal heart rate in labor (fetal electrocardiography). Since the equipment is very expensive and still for the most part in the proto-type stage, its use has been limited mostly to gathering information for research purposes rather than everyday clinical activity. However, some medical centers are fortunate to have their use daily. Valuable information has been obtained regarding the physiology and functional pathology of labor as well as the effects of drugs in labor. Fetal electrocardiography is useful in detecting fetal existence (as early as 11 weeks), diagnosing presentation, multiple pregnancy, determining the effects of drugs and anesthesia, and the status of the baby as it progresses down the birth canal (see Fig. 12-7). In this case fetal hypoxia can now be detected and treatment instituted so that minor degrees of brain damage can be prevented.

Other Aspects of Care

Temperature, Pulse and Respiration. The pulse in normal labor is usually in the 70's or the 80's and rarely exceeds 100. Sometimes the pulse rate on admission is slightly increased because of the excitement of coming to the hospital, but this returns to normal shortly thereafter. A persistent pulse rate over 100 suggests exhaustion or dehydration. The temperature and respiration should also be normal. If there is an elevation of temperature over 37.2° C. or 99° F. (orally), or the pulse and respiration become rapid, the physician should be notified. The temperature should be recorded every 4 hours, or more frequently if indicated. On the other hand, the pulse and respiration should be taken every hour.

Blood Pressure. The blood pressure should be recorded every hour during labor. During the first stage of labor there is little change in blood pressure between contractions, but during contractions an average increase of 5 to 10 mm. Hg may be expected. For this reason the blood pressure readings should be taken between the contractions. Any unusual recordings of either systolic or diastolic pressure should be reported immediately.

Fluid and Food Intake. The practice here varies greatly among different physicians and in different institutions. Therefore, the wishes of the physician in charge should be ascertained before proceeding. In general, it is customary to urge the mother to take water or clear fluids, such as tea with sugar, during the early phase of the first stage of labor, but she should not be given solid or liquid foods because digestion is delayed during labor. Evidence that the powers of digestion are impaired at this time is demonstrated by the fact that it is not unusual for nausea and/or vomiting to occur near the end of the first stage of labor. It may be necessary to administer a general anesthetic for the delivery, so that if the patient takes fluid or food shortly before delivery, vomiting and consequent aspiration may occur. On the other hand, in a prolonged labor, it is most important to maintain adequate fluid and caloric intake in order to forestall dehydration and exhaustion, in which case the physician may

Fig. 13-8. Dystocia due to bladder distention. The tremendously distended bladder is plainly seen in the photograph. This patient was sent to the hospital after 3 days of ineffectual labor at home. The cervix had been dilated, it is believed, for 24 hours, yet no progress had been made. Catheterization of the greatly distended bladder yielded 1,000 cc. of urine. Following this, the infant's head descended at once, and delivery was easy. (Eastman: Williams' Obstetrics, ed. 11, New York, Appleton)

find it desirable to administer intravenous glucose solutions.

Bladder. The patient should be asked to void at least every 3 or 4 hours. The mother in labor often attributes all of her discomfort to the intensity of uterine contractions and therefore is unaware that it is the pressure of a full bladder which has increased her discomfort. In addition to causing unnecessary discomfort, a full bladder may be a serious impediment to labor (Fig. 13-8) or the cause of urinary retention in the puerperium. If the distended bladder can be palpated above the symphysis pubis, and the patient is unable to void, the physician should be so informed. Not infrequently he will order catheterization in such cases. Various techniques are used, all designed at maintaining strict asepsis. One technique employs sterile tissue forceps to hold the catheter.

Analgesia. (See Chap. 12, Analgesia and Anesthesia.) Before administering the medication prescribed to promote analgesia, the nurse informs the mother that she is going to give her medication which will make her more comfortable and help her in labor. She should encourage the mother to try to rest and assure her that she will not be left alone. It is also wise to tell her that you will remain quietly at the bedside and keep conversation at the very minimum in order for her to get the maximum benefit from the medication. Her bladder should be emptied prior to administering the drugs, and the fetal heart tones and the mother's vital signs can be recorded before and after such medication is given. Once analgesic therapy has been instituted, the mother should not receive fluids or food by mouth and should remain in bed. The environment should be conducive to rest, the room quiet and darkened but with sufficient light to permit accurate observation of the patient. Many institutions require that side rails be applied when the patient is medicated, even though there is someone in attendance. The necessity of this can be explained to both the patient and her husband, so that any undue fears or misinterpretations are avoided. The father, especially, should be alerted to the importance of keeping the rails up if he is attending to any of his wife's needs, since he is not used to their presence and is apt to forget to reapply them if he steps away from the bedside for a time. This can

FIG. 13-9. Mother is encouraged to relax and sleep between contractions (cervix 10 cm. dilated but fetal head needs to descend further). (MacDonald House, University Hospitals of Cleveland)

be a difficult experience for the husband. Thus, if he shows the strain at this time, he may welcome the suggestion of having a cup of coffee and a change of scene for a while. If the mother has received scopolamine or other drugs in dosage sufficient to cause her to be heavily sedated, she *never* should be left unattended.

Signs of Second Stage. There are certain signs and symptoms, both behavioral and physical, which herald the onset of the second stage of labor. These signs and symptoms are to be watched for carefully. They are as follows: (1) The patient begins to bear down of her own accord; this is caused by a reflex when the head begins to press on the perineal floor. (2) Her mood of increasing apprehension, which has been building since the contractions became well established, deepens; she becomes more serious and may appear bewildered by the force of the contractions. (3) There is usually a sudden increase in show that is more blood-tinged. (4) The patient becomes increasingly irritable and unwilling to be touched; she may cry if disturbed. (5) The mother thinks that she needs to defecate. This symptom is due to pressure of the head on the perineal floor and consequently against the rectum. (6) Although she has been "working" successfully with her contractions during most of her labor, the uncertainty that she has been experiencing (since 4 to 8 cm. cervical dilatation) as to her ability to cope with the contractions becomes overwhelming; she is frustrated and feels unable to manage if left alone. (7) The membranes may rupture, with discharge of amniotic fluid. This, of course, may take place any time but occurs most frequently at the beginning of the second stage. (8) The mother may be eager to be "put to sleep"; or if she is given appropriate help, she may narrow her concentration to trying to cope with the contractions and/or pushing according to instructions. It is important to remember that the mother's consciousness is somewhat altered because of the pain, her enforced concentration and possibly medication; therefore, any coaching should be short and explicit and may need to be repeated with each contraction. The nurse also must be firm but gentle in setting limits with the mother, so that she can conserve her energy for the second stage. Thrashing about and continued crying only lead to exhaustion, and the mother needs the firm guidance of a skillful person to help her to maintain control. (9) The perineum begins to bulge and the anal orifice to dilate. This is a late sign, but if signs numbered 1, 3, 5, and 7

occur, it should be watched for with every contraction. Only rectal or vaginal examination (or the appearance of the head) can definitely confirm the suspicion. Emesis at this time is not unusual.

In order to spare the mother a hurried trip to the delivery room and permit adequate time to cleanse and drape her properly for the delivery without unnecessary rush, the nurse should report promptly any or all of these symptoms which she observes. If these signs are overlooked, a precipitate delivery may occur without benefit of medical attention. In general, primigravidas are usually taken to the delivery room when the cervix is fully dilated, and multiparas when it is 7 or 8 cm. dilated.

CONDUCT OF THE SECOND STAGE

The second stage of labor (expulsion stage) begins with the complete dilatation of the cervix and ends with delivery of the baby. The complete dilatation of the cervix can be confirmed definitely only by rectal or vaginal examination. However, the nurse often is able to make a nursing diagnosis on the basis of her observations of the progress of labor, particularly if she correlates these findings with knowledge of the mother's parity, the speed of any previous labors, the pelvic measurements, etc., noted in the antepartal record. Although the general rule regarding the optimal time for taking a mother to the delivery room has been stated, it must be remembered that, in addition, the physician will be guided in his decision to give such an order by such factors as the station of the presenting part and the speed with which labor is progressing. If on examination of a primigravida, the physician finds the cervix to be fully dilated but the presenting part of the fetus only descended to the level of the ischial spines (midpelvis), he undoubtedly will want the mother to remain in the labor room to permit the forces of labor to bring about further descent of the fetus before taking the mother to the delivery room. During this period he may want the patient to exert her abdominal forces and "bear down." In most cases bearing-down efforts are reflex and spontaneous in the second stage of labor, but, occasionally, the mother does not employ her expulsive forces to good advantage, particularly if she has had caudal analgesia. The nurse will be asked to coach and encourage the mother in this procedure. The thighs should be flexed on the abdomen, with hands grasped just below the knees when a contraction begins. Instructions should be given to take a deep breath as soon as the contraction begins and, with her breath held, to exert downward pressure exactly as if she were straining at stool. Pulling on the knees at this time, as well as flexing the chin on the chest, is a helpful adjunct to maintain downward pressure of the diaphragm and to stabilize the chest and the abdominal musculature. In addition, maintaining the legs flexed as for the "push" position deters the mother from pushing her feet against the table or bed. Avoiding such pressure on the feet is important, because it discourages tensing of the gluteal muscles and thus contributes to further relaxation of the pelvic floor. The "bearing down" effort should be as long and sustained as possible, since short "grunty" endeavors are of little avail. If at this time the mother is in the delivery room, but her legs as yet have not been put up in stirrups or leg holders, she can be coached in the same manner. In most hospitals the delivery tables have firmly attached hand grips which can be adjusted in position so that the mother can reach them comfortably to pull against, if she wishes. However, in doing so her hands are not free to pull up on her knees with the contraction, so that the nurse or other person in attendance needs to assist her. This can be accomplished by assisting the mother to bring her legs up into position and exerting proper pressure against her knees as she bears down with the contraction. Care should be exercised to grasp the mother's knees from above, since doing so under the knees could exert undesirable pressure on the popliteal veins. At the end of each contraction the mother is assisted to put her legs down and encouraged to rest until the next contraction begins. Usually, these bearing-down efforts are rewarded by increased bulging of the perineum, that is, by further descent of the head. The patient should be informed of such progress, for encouragement is all-important. In certain instances it may be undesirable for the mother to bear down; thus the nurse should not encourage the mother to do so without the physician's request. In these cases, if the mother has an urge to bear down, she can be instructed to pant during each contraction; this will obviate her bearing down since it is impossible to push while panting.

When the mother is ready to be transferred to the delivery room, it is more helpful if the same nurse who has been attending her in labor accompanies her to the delivery room. This transfer will mean a new environment for the patient to cope with under very stressful circumstances.

There may be great physical and mental exertion called for with little preparation or practice. To the mother in labor who is unfamiliar with such surroundings, the "sterile" atmosphere of the delivery room can be strange, cold and uninviting, with its obstetric furnishings and supplies that become even more foreboding as they reflect the glittering lights of the room. Under such circumstances the sight and the sound of familiar faces and voices, even though partially concealed and muffled by the surgical caps, masks and gowns, do give the patient some sense of continuity and security. Furthermore, by this time the nurse and the patient should have established a communication pattern, each able to pick up the other's more covert cues. Thus, the coaching, guidance and follow-through necessary in the second stage of labor will be expedited if the same person continues with the care.

The nurse will notice that the mother has become increasingly involved in the whole birth process. The seemingly panicky frustration of the late active phase subsides a bit (with appropriate coaching and reassurance), and the patient may experience a sense of relief that the expulsive stage has begun. The desire to push and to bear down is very strong now—uncontrollable, in fact —and the patient generally gets enormous satisfaction with each push. Some patients, however (e.g., those with a highly charged emotional labor), experience acute pain and need all available help and encouragement to continue bearing down. The nurse will note that in most instances there is complete exhaustion after each expulsive effort, and the mother often drops off to sleep, only to be roused by the next contraction. Since consciousness is still altered, it may be difficult for the mother to follow directions readily even though she may want to. Again, repeated, short, explicit directions are required to encourage her to rest or to work, but especially to prepare the mother for the expulsive effort if she is sleeping between contractions and awakens abruptly.

Muscular cramps in the legs are common in the second stage because of pressure exerted by the baby's head on certain nerves in the pelvis. To relieve these cramps, the leg can be straightened and the ankle dorsiflexed by exerting pressure upward against the ball of the foot until the cramp subsides (see Fig. 8-15). Meanwhile, the knee is stabilized with the other hand. These cramps cause excruciating pain and must never be ignored.

FIG. 13-10. The delivery room. Nurse is preparing instrument table.

Good obstetric care during the second stage of labor demands the closest teamwork among physician, nurse and anesthetist. By previous understanding, or more often by established hospital routine, each has his or her own responsibilities in the delivery room, and, if the best interests of the mother and her infant are to be fulfilled, the responsibilities of each must be carried out smoothly and efficiently.

Up to now, the primary focus for the nurse has been on direct patient care. Now she must enlarge her focus to include the obstetrician and other allied professionals; that is, there will be more activities which will require the actual assistance of these persons than was necessary during the first stage of labor. Thus, the nurse must be sensitive not only to the cues sent by the mother but also to those relayed by the other personnel.

Preparation for Delivery

Preparation of the Delivery Room. There are no two hospitals in which the set-up of a delivery room or the procedure for delivery is precisely the same, and this is one phase of the nurse's work which she must learn wholly from actual observation and experience in her own institution. Nevertheless, she can obtain a general idea of the main equipment used from Figure 13-10.

The delivery table is designed so that its surface is actually composed of two adjoining sections, each covered with its own mattress. This permits the patient to lie in the supine position until it is desired to put her legs up into stirrups, that is, put her in the lithotomy position. At this time the table is "broken" by a mechanical device. The retractable or lower end of the table drops and is rolled under the main section of the table. Thus ready access is given to the perineal region. Or, if it is desired to deliver the patient in the dorsal recumbent position, the lower portion of the table can be allowed to remain in place.

The instrument table opposite the foot of the delivery table contains the principal sterile supplies and instruments needed for normal delivery, including, among other articles, towels, sponges, catheter, solutions, basins and the "cord set." The cord set is a group of instruments used for clamping and cutting the umbilical cord, namely, 2 hemostats, a pair of scissors and a cord tie or clamp. Other instruments often are included, because it may be necessary for the physician to perform an episiotomy or to repair lacerations (p. 283). Other instruments frequently included are 2 hemostats, 2 Allis clamps, 1 mouse-tooth tissue forceps, 2 sponge sticks, 1 vaginal retractor, 2 tenaculae, 1 needle holder, assorted needles and a pair of obstetric forceps.

A double-bowl solution stand or basin rack generally is used to hold the basins, one for wet sponges and the other to receive the placenta. Emergency instruments, a crib and a resuscitator are part of standard delivery room equipment. Even if the infant does not require resuscitation, the resuscitator affords him a warm, protected environment, and it is a convenient place in which to give him care. To facilitate the delivery, all equipment should be in readiness at all times.

Asepsis and Antisepsis. Persons who have a communicable disease or persons who have been in contact with a communicable disease should be excluded from maternity service until examined by a physician. The examining physician should certify that the employee is free from infections before he or she is allowed to return to duty. Personnel with evidence of upper respiratory infections or open skin lesions, diarrhea or any other infectious disease also should be excluded. Furthermore, all persons working in the maternity area should have a pre-employment physical examination and thereafter an annual physical examination and such interim examinations as may be required by the hospital.[6]

Of prime importance in the conduct of the second stage are strict asepsis and antisepsis throughout. To this end everyone in the delivery room wears a clean cotton uniform, cap and mask, and those actually participating in the delivery are in sterile attire. Masking must include both nose and mouth. Caps should be so adjusted as to keep *all* hair covered (Fig. 13-11). If the nurse scrubs to assist the doctor, the strictest aseptic technique must be observed. The hands are disinfected as carefully as for a major surgical operation. Scrubbing the hands should be started sufficiently early so that full time may be allotted for the scrub, as well as to don gown and gloves.

Transfer of the Mother to the Delivery Room. When the physician deems the birth to be im-

---

[6] Recommendations from the Manual of Standards in Obstetric-Gynecologic Practice, p. 11, Chicago, The American College of Obstetricians and Gynecologists, 1963.

FIG. 13-11. (*Left*) *Incorrect* method of wearing cap. Bacteria, hairs and other infectious particles can readily fall from exposed hair and contaminate sterile fields. (*Right*) *Correct* method of adjusting cap so that *all* hair is covered.

minent, he will ask that the mother be transferred to the delivery room and prepared for delivery. If the mother is awake, she can be told what is happening and be informed in advance about any procedure. If the husband will not be accompanying his wife to the delivery room, then time is allowed, if possible, for them to bid each other a temporary goodbye. This kind of planning not only is supportive but also enables both to cooperate more fully. Care should be taken to have only one person instruct or coach the mother at any one time. When delivery is imminent, her attention will be limited necessarily, as already illustrated, and the sound of several voices at one time is confusing. If the physician, for example, is coaching, it is well for nurse not to participate verbally; however, she should remain alert and ready to step into the role whenever it is appropriate.

Prior to the actual transfer to the delivery room the nurse should find out what type of anesthesia the physician is planning to use. Since the immediate positioning of the patient in the delivery room will depend on the type of anesthesia used, this preplanning will expedite activities during delivery and promote smoother functioning of the team.

Fig. 13-12. Proper draping for delivery showing appropriate placement of sterile towels, one of which covers the anus. (The Johns Hopkins Hospital, Baltimore, Md.)

Delivery

If spinal anesthesia is to be administered, the patient is turned on her side for the administration. If she is given a saddle block, she may be placed on her side or assisted to a sitting position on the side of the delivery table, with her feet supported on a stool and her body leaning forward against the nurse. Her back should be toward the operator and bowed (the position requires flexion of the neck and the lumbar spine). This principle of cervical and lumbar flexion is used also in the side lying position (see Chap. 12).

Although the positioning and the administration of the anesthesia take only a few minutes, the mother undoubtedly will be extremely uncomfortable due to the severity of the contractions at this time; she should be assured that this discomfort is only temporary, and soon she will be pain-free. The fetal heart tones and the maternal blood pressure should be checked frequently—every 5 minutes or so. In addition, the mother should have her head elevated with two small pillows to help prevent the anesthetic level from rising beyond the desired height. So that the anesthetic level may stabilize, the nurse waits for instructions from the anesthetist before putting the mother's legs in stirrups or performing any other manipulations. If the mother is to receive general anesthesia, she lies supine on the table. Local or pudendal anesthesia is administered with the mother in the lithotomy position (see Chap. 12).

As has been previously stated, anesthesia should be administered only by a qualified physician or a nurse anesthetist. This entire subject is discussed in more detail in Chapter 12, Analgesia and Anesthesia for Labor.

During the time that the anesthesia is being administered, the circulating nurse can uncover the sterile tables, check the resuscitator and attach a sterile suction catheter and oxygen mask, and perform other duties for which she is responsible. Once the anesthesia has been administered, the nurse resumes checking the fetal heart tones every 5 minutes.

Before elevating the mother's legs into the stirrups, cotton flannel boots which cover the entire leg are put on. In putting the legs of the patient up into stirrups or leg holders, care should be used not to separate the legs too widely or to have one leg higher than the other. Both legs should be raised or lowered at the same time, with a nurse supporting each one if the mother is unable to help in the positioning. Failure to

FIG. 13-13. Scalp of the infant detected through a slitlike vulvar opening as the perineal region begins to bulge and the skin over it becomes tense and glistening. Pressure of the descending head causes the anus to become patulous and everted. For purposes of showing changes which take place in the anus the lower towel has been removed from this photograph and the succeeding ones of this series, but this is for illustrative purposes only. (The Johns Hopkins Hospital, Baltimore, Md.)

observe these instructions may result in straining the ligaments of the pelvis, with consequent discomfort in the puerperium. Care should be taken to avoid pressure on the popliteal space, and to angle the stirrups so that the feet are not dependent. The mother also is given handles to grip and pull on, which aid her in her bearing-down efforts. Wrist straps usually are attached to these, which are secured about the wrist and allow some limited movement but prevent her from reaching up to touch the sterile drapes. The purpose of the handles and the cuffs should be explained to the mother, since many patients often complain about being "strapped down."

With the patient in the lithotomy position, the nurse carries out the procedure for cleansing the vulva and the surrounding area. If the delivery is to be conducted with the mother in the recumbent position, this may be carried out with the knees drawn up slightly and the legs sepa-

FIG. 13-14. Appearance of the infant's head with subsequent contractions. The vulva becomes more dilated and distended by the infant's head so that the opening is gradually converted into an ovoid. (The Johns Hopkins Hospital, Baltimore, Md.)

rated. Then, the physician, who meanwhile has scrubbed his hands and donned sterile gown and gloves, drapes the patient with towels and sheets appropriate for the purpose (Fig. 13-12).

After the patient has been prepared for delivery, catheterization, if done, is carried out by the physician. Sometimes it is difficult to catheterize a patient in the second stage of labor, since the infant's head may compress the urethra. If the catheter does not pass easily, force never should be employed. Whenever it is possible and appropriate, all procedures, of course, should be explained to the mother as they occur.

As the infant descends the birth canal, pressure against the rectum may cause fecal material to be expelled. The physician will employ sponges (as a rule soaked with saline solution) to remove any fecal material which may escape from the rectum.

Fundal pressure should not be used to accomplish spontaneous delivery or to bring the head deeper into the birth canal. Severe fundal pressure may cause uterine damage or rupture of the uterus.

As soon as the head distends the perineum to a diameter of 6 or 8 cm., the physician often will place a towel over the rectum and exert forward pressure on the chin of the baby's head while the other hand exerts downward pressure on the occiput (Figs. 13-13 to 17). This is called Ritgen's maneuver, and allows the physician to control the egress of the head; it also favors extension so that the head is born with the smallest diameter presenting. The head usually is delivered between contractions and as slowly as possible (Fig. 13-18). At this time the mother may complain about a "splitting" sensation due to the extreme vaginal stretching as the head is born. All these measures (control of head by Ritgen's maneuver, extension and slow delivery between contractions) help to prevent lacerations. If a tear seems to be inevitable, an incision which is called an episiotomy may be made in the perineum. This will not only prevent lacerations but also will facilitate the delivery (see p. 281). Immediately after the birth of the infant's head the physician passes his finger along the occiput to

FIG. 13-16. Farther advanced extension of the head. The left hand is used to prevent sudden expulsion of the head as it crowns, while pressure on the infant's chin through the perineum by the right hand expedites extension and delivery. This is Ritgen's maneuver. (The Johns Hopkins Hospital, Baltimore, Md.)

FIG. 13-15. Control of the progress of the head to preserve the perineum from tearing. (The Johns Hopkins Hospital, Baltimore, Md.)

Fig. 13-17. Ritgen's maneuver, as it appears in median section. Arrow shows direction of pressure.

the infant's neck in order to feel whether a loop or more of umbilical cord encircles it. If such a coil is felt, it should be gently drawn down and, if loose enough, slipped over the infant's head. This is done to prevent interference with the infant's oxygen supply, which could result from pressure of his shoulder on the umbilical cord. If the cord is too tightly coiled to permit this procedure, it must be clamped and cut before the shoulders are delivered; then the infant must be extracted immediately before asphyxiation results. As shown in Figure 13-19, the anterior shoulder usually is brought under the symphysis pubis first and then the posterior shoulder is delivered, after which the remainder of the body follows without particular mechanism (Figs. 13-20, 21). The exact time of the baby's birth should be noted. The infant usually cries immediately, and the lungs become expanded; about this time the pulsations in the umbilical cord begin to diminish. The physician usually will defer clamping the cord until this occurs, or for a minute or so if practicable, because of the marked benefit of the additional blood to the infant. Using sterile instruments, he cuts the cord between the 2 Kelly clamps, which have been placed a few inches from the umbilicus, then the umbilical clamp or tie is applied. The tie, a sterilized linen tape ligature, is usually applied about an inch from the abdomen, with care to secure it tight enough to prevent bleeding without its cutting into the cord

(Figs. 13-22, 25). A second ligature may be applied for further protection if it is desired, or if it is necessary because of any bleeding. There are several types of umbilical clamps, such as the Kane, the Zeigler and the Hesseltine, which are

Fig. 13-18. Birth of the head. The full hand is used to control the progress with emergence of the forehead and face. (The Johns Hopkins Hospital, Baltimore, Md.)

Fig. 13-19. Delivery of the shoulders. (*Left*) The anterior shoulder is brought under the symphysis pubis. (*Right*) Delivery of the posterior shoulder. (The Johns Hopkins Hospital, Baltimore, Md.)

Fig. 13-20. Delivery of the infant's body. (The Johns Hopkins Hospital, Baltimore, Md.)

used extensively in many institutions (Fig. 13-24). With these the possibility of hemorrhage is minimized.

The first 15 minutes after the infant's birth is the most hazardous period of life, when more infants succumb than during any subsequent time. The responsibility for much of the care during this period is delegated to the nurse, so that the physician may devote his attention to the mother during the third stage of labor (see p. 274 and Chap. 16).

CONDUCT OF THE THIRD STAGE
Delivery of the Placenta

The third stage of labor (placental stage) begins after the delivery of the baby and terminates with the birth of the placenta. Immediately after delivery of the infant the height of the uterine fundus and its consistency are ascertained. The physician may do this by palpating the uterus through a sterile towel placed on the lower abdomen, but it is a duty which often is delegated to the nurse, at least while the physician is engaged in clamping and cutting the umbilical cord. The nurse may do so by placing her hand on the abdomen *under* the sterile drape. The uterus should be held very gently with the fingers behind the fundus and the thumb in front. So long as the uterus remains hard, and there is no bleeding, the policy is ordinarily one of watchful waiting until the placenta is separated; no massage is practiced, the hand simply resting on the fundus to

Fig. 13-21. (*Left*) Upon delivery the infant is held in the head-down position to promote drainage of secretions from the respiratory passage. Mucus is gently wiped from the infant's face, then suctioned from the nostrils and the mouth with an ear bulb syringe or other suction device. Note that there is no traction on the cord, which is still attached to the placenta. (The Johns Hopkins Hospital, Baltimore, Md.)

Fig. 13-22. (*Right*) The cord is cut between the two Kelly clamps, which have been placed a few inches from the umbilicus. (The Johns Hopkins Hospital, Baltimore)

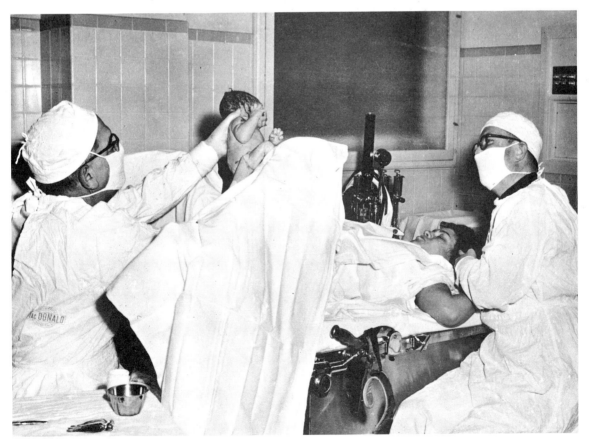

Fig. 13-23. Doctor lifts baby for parents to see immediately upon delivery.

Fig. 13-24. Umbilical cord clamp. A double-grip cord clamp in the opened and closed positions. (Hollister, Inc., Chicago, Ill.)

make certain that the organ does not balloon out with blood. Since attempts to deliver the placenta prior to its separation from the uterine wall are not only futile but may be dangerous, it is most important that the signs of placental separation be well understood. If the responsibility of

"guarding" the fundus is delegated to the nurse, she should watch for signs of placental separation and report such to the physician. The signs which suggest that the placenta has separated are as follows:

1. The uterus rises upward in the abdomen; this is due to the fact that the placenta, having been separated, passes downward into the lower uterine segment and the vagina, where its bulk pushes the uterus upward.

2. The umbilical cord protrudes 3 or more inches farther out of the vagina, indicating that the placenta also has descended.

3. The uterus changes from a discoid to a globular shape and becomes, as a rule, more firm.

4. A sudden trickle or spurt of blood often occurs.

These signs are apparent sometimes within a minute or so after delivery of the infant and usually within 5 minutes. When the placenta has certainly separated, the physician first ascertains that the uterus is firmly contracted. He then may ask the patient, if not anesthetized, to "bear down," and the intra-abdominal pressure so produced may be adequate to expel the placenta (Fig. 13-26). If this fails, or if it is not practicable because of anesthesia, the physician, again having made certain that the uterus is hard, exerts gentle pressure downward with his hand on the fundus and, employing the placenta as a piston, simply moves the placenta out of the vagina.

Fig. 13-25. Tying umbilical cord. Note the knuckles are kept together. This gives a better controlled tie and is a safeguard against jerking and tearing the cord in case one hand should slip. (*Bottom*) Square knot: first and second steps in tying.

FIG. 13-26. Waiting for the separation of the placenta.

FIG. 13-27. Expression of placenta is usually done by the physician, if necessary, but *on his instructions* may be done by an assistant. The *uterus must be hard* if this is attempted. Note that the uterus is not squeezed.

FIG. 13-28. Third stage of labor. The delivery of the placenta. (The Johns Hopkins Hospital, Baltimore, Md.)

This procedure, known as placental "expression," must be done gently and without squeezing (Fig. 13-27). It never should be attempted unless the uterus is hard; otherwise the organ may be turned inside out. This is one of the gravest complications of obstetrics and is known as "inversion" of the uterus (p. 491). The physician carries out a careful inspection of the placenta to make sure that it is intact (Fig. 13-29); if a piece is left in the uterus, it may cause subsequent hemorrhage.

Oxytocin and/or ergonovine, or their derivatives, may be administered at the physician's request to increase uterine contractions and thereby to minimize bleeding. These agents are employed widely in the conduct of the normal third stage of labor, but the timing of their administration differs greatly in various hospitals. These oxytocics are not necessary in most cases, but their use is considered ideal from the viewpoint of minimizing blood loss and the general safety of the mother.

The Oxytocics. Ergonovine is an alkaloid of ergot. It is a powerful oxytocic; it stimulates uterine contractions and exerts an effect which may persist for several hours. When administered intravenously, the uterine response is almost immediate, and within a few minutes after intramuscular or oral administration. This response is sustained in character with no tendency toward relaxation and so is ideal for the prevention and the control of postpartal hemorrhage. This drug will cause an elevation of blood pressure. More recently a semisynthetic derivative of ergonovine, methylergonovine tartrate, has been widely employed because it possesses several advantages

FIG. 13-29. Inspecting the placenta: (A) the fetal side, (B) the maternal side. (The Johns Hopkins Hospital, Baltimore, Md.)

Fig. 13-30. Proper method of palpating fundus of uterus during first hour after delivery to guard against relaxation and hemorrhage. The right hand is placed just above the symphysis pubis to act as a guard; meanwhile the other hand is cupped around the fundus of the uterus.

over the parent drug. Usually called by its trade name, Methergine, it has the ability to produce stronger and longer contractions and is less likely to cause elevation of the blood pressure. Both drugs when given intravenously may cause transient headache and, to a lesser extent, temporary chest pain, palpitation and dyspnea. These side-effects are less likely to occur with intramuscular administration of the drugs.

Oxytocin is another agent which, like ergonovine, causes a marked contraction of the uterus. However, the response of the uterus to oxytocin resembles the response to ergonovine for only the first 5 to 10 minutes; then normal rhythmic contractions of amplified degree return, with intermittent periods of relaxation. The oxytocic fraction separated from posterior pituitary extract is referred to by the name oxytocin; it is widely used because it does not possess the strong vasopressor effects of Pituitrin which was used more extensively in former years. Oxytocin's most important side effect is its antidiuretic effect which can cause water intoxication if administered intravenously in a large volume of electrolyte-free aqueous dextrose solution. Fortunately the antidiuretic effect disappears within a few minutes after the infusion is discontinued. Recently, a synthetic oxytocin injection has been developed and marketed under the brand name of Syntocinon. Its action, dosage and indications are similar to those of oxytocin. Another drug which recently has been developed is sparteine sulfate (Tocos-

amine). It is used primarily in dysfunctional types of labor and for induction of labor. When used as recommended, it usually produces a gradual onset of regular uterine contractions similar to that encountered in normal labor. The quality of uterine response cannot always be predicted, however, and cases of uterine rupture following its use have been reported. Increasingly, the use of I.M. oxytocic preparations during labor is being discarded in favor of the more easily controlled I.V. route by drip.

On the obstetrician's order the nurse administers the oxytocic intramuscularly, the intravenous medications being administered by a physician. The average doses of the drugs are as follows: oxytocin, 10 units (1 cc.) intramuscularly or intravenously; Syntocinon, 10 units (1 cc.) intramuscularly or intravenously; Tocosamine, 150 mg. (1 cc.) intramuscularly, administered at 1½ to 2 hour intervals to maintain satisfactory uterine stimulation until a total of 4 doses (600 mg.) has been given; ergonovine, 0.2 mg. ($\frac{1}{320}$ gr.) or 1 cc. intramuscularly or intravenously; and Methergine, 0.2 mg. ($\frac{1}{320}$ gr.) or 1 cc. intramuscularly or intravenously. Various institutions use the drugs separately or in conjunction as is necessary to produce the desired results. The choice of the oxytocic usually will depend on the anesthetic agent administered. Oxytocin is contraindicated for use with drugs that have a sympathomimetic action.

Immediate Postpartal Care

Physical and Psychological Care. Constant massage of the uterus during the period after the delivery of the placenta is unnecessary and undesirable. However, if the organ shows any tendency to relax, it is to be massaged immediately with firm but gentle circular strokes until it contracts effectively, in order to prevent blood loss.

After the delivery has been completed, the drapes and the soiled linen under the mother's buttocks are removed, and the lower end of the delivery table is replaced. The mother's legs are lowered from the stirrups simultaneously, and after a sterile perineal pad is applied, she should be covered with a blanket to avoid chilling. She is now ready to be transferred to her own bed. Many delivery suites have a designated postpartum recovery area or adjacent recovery room where the mother remains for an hour or so or until she has recovered from the anesthesia, her vital signs have stabilized, and there is no unusual bleeding from the birth canal.

If the mother is awake at this time, she will be eager to have a closer look at her baby and hold it, if this is possible. One should remember that although she is quite exhausted, she is usually elated, proud of her accomplishment of giving birth, and eager to share this with her husband. Whenever possible, all efforts should be made to allow the father, the mother and the infant to share this momentous time together. At one hospital the baby is placed in the mother's arms as soon as she is transferred to her bed, and the husband is permitted to remain at her bedside while she is in the recovery area. This arrangement provides an excellent opportunity to let both mother and father have a close, thorough look at their baby and to let them begin the necessary process of incorporating him into their family unit. Since all three are under the watchful (but unobtrusive) eye of the nurse, there is little danger to the infant from undue exposure, choking on mucus, smothering, etc.

Immediately after delivery, or perhaps later, the parents, particularly the mother, may relieve tension by giving way to some emotional displays such as laughing, crying, incessant chatter or anger (if all has not gone well or as expected). These emotions often are quite unexpected and shock and embarrass those involved. A calm, accepting, nonjudgmental attitude on the part of the nurse is very effective in allaying any embarrassment and in helping the patient to gain control.

The nurse must remember that the patient is beginning a period that is enormously important; she is, in fact, now a "mother" with all its concomitant responsibilities; glimmerings of this already are reaching the consciousness. This is not the "end" but only the beginning of a whole new role! In addition, she is physically and emotionally exhausted from the great effort she has put forth; thus, there may be a temporary emotional upheaval.

Several comfort measures can be employed to restore calm and to help the mother to relax enough to get some much needed rest and sleep. A soothing backrub, change of gown and linen, a quiet conversation with the nurse and/or the husband in which the patient is allowed to ventilate her feelings, an environment conducive to rest, all are helpful. In addition, a warm beverage can be offered to help to allay undue excitement; since the mother is apt to be extremely hungry and thirsty, this is welcome nourishment as well as a therapeutic soporific.

Many mothers, of course, do not have an emotional outburst per se, although the majority do experience some degree of excitement and elation when the delivery is accomplished. Any of the above nursing activities are suitable also for them. Some patients experience a great need for sleep and drop off as soon as they ascertain that the baby is "all right." If the patient is sleeping continuously or intermittently, she should be allowed to do so, being disturbed only for those nursing observations that are necessary. When she indicates readiness (after the first hour after delivery), her baby should be presented, and she should be allowed to examine and to explore to her heart's content.

The mothers who have not been conscious during the delivery have rather different reactions than those patients who have participated in the birth process. Often they do not seem to believe that delivery has taken place, or that the baby shown them "is really mine." They will question again and again: "Is it really all over?" "What is it again?" (This refers to the sex of the child.) "Did I have the baby?" The apparent alteration in awareness seems to be related to the anesthesia and the unconsciousness. These patients need more firm reassurance and contact with their infants to help them realize that they have had a baby. Even though the repeated questioning may become annoying, the nurse should recognize that this is necessary for the mother so that she can begin the important process of disengagement from the symbiotic relationship that she had with her infant during pregnancy. She must now establish the baby as a real entity outside her body rather than inside. All mothers have this task to perform, but it is harder for the mother who has been delivered under heavy anesthesia, for as far as she is concerned, she was not "there" when it all happened.

Maternal feelings, as we know, do not spring unbound at the time of delivery. Rather they are developed, often slowly, as is the case in any other developmental process (see Chap. 16). The early encounters and care that the mother receives in the delivery area help to pave the way for later responses in the postpartal period.

The first hour following the delivery is a most critical one for the mother. It is at this time that postpartal hemorrhage is most likely to occur as the result of uterine relaxation. Thus, it is mandatory that the uterus be watched constantly throughout this period by a competent nurse who keeps her hand more or less constantly on the fundus and at the slightest sign of diminishing contraction massages it, to make sure that it does not relapse and balloon with blood (Fig. 13-30). It is important for the nurse to be constantly alert not only to the condition of the mother's uterus but also to any abnormal symptoms related to her general condition. Checking of the maternal vital signs is usually included in the nursing observations. These signs are checked as often as necessary until they become stable, as previously stated.

IMMEDIATE CARE OF THE INFANT

As soon as the infant is born, measures are taken to promote a clear air passage before the

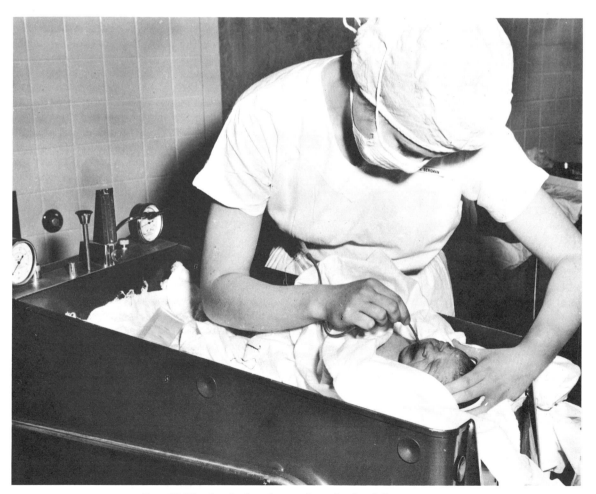

Fig. 13-31. Suctioning the newborn in the delivery room.

onset of respiration. Often, as the head is delivered, it is necessary to wipe the mucus and fluid from the infant's nose and mouth before he has a chance to gasp and aspirate with this first breath. From the moment of delivery the infant should be kept in the head-down position until his upper respiratory passage is cleared of mucus, amniotic fluid, etc. A small rubber bulb syringe, or a soft rubber suction catheter attached to a mechanical suction or mouth aspirator, is used promptly to suction the oropharynx and to remove fluids which may be obstructing the airway. If there seems to be much mucus present, the physician will hold the infant up by his ankles to encourage more mucus to drain from the throat. The mucosal surfaces of the palate and the posterior pharynx should not be wiped with gauze, since its rough texture can lead to abrasions and thus provide a portal of entry for pathogenic organisms. A flexible rubber may be passed by the physician to suction the larynx if the above measures do not clear the mucus well enough.

The baby may not "cry" at once, but he usually gasps or cries after the mucus has been removed, as he now needs oxygen by way of the lungs, since the accustomed supply was cut off when the placental circulation stopped. If crying has to be stimulated, it must be done with extreme care. As the infant is being held in the head-down position to promote the drainage of mucus from the respiratory passages, gentle rubbing of the infant's back is usually sufficient stimulus to initiate crying. And, in the act of crying, mucus is forced from the nose and the throat, thus enabling the infant to be better able to breathe. Vigorous, external irritants are *unnecessary* and *dangerous* and should not be employed. These include spanking the soles of the feet and/or buttocks, forcible rubbing of the skin along the spine, alternate hot and cold tubbing of the infant, and dilatation of the anal sphincter. These procedures are obsolete and shocking to the infant.

A sterile receiver should be available for the physician to wrap around the infant until it can be placed in a warm crib or incubator. It must be remembered that any room is much cooler than the mother's body, and the infant never should be exposed to chilling. As soon as the physician has clamped and cut the cord, he usually places the infant in a heated crib or resuscitator (previously draped with a sterile receiver to avoid contaminating his gloves) so that he may devote his attention to the mother during the third stage of labor. As mentioned previously, even for the infant who requires no resuscitation, the resuscitator or incubator affords a warm protected environment for the infant and, in addition, a convenient place for the nurse now to proceed with the infant's care. If a circulating nurse is responsible for the infant's care in the delivery room, she will have cleansed her hands thoroughly with some agent such as pHisoHex or surgical soap in preparation, preferably while the physician is delivering the infant's head.

Appraisal of the Newborn Infant

Once the physician has placed the infant in the heated crib (or incubator or resuscitator) in the delivery room, the responsibility for the infant's care usually is delegated to the professional nurse. It is imperative that the infant's condition be evaluated accurately immediately after birth, and that close observation be continued by the nurse. As she makes her observations, her interpretation of the baby's responses will result in a nursing diagnosis and consequent plan for nursing intervention.

Suctioning. Since it is important to maintain a clear airway for the infant, it may be necessary to suction further mucus from the oropharynx. It is important *not to oversuction* at any time, because this merely deprives the infant of oxygen and irritates the mucous membrane. If further suctioning is necessary, the nurse may use the suction apparatus on the electric infant resuscitator, a bulb syringe, or a soft rubber catheter attached to a De Lee glass trap, which was designed especially for aspirating mucus in the treatment of newborn infants (Fig. 13-31). Care should be taken not to traumatize the tissues of the oropharynx with the tip of the catheter or with forceful suction. When the nasopharynx is obstructed by mucus which must be removed via the nostrils, the nurse may safely pass a small French catheter into the nostril if she avoids using force. The catheter must *not* be inserted far back. If the catheter is directed horizontally, as if passing over the roof of the mouth, instead of directing it upward as for the adult patient, it usually slips into the tiny infant nostril with more ease. If a bulb syringe is used, it should be collapsed before it is inserted in the baby's mouth; otherwise the material in the oropharynx will be forced into the bronchi and lungs when the bulb is collapsed.

The Apgar Scoring System. The Apgar score provides a valuable index for evaluating the newborn infant's condition at birth. Every nurse who is responsible for the care of newborn infants, not merely those in the delivery room, should be familiar with the principles set forth by Apgar for infant evaluation because they provide a simple, accurate and safe means of quickly appraising the infant's condition. The Apgar scoring system is based on the following five signs (ranked in order of importance). In general, they are made at 1 minute of life and repeated again in 5 minutes. Each sign is evaluated according to the degree to which it is present and is given a score of 0, 1, or 2 (see Table 13-3). The scores of each of the signs then are added together to give a total score (10 is maximum).

HEART RATE. This sign is the most important and the last to be absent when the infant's condition is grave. It may be evaluated by palpating the pulsation of the cord or by observing the pulsation where the cord joins the abdomen. Listening to the heartbeat with a stethoscope is surely the most accurate method of ascertaining the beat. The beat may range from 150 to 180 beats per minute during the first few minutes of life; later, within the hour, it usually slows to between 130 and 140 beats per minute. Crying or increased activity will increase the number of beats. If the rate is 100 per minute or under, asphyxia is present, and resuscitation is indicated.

RESPIRATORY EFFORT. A baby who is responding well cries vigorously and has no difficulty in breathing. "Regular" respiration usually is established in a minute or so. Depressed, irregular respiration or apnea indicates that respiratory difficulty is present, and these signs should be reported immediately so that prompt treatment may be instituted (see p. 536).

MUSCLE TONE. An infant who has excellent tonus will keep his extremities flexed and resist efforts to extend them. A baby who does not keep his extremities flexed consistently usually has only moderate tonus; one who is flaccid is in extremely poor condition.

REFLEX IRRITABILITY. Although there are several ways to test this sign, the one most frequently used is a slap on the sole of the infant's foot. This sign can be observed when a vigorous infant is suctioned for mucus by the way in which he resists the catheter. A baby who is in excellent condition will respond with a vigorous cry. He is judged to have a poor response if he cries weakly or merely makes a grimace. If there is a good deal of central

TABLE 13-3. THE APGAR SCORING CHART*

SIGN	0	1	2
Heart rate	Absent	Slow (less than 100)	Over 100
Respiratory effort	Absent	Slow, irregular	Good, crying
Muscle tone	Flaccid	Some flexion of extremities	Active motion
Reflex irritability	No response	Cry	Vigorous cry
Color	Blue, pale	Body pink, extremities blue	Completely pink

* Special Committee on Infant Mortality of the Medical Society of the County of New York: Resuscitation of the Newborn, Philadelphia, Smith Kline & French Laboratories, 1963.

nervous system depression, the infant will not respond at all.

COLOR. Cyanosis is seen in all infants at the moment of birth. As the infant's circulation makes the change from fetal to extra-uterine existence, and he begins to breathe, the body of a healthy infant usually will become pink within 3 minutes (see Chap. 4). Since acrocyanosis usually is present for a short while, even in infants who are in excellent condition, those who have scored 2 for each of the other signs may receive only a score of 1 for this part of the evaluation. This will, of course, influence his total score.

INTERPRETATION. An Apgar score of 7 to 10 indicates that the infant's condition is good. If he breathes and cries (or coughs) seconds after delivery, there are usually no special procedures necessary other than those of routine close observation, maintaining a clear airway, and supplying warmth as necessary. A score of 4 to 6 means that the baby is in fair condition. There may be moderate central nervous system depression, some muscle flaccidity, cyanosis, and respiration will not establish readily. *These infants must have their air passages cleared and be given oxygen promptly.* Administration of oxygen can best be done by mask, and the flow should not exceed 4 liters. Gentle patting and rubbing with the receiving blanket to dry the infant's body usually acts as an additional stimulus. A score of 0 to 3 denotes an extremely poor condition. Resuscitation is needed immediately (see Chap. 23).

Other Aspects of Care

Care of the Cord. In many hospitals no dressing is applied after the cord has been clamped or ligated and cut; in others a sterile plain gauze dressing is applied around the cord stump and secured with a binder, which is removed at appropriate times. Regardless of the technic employed, it is imperative that frequent inspection be done to note any signs of bleeding and that strict aseptic precautions be utilized in caring for the cord stump. The method of leaving the cord stump exposed has proved to be very satisfactory. If it is left free, it apparently dries and separates more quickly than when it is kept covered. There is also less irritation of the abdomen and the back, which sometimes results from a moist binder. Some pediatricians think that the abdominal muscles become stronger by not being bound.

Care of the Eyes. As soon as the cord is cared for and the infant's respiration is well established, the eyes should receive prophylactic treatment for protection against ophthalmia neonatorum (see Chap. 23, Disorders of the Newborn). This treatment is so important that at the present time the use of some antibacterial agent is mandatory by statute in all states. Penicillin and silver nitrate are the usual agents employed, although a non-irritating solution of 15 per cent sulphacetamide is preferred by some physicians. When silver nitrate is used, it is supplied in wax ampules containing a 1 per cent solution especially prepared for eye instillation (Fig. 13-32).

Instilling drops in the infant's eyes is more easily accomplished if the nurse shades the eyes from the light while putting the drops first in one eye, allowing time for the baby to recover from the shock and the smarting before she puts the drops in the other eye. One of the best methods is to draw down the lower lid gently and carefully instill 2 drops of the solution in the conjunctival sac, using great care not to drop it on the cornea. After 2 minutes, when it will have diffused itself over the entire conjunctiva, the lids should again be held apart and the conjunctival sac of each eye flushed gently with normal saline solution or sterile distilled water (Fig. 13-33). The prompt irrigation of the eyes following instillation of silver nitrate drops is said to reduce the incidence of chemical conjunctivitis without affecting the prophylactic efficacy. The nurse must take especial precautions against allowing any contamination of the eyes and against dropping any silver solution upon the face. Silver nitrate prophylaxis may cause signs of irritation, such as redness, edema or discharge, but these manifestations are transient and in no way cause permanent damage if the silver nitrate solution used is in correct concentration.

If penicillin is to be used, it can be obtained in ophthalmic drops or ointment. The technique for instillation is similar to that for silver nitrate, except that there is no flushing with saline or water. Penicillin is also given intramuscularly for both prophylaxis and treatment of ophthalmia neonatorum. When gonorrheal ophthalmia does develop, it can be cured by penicillin within a few hours, whereas silver nitrate has long since been abandoned for treatment purposes. The incidence of chemical irritation with penicillin ointment or intramuscular injection is much less than with silver nitrate, and the irritation is generally milder. However, some sensitivity reactions have been reported, thus, silver nitrate continues to be used.

Hypoprothrombinemia Prophylaxis. Many physicians prescribe that a single dose of phytonadione solution (Aquamephyton) 1.0 mg. (0.5 cc.) be administered intramuscularly during the course of the immediate care of the newborn after delivery. This water-soluble form of vitamin K_1 acts as a preventative measure against neonatal hemorrhagic disease. Amounts of the medication in excess of 1.0 mg. may predispose to the development of hyperbilirubinemia and should be avoided.

Fig. 13-32. (*Left*) Silver nitrate 1 per cent solution for the care of the eyes of newborn babies; needle puncture of wax ampule. (*Right*) Showing how to manipulate the ampule in administering the drug. (Eli Lilly and Company)

FIG. 13-33. Silver nitrate prophylaxis. (*Top*) Instillation of 2 drops of silver nitrate 1 per cent solution from a wax ampule into the conjunctival sac of each eye. (*Bottom*) After the medication has diffused over the entire conjunctiva (2 minutes), the conjunctival sac of each eye is gently flushed with sterile distilled water or normal saline solution to remove the excess silver nitrate.

Identification Methods. Some method of identification of the newborn is applied before the cord is cut or before the baby is removed from the delivery room. There are several satisfactory methods in use. Some hospitals use the linen tapes marked with the mother's name and hospital number, fastening one to the baby's arm or ankle and the other to the mother's wrist. The identification beads are made up with the mother's surname and initials and sealed with a lead bead. This bracelet or anklet is applied before the baby leaves the delivery room (Fig. 13-34). The pliable plastic bracelet or anklet has space for the mother's name and initials as well as a permanent lock which has to be cut to be removed.

The palmprint and footprint method of identification consists of a stainless procedure made on chemically treated sensitized paper. It is designed to take the palmprints or footprints of the baby and the thumbprint of the mother at the time of delivery and may be repeated at the time of discharge from the hospital. It is a simple, quick and permanent method.

The following editorial comment presents the recommendations of the American Hospital Association.

> Mix-ups involving two or more babies are quite rare in hospital nurseries, but they still can happen. In one state alone in a period of 18 months eight mix-ups or alleged mix-ups occurred. When such a mix-up, alleged or actual, does occur, a torrent of unfavorable publicity is unloosed and the parents concerned may be haunted by a lifetime of doubt

FIG. 13-34. Identification method, using strand of beads. If surname is at all common, use initial of mother's first name also, as shown above. The beads must be sealed around baby's wrist or ankle before he leaves the delivery room.

about their child. The confusion sometimes arises because two mothers in a hospital at the same time have the same surname; it sometimes arises because a single identification becomes detached from the baby; or it may even arise because parents get to wondering after they leave the hospital how the attendants maintained the identity of the babies. Sometimes the confusion is easily straightened out, and sometimes it leads to giving the wrong baby a harmless prescription; only rarely does it lead to an actual exchange of babies. The American Hospital Association has long been aware of this problem, and, because it has been found that photographs, footprints, handprints, and fingerprints are adjuncts but cannot yet be considered reliable as the sole means of identifying the newborn infant, the Association has urged the adoption of a standard operating procedure that if applied would reduce mix-ups to the vanishing point.

> The main features of this procedure are as follows: (1) Each baby should be marked in the delivery room with two items of identification. (2) The identification items should show the mother's full name, date and time of birth, and some correlation with the mother, such as her fingerprint or number. (3) Each time the baby comes to the mother, the mother should be informed that it is her responsibility to identify her baby by the marking. (4) When the baby and mother are discharged, one of the bands should be removed, preferably by the mother, and, after the mother has properly identified her baby, the removed identification should then be pasted to the baby's chart. The mother should acknowledge in writing that this is how her baby was marked, and that she identified it as hers. The leaflet that gives the full procedure in detail has been available since December, 1949. Once established as a routine, this procedure, far from being a burden, would prevent a type of mistake that would otherwise be easy to make but is nonetheless inexcusable.[7]

Current practice emphasizes that the newborn should be discharged without removing the identification band. Several states now have laws making it mandatory not to remove the identification bands on hospital premises. The mother should be taught how to remove the band as part of the discharge instructions.

As already discussed in Chapter 1, the registration of the infant's birth is a legal responsibility. It is mandatory that a birth certificate, such as that shown in Figure 1-5, be filled out on every birth and submitted promptly to the local registrar.

[7] Editorial Comment: Identification of the newborn infant. J.A.M.A. 162:44, 1956.

After the Delivery. After caring for the infant, the nurse will continue to assist the physician with the care of the mother and her infant. If the mother is awake, she may be anxious to have her baby brought near so that she may see it at close range. If she is drowsy, it may be better to wait until she is more alert. The nurse will be governed by each mother's response at this time. Some mothers want to touch their babies; others are eager to hold their babies at this time, and if this is sanctioned by the physician, there is no reason that it should not be permitted for a brief period. In this instance the nurse should be careful to keep her hand under the infant for support and added protection, should this be necessary, because of the mother's excitement in her first contact with her newborn.

If the infant is well wrapped and warm, he may be kept in a crib at the mother's side until the mother leaves the delivery room. He should be kept in a modified Trendelenburg position (at an angle of 30°) to promote drainage of mucus, and on his side to avoid aspiration of this mucus. Care should be taken to avoid placing the infant in an exaggerated Trendelenburg position (almost directly downward), since the relatively large amount of abdominal contents will press against the diaphragm and the partially expanded lungs and may impede the infant's respiratory efforts.

The nurse observes the infant at frequent intervals to make sure that he is breathing properly, that the mouth and the nose are free from mucus, and that there is no bleeding from the cord. Because this period may be a critical one for the infant, many hospitals have facilities, such as a receiving nursery on the labor and delivery division, where the infant is transferred at this time. This not only provides closer supervision and care for the infant but also permits the nurse in the delivery room to devote her undivided attention to the mother.

Baptism of Infant. If there is any probability that the infant is in imminent danger and may not live, the question of baptism should be considered in cases in which the religion of the family is Roman Catholic; this also applies to some of the other denominations of the Christian church. This is an essential duty and means a great deal to the families concerned, and thoughtfulness in this matter will never be forgotten by them. (It is to be understood that such baptism would be reported to the family.)

The following simple instructions were given by the late Rev. Paul L. Blakely, S.J., Ph.D.

> The Catholic Church teaches that in case of emergency, any one may and should baptize. What is necessary is to make the intention of doing what the Church wishes to do and then to pour the water on the child (the head by preference) saying at the same time, "I baptize thee in the name of the Father and of the Son and of the Holy Ghost." The water may be warmed if necessary but it must be pure water and care should be taken to make it flow. If there is any doubt whether the child is alive or dead, it should be baptized, but conditionally (i.e., "If thou art alive, I baptize thee . . .").

On page 281 of the Book of Common Prayer of the Protestant Episcopal Church, it is stated: "In cases of extreme sickness, or any imminent peril, if a Minister cannot be procured, then any baptized person present may administer holy Baptism, using the foregoing form" (i.e., the form given above).

EMERGENCY DELIVERY BY THE NURSE

In the course of labor one occasionally encounters the so-called *precipitate delivery,* a rapid spontaneous delivery in which the infant is born without adequate preparations on the part of the physician or the nurse, sometimes even without benefit of their immediate care. This may occur in certain multiparous women, particularly if the soft parts of the pelvis offer little resistance, if the contractions are unusually strong and forceful, or if the mother does not experience painful sensations during labor and thus has inadequate warning that the delivery is approaching. The mother, of course, may suffer lacerations of the tissues as the result of tumultuous labor. The infant is endangered because, in its rapid progress through the birth canal, it may suffer cerebral trauma; or the umbilical cord may be torn in the process of the delivery. In addition, if the mother is unattended, the infant may be in jeopardy from lack of care during the first few minutes of life.

Whether the nurse is caring for a mother in the hospital labor room, making a home visit, or involved in some emergency situation, it is well for her to be prepared for a precipitate delivery. It seldom happens that the nurse is alone with her patient in the hospital when the delivery is imminent; but knowing what to do in such a situation, in the event that the physician is not present, is advantageous for all concerned. In the excitement which may ensue, the nurse's concern for the

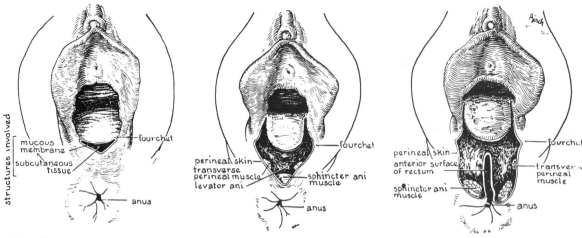

FIG. 13-35 A. First-degree tear.   FIG. 13-35 B. Second-degree tear.   FIG. 13-35 C. Third-degree tear.

immediate safety of the mother and the baby usually demands all of her attention.

However, it should be stressed that the nurse's composure and her ability to convey this is one of the cornerstones in a successful delivery. Whenever possible, the nurse is to let the mother know what to anticipate and instruct her as best she can in what she can do to cooperate effectively. Here teamwork with the mother is essential and can be accomplished if the nurse instills confidence by demonstrating her competence in both the physical and the emotional aspects of care. If the father is present, he can be utilized in the care of his wife in whatever capacity seems most appropriate and in accord with his ability. He might help best by taking care of the other children or by calling the physician, or he might be involved directly in some aspect of the delivery. If it seems more desirable that he be away from the immediate vicinity, then the reasons for his leaving should be given. He should not be dismissed summarily from the situation.

The nurse who is consistently conscientious about applying principles of asepsis and antisepsis will automatically apply them in this instance, to the best of her ability. Usually, there is inadequate time for proper cleansing of the vulva, or scrubbing her own hands and donning sterile gloves, or draping the mother, all of which would be ideal. However, a clean delivery area should be maintained, and, if time and facilities permit, the nurse's hands should be cleansed.

Delivery of the Head. As the head distends the perineum at the acme of a contraction, gentle pressure is exerted against the head to control its progress and thereby to prevent undue stretching of the perineum. This kind of *control* applied to the descending head during each contraction will prevent its sudden expulsion through the vulva, reducing the possibility of consequent complications. *The head must never be held back.* The mother should be encouraged to pant during the contraction to deter bearing down efforts on her part, particularly as the head, which will be supported by the nurse, is being delivered. Whenever possible, the infant's head should be delivered between contractions.

Rupture of the Membranes. If the membranes have not ruptured previously, they may remain intact until they appear as a smooth, glistening object at the vulva. If they protrude, they may rupture with the next contraction. But if the membranes have not ruptured before the head is delivered, they must be broken and removed immediately (by nipping them at the nape of the infant's neck) to prevent aspiration of fluid when the infant takes its first breath.

Precautions Concerning the Cord. As soon as the head is delivered, the nurse should feel for a loop or loops of cord around the neck and, if any is found, gently slip it over the baby's head, if this can be done easily. But, as stated on page 265, if the cord is coiled too tightly to permit this, it must be doubly clamped and cut (between the clamps) before delivery of the rest of the body. One or more loops of cord around the fetal neck occur in about a quarter of all deliveries.

Delivery of the Infant's Body. After external rotation of the head, which is usually spontaneous, there is no occasion for haste in the delivery of the body. Gentle downward pressure with the hands on either side of the head may be exerted to direct the anterior shoulder under the symphysis pubis, then reversed upward in order to deliver the posterior shoulder over the perineum. The infant's body now will follow easily and quickly and should be supported as it is born.

Immediate Care of the Infant. As soon as the face appears, mucus and fluids should be wiped from the nose and the mouth. Then, after the infant is born, if he does not cry spontaneously, or if there seems to be mucus in the respiratory passages, the infant should be held up by his ankles to encourage the mucus to drain from his nose and mouth. In doing this, care must be exercised to avoid any traction on the umbilical cord and, at the same time, to prevent the infant's head from pressing down against the bed. Drainage of mucus is stimulated when the infant cries but can be encouraged by "milking the trachea" (i.e., with the forefinger, stroking the neck from its base toward the chin). Further stimulation by gentle rubbing of the back may stimulate breathing.

Care of the Cord. There is *no* hurry to cut the cord, so this should be delayed until proper equipment is available. It is a good plan to clamp the cord after pulsations cease (but not imperative at the moment) and to wait for the physician to cut the cord after he arrives. One must always bear in mind that sterile conditions must exist for the cord-cutting procedure; otherwise the infant's safety is jeopardized. Also, the technique for applying the cord tie or umbilical clamp must be assiduously carried out to prevent bleeding from the umbilical stump (see p. 265).

Delivery of the Placenta. When signs of placental separation are apparent, the mother can be asked to bear down with the next contraction to deliver the placenta. Since the danger of hemorrhage is always to be guarded against, the fundus should be massaged after the delivery of the placenta if there is the slightest tendency toward relaxation of the uterine muscles.

When the infant is breathing satisfactorily, he can be placed on his side across his mother's abdomen (with his head kept low to promote postural drainage and his body covered to prevent chilling). This accomplishes several things: the mother is given her baby, she can touch him and is usually enthralled by the close physical contact with him; the warmth of the mother's body prevents the infant from being chilled; and

the pressure exerted on the uterus by the weight of the infant helps it to contract.

One must remember to proceed slowly and carefully throughout the delivery. As stated earlier, the nurse's reaction to the situation undoubtedly will be transferred to the mother; if the nurse remains poised and unfaltering, the mother and other people involved are more likely to do so.

LACERATIONS OF THE BIRTH CANAL

During the process of a normal delivery lacerations of the perineum and the vagina may be caused by rapid and sudden expulsion of the head (particularly when it "pops" out), the excessive size of the infant and very friable maternal tissues. In other circumstances they may be caused by difficult forceps deliveries, breech extractions or contraction of the pelvic outlet in which the head is forced posteriorly. Some tears are unavoidable, even in the most skilled hands.

Perineal lacerations usually are classified in 3 degrees, according to the extent of the tear.

First-degree lacerations are those which involve the fourchet, the perineal skin and the vaginal mucous membrane without involving any of the muscles (Fig. 13-35 A).

Second-degree lacerations are those which involve (in addition to skin and mucous membrane) the muscles of the perineal body but not the rectal sphincter. These tears usually extend upward on one or both sides of the vagina, making a triangular injury (Fig. 13-35 B).

Third-degree lacerations are those which extend completely through the skin, the mucous membrane, the perineal body and the rectal sphincter (Fig. 13-35 C). This type is often referred to as a complete tear. Not infrequently these third-degree lacerations extend a certain distance up the anterior wall of the rectum.

First- and second-degree lacerations are extremely common in primigravidas; their high incidence is one of the reasons that episiotomy is widely employed. Fortunately, third-degree lacerations are far less common. All three types of lacerations are repaired by the physician immediately after the delivery to ensure that the perineal structures are returned approximately to their former condition. The technique employed for the repair of a laceration is virtually the same as that used for episiotomy incisions (see p. 283), although the former is more difficult to do because of the irregular lines of tissue which must be approximated.

FIG. 13-36. Episiotomy. Showing lines of incision for median and mediolateral episiotomy.

(Technic employed at the Johns Hopkins Hospital. Many other methods are equally satisfactory.)

FIG. 13-37. Episiotomy. "Tail-sponge" in vagina to occlude bleeding, continuous suture in vaginal mucosa.

FIG. 13-38. Episiotomy. After the levator ani muscle has been united by two or more sutures (shown tied and cut), the fascia covering the muscle is sutured. Note the "tail-sponge."

FIG. 13-39. Episiotomy. After suturing to the lowermost angle of the fascia, the round needle is replaced by cutting needle and the running suture continued upward in subcuticular fascia.

EPISIOTOMY AND REPAIR

An episiotomy is an incision of the perineum made to facilitate delivery. The incision is made with blunt-pointed straight scissors about the time that the head distends the vulva and is visible to a diameter of several centimeters. The incision may be made in the midline of the perineum—a median episiotomy. Or it may be begun in the midline and directed downward and laterally away from the rectum—a mediolateral episiotomy (Fig. 13-36). In the latter instance the incision may be directed to either the right or to the left side of the mother's pelvis.

As the infant's head distends the vulva, if a laceration seems to be inevitable, the physician undoubtedly will choose to incise the perineum rather than allow that structure to sustain a traumatic tear. This operation serves several purposes:

1. It substitutes a straight, clean-cut surgical incision for the ragged, contused laceration which otherwise is likely to ensue; such an incision is easier to repair and heals better than a tear.

2. The direction of the episiotomy can be controlled, whereas a tear may extend in any direction, sometimes involving the anal sphincter and the rectum.

3. Inordinate stretching and tearing of the perineal musculature is avoided and the incidence of subsequent perineal relaxation with cystocele-rectocele may be reduced. It spares the baby's head the necessity of serving as a "battering ram" against perineal obstruction; if prolonged, this "pounding" of the infant's head against the perineum may cause brain injury.

4. The operation shortens the duration of the second stage of labor.

In view of these several advantages of episiotomy, many physicians employ it routinely in the delivery of the primigravida.

There are many equally satisfactory methods utilized by different physicians for episiotomy repair. The suture material ordinarily used is a fine chromic catgut, either 00 or 000. The technique employed at the Johns Hopkins Hospital is shown in Figures 13-37 through 39. A round needle and continuous suture is used to close the vaginal mucosa and fourchet, and then laid aside while several interrupted sutures are placed in the levator ani muscle and the fascia. Then the continuous suture is again picked up and used to unite the subcutaneous fascia. Finally, the round needle is replaced by a large, straight cutting needle, and the running suture is continued upward as a subcuticular stitch.

SUGGESTED READING

Allen, S.: Nurse attendance during labor. Am. J. Nurs. 64:70-74, July, 1964.

Anderson, B.: Training course for obstetric technicians. Pediatric Nursing Currents, Ross Laboratories 12:1-2, May, 1965.

Bernstine, R. L.: Fetal Electrocardiography and Electroencephalography. Springfield, Charles C Thomas, 1961.

Bishop, E. H.: The obstetric uses of ultrasound. J. International Fed. Gynec. Obstet. 4:190-196, July, 1966.

Blaylock, J.: The psychological and cultural influences on the reaction to pain: a review of the literature. Nurs. Forum 7:262-274, 1968.

Bradford, W. D.: The case for careful examination of the placenta. Clin. Pediat. 7:716-719, December, 1968.

Bradley, R. A.: Fathers' presence in delivery rooms. Psychosomatics 111:474-479, November-December, 1962.

Brady, J. P., and James, L. S.: Heart rate changes in the fetus and newborn infant during labor, delivery and the immediate neonatal period. Am. J. Obstet. Gynec. 84:1-13, July, 1962.

Buxton, C. L.: Study of Psychophysical Methods for Relief of Childbirth Pain. Philadelphia, W. B. Saunders, 1962.

Carbary, L. J.: The fetal heart monitor. Nurs. Outlook 11:835, November, 1963.

Chambers, W.: Nursing Diagnosis. Am. J. Nurs. 62:102-104, November, 1962.

Chambers, W. G., and Price, G. G.: Influence of the nurse upon effects of analgesics administered. Nurs. Research 16:228-233, Summer, 1967.

Christian, J. R.: Comparison of ocular reactions with the use of silver nitrate and erythromycin ointment in opthalmia neonatorum prophylaxis. J. Pediat. 57:55-60, July, 1960.

Cibils, L. A., and Hendricks, C. H.: Normal labor in vertex presentations. Am. J. Obstet. Gynec. 91:385-395, February 1, 1965.

Clark, A. L.: The adaption problems and patterns of an expanding family: the neonatal period. Nurs. Forum 5, 1:92-109, 1966.

Committee on Fetus and the Newborn: Standards and Recommendations for Hospital Care of Newborn Infants. Evanston, American Academy of Pediatrics, 1964.

Crowley, D. M.: Pain and Its Alleviation. The Regents of the University of California, 1962.

Cummins, H., and Midlo, C.: Fingerprints, Palms and Soles. New York, Dover, 1962.

De Agustina, J., et al.: Ward study: The meaning of touch in intrapersonal communication in Burd, S., and Marshall, M.: Some Clinical Approaches to Psychiatric Nursing. New York, Macmillan, 1963.

Donald, I.: Diagnostic uses of sonar (ultrasonic echo sounding) in obstetrics and gynecology. Advances in Obstet. Gynec. 1:314-329, 1967.

Durand, M., and Prince, R.: Nursing diagnosis: process and decision. Nurs. Forum 5, No. 4: 50-64.

Dwyer, J. M., and Lynch, W. A.: Nursing responsibility for decreasing maternal and perinatal mortality and morbidity. Hosp. Progr. 48:66-67, January, 1967.

Eastman, N. J., and Hellman, L. M.: Williams Obstetrics, ed. 13, New York, Appleton, 1966.

Estey, G. P.: Word from a mother. Am. J. Nurs. 69:1453-1454, July, 1969.

Gaisford, W.: Changing fashions in infant care. J. Pediat. 64:913, June, 1964.

Goodman, R. R.: Psychological support in labor, a supervisor's view. Hosp. Topics 42:99-100, August, 1964.

Hamilton, P. M.: Basic Maternity Nursing. St. Louis, C. V. Mosby, 1967.

Hellman, L. M.: Electronics in obstetrics and gynaecology. J. Obstet. Gynec. British Commonwealth 72:896-906, December, 1965.

Hellman, L. M., et al.: Some factors affecting the fetal heart rate. Am. J. Obstet. Gynec. 82:1055-1063, November, 1961.

Hendricks, C. H., and Pose, S. V.: Intranasal oxytocin in obstetrics. J.A.M.A. 175:384-387, February 4, 1961.

Hoff, F. E.: How any nurse can help. Am. J. Nurs. 69:1451-1453, July, 1969.

Hommel, F.: Nurses in private practice as monitrices. Am. J. Nurs. 69:1446-1450, July, 1969.

Hon, E. H.: Electronic evaluation of fetal heart rates. Am. J. Obstet. Gynec. 83:333-338, February 1, 1962.

Ioris, J.: Effective support during labor and delivery. R. N. 25:70-78, 88, February, 1962.

Johnson, B. S.: Meaning of touch in nursing. Nurs. Outlook 65:59-60, February, 1965.

Jones, J. A.: Examining the newborn's eyes, a satisfactory method. Clin. Pediat. 7:124, February, 1968.

Jourard, S.: The bedside manner. Am. J. Nurs. 60: 63-66, January, 1960.

Kachelski, A.: The nurse-patient relationship. Am. J. Nurs. 61:76-81, May, 1961.

Karmel, M.: Thank You, Dr. Lamaze. Philadelphia, J. B. Lippincott, 1959.

Karmorita, N.: Nursing diagnosis. Am. J. Nurs. 63: 83-86, December, 1963.

Kelly, J. V.: Effect of fear on uterine motility. Am. J. Obstet. Gynec. 83:576-581, March 1, 1962.

————: Effect of hynotically induced anxiety on uterine muscle. Am. J. Obstet. Gynec. 83:582-587, March 1, 1962.

Kendall, B., and Farell, D. M.: Use of fetal electrocardiography. Am. J. Nurs. 64:75-79, July, 1964.

Larks, S. D.: Electrohystereography. Springfield, Charles C Thomas, 1960.

————: Fetal Electrocardiography. Springfield, Charles C Thomas, 1961.

La Fever, J.: View from the side of the table. Am. J. Nurs. 63:67-69, June, 1963.

Lesser, M., and Keane, V.: Nurse-Patient Relationships in a Hospital Maternity Service, St. Louis, C. V. Mosby, 1956.

Levine, M. E.: Adaption and assessment, a rationale for nursing intervention. Am. J. Nurs. 66:2450-2453, November, 1966.

Ludemann, R. S.: Empathy—a component of therapeutic nursing. Nurs. Forum 7:275-288, 1968.

McCabe, G. S.: Cultural influences on patient behavior. Am. J. Nurs. 60:1101-1102, August, 1960.

McLennan, C. E.: Synopsis of Obstetrics. St. Louis, C. V. Mosby, 1966.

Manning, R. E.: To do or not to do—a critical review of vaginal examination during labor. Am. J. Obstet. Gynec. 82:1356-1358, December, 1961.

Miller, J. S.: Childbirth. New York, Atheneum, 1963.

Montgomery, T. L.: Immediate care of the newborn. Clin. Obstet. Gynec. 5:30-43, March, 1962.

Moss, F. T., and Meyer, B.: The effects of nursing interaction upon pain relief in patients. Nurs. Research 15:303-306, Fall, 1966.

Newman, M. A.: Identifying and meeting patient's needs in short-span nurse-patient relationships. Nurs. Forum 5:76-86, 1966.

Newton, M.: Where is childbirth education going? Convention Report of the International Childbirth Education Association, Chicago, 1964, pp. 35 a-c, 41, Milwaukee, The Association, 1964.

Newton, N., and Newton, M.: Mothers' reactions to their newborn babies. J.A.M.A. 181:206-210, July 21, 1962.

Novack, J.: Psychological support and labor—a nursing educator's views. Hosp. Topics 42:97-98, August, 1964.

Pettit, R.: Palliation of common obstetrical discomfort. Am. J. Obstet. 85:125, January, 1963.

Psychophysical Preparation for Childbearing: Guidelines for Teaching, ed. 2, New York, Maternity Center Association, 1965.

Read, G. D.: Childbirth Without Fear, rev. ed., New York, Harper, 1953.

Reeder, S.: Becoming a mother, Nursing implication in a problem of role transition, A.N.A. Regional Clinical Conferences, 204-210, New York, Appleton-Century-Crofts, 1968.

Reiter, F. K.: The clinical nursing approach. Nurs. Forum 5:39-44, 1966.

Reynolds, S. R. M., et al.: Clinical Measurement of Uterine Forces in Pregnancy and Labor. Springfield, Charles C Thomas, 1954.

Rich, O. J.: Hospital routines as rites of passage in developing maternal identity. Nurs. Clinics of North America 4:101-109, March, 1969.

Riker, A. P.: How it feels to be a maternity patient. R.N. 26:47-50, October, 1963.

Rosengren, W. R.: Some psychological aspects of delivery room difficulties. J. Nerv. Ment. Dis. 132: 515-521, June, 1961.

Saltenis, I. J.: Physical Touch and Nursing Support in Labor, unpublished master's thesis. Yale University, New Haven, Conn., 1962.

Smoyak, Shirley: Cultural incongruence: the effect on nurses' perceptions. Nurs. Forum 7:234-247, 1968.

Taylor, P. M., et al.: Venous hypertension in the newborn associated with delayed clamping of the umbilical cord. Acta Pediat. 50:149-159, March, 1961.

Travelbee, J.: What do we mean by rapport? Am. J. Nurs. 63:70-72, February, 1963.

Tryon, P. A., and Leonard, R. C.: The effect of the patient's participation on the outcome of a nursing procedure. Nurs. Forum 3:79-89, 1964.

Turner, R. H.: Role taking: process versus conformity, in Rose, A. M. (ed.): Human Behavior and Social Processes, pp. 20-40, Boston, Houghton Mifflin, 1962.

————: Role taking, role standpoint and reference group behavior. Am. J. Sociology 61:316-328, January, 1956.

Ulin, P. R.: The exhilarating moment of birth. Am. J. Nurs. 63:60-67, June, 1963.

Van Auken, W. B. B.: Preparing the patient for labor. Obstet. Gynec. 24:318-321, August, 1964.

Vellay, P., et al.: Childbirth without Pain, translated by D. Lloyd, New York, Dutton, 1959.

Walike, B. C., and Meyer, B.: Relation between placebo reactivity and selected personality factors. Nurs. Research 15:119-123, Spring, 1966.

Wessel, H. S.: Natural Childbirth and the Christian Family. New York, Harper and Row, 1963.

Wiedenbach, E.: Family-Centered Maternity Nursing. New York, G. P. Putnam, 1967.

Wright, E.: New Childbirth. New York, Hart, 1966.

Yeaworth, R. C.: Identification and maternity nursing. Nurs. Forum 7:248-261, 1968.

Zborowski, Mark: Cultural components in responses to pain. J. Social Issues 8:21-25, 1952.

CONFERENCE MATERIAL

1. A mother who is contemplating the delivery of her first child is worried for fear that she may not get her own baby if another infant is born at the same time she is delivered. How would you reassure this mother concerning the identification methods for newborn infants?

2. An 18-year-old mother having her first baby is admitted to the hospital in early labor. It is obvious from her behavior that she has had no preparation for this experience and is frightened and apprehensive. What specific measures would you include in your nursing plan for her care?

3. An unwed mother goes into labor, having made no arrangements for the care of her 2-year-old girl and her 12-year-old boy. What resources could you suggest in this situation? What is the responsibility of hospital and community agencies in this case?

4. How do the public health organizations and hospitals in your community help the patient and her family to prepare for the delivery?

5. Why is prophylaxis for the eyes of the newborn required by law in all states? How would you go about securing the desired information concerning such legislation in the various states of the United States?

6. You are caring for a mother having her fourth child who is in very active labor. Suddenly, the membranes rupture, and she begins to bear down. As you observe the perineum, you see the infant's head crowning. Since you are alone with this mother at the time, what will you do?

7. A 21-year-old mother at term, who has attended "natural childbirth" classes for a previous pregnancy, comes to the hospital on her physician's instructions because her membranes have ruptured. She is apologetic because her contractions are only 10 to 12 minutes apart, of mild intensity, lasting about 35 seconds and "not really good enough yet to come to the hospital." On examination, her cervix is found to be 2 cm. dilated and 10 per cent effaced. Discuss the nursing care you would plan for this mother if she were assigned to your care.

Study Questions

Unit Three: Nursing During Labor and Delivery

Read through the entire question and place your answer on the line to the right.

1. Give the term of the phrase which best fits each of the following statements:

   A. Enlargement of the external os to 10 cm. in diameter.
   B. Maximum shortening of the cervical canal.
   C. A type of drug used in obstetrics which blots out memory of whatever occurs under its influence.
   D. A condition caused by failure of the uterine muscle to stay contracted after delivery.
   E. A surgical incision of the perineum during second-stage labor.
   F. Settling of the baby's head into the brim of the pelvis.

dilatation
effacement
amnesia(?)
uterine atony
hemorrhage
episiotomy
lightening

2. The character and the frequency of uterine contractions and the location of the discomfort experienced by the mother during labor often provide pertinent information regarding the labor.

   SITUATION No. 1: In the case of a multipara who is having discomfort but is not in real labor, which of these symptoms would most probably serve to identify false labor contractions?

   A. Discomfort may begin as early as 3 or 4 weeks before the onset of true labor.
   B. Discomfort occurs 3 or 4 days before the onset of true labor.
   C. Contractions occur at regular intervals.
   D. Contractions occur at irregular intervals.
   E. Discomfort is confined to the lower abdomen and the groin.
   F. Discomfort is felt in the upper abdomen and the back.

   Select the number corresponding to the correct letter or letters.
   1. A only
   2. A and C
   3. A, D and E
   4. All of them   *3*

   SITUATION No. 2: In the case of a primigravida in the beginning of the first stage of labor, which of the following symptoms would most probably describe her labor contractions?

   A. Contractions occur at regular intervals.
   B. Contractions occur at irregular intervals.
   C. Discomfort is confined to the lower abdomen and the groin.
   D. Discomfort is located in the lower back and the abdomen.
   E. Contractions occur at intervals of from 2 to 3 minutes.
   F. Contractions occur at intervals of from 10 to 15 minutes.

   Select the number corresponding to the correct letters.
   1. A and C
   2. A, D and F
   3. B, C and E
   4. All of them   *2*

SITUATION NO. 3: In the case of a primigravida approaching the end of the first stage of labor, which of the following symptoms would most probably give an accurate description of her labor?
A. Contractions occur at regular intervals.
B. Contractions occur at irregular intervals.
C. Contractions occur at intervals of every 1 to 1½ minutes.
D. Contractions occur at intervals of from 2 to 3 minutes.
E. Duration of contraction is from 45 to 60 seconds.
F. Duration of contraction is from 50 to 70 seconds.

Select the number corresponding to the correct letters.
1. A, C and E
2. A, D and F
3. B, D and E
4. All of them   2

3. Labor is divided into the first, the second and the third stages.
    A. When is the first stage of labor considered to be terminated?
        1. When contractions occur at 10- to 15-minute intervals.
        2. When the cervix is completely dilated.
        3. When the baby is delivered.   2
    B. When is the second stage of labor considered to be terminated?
        1. When the cervix is completely dilated.
        2. When contractions occur at 2- to 3-minute intervals.
        3. When the baby is delivered.   3
    C. When is the third stage of labor considered to be terminated?
        1. When the baby is delivered.
        2. When the placenta is delivered.
        3. After the uterus has remained firm for 1 hour.   2

4. The nurse is caring for a mother during the first stage of labor. Which of the following observations would she report promptly to the physician?
A. Small amounts of bright blood in the vaginal discharge.
B. Plugs of blood-streaked mucus in the vaginal discharge.
C. Sudden gush of amniotic fluid from the vagina.
D. Mother has a frequent desire to urinate.
E. Fetal heart rate slows during uterine contractions but returns to its usual rate 10 to 15 seconds following the contractions.

Select the number corresponding to the correct letters.
1. A and C
2. A, C and E
3. B, D and E
4. All of them   1

5. On admission of the mother to the labor suite, which of the following procedures are usually carried out routinely?
A. Check mother's temperature, pulse, respirations and blood pressure.
B. Take the mother to the bathroom and have her void.
C. Cleanse and shave the vulvar and perineal area.
D. Listen to the fetal heart sounds.
E. Prepare the mother for vaginal examination.

Select the number corresponding to the correct letter or letters.
1. A only
2. A and E
3. A, C and D
4. All of them   3

6. Why is an enema frequently given to a mother during the early part of the first stage of labor?
   A. To obtain a stool specimen.
   B. To avoid straining as the mother bears down with contractions.
   C. To cleanse the lower bowel and/or stimulate labor contractions.   <u>C</u>

7. After the cervix is dilated, and particularly if the membranes have ruptured, what facilities would provide the mother with the greatest degree of comfort and safety to expel an enema?
   A. Use of toilet facilities in bathroom.
   B. Remain in bed and use the bedpan.
   C. Use the bedpan on a chair close to the bed.   <u>B</u>

8. Often it is the nurse's responsibility to decide when the mother is ready to be moved from the labor room to the delivery room. Which of the following signs would signify to the nurse that the time of delivery is near?
   A. Mother has a desire to defecate.
   B. Increase in frequency, duration and intensity of uterine contractions.
   C. Mother begins to bear down spontaneously with uterine contractions.
   D. Bulging of the perineum.
   E. Increase in amount of blood-stained mucus from the vagina.

   Select the number corresponding to the correct letter or letters.
   1. D only
   2. A, C and E
   3. B, D and E
   4. All of them   <u>4</u>

9. A physician was busy draining mucus from the mouth of the baby immediately after its birth and asked the nurse to let him know as soon as the placenta seemed to be separated. Which of the following would indicate that it was separated?
   A. Gradual descent of the uterus farther into the pelvis.
   B. Protrusion of several more inches of umbilical cord.
   C. Uterus becomes more firm and rounded.
   D. A sudden gush of blood from the vagina.
   E. Large clots of blood slip out of the vagina.

   Select the number corresponding to the correct letters.
   1. A and C
   2. B, C and D
   3. B, C and E
   4. All of them   <u>2</u>

10. As soon as the physician had clamped and cut the umbilical cord, he handed the infant over to the nurse to care for. Which of the following acts would the nurse perform in the immediate care of the infant?
   A. Place the infant so that he lies in a modified Trendelenburg position in a heated crib or resuscitator.
   B. Wipe the mucus out of the infant's mouth with sterile gauze.
   C. Slap the infant's back and soles of the feet sharply to stimulate crying.
   D. Gently remove all vernix caseosa and blood in drying the infant's body with the receiving blanket.
   E. "Label" infant with required item of identification as soon as he is transferred to the nursery.

   Select the number corresponding to the correct letter or letters.
   1. A only
   2. A and C
   3. B, D and E
   4. All of them   <u>1</u>

11. After the delivery the infant is cared for by a nurse in the receiving nursery. The nurse who is caring for the mother during the first hour after the delivery of the placenta would include which of the following in her nursing care plan?
    A. Keep the mother warm and out of drafts.
    B. Express blood clots if they should accumulate in the uterus.
    C. Massage the fundus continuously.
    D. Administer ergotrate 0.2 mg. intramuscularly.
    E. Check the mother's vital signs at frequent intervals.

    Select the number corresponding to the correct letter or letters.
      1. B only
      2. A and C
      3. A, B and E
      4. All of them   3
      _____

12. Possibly the most dangerous stage of labor for the mother is the third stage because of the possibility of postpartal hemorrhage and shock.
    A. Because there is a certain amount of blood loss, hemorrhage is said to take place when the loss exceeds what amount of blood?
      1. 100 cc.
      2. 300 cc.
      3. 500 cc.   3
      _____
    B. The most common cause of postpartal hemorrhage is atony of the uterus. What is the first thing to do as a preventive measure if the uterus appears to be atonic?
      1. Take a firm grasp on the uterus.
      2. Massage the uterus firmly.
      3. Administer an oxytocic drug.   2
      _____

13. The physician told the nurse to watch a mother during labor for evidence of a prolapsed cord which he feared might occur.
    A. When would the nurse consider that a prolapsed cord would be most likely to occur?
      1. During the second stage of labor.
      2. In breech presentation.
      3. If the presenting part was not engaged in the pelvic brim.
      4. If the amniotic sac were intact.
      5. If the mother were particularly fatigued.   3
      _____
    B. If the nurse did suspect the cord to be prolapsed, what position should she put the mother in, with the hope of relieving the pressure on the cord?
      1. Knee-chest position.
      2. Fowler's position.
      3. Sims' position.
      4. A prone position.   1
      _____
    C. In addition to changing the mother's position to relieve pressure on the cord, what other measures may the nurse employ if she observes the umbilical cord prolapsed out of the vagina?
      1. Immediately wash the cord with warm antiseptic solution and replace in vagina.
      2. Cover the cord with a wet sponge.
      3. Apply a clamp to the exposed cord and cover with a sterile towel.
      4. Keep the cord warm and moist by continuous applications of sterile saline compresses.   4
      _____

    D. What are the chief objectives of the emergency care given when prolapsed cord occurs?
      1. To prevent cold air from prematurely stimulating respiration.
      2. To prevent drying of the cord while it is still pulsating.
      3. To stimulate and restore circulation in the cord by vasodilation.
      4. To prevent or relieve pressure on the cord.   4
      _____

    Note: The key to the correct answers to these questions is given on page 613.

UNIT FOUR
Nursing in the Normal Puerperium

The Physiology of the Puerperium
Nursing Care During the Puerperium

The Physiology of the Puerperium

14

Anatomic Changes • Clinical Aspects • Postpartal Examinations

INTRODUCTION

This chapter deals with the study of the anatomic and the physiologic changes that normally occur during the puerperium. Knowledge and understanding of the reproductive process concerning pregnancy and labor will serve as a basis for understanding how the generative organs and the various systems of the human body adapt following the delivery.

The term puerperium (from *puer,* a child; and *parere,* to bring forth) refers to the 6-week period elapsing between the termination of labor and the return of the reproductive organs to their normal condition. This includes both the *progressive changes* in the breasts for lactation and *involution* of the internal reproductive organs. Although the changes brought about by involution are considered to be normal physiologic processes, they border closely between a condition of health and disease, for under no other circumstances does such marked and rapid involution of tissues occur without a departure from a state of health. For this reason, the quality of the mother's care at this time is essential to ensure her immediate as well as her future health.

ANATOMIC CHANGES

Uterus

Involution of the Uterus. Immediately following the delivery of the placenta the uterus becomes an almost solid mass of tissue, about the size of a grapefruit. Its thick anterior and posterior walls lie in close opposition, so that the center cavity is flattened. The uterus remains about the same size for the first 2 days after delivery but then rapidly decreases in size by an atrophic process called involution. This is effected partly by the contraction of the uterus and partly by autolytic processes in which some of the protein material of the uterine wall is broken down into simpler components which then are absorbed and eventually cast off through the urine.

THE PROCESS OF INVOLUTION. The separation of the placenta and the membranes from the uterine wall takes place in the outer portion of the spongy layer of the decidua, and, therefore, a remnant of this layer remains in the uterus to be cast off in part in the lochia. Within 2 or 3 days after labor this remaining portion of decidua becomes differentiated into two layers, leaving the deeper or unaltered layer attached to the muscular wall from which the new endometrial lining is generated. The layer adjoining the uterine cavity becomes necrotic and is cast off in the lochia. The process is very like the healing of any surface; there is oozing of blood from the small vessels on this surface. The bleeding from the larger vessels is controlled by compression of the retracted uterine muscle fibers. The process of regeneration is rapid, except at the site of former placental attachment, which requires 6 or 7 weeks to heal completely. Elsewhere, the free surface of the endometrium is restored in half that time.

THE PROGRESS OF INVOLUTION. The normal process of involution requires 5 or 6 weeks, and at the end of that time the uterus regains its normal size, although it never returns exactly to its virgin state. One can realize more fully the rapidity of this process by comparing the changes which occur in the weight of this organ. Immediately following the delivery the uterus weighs approximately 2 pounds; at the end of the first week, about 1 pound; at the end of the second week, about 12 ounces; and by the time that involution is complete, it should weigh only about 2 ounces. By observing the height of the fundus, which may be felt through the abdominal wall, the nurse is able to appreciate more fully these remarkable changes. Immediately after the birth of the placenta the uterus sinks into the pelvis, and the fundus is felt midway between the umbilicus and the symphysis, but it soon rises to the level of the umbilicus (5 or 5½ inches above the pubes); and 12 hours later it probably will be found a little higher. Day-by-day careful measurements will show that it is diminishing in size, so that at the end of 10 days or so it cannot be detected by abdominal palpation. The approximate rate of decrease in the height of the fundus is a little over half an inch or one fingerbreadth a day. Observation of this rate of involution is very important; the physician will want to be informed about any marked delay, especially if accompanied by suppression of the lochia or retention of clots. In measuring the height of the uterus, care should be taken that the observations are made after the bladder is emptied, as a full bladder will raise the height of the fundus.

Apparent indications that involution is not occurring satisfactorily are: the uterus fails to decrease progressively in size, it remains "flabby" and causes the mother much discomfort (see Subinvolution in Chap. 21, Complications of the Puerperium).

Changes in the Cervix. After the delivery the cervix is a soft, flabby structure but, because it is retracting, by the end of the 1st week it becomes so narrow that it would be difficult to introduce anything the size of a finger. Unlike the process of involution which is now occurring in the body of the uterus, a very considerable new formation of muscle cells is taking place in the cervix and, simultaneously, any lacerations are healing. Once a mother has delivered a child vaginally, the cervix does not assume its pregravid appearance, but the external os remains open in varying degrees, although the internal os is closed. This is one of the characteristics of the uterus of a multiparous woman.

The Lochia. A knowledge of the healing process by which the lining of the uterus becomes regenerated is a valuable adjunct to the nurse in understanding and interpreting the lochial discharge. At first the discharge consists almost entirely of blood with a small amount of mucus, particles of decidua and cellular debris which escape from the placental site. It should not contain large clots or membrane or be excessive in amount. This discharge lasts about 3 days and is called *lochia rubra*. As the oozing of blood from the healing surface diminishes, the discharge becomes more serous or watery and gradually changes to a pinkish color, the so-called *lochia serosa*. Toward the 10th day the lochia is thinner, greatly decreased in amount and almost colorless, the so-called *lochia alba*. By the end of the 3rd week the discharge usually disappears, though a brownish mucoid discharge may persist a little longer. Lochia possesses a peculiar animal emanation which is quite characteristic and should never, at any time, have an offensive odor.

The quantity of lochia varies with individuals, but, generally speaking, it is more profuse in multiparas. It is to be expected that when a mother is out of bed for the first time there may be a definite increase in the amount of discharge. Nevertheless, the recurrence of fresh bleeding after the discharge has become dark and diminished in amount, or the persistence of bright blood in the lochia or the suppression of the discharge (which may be caused by cold, fright, grief or other emotion) should be reported to the obstetrician. The daily observation of the amount and the character of the lochia is of the greatest importance as an index of the progress of healing of the endometrial surface.

The Pelvis

The vaginal walls, the vulva and all other tissues which have become hypertrophied during pregnancy also undergo a process of involution in their return to normal. The *vagina* requires some time to recover from the distention brought about by the delivery. This capacious passage gradually diminishes in size, although rarely returns to its nulliparous condition. The *labia majora* and the *labia minora* become flabby and atrophic as compared with their condition before childbearing. Any abrasions and lacerations of the genital canal caused by the passage of the fetus should heal completely during the puerperium. The *ligaments* that support the uterus, the ovaries and the tubes, which have also undergone great tension and stretching, are now relaxed and will take considerable time to return almost to their normal size and position. This is one of the reasons that the mother must be given intelligent interpretation of early ambulation.

Abdominal Wall

The abdominal wall recovers partially from the overstretching but remains soft and flabby for some time. The striae, due to the rupture of the elastic fibers of the cutis, usually remain but become less conspicuous because of their silvery appearance. The process of involution in the abdominal structures requires at least 6 weeks. Provided that the abdominal walls have retained their muscle tone, they gradually return to their original condition. However, if these muscles are relaxed because they have lost their tone, there may be a marked separation or *diastasis of the recti muscles,* so that the abdominal organs are not properly supported. Rest, diet, prescribed exercises, good body mechanics and good posture may do much to restore the tonicity of these muscles.

The Breasts

During pregnancy progressive changes occur in the breasts in preparation for lactation (see Chap. 6). After the delivery the breasts continue much the same for about 2 days. The breasts secrete a small amount of *colostrum,* which appears as a thin yellowish fluid. It will be remembered that colostrum is formed at the end of pregnancy, and women who carry out special breast care preparation during the last weeks of pregnancy often are able manually to express small amounts of it before the birth of the baby. The nutritive value of colostrum is low in comparison with that of normal breast milk. Colostrum contains more protein (lactalbumin) and inorganic salts but less fat and carbohydrate than human breast milk. During these first days after the delivery breast-feeding is advantageous for both mother and infant. The infant's sucking at the breast helps to stimulate lactation, and, in addition, it stimulates the uterus to contract. These early breast feeding experiences simultaneously fulfill the infant's need for sucking.

On the 3rd or the 4th day postpartum the breast milk usually "comes in." There is an obvious change in the color of the secretion from the nipples; it becomes bluish white, the usual color of normal breast milk. At this time the breasts suddenly become larger, firmer and more tender as the lacteal secretion is established, causing the mother to experience throbbing pains in the breasts, extending into the axillae. This congestion, which usually subsides in 1 or 2 days, is caused in part by the pressure from the increased amount of milk in the lobes and the ducts but even more by the increased circulation of blood and lymph in the mammary gland, producing tension on the very sensitive surrounding tissues. This is sometimes referred to as *primary engorgement.*

Breast milk varies markedly in its quality and quantity, not only in different individuals, but also in the same individual at various times. In general, the amount of breast milk increases as the infant's need for it increases. Nature seems to have coordinated carefully the mother's need for rest and the infant's need for food during the first 2 days, when only colostrum is secreted. But during this time lactation is definitely stimulated by the infant's sucking, and although the secretion of breast milk would occur naturally, without this stimulation and the complete emptying of the breasts the secretion of breast milk would not continue for more than a few days. If the infant is put to breast consistently, by the end of the first week a healthy mother usually has about 6 to 10 ounces of breast milk a day. By the end of 4 weeks this amount almost doubles, so that she produces about 20 ounces a day. Breast milk is produced on the basis of "supply and demand" (i.e., the amount secreted gradually adjusts in relation to what the baby takes at an average feeding). In time, as the baby grows, the mother may have about 30 ounces of breast milk a day.

The supply of breast milk is dependent on several factors, such as the mother's diet, the amount of exercise and rest she gets, and her level of contentment. An adequate diet for lactation requires increased amounts of protein, calcium, iron and vitamins as well as an ample fluid intake (see p. 328). The mother who is breast-feeding needs a good night's sleep, a rest period in the middle of the day and normal exercise. Worry, emotional tension and too much activity (overexertion and fatigue) have an adverse effect on lactation (see Chaps. 8 and 16). In relation to lactation, the actual size of the breast is not as important as the amount of glandular tissue, since the secreting tissues of the mammary gland produce the breast milk and not the fat. It has been verified that certain drugs, if administered to the lactating mother, are excreted in the breast milk, for example, large doses of salicylates, certain cathartics, iodides, bromides, quinine, atropine, opium, etc.

CLINICAL ASPECTS

Temperature

Slight rises in temperature may occur without apparent cause following the delivery, but, in general, the mother's temperature should remain within normal limits during the puerperium, that is, below 38° C. (100.4° F.) when taken by mouth. Any mother whose temperature exceeds this limit in any two consecutive 24-hour periods of the puerperium (excluding the first 24 hours postpartum) is considered to be febrile.

It was formerly believed that an elevation of temperature naturally occurred with the establishment of lactation on the 3rd or the 4th day after the delivery, and the so-called *milk-fever* was considered to be a normal accompaniment of this process. At the present time this is considered to be a fallacy. On rare occasions a sharp peak of fever for several hours may be caused by extreme vascular and lymphatic engorgement of the breasts, but this does not last longer than 12 hours at the most.

In judging the significance of a rise in temperature, the pulse rate provides a helpful guide, for in a puerperal patient with a slow pulse, a slightly elevated temperature is not likely to signify a complication. Nevertheless, any rise of temperature in the puerperium should excite the suspicion of endometritis (see Chap. 21, Complications of the Puerperium).

Pulse

In the early puerperium a pulse rate which is somewhat slower than that at other times is a favorable symptom. The rate usually averages between 60 and 70 but may even become a little slower than this in 1 or 2 days after the delivery. This is merely a transient phenomenon, so that by the end of the 1st week or 10 days the pulse returns to its normal rate. On the other hand, a rapid pulse after labor, unless the mother has cardiac disease, may be an indication of shock or hemorrhage.

Blood

Most of the blood and metabolic alterations characteristic of normal pregnancy disappear within the first 2 weeks of the puerperium.

After-pains

Normally, after the delivery of the first child, the uterine muscle tends to remain in a state of tonic contraction and retraction. But if the uterus has been subjected to any marked distention, or if tissue or blood clots have been retained in the cavity, then active contractions occur in an effort to expel them, and these contractions may be painful. In multiparas a certain amount of the initial tonicity of the uterine muscle has been lost, and these contractions and retractions cannot be sustained. Consequently, the muscle contracts and relaxes at intervals, and these contractions give rise to the sensation of pain, the so-called "after-pains." These after-pains are more noticeable after a pregnancy in which the uterus has been greatly distended, as with multiple births or hydramnios. They are particularly noticeable in the breast-feeding mother, when the infant is put to breast (because sucking stimulates the uterus to contract), and they may last for days, although ordinarily they become quite bearable in about 48 hours after delivery. They also occur with increased intensity, following the administration of oxytocic agents such as ergotrate. Often after-pains become so sharp that the administration of a sedative is necessary. Any time that they are severe enough to disturb the mother's rest and peace of mind, the physician should be notified.

Digestion

Although the mother's appetite may be diminished the first few days after labor, the digestive tract functions normally in the puerperium. Her thirst is considerably increased at this time due to the marked diaphoresis and loss of fluids associated with the puerperium. Moreover, the fact that the mother has probably gone without fluids for some hours in labor undoubtedly increases her thirst.

Loss of Weight

In addition to the 10- or 11-pound loss of weight which results at delivery, there is generally a still further loss of about 5 pounds of body weight early in the puerperium due to the marked diuresis, with its associated loss of body fluid.

Kidneys

The amount of urine excreted by the kidneys in the puerperium is of particular significance. As previously stated, during pregnancy there is an increased tendency of the body to retain water, so that now the tremendous output of urine represents the body's effort to return its water metabolism to normal. Diuresis regularly occurs between the 2nd and the 5th days after delivery, sometimes reaching a daily output of 3,000 cc. After the delivery, in particular, the bladder may distend without any awareness on the part of the mother, especially if she has received any form of analgesia. Therefore, it becomes a major responsibility of the nurse to be alert to signs of a full bladder and thus to prevent distention from occurring.

During the first few days after labor there may be an increase in the amount of nitrogen in the urine. This excretion is due to the breakdown of protein material of the uterine wall during involution (p. 293). Concerning acetone in the urine— as long as the regimen of "starvation" is not included in the management of labor, the presence of acetone in the urine, related to the incomplete metabolism of body fat, would not occur. Occasionally, during the first weeks of the puerperium the urine contains substantial amounts of sugar, which has no relationship to diabetes but is due to the presence of lactose, milk sugar, which is absorbed from the mammary glands.

Intestinal Elimination

The mother is nearly always constipated during the first few days of the puerperium. This is due to the relaxed condition of the intestinal and the abdominal muscles, in particular, and to the inability of the abdominal wall to aid in the evacuation of the intestinal contents. In addition, if hemorrhoids are present, the mother often is afraid to have a stool because of the discomfort these varicosities cause during elimination.

Skin

It is to be expected that elimination of waste products via the skin is accelerated in the early puerperium, often to such a degree that the mother is drenched with perspiration. These episodes of profuse sweating, which frequently occur in the night, gradually subside and do not require any specific treatment aside from protecting the mother from chilling at such times as they occur.

Menstruation

If the mother does not breast-feed her infant, the menstrual flow probably will return within 8 weeks after delivery. Ordinarily, menstruation does not occur so long as the mother is breast-feeding, but this is not a certainty. During lactation the first menstrual period may occur as early as the 2nd month but usually occurs about the 4th month following the delivery. It has been known not to reappear until as late as the 18th month. Studies have shown that failure to menstruate during lactation is due to suppression of ovulation, but, since some mothers have been known to become pregnant in the course of breast-feeding an infant, we know that this is not always the case.

POSTPARTAL EXAMINATIONS

The condition of the mother is confirmed before she is discharged from the hospital to make sure that her progress has been satisfactory during the early puerperium. In addition to verifying her vital signs and present weight, observations are made to determine the condition of her breasts, the progress of involution and the healing of the perineal wound. A pelvic examination is deferred, since findings made by palpation of the uterus and inspection of the lochia will give satisfactory evidence as to the progress of involution at this time.

Follow-up Examinations

As has been mentioned previously, the reproductive tract should return to its normal condition by the end of the puerperium. In order to investigate the general physical condition of the mother and determine with what normalcy she has completed her maternity experience, she should return to her physician for examination about 6 weeks postpartum. During the visit the weight and the blood pressure are taken, the urine is examined for albumin, and a blood count may be done. The condition of the abdominal walls is observed, and the breasts are inspected. If the mother is breast-feeding, the condition of the nipples and the degree of lacteal secretion are a significant part of the observation. If the mother is not breast-feeding, the breasts should be observed to see that physiologic readjustments have occurred. A thorough pelvic examination is carried out to investigate the position of the uterus, the healing of perineal wounds, the support of the pelvic floor, and whether involution is complete. In addition, this return examination provides an opportunity for the mother and the obstetrician to discuss any other problems relating to this maternity experience and to discuss methods of family planning (see Chap. 15). If abnormalities are found, they may be treated at this time and arrangements made for further examinations and treatments as necessary. Regardless, most physicians instruct their patients to return in 6 months for a check-up examination. Many encourage the mothers to return for a check-up again at the end of 1 year.

SUGGESTED READING

Eastman, N. J., and Hellman, L. H.: Williams Obstretrics, ed. 13, New York, Appleton, 1966.

Greenhill, J. P.: Obstetrics, ed. 13, Philadelphia, W. B. Saunders, 1965.

Hendricks, C. H.: Uterine contractility changes in the early puerperium. Clin. Obstet. Gynec. 11:125-144, March, 1968.

Moawad, A. H., and Hendricks, C. H.: Spontaneous and pharmacologically induced disruption of myometrial activity in the early puerperium. Am. J. Obstet. Gynec. 98:1091-1098, August 15, 1967.

Sharman, A.: Reproductive Physiology of the Post-Partum Period. Edinburgh and London, E. & S. Livingstone, 1966.

Nursing Care During the Puerperium

15

*Changes and Reactions During the Puerperium • Immediate Care
General Physical Care • Special Physical Care Aspects
The Mother Who Is Nursing • Parental Guidance and Instruction*

INTRODUCTION

During the last two decades the constantly expanding dimensions of maternity nursing have redirected the emphasis and given new significance to what had become a rather routinized kind of care for the mother, as well as for those who provided the nursing care.

The newly delivered mother is usually a healthy patient who is adjusting physically and emotionally from the experiences of pregnancy and labor. However, in addition, a vastly important developmental phase begins for the mother and her newborn, and she must adapt to her infant, as well as to a new family structure.

In the context of total health care, on a continuum, "optimal maternal care can be defined as the accomplishment of those measures which are necessary to achieve a state of physical, mental and social well-being, and the maintenance of this state prior to planned conception, during pregnancy, and throughout the postpartal period, not just for the mother and child but for the whole family."[1]

In Chapter 1 it is stated that providing optimal maternal care requires a thoughtful approach to the many facets and factors responsible for high-level wellness of the maternity patient. Her needs for physical care have been greatly modified by the advent of early ambulation following delivery and the subsequent evolution of more simplified maternity nursing procedures. Newly delivered mothers need certain kinds of physical care; for example, in relation to evaluating the progressive changes which occur in the breasts for lactation, as well as the involutional changes of the internal reproductive organs to regain the normal nonpregnant condition. New mothers need nourishment, rest and sleep, and activity tempered with purposeful use of early ambulation.

Increased insight into the psycho-social needs of the newly delivered mother has resulted in greater attention to the emotional aspects of her care. This does not in any sense negate the need for physical care. As has been emphasized previously, the mother, the infant, the father and other children are considered as a family unit. In the hospital the same nurse may not necessarily have the responsibility for caring for the mother and her new baby at the same time (the baby might be cared for by nurses assigned primarily to the nursery). Nevertheless, the infant's care must be considered in relation to his mother's care, and their care in turn must be related to the total family constellation. A very important consideration is the need that the mother and her newly born infant have for each other; and in today's highly organized hospitals, such times do not always coincide with hospital policy or routine.

The simplification of certain aspects of physical care in no way diminishes the need for professional nursing care, for the astute nurse can use

---

[1] Peckham, B. M.: Optimal maternal care. Obstet. Gynec. 33:862-868, June, 1969.

physical care activity as a valuable entree in developing a productive nurse-patient relationship (see Chap. 13). Moreover, she needs to use her observational and communicative skills continuously. The mother's physiological functioning must be observed accurately, her dependency needs must be met, anticipatory guidance and health teachings must be given according to the mother's readiness to learn, and the developing relationship between the mother and infant should be appropriately observed, guided and nurtured. This may appear to be a gigantic challenge to the nurse. However, the shortened hospital stay for the mother who has had an uncomplicated delivery makes it all the more important to see that she receives the support and kind of teaching she requires concerning the care of her baby and herself, before being discharged to face her new responsibilities. Truly, this is a period when nursing assessment can be utilized most fruitfully.

High-level wellness (see page 5) might well be paraphrased; High-level wellness for the mother and her newly born infant is an integrated method of functioning (interacting) which is oriented toward maximizing the potential of the mother-infant relationship of which this mother-infant 'couple' is capable. This requires that the mother-infant adaptation be dynamic, but maintains a continuum of balance and purposeful direction within the environment (family) where they are functioning (see Chap. 16).

CHANGES AND REACTIONS DURING THE PUERPERIUM

As stated in Chapter 13, immediately after labor, the mother experiences a sense of complete fatigue which is comparable to that which would normally follow any strenuous muscular activity. At the same time, if she has been awake during the delivery of her infant, she may be so exhilarated by the experience and the feeling of relief which accompanies it that she is not aware of being exhausted. She is interested in seeing and holding her baby and visiting with her husband. Although this first visit of the family together may be rather

Fig. 15-1. Parents and baby having first visit after delivery.

Fig. 15-2. Mother observes umbilical cord stump of her newborn. (MacDonald House, The University Hospitals of Cleveland, Cleveland, Ohio)

brief, it is an experience which is particularly gratifying to the parents. Following this, every effort should be made to help the mother to rest, and with little encouragement she usually passes off into a sound natural sleep. The discomforts and activities which may interfere with sleep, such as soreness of the vulva, hemorrhoids, "after-pains," and frequent postpartal observations, should be expedited and/or mitigated as much as possible.

Fig. 15-3. Mother learning ways to change her baby's position. (MacDonald House, The University Hospitals of Cleveland, Cleveland, Ohio)

Many mothers complain of feeling chilled immediately after labor; a few even appear to have a shaking chill. Such chills may be due in part to nervous reaction and exhaustion. There is some disturbance of equilibrium between internal and external temperature caused by excessive perspiration during the muscular exertion of labor. Some authorities believe that the "chill" may be due partly to the sudden release of intra-abdominal pressure which results as the uterus is emptied at delivery. This reaction may be alleviated if the mother is made comfortable in a warm bed and given a warm beverage when possible (see Chap. 13). If her body does begin to quiver, an extra cotton blanket should be placed over her or tucked close around her body for comfort. Many mothers (and their husbands) are frightened or disturbed by the chill; thus, reassurance by the nurse that this is not an unusual occurrence following delivery is extremely helpful.

Physiologic and Psychological Changes

Specific anatomic and physiologic changes already have been discussed in Chapter 14. However, it is well to keep in mind that these alterations occur abruptly and are sizable. They involve profound diminution in circulating blood volume, a weight loss, displacement of internal organs, etc. It is truly marvelous that the new parturient copes so adequately, and that she complains so little (see Suggested Reading).

The normal puerperal course follows a predictable healing and regenerative pattern, one that is not confined to the physical aspects of the patient. A new role must be assumed along with all of its concomitant tasks, new attitudes must be formed, and these adjustments must be undertaken before physical restoration is complete.

As with any regenerative process, energy is involved—energy that is needed to survive and to meet the everyday obligations of the mother's social and individual role. During the time that the mother coped with the increasing demands of labor there was a progressive withdrawal of social energy (i.e., a narrowing of attention and an inward turning. See Chap. 13). During the postpartal period the reverse process occurs: the mother is slowly able to extend the sphere of physical and psychic energy from herself to others in the immediate environment and then to events and persons outside her immediate environment.

Phases of the Restorative Period of the Puerperium. "TAKING-IN" PHASE. One author[2] has described certain phases that occur during the restorative period of the puerperium. The first of these seems to be a "taking-in" period (this lasts 2 or 3 days), in which the mother is passive and dependent. She tries to do what she is told, she gratefully accepts what she is given, and she initiates little or no action; rather she awaits the action of others. She seems to be grateful when decisions are made for her, and even simple decision-making as well as slight physical activity

seems to fatigue her. It becomes apparent to the nurse that the needs she expresses are more in relation to herself than in relation to her baby. The wise nurse attempts to meet these needs to the mother's satisfaction, thus enabling her to move on to the more complex tasks of mothering her baby.

Sleep and food play an important part during this phase. The mother is far more able to begin the activities required of her if she is allowed to have a well-earned refreshing sleep. If this necessary rest is disrupted, the mother may experience a "sleep-hunger" which may last for several days; this results in irritability, fatigue and general interference with the normal restorative process. Thus, the necessity of appropriate intervention by the nurse to allow the mother to get adequate sleep cannot be stressed enough.

The nurse will note, also, that the mother usually has a good appetite and, in fact, may talk a good deal about food, about either the adequacy or the inadequacy of her meals. In-between nourishment is appreciated and needed (especially by nursing mothers). The concern about food seems to be a part of the mother's general need to be restored. Food, as we know, has tremendous psychological significance in terms of care-asking and care-giving (see Chap. 8). The nurse should be especially cognizant of the mother's need for hearty meals and should expedite extra nourishment whenever possible. Moreover, she should be aware that a poor appetite often is one of the first symptoms that all is not proceeding normally in the puerperal period.

Psychological Adjustment. During the "taking-in" phase the mother begins to relive the delivery experience in order to integrate it fully with reality. She is apt to be very talkative at this time, and she may want to know certain specifics and details so that she can form a total picture of what "really happened" during delivery. As she obtains this information, she is able to realize more fully that the pregnancy and the delivery are truly over, and that her baby now is born and is an individual outside of and separate from herself. This is a considerable task and involves rather profound changes in attitudes and feelings. The symbiotic relationship between mother and infant during pregnancy is at an end, and the mother now must identify her child as a separate individual (see Chap. 16).

TAKING-HOLD PHASE. The second phase in the puerperal period has been described as a "taking-

[2] Rubin, R.: Puerperal change. Nurs. Outlook 9:753-755, December, 1961.

Fig. 15-4. Mother enfolds her newborn. (MacDonald House, The University Hospitals of Cleveland, Cleveland, Ohio)

hold" phase; that is, the mother strives for independence and autonomy and finally begins to be the initiator. One of her main concerns at this point seems to be her ability to control her bodily functions; her bowels and bladder must perform well, and she takes an active part in seeing that they do. If she is nursing her infant, she is concerned about producing an acceptable quantity and quality of milk. She often will ask the nurses and the doctors anxiously (referring to the milk),

"Has it come in yet?" And later she wants to know: "Do you think I have enough?" She cannot have enough explanation and reassurance that she is "performing" well at this time. She wants to walk, to sit, to move as she did before delivery and is very anxious and impatient if she cannot make her body behave as it once did. It is as though she is thinking, "How can I possibly assume all my responsibilities for others if I cannot control my own body?"

Her first mothering tasks are especially important to her, and "failures" (inability to elicit a bubble from her infant, poor sucking response on the part of the baby, her awkwardness in handling her child), no matter how small and expected (by the staff), can send her to the depths of despair. Even the skillful intervention of the nurse seems only to point up her "inadequacy" as a mother. She often will voice her feelings with an "Oh, I'll never be able to bathe him as easily as you do." Or she says: "He always seems to take his milk better when *you* feed him." Conversely, when she succeeds at a task, her delight and relief are wonderful to behold. It is difficult to imagine (for anyone other than a new mother) how thrilling a hearty bubble from a small infant can be.

Since there is a good deal of anxiety as well as activity in this phase, fatigue and exhaustion may occur if the mother is not helped to set realistic expectations and limits for herself. Since this "taking-hold" phase lasts about 10 days, much of it will take place at home.

The nurse can be invaluable in giving the mother, as she appears able and ready to accept it, anticipatory guidance about what to expect and how to manage. During the hospital stay the mother profits greatly from reassurance and explanation regarding the various processes and hour-by-hour events. She finds guidance and reinforcement of appropriate behavior by the nurse particularly helpful when she attempts to perform her mothering tasks.

When assisting the mother, the nurse must be careful not to impose herself between the mother and her baby (no matter how awkward or maladroit the mother seems). Rather, the nurse should allow the mother to perform the actual task (after necessary demonstration or instruction) and then encourage or reinforce whatever behavior was appropriate. In this way she demonstrates that she has confidence in the mother's ability to cope with new tasks. In order to gain skill and confidence in her mothering ability, the mother needs the opportunity to make decisions about the baby's needs as well as guidance regarding his physical care. When she is allowed to find answers to her questions (again with guidance as necessary) and is reassured that her judgment is correct, she is able to feel confident in her ability to perceive needs accurately and to make decisions. Thus, she is better able to meet problems in the future. (See Suggested Reading for a more thorough discussion of changes and behavior during the puerperium.)

Postpartal Blues. Sometime during the puerperium, for no apparent reason, the mother quite suddenly may experience a "let-down" feeling. She may become irritable and tearful, may even lose her appetite and find it difficult to sleep. These are the usual manifestations of the so-called "postpartal blues"; they usually are very temporary and may occur while the mother is in the hospital or after her discharge. This temporary depression is thought to be related to the hormonal changes that occur during this time and the ego regression that can accompany the increased dependency needs and responsibilities. Discomfort, fatigue and exhaustion certainly contribute to this condition, if they do not actually precipitate it. The mother may release tension by crying and thus become more comfortable. However, since she usually does not know exactly why she is crying, she may feel guilty about this somewhat unaccustomed emotional display.

The nurse can help the mother most effectively if she is able to recognize and to interpret the mother's behavior and, in turn, is kind and understanding. If the mother does want to cry, her privacy should be respected, and she should be assured that this behavior is not only acceptable but therapeutic. Accurate reporting and recording of the mother's emotional state is important at all times. Occasionally a more serious and pathologic psychological upheaval occurs, and the prodromal signs may become apparent during the hospital stay (see Chap. 21).

Summary. It is well to keep in mind during the early days of the puerperium that although the mother appears to recover with amazing rapidity after the delivery, she is still going through a period of transition. Therefore, she is more vulnerable to stress at this time. Problems that she otherwise might handle with relative ease may stimulate emotionally charged situations as she faces the increased responsibilities for the nurturing and the care of her new baby, her family and home. At the same time, the mother's own need for affection and attention may bring about feelings of jealousy and guilt when the major attention more often than not is directed to the infant. Therefore, care should be focused on providing physical rest for the mother as well as an environment that is as free from tension and worry as possible. In addition, the mother should be given as much help as she needs to gain self-confidence

FIG. 15-5. Nurse palpating fundus.

in caring for her baby and perceiving his needs. This will mean that the old cliché "routine post-partum care" is not to be taken literally. Nursing care during the puerperium, as during any other period of the childbearing cycle, must be "tailored" to meet the needs of each individual patient.

IMMEDIATE CARE

Intelligent interpretation of the patient's physi-ologic and behavioral responses is essential to the mother's safety and welfare. Paramount among the physiologic responses is the condition of the uterus. The mother must be observed carefully for bleeding during the first 6 hours after labor and particularly during the 1st hour after delivery (see Chap. 13).

Considerable information can be gained by palpating the fundus through the abdominal wall

to be assured that the uterus remains firm, round and well contracted. At the same time it is also important to inspect the perineal pad for obvious signs of bleeding, as well as to take the pulse and the blood pressure. During the first hour these observations should be made at least every 15 minutes, or more often if indicated. In some hospitals it is customary to have a nurse (or a properly prepared nurse's aide) sit at the bedside during this hour, with her hand on the mother's abdomen so that she can feel the fundus con-stantly. As long as the bleeding is minimal, and the uterus remains firm, well-contracted and does not increase in size, it is neither necessary nor desirable to stimulate it. However, if the uterus becomes soft and boggy because of relaxation, the fundus should be massaged immediately until it becomes contracted again. This can be best accomplished if one hand is placed just above the symphysis pubis to act as a guard, as the other hand is cupped around the fundus and rotated gently. It should be remembered that the uterus is a sensitive organ which, under normal circumstances, responds quickly to tactile stimulation. Care must be taken to avoid overmassage, because, in addition to causing the mother considerable pain, this may stimulate premature uterine contractions and thereby cause undue muscle fatigue. Such a condition would further encourage uterine relaxation and hemorrhage. If the uterus is atonic, blood which collects in the cavity should be expressed with firm but gentle force in the direction of the outlet, but only after the fundus has been first massaged (Fig. 15-5). Failure to see that the uterus is contracted before pushing downward against it could result in inversion of the uterus, an exceedingly serious complication.

During the 1st hour the mother should be kept clean, dry and comfortable but allowed to rest as much as possible. At the end of this hour it is usually customary to give the mother a partial bath as necessary and take the temperature, in addition to other vital signs, before transferring her to the postpartal division. The nurse must be constantly alert for any changes in the mother's condition, such as her color, character of the pulse, respiration and blood pressure, the status of the fundus and the amount of vaginal bleeding.

GENERAL PHYSICAL CARE

The daily routine procedures for the postpartal patient vary in different hospitals, but the principles of care are essentially the same. Certain observations should be made and recorded daily. These would include such findings as temperature, pulse and respiration; urinary and intestinal elimination; the physical changes which occur normally in the puerperium. One should note the changes in the breasts, the height and consistency of the fundus, the character, the amount and the color of the lochial discharge and the condition of the episiotomy (see Chap. 14). Furthermore, it is equally important for the nurse to be alert to the mother's general comfort and well-being—how she rests and sleeps, her activity, her appetite, her emotional status and, particularly, because of its vast influence, how she is adjusting to her role as a new mother (see Chap. 16).

Temperature, Pulse and Respiration

The temperature should be carefully watched during the first 2 weeks of the puerperium, as fever is usually the first symptom of an infectious process. And, as has been stated previously, the pulse rate provides a helpful guide in determining the significance of a rise in temperature. These observations are usually made and recorded every 4 hours for the first few days after delivery, omitting the 2 A.M. observations, which would disturb the mother's sleep. Thereafter, they are made every night and morning, as long as the mother is progressing normally. If the temperature rises above 37.8° C. (100° F.) or the pulse rate above 100, the physician should be notified immediately. Usually, the blood pressure is not checked regularly unless there has been some abnormality. Then observations and recordings are made every 2 to 4 hours or more frequently, as indicated.

Nutrition

Very shortly following the delivery, after having gone without food or fluids for some hours, the mother may express a desire for something to eat. However, when food is put before her, she may have little appetite. Unless she has received a general anesthetic or is nauseated, there is usually no contraindication to giving her some nourishment. It may be prudent to give her small amounts of easily digested foods, such as tea and toast, jello or custard, for this first meal. Thereafter, she enjoys a normal diet.

The two factors which the nurse must bear in mind when considering the mother's diet are (1) providing for her general nutrition and (2) providing enough nourishing foods to supply the additional calories and nutrients required during lactation. If these nutritional requirements are provided for, the mother's convalescence will be more rapid, her strength will be recovered more quickly, and the quality and quantity of her milk will be better. She will also be more able to resist infections.

Mothers in general, and particularly mothers who are breast-feeding, usually have good appetites and become hungry between meals. For this reason it is advisable to see that they receive intermediate nourishment consisting of a nourishing beverage or a snack 3 times a day. If the nourishment is in the form of a glass of milk or some milk product, this helps to incorporate the additional milk requirement for the nursing mother.

Rest and Sleep

During the puerperium the mother needs an abundance of rest and should be encouraged to relax and sleep whenever possible. This can best be accomplished if she is comfortable and free from worry and other anxiety-producing situations. The need for rest has even more significance for the mother who is breast-feeding, because worry and fatigue inhibit her milk supply. With the exception of the husband, visitors should be limited during the first week or so because they can be tiring. A mother who is not getting sufficient rest is usually anxious, and worries over minor things that otherwise might cause her little concern. Furthermore, many emotional problems are often precipitated by sleeplessness and fatigue.

It becomes the nurse's responsibility to adjust the hospital routine whenever possible to provide the mother with uninterrupted periods of rest. Routine procedures can be delayed or rearranged to meet the mother's needs. A bottle-fed infant may be fed occasionally by the nurse if the mother is sleeping and does not want to be awakened. If the mother is unable to nap during the day (and she may not, due to excitement and fatigue), she can be encouraged to rest as quietly as possible for certain continuous periods. The need for rest and sleep may have to be explained and reiterated to her, especially during the "taking-hold" phase, as she is eager to be up and about and may tend to overdo.

Early Ambulation

Although early ambulation of the so-called "normal" mother had its inception out of necessity during World War II, experience with this aspect of management of the puerperium has shown that it possesses certain intrinsic advantages to the mother, and as a result it is almost generally accepted today. The mothers seem to get their strength back more quickly and appear to be stronger on the 5th or 6th day than they used to be at the time of discharge under the old regimen. This is proved by multiparas who were kept on bed rest for 7 to 14 days following previous deliveries, who state that they feel better and stronger with early ambulation. With this increase in exercise for the newly delivered mother, her circulation is stimulated, and there are fewer complications of thrombophlebitis. Moreover, bladder and bowel functions are improved, with the result that bladder complications leading to catheterization are greatly reduced. Abdominal distention and constipation occur less frequently. The majority of healthy mothers are allowed out of bed in 8 to 24 hours.

If the patient has had a conduction anesthesia which involves entering the dura, she may be kept in a recumbent position for about the first 8 hours. It is felt by many physicians that keeping the patient flat in bed for this time helps to prevent the occurrence of a postspinal headache, since headache is precipitated and aggravated when the head is elevated. Postspinal headache is thought to be due to a leakage of the spinal fluid through the puncture hole of the dura, with subsequent decrease in cerebrospinal fluid volume and pressure. Therefore, the use of a small gauge needle for making the puncture, a recumbent position while the puncture hole is sealing, and encouraging the patient to force fluids (to hasten fluid replacement) are all measures which may be helpful in the prevention of this condition.

The first time that the mother is out of bed she should "dangle" for a short time before actually getting up. Then usually she can walk a few steps from the bed and sit in a chair for a brief period. On succeeding times up, she can increase her activity gradually. The newly delivered mother needs someone to assist her in and out of bed and to go with her when she walks to the bathroom. The nurse should remain close at hand while the mother is in the bathroom so that she can give immediate assistance if the mother becomes weak or faint.

It is important that the nurse explain the purposes of early ambulation to the mother and help her to learn how she can achieve an effective combination of sitting, walking and lying in bed. All too many mothers feel that once they are out of bed they are "on their own" and expected to take care of themselves entirely. Most of them are afraid of being a nuisance and hesitate to ask for help, whereas others do not realize that help is available. The nurse's attitude is important, for if she acts friendly and interested in the mother, demonstrates a desire to help her and makes her feel comfortable, the mother is more likely to ask for help. New mothers, in particular, are sensitive to the attitudes of those responsible for their care. Many of them are experiencing an enforced dependency for the first time in their adult lives and find this difficult. Others become resentful because they feel that they are being forced toward independence too quickly. It is only as the nurse recognizes each patient as an individual that she is able to gain insight in providing for the mother's total nursing needs.

Although it is customary for mothers to be discharged home on the 5th to the 7th day, and in some instances as early as the 3rd or the 4th, it should be remembered that early ambulation and the duration of hospital stay are two entirely different matters. Regardless of the day of discharge, mothers should be cautioned to proceed slowly at home during the puerperium, resting a large part of the time. If teaching about "getting back to routine gradually" was begun early in the antepartal period, the mother will be better prepared.

Bathing

As previously mentioned, the mother is prone to have marked diaphoresis in the early puerperium, so that she will find the daily bath or shower refreshing and a source of comfort. The first complete bed bath after delivery should be given by the nurse, even if the mother has already been allowed out of bed for a brief period. This not only conserves a considerable amount of the mother's energy but permits the nurse on the postpartal division, who may be caring for the mother for the first time, to have an opportunity to make certain observations. If the mother is not fatigued, this may be an opportune time also to include some appropriate health teaching. The nurse will be guided in her teaching by the "readiness" of the mother to learn and should remember that she can absorb only so much information at one time. In addition to answering specific questions asked by the mother, the nurse might include information about breast care, perineal hygiene, elimination, general activity and hospital routines.

After the first bath the mother usually is able to shower or, if she is on bed rest, to bathe herself at least partially. Nevertheless, help should be given as necessary. Showers usually are permitted as soon as the patient becomes ambulatory, if such facilities are available. The first time or two that the mother takes a shower, the nurse or the attendant should remain nearby for safety. It is particularly important that a patient who has had a cesarean section be instructed regarding her bathing. Usually, these patients are not allowed to shower even though they are ambulatory, since the incision should be kept dry until it has closed, and/or the sutures have been removed.

Tub baths usually are allowed in 2 weeks, and some physicians permit tub bathing earlier (see Suggested Reading).

Urinary Elimination

The newly delivered mother does not usually express a desire to void, in part because the bladder capacity is increased as a result of reduced interabdominal pressure. In addition, if the mother has received analgesia or anesthesia during labor, the sensation of a full bladder may be further diminished. The mother should be encouraged to void within the first 6 to 8 hours following the delivery. It is not prudent, however, to adhere to a designated lapse of time to indicate when the mother should empty her bladder, but rather on evidence indicating the degree of bladder distention. It should be kept in mind that there is an increased urinary output during the early puerperium. Moreover, mothers who have received intravenous fluids, or who are having them, are very likely to develop a full bladder. As the bladder fills with urine, it gradually protrudes above the symphysis pubis and can be observed bulging in front of the uterus. If the bladder is markedly distended, the uterus may be pushed upward and to the side and may be somewhat relaxed. When a hand is cupped over the fundus to massage it and to bring the uterus back to its midline position, the bladder will protrude still further. When the hand is removed, the uterus will return to its displaced position. Further evidence of bladder distention can be gained by palpation and percussion of the lower abdomen, which will reveal a difference in consistency between the uterus and the bladder. The latter will be ballotable and filled with liquid in contrast with the uterus, which will have a firm tone. Such observations are of extreme importance and demand immediate attention, first, because a full bladder is considered to be one of the causes of postpartal hemorrhage, and, second, because if the bladder is permitted to become distended, urinary retention will follow inevitably.

Some mothers have difficulty in voiding at first. As a result of the labor itself, the tone of the bladder wall may be temporarily impaired, or the tissues at the base of the bladder and around the urethra may be edematous. Often the patient's inability to void is due to the fact that she is not accustomed to using the bedpan and would have this same difficulty using one any time. If the mother is allowed early bathroom privileges, urinary elimination may present no problem. On the other hand, some efforts may be needed to excite normal urination. First of all, a positive approach, asking the mother, "Will you try . . ."

rather than "Do you feel as if you want to . . ." is often helpful to get the mother to void. Also, making her feel at ease by helping her to assume a comfortable position, providing privacy and giving her assurance will help to avoid building up tensions which might further inhibit normal urination.

The nurse should offer the mother a bedpan at intervals of 2 to 3 hours at first and measure the urine at each voiding during the first day or days or until it has been established that the mother is emptying her bladder completely. A voiding must measure 100 cc. to be considered satisfactory. At the first attempt the mother may void a small amount of urine and obviously not empty her bladder. If the bladder is not distended, she may be allowed to wait an hour or so before trying again to empty it, because then she may do so. But if she continues to void in small amounts at frequent intervals, one may suspect that she has a residual urine, and thus these voidings are merely the overflow of a distended bladder. Every effort should be made to encourage the mother to void in sufficient amount so that catheterization will not have to be resorted to, but any time she is unable to do so, and there is evidence of bladder distention, she should be catheterized immediately.

Catheterization. Although the procedure for catheterization varies to some degree in different hospitals, the principles involved are essentially the same. Aseptic technique must be maintained throughout to avoid introducing bacteria into the bladder or contaminating the birth canal. If the mother is given routine perineal care prior to beginning the catheterization procedure, the potential danger of infection is further reduced.

Because there is a certain amount of soreness of the external genitalia, the nurse should proceed with extreme gentleness and convey to the mother the impression that she is aware of the additional tenderness. As the labia are separated to expose the vestibule, care should be exercised to prevent pulling on the perineal sutures. The nurse will find that the meatus may be difficult to locate due to the edema and consequent distortion of the tissues; therefore a good light is imperative.

The urinary meatus and surrounding area are cleansed prior to the insertion of the catheter; the nurse should proceed gently, but remember all the while that a certain degree of friction is necessary for proper cleansing of the area. None of the cleansing solution should be permitted to run into the vaginal orifice because of the danger of contaminating the birth canal. Immediately following the cleansing, a dry cotton ball should be placed at the introitus to prevent excretions from the vagina (i.e., blood or lochia) from spreading upward to the urinary meatus, from whence it can be carried into the bladder when the catheter is inserted.

Intestinal Elimination

Because the bowel tends to remain relaxed in the early puerperium (as in pregnancy), intestinal elimination may be somewhat of a problem. In view of the sluggishness of the bowels during this time, constipation can be anticipated unless certain measures are instituted to prevent it. Although obstetricians' orders vary, it is common to give a stool softener each night after delivery and/or a laxative or mild cathartic on the evening of the 2nd day following delivery. If a bowel evacuation has not occurred by the morning of the 3rd day, a cleansing enema or a suppository may be prescribed. The latter is very effective and less traumatic for most patients.

If there has been no elimination for several days, and especially if the mother has had more extensive perineal repair done, an oil retention enema, followed some hours later by a cleansing enema, sometimes is ordered.

The mother who is breast-feeding should be advised to follow her physician's prescription if laxatives are required to encourage proper elimination after she is discharged from the hospital. Certain laxatives are excreted in breast milk and therefore, affect the infant. In addition, the usual measures employed to encourage good bowel habits (i.e., adequate fluid intake, roughage foods in the diet, establishing a habit time, etc.) should be included in the health teaching.

SPECIAL PHYSICAL CARE ASPECTS

Throughout the care of the maternity patient, emphasis has been directed to the prevention of infection by application of principles of antiseptic and aseptic techniques. In view of this, the special procedures employed in the care of the mother during the puerperium should be planned so that individual care techniques can be maintained whenever possible. Disposable equipment for such purposes is safe, it utilizes simplified procedures, and it is economical.

Each mother should have her own supplies and equipment kept in a designated place, for her convenience. This is facilitated in hospitals where the physical plan of the postpartal unit provides a bathroom adjoining each room, in which separate shelves are provided for each mother's equipment and supplies. Such practices are important in the over-all effort to prevent cross contamination.

Breast Care

The care of the breasts during pregnancy has been discussed in Chapter 8, Antepartal Care. Although some aspects differ after the delivery, depending on whether or not the mother is breast-feeding, the principles of good breast hygiene continue to be of primary importance.

The routine care is directed to maintain cleanliness and adequate breast support necessary for the normal function of the breasts and the comfort of the mother. Precautions should always be exercised to handle the breasts gently, and above all to avoid rough rubbing, massage or pressure on these organs.

The mother who is bottle-feeding her infant should bathe her breasts daily with mild soap and water; this is done most conveniently at the time of the daily shower or bath. No other special care need be given. Research[3] has indicated that the mother who is breast-feeding should avoid the use of soap on her nipples, since this substance removes the protective skin oils and leaves the nipple more prone to damage. It is recommended that she wash her breasts daily with plain water at the bath or shower time. No further cleansing before each nursing need be done (see Chap. 16). However, the hands should be washed in soap and water if they are to come in contact with the breast. The nurse often has an excellent opportunity for health teaching about postpartal care of the breasts while she is giving the mother her first bath after the delivery.

Some kind of breast support should be worn 24 hours a day after delivery. Various types of binders or brassières may be used as long as they support the entire breast in the natural position. When a breast is well supported, it is not only more comfortable, but also, if it is pendulous, proper support aids in preventing congestion caused by interference with circulation. Following the delivery, the breasts are soft, but by the 3rd or the 4th postpartal day, as milk replaces colostrum in the breasts, they become heavier, firmer and more tender. The mother may experience throbbing pains in her breasts, which extend back into the axillae. During this time, analgesic medication may be required for pain relief until the congestion subsides in 1 or 2 days. Even the mother who is breast-feeding experiences temporary discomfort when the breasts become full.

The mother who is breast-feeding should wear a nursing brassière not only for support of the breasts but also to ensure further cleanliness. Since the milk secretion is likely to leak from the nipples, they should be directly covered with breast squares, such as sterile 4 x 4 gauze dressings. During the mother's hospital stay she may wear a binder which is convenient for breast-feeding (such as the bikini), unless her breasts are pendulous. Heavy breasts require the additional support afforded by the more conventional type brassière. Many mothers prefer to wear a nursing brassière even before the milk comes in. But

[3] Newton, M., and Newton, N.: The normal course and management of lactation. Clin. Obstet. Gynec. 5:44-63, March, 1962.

Fig. 15-6. Breast binder made from straight binder, 10 inches wide. Shoulder straps are attached. (MacDonald House, The University Hospitals of Cleveland, Cleveland, Ohio)

regardless of which one is used, it should provide uplift support and be well fitted so that it is not too tight and avoids undue pressure on the nipples.

Lactation

The process of lactation is thought to be initiated by the sudden change in the proportion of estrogen and progesterone in the mother's blood level following delivery of the placenta. Thus, placental expulsion is said to stimulate the release of *prolactin,* the lactogenic hormone, from the anterior pituitary. After the infant is put to breast, the stimulation of the nipples by the infant's sucking aids the further release of prolactin. Prolactin, in turn, stimulates milk secretion in the alveoli. The regular, periodic emptying of the milk from the alveoli by the infant's sucking stimulates the continuation of the process of lactation. When the infant is not put to breast, or the sucking stimulus is suddenly interrupted, suppression of lactation is initiated and the breasts become engorged with milk, and very painful.

Suppression of Lactation. The breasts fill with milk initially, unless lactation is suppressed, whether or not the mother nurses her infant. Tenseness and engorgement result as milk fills the breasts (see Chap. 16). Since the accumulation of milk in the breast inhibits further secretion, engorgement generally subsides in a day or two. However, until the breasts soften the mother may experience considerable discomfort.

In the event that the mother is not going to breast-feed, the physician will prescribe orders accordingly. Many physicians use estrogenic hormones to suppress the production of the lactogenic hormone. Diethylstilbestrol, an estrogenic hormone, is one of the drugs in use today for this purpose. It usually is given orally in relatively large doses during the early postpartal period and is decreased gradually.

Lactation is not always effectively suppressed by the administration of hormones such as diethylstilbestrol and premarin, and there may be a mild transient filling or engorgement either a few days after delivery or later, in 1 or 2 weeks. This soon disappears spontaneously. It is important for the nurse to remember that side effects sometimes accompany the administration of hormones. For instance, the androgens have the potential for retarding the onset of menstruation. Uterine bleeding may follow a prolonged course of estrogen therapy. The nurse will observe that after a course of stilbestrol the lochial discharge is heavier and contains a greater proportion of bright red blood.

A combination of hormones such as estrogens and androgens has been widely used to suppress lactation (it suppresses the release of prolactin), prevent engorgement, and reduce the tenderness of the breasts. In addition, these hormones in combination counteract the undesirable side effects of each other. Deladumone-OB is an example of a long-acting estrogen-androgen combination and is given intramuscularly; one injection is all that is necessary. To achieve maximum effectiveness, the antilactogenic hormones must be given immediately after (or just prior to) delivery, since the anterior pituitary begins production of the lactogenic hormone immediately.

If hormones are not used, the breasts usually become engorged 2 to 3 days after delivery, and the tenseness and discomfort last from 24 to 48 hours. Since the breasts are not emptied, the accumulated milk suppresses further secretion of milk. As secretion subsides, engorgement wanes, and the breasts become more comfortable.

During the period of engorgement, discomfort may be considerable, and the mother should receive as much symptomatic relief as possible. A well-fitting uplift brassière or a correctly applied breast binder relieve discomfort from the weight of the breasts and wearing it before the milk "comes in" is helpful. The breast binder should fit snugly but not to the extent that in itself it causes discomfort. The mother can assist by supporting her breasts in the normal position while the binder is being applied. To encourage uplift support, the binder should be pinned from the bottom up. A good principle to remember in providing support for the breasts is that a variety of methods may be adequate as long as they lift the breasts, suspend the weight from the shoulders and do not exert pressure on any area.

One author reported from her study of a group of 38 subjects that a supporting brassière or breast binder was found to be more effective than a compression binder in reducing breast tenderness in the non-nursing mother.[4] No significant differences were found between the two groups in the other symptom categories. Furthermore, the findings suggested that the supportive brassière or binder was just as effective as the compression binder in preventing engorgement and suppressing lactation. The application of ice caps to the breasts also may contribute to the mother's comfort when the

---

[4] Bristol, W. M.: Comparative effectiveness of compressional and supporting breast binders in suppressing lactation. Nurs. Res. 15:203-206, Summer, 1966.

breasts are full and tender. Analgesics such as aspirin or a similar compound are helpful in relieving discomfort. The nurse must remember that the milk should not be pumped or expressed from the breasts, since this only stimulates the secretion of more milk. In the past it was thought that the application of very tight binders, restriction of fluids and the administration of diuretics all suppressed lactation; these practices are no longer in general use and have been found to be of little value (see Suggested Reading).

Care of the Perineum

Perineal care is a procedure employed to cleanse the vulva, the perineum and the anal region as a means of preventing infection, promoting healing of the perineum and making the mother comfortable. In addition, it provides an opportunity for the nurse to inspect the area and the lochial discharge. Regardless of whether or not an episiotomy has been performed, perineal care should be done as a routine part of morning care, each time that the mother voids, and after each bowel evacuation. The nurse usually attends to this aspect of care until the mother becomes ambulatory; then, after proper instruction, the mother herself may assume this care. However, it should be emphasized that even though the nurse may not be performing the actual procedure, she should make a point of inspecting the mother's perineum daily, preferably in the morning, to ascertain whether the stitches are healing properly and to check the character and the amount of lochia. If the mother is allowed to shower, these observations should be made first so that the nurse can observe the lochial discharge more accurately.

There has been much discussion concerning the "best way" for the nurse to give perineal care in the time immediately following delivery. The technique for individual care has simplified the procedure to a large measure, but procedures will vary according to hospital routines. Most hospitals maintain that this is a "clean" procedure rather than a sterile one, and that the safety of the mother is ensured if antiseptic precautions are adhered to conscientiously.

Disposable washcloths, cotton balls or gauze sponges may be used for cleansing. When the pubic hair begins to appear, cotton balls tend to catch on the stubble, and particles of cotton remain unless they are picked off. Another variation found is in relation to the cleansing agent, which might be a mild soap or detergent solution.

In preparation for the procedure, the nurse should wash her hands thoroughly. After preparing the mother, remove the perineal pad, noting the amount, the odor and the appearance of the lochia and discard the pad in a paper bag. Whether removing the perineal pad or in using the sponges or washclothes in the actual cleansing process, always proceed from the front toward the back to avoid contamination of the vestibule from the anal region.

The labia is cleansed first, working from the pubis to the perineum, taking care not to separate the labia with the fingers. The cleansing is done by using a single downward stroke with each sponge, which then is discarded in the paper bag. This cleansing is repeated with as many sponges as necessary. The area then is dried in the same manner.

The cleansing of the anal region can be accomplished most effectively if the mother is turned on her side and the buttocks separated before wiping from the perineum to the anus. If the mother's thighs or buttocks are soiled with profuse lochia, these areas should be bathed with soap and water, for these parts do not have to be cleansed in the same manner as the vulva.

When disposable washcloths are used, the first cloth is soaped and the labia washed down on one side to the perineum and then on the other side. Then the anus is washed last, and the soaped washcloth is discarded. The area is rinsed in the same manner with a second washcloth and dried with a third one. The perineum should be kept clean and dry to promote healing.

The nurse must be mindful of the potential danger of infection if pathogenic organisms ascend the birth canal to the uterus. Care should always be exercised to see that none of the cleansing solution seeps into the vagina because of the possibility of contamination. If the washcloths or moist sponges are used, they should not be dripping wet.

The clean perineal pad should be grasped on the outside so that the nurse's fingers do not touch the side which will come in contact with the mother's perineum. Then the pad is applied to the vulva (front to back) and secured to the sanitary belt in front before turning the mother to her side to secure the back tab.

Perineal Self-Care. The first time the mother is allowed up to the bathroom, the nurse should take her and show her where her equipment is kept and how to do perineal self-care. The principles of personal hygiene which were stressed

FIG. 15-7. Perineal heat lamp. (Dann Manufacturing Company, Cleveland, Ohio)

when the nurse gave the mother perineal care in bed should be reviewed again. Instruct the mother to wash her hands carefully before and after carrying out the procedure. Show her how to assemble the necessary equipment, the paper bag, box of small cleansing tissues and wrapped perineal pad, all of which can be placed on a small stool or table adjacent to the toilet. A box of small cleansing tissues is preferable to a roll of tissue for obvious reasons. Have the mother unfasten the perineal pad she is wearing, and instruct her to grasp it by the tabs and remove it from front to back. This perineal pad is placed in the paper bag, which will be disposed of in a step-on can or other covered waste receptacle. After the mother voids, instruct her to cleanse herself from front to back with tissues, using fresh tissues for each stroke and discarding them in the toilet. The mother should again be instructed how to handle the clean perineal pad so that the inner surface is not contaminated by her fingers and to put it on from front to back. It should be fastened immediately to prevent the pad from moving forward. The toilet should be flushed after the mother assumes a standing position to avoid having any of the flushing water spray the perineum.

Perineal Discomfort. Following a spontaneous vaginal delivery without laceration, mothers usually do not experience perineal discomfort. It is most likely to be present if an episiotomy has been performed, or if lacerations have been repaired, particularly if the perineum is edematous, and there is tension on the perineal sutures. Almost all primigravidas experience some degree of discomfort from an episiotomy, depending largely on the extent of the wound and the amount of suturing done. For the most part during the first few days, local treatment in the form of dry heat, analgesic sprays or ointments is all that is necessary to alleviate the discomfort. But if the pain is more severe in the first day or so, such treatment may not be sufficient, and analgesic medications may have to be administered by mouth or hypodermic injection. Later on, sitz baths may be ordered if the discomfort persists.

Exposure of the perineum to heat from the perineal lamp not only provides a considerable measure of comfort to the mother but also supplies a safe amount of heat to promote local healing of the perineal wound. The physician may prescribe such treatment for 20- to 25-minute periods, 2 or 3 times a day. If a lamp such as the one shown in Figure 15-7 is used, the mother can recline in bed with the lamp between her knees during the treatment, without spreading the thighs too far apart. This lamp is so constructed that the frame can be completely covered with a pillowcase. The excess cover is brought forward over the arch of the frame and tucked securely between it and the shield which is around the bulb. The heat is provided by an ordinary 25-watt light bulb. When the mother has assumed the dorsal recumbent position, the lamp can be easily slipped between her legs and placed about 10 to 12 inches from the perineum. After the perineum is exposed, the bulb should be adjusted so that the light shines directly on it. The mother can be completely covered during the treatment, because the arch of the lamp frame acts as a cradle to support the top bedclothes.

Mothers who have discomfort from perineal sutures usually will find it uncomfortable to sit for the first few days. Many of them will be observed sitting in a rigid position, bearing their weight on one side of the buttocks or the other, with obvious discomfort to the back as well as the perineum. Therefore, it is important to teach the mother how to sit comfortably with her body erect. In the sitting position, the perineum is suspended at the lowermost level of the ischial tuberosities, which bear the weight of the body. Thus, in order to achieve a greater measure of comfort, the mother must bring her buttocks together to relieve pressure and tension on the perineum, in the same manner as that described in the exercise for contraction and relaxation of pelvic floor muscles (see p. 199). After assuming a sitting position the mother should be instructed to raise her hips very slightly from the chair, only enough to permit her to squeeze her buttocks together and contract the muscles of the pelvic floor, and hold them this way momentarily until after she has let her full weight down again. This exercise will also prove to be helpful to the mother when she is reclining in bed.

Abdominal Support

At the present time there is general agreement that an abdominal binder is unnecessary. It was formerly routine practice to apply one to the newly delivered mother because it was thought that it aided involution and helped to restore the mother's figure. Actually, a binder is of no value for such purposes, and because it inhibits the movements of the abdominal wall, it may actually retard the soft, flabby structures in regaining tone. However, the physician may advise the use of a binder if the mother's abdomen is unusually flabby or pendulous, particularly if the mother believes that she would feel more comfortable with some support. If the mother is ambulatory, the straight abdominal binder may be preferable to the scultetus binder because it is more likely to stay in place when the mother moves about. It must be remembered that the binder is applied from the waist down to avoid pushing the uterus upward.

THE MOTHER WHO IS NURSING

Making the Decision

The type of infant feeding is an important decision for the parents to make. Their ultimate choice will be influenced by a variety of factors, physical and psychological as well as social. Ideally, the subject of the method of infant feeding will be raised during the antepartal period, and the parents will have time and guidance from the doctor and the nurse in making a decision that is most suitable for them.

It is no longer essential that the mother breast-feed her infant to ensure his survival or well-being. The development of modern methods of artificial feeding adequately meet the infant's needs for nutrition and growth (see p. 377). However, breast-feeding has several advantages (see p. 378). Particularly important is the fact that if the mother wants to nurse her infant, this method of feeding can enhance a close relationship between her and her baby.

A variety of factors will influence the couple's decision to breast-feed the infant. The term *couple* is used here deliberately, since the husband's attitudes, feelings and behavior may be as important in terms of decision-making as the mother's. Moreover, they usually have a profound influence on the outcome of the nursing experience. It is wise for the physician and the nurse to explore adequately with the mother (and the father, if necessary) their mutual attitudes, since they are so relevant.

The nurse will note that there seems to be a wide range of commitment to breast-feeding. For instance, some mothers are very eager to nurse their infants; others want to breast-feed but do not feel bad (or "inadequate") if for some reason they cannot. Others try to nurse in spite of the fact that they would prefer to give the baby a bottle; still others flatly refuse to attempt to nurse. Some mothers feel that breast-feeding is too tiring, confining or simply repulsive; many are afraid that it will disfigure their breasts. The mores and pressure of the mother's class and peer group also are important. Bottle-feeding may be the acceptable practice in the community or neighborhood; relatives, friends, etc., may be either very much for or against breast-feeding. Return to employment for the mother may be a very significant factor.

Certain conditions in both the mother and the infant also can have a bearing on the decision and outcome. The mother's physical condition is particularly important. Diseases and infection (i.e., syphilis, tuberculosis, heart and kidney disease, staphylococcal infections, communicable diseases) generally are contraindications for breast-feeding. Similarly, certain infections and anomalies in the infant may make nursing impossible, or at least temporarily impossible (see Chap. 23). Breast infection or painful, cracked or fissured nipples also may require temporary discontinuance of nursing. Pregnancy usually is considered to be an indication for weaning because of the physiologic strain that it places on the mother.

The attitudes of the doctor and nurse influence the couple a good deal; so do the amount and the kind of help that the mother gets in the hospital when she is first attempting to nurse. The willingness on the part of the staff to impart information and to give assistance helps the parents immensely, especially if they have little information about the process or are actually misinformed about it. However, it is unwise to try to persuade a mother to nurse if she has very negative feelings about breast-feeding. This situation often leads to emotional conflicts in the mother and may impede the adjustment between mother and infant.

Mechanisms in Lactation

The anatomy of the breasts and the physiology of lactation have been discussed in Chapters 2 and 14, to which the student is referred for a renewal of background understanding of the subject.

Secretion of Milk. Two major mechanisms are involved in lactation. The first of these is the secretion of milk. It is believed, as was previously stated, that the hormone luteotrophin (prolactin, LTH, the lactogenic or mammogenic hormone) is responsible for the initiation of lactation. It is thought that the release of this hormone is enhanced by the sucking of the infant. The milk itself is secreted by the alveoli or acini cells. This secretion commences 3 to 4 days postpartum and continues for as long as the breasts are sufficiently emptied. Frequency of emptying the breasts also is a very important factor, especially when lactation is becoming established. Thus, both the production of milk and the quantity produced are dependent on *frequent* and *complete* emptying of the breasts. The nurse will recall that if the breasts are not entirely emptied, and the back pressure in the alveoli is not relieved, milk secretion decreases and eventually stops (see p. 312).

When lactation is becoming established, milk secretion can be stimulated by having the infant nurse both breasts at each feeding and by increasing the frequency of the feedings. Care should be taken not to tire the mother unduly. Milk production is slow in some mothers, but it can be stimulated by allowing the infant to nurse both breasts every 3 to 4 hours.

Milk-Ejection Reflex. This is the second mechanism involved in lactation. This reflex has been called also expulsion mechanism, the let-down reflex and the draught reflex. It is postulated that the mechanism works in the following way: Impulses from the baby's sucking cause release of oxytocin from the posterior portion of the pituitary. This hormone causes the contractile tissue (myoepithelial cells) around the alveoli to squeeze the milk into the larger ducts and eventually to propel it to the ducts leading to the nipples. Then the milk is removed by the compression and suction action of the baby's nursing. It is important to remember that the let-down reflex can be influenced profoundly by psychic factors and the emotions of the mother. For instance, some mothers find that the let-down reflex is elicited (i.e., their breasts begin to drip milk) by an infant's cry or some other sound, sight, etc., that has become associated with nursing. Often they will say that they can feel their milk "come down" in anticipation of nursing. Fear, worry, pain and tension, all may affect the expulsion mechanism adversely. Thus, it is particularly important for the nurse to help the mother to avoid these emotional disturbances whenever possible. A relaxed atmosphere for nursing, adequate assistance, effective pain relief, and a supportive attitude on the part of the nurse are essential components of effective nursing care for the mother who is breast-feeding. Sometimes oxytocin is given the mother during early lactation to facilitate the milk flow. It may be administered by injection or by a nasal spray (40 U.S.P. units per ml. of solution). This hormone assists the ejection of milk when the let-down reflex is inhibited (as in times of stress) and also is effective in facilitating the milk flow when the breasts are engorged.

Engorgement

Breast discomfort several days after delivery has been attributed to venous and lymphatic engorgement, which mothers experience in relation to initiation of lactation. More recently it has been proposed that postpartal breast discomfort is attributed to two factors: (1) venous and lymphatic engorgement and (2) filling of the acini with milk. Most studies indicate that breast discomfort occurring during the first 3 or 4 postpartal days, the "initial breast engorgement," is due to venous engorgement. The breast discomfort appearing after the 3rd or 4th postpartal day is due to filling of the acini with milk, the so-called "late engorgement." Thus, any treatment during the first few days is directed toward symptomatic relief of engorgement.[5]

The peak incidence of discomfort seems to occur on the 4th or the 5th day postpartum. It is believed that the engorgement is caused by the pressure from the increased amount of milk in the lobes and ducts.

Symptoms. When the milk "comes in," the breasts suddenly become larger, firmer and more tender; consequently, many mothers experience varying degrees of discomfort. Some do not seem to be bothered by this transitory condition (and produce a large quantity of milk), but the majority usually have at least a moderate amount of tenderness and pain. A few experience a great deal of discomfort, with throbbing pains in the breast, extending to the axilla.

The engorgement may distend the breasts so much that the skin appears to be shiny. The tissue surrounding the nipple may also become taut to the extent that it actually retracts the nipple, making it extremely difficult for the baby to grasp the nipple and the areola adequately. It used to be thought that fever was a normal consequence of this condition; however, engorgement is *not* an inflammatory process, and if fever occurs, some other cause should be suspected. Still the breasts may be reddened and feel warm to the touch. They can be very painful, and they become more so when touched or moved.

Although this condition is transitory and usually disappears in 24 to 48 hours, prompt treatment should be instituted, not only for the mother's comfort but also to prevent the condition from progressing. If engorgement is allowed to become marked, then emptying of the breasts (which is the basis of treatment) becomes very difficult because of the occlusion of the ducts by the surrounding congested tissues and the thick and tenacious character of the retained secretions. Secondary lymphatic and venous stasis may occur because the milk cannot be emptied.

Until this time it has been somewhat difficult to find an objective means for evaluating venous engorgement of the breast. Menczer and Eskin have made a study evaluating venous engorgement of the breast by means of thermography. It is known that the amount of infrared emission from the skin is proportional to its temperature. In this study the infrared emission from the skin of the breast is recorded on a polaroid photographic film. The image is recorded in different shades of gray and black, thus the lighter area of the film corresponds to the skin areas of the breast with increased infrared emission (hot areas).[6]

Treatment usually consists of removal of the milk, support of the breast, hot packs and/or ice bags and analgesics for the relief of pain. Removal of the milk may be facilitated by the use of oxytocin before the baby nurses to encourage the let-down reflex. Interestingly enough, this drug sometimes is used to relieve discomfort from

[5] Menczer, J., and Eskin, B.: Evaluation of postpartum breast engorgement by thermography. Obstet. Gynec. 33: 260-263, February, 1969.

[6] Ibid., p. 262.

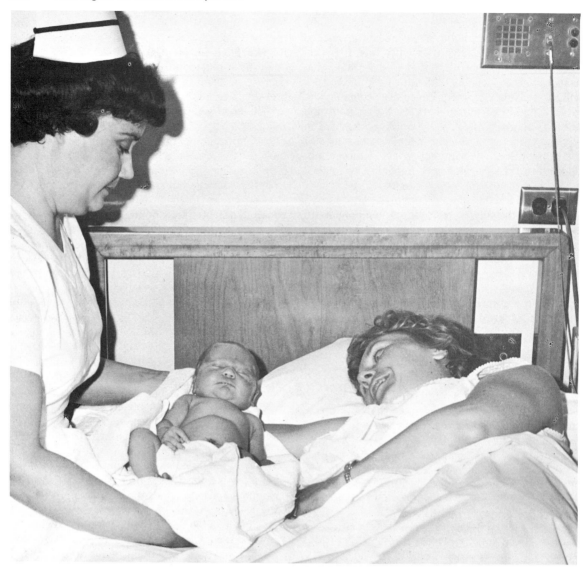

Fig. 15-8. Baby handed to mother for feeding. Mother enjoys a brief look at her baby, a part of the identification processes in maternal claiming. (MacDonald House, The University Hospitals of Cleveland, Cleveland, Ohio)

engorgement in mothers who are *not* nursing. The way in which the drug relieves pain in breasts that are not being emptied is unclear. In addition, manual expression of the milk and pumping (see p. 325), as well as the use of a nipple shield (to help the baby to grasp the nipple), may be recommended. Some mothers find the use of hot packs 15 to 20 minutes before nursing beneficial in improving the flow of milk. Often ice packs between nursing periods are very useful in alleviating discomfort. A good uplift support for the breasts cannot be stressed enough (see p. 156), particularly during the period of engorgement, and a

well-fitting brassière should be worn night and day. Analgesics such as aspirin, Darvon or codeine frequently are used for pain relief. These should be given in adequate dosage and with appropriate timing so that the mother can be relatively comfortable during nursing. Since engorgement is transitory, the drugs are needed for a very short time; hence any danger to the infant is minimal.

Initiation of Breast-Feeding

Depending on the condition of both the mother and the infant, breast-feeding usually is started from 8 to 24 hours after delivery. Since the assessment of relevant data is a part of every nursing care plan, such observations as the readiness of both mother and baby for breast feeding is of primary importance. The mother should be encouraged to participate in decision-making which determines breast feeding practices, insofar as they concern her baby and herself.

Some physicians prefer to give the baby one or two bottle feedings of water before he begins to breast-feed. It is felt that this helps the infant to regurgitate any mucus or secretions that have been swallowed during delivery. If mucus is a problem with the baby, postponement of nursing is thought by some to be beneficial until the baby can rid himself of it. Usually, the baby is clear of mucus in 24 hours.

Rather than delaying the initiation of breast-feeding for all babies, it is better to maintain close supervision and guidance of mothers and babies during the early feeding periods.

Many infants indicate their readiness to suck from birth. However, others do not seem to be so eager; these infants need a short period of rest before they demonstrate their readiness. Similarly, the mother may be rested enough a few hours after the baby's birth to commence breast-feeding, or she may need several hours or a day in which to restore herself after delivery. Usually in 24 hours or so both mother and baby are ready for the nursing experience.

Colostrum will be the chief source of the infant's nourishment until the milk comes in. Putting the infant to breast early is advantageous for both mother and baby, since the sucking stimulates the milk production and helps the uterus to contract; moreover, nursing satisfies the infant's need for sucking. It is important for the nurse to remember that *both* mother and baby must learn how to work as a team in the nursing process. Hence, practice is essential. Even though the mother has breast-fed before, there is a wide range in nursing behavior[7] among infants, and the experience of breast-feeding each infant can be somewhat "new." The mother will need to learn how to handle the infant appropriately, how to interpret his cues of hunger and satiety, and how to help him to grasp the nipple and to withdraw the milk successfully. The infant, in turn, must learn to associate the nipple with food and to coordinate his grasping of the nipple with his sucking and swallowing in such a way as to get his food successfully. No wonder that mother and baby often take a few days to become adept at this process!

An interested and experienced nurse should be immediately available to mothers in their first experiences with their new babies. Maternity nurses in the hospital can play a major role in facilitating the mothers' efforts to breast-feed their babies. "Many of the problems associated with unsuccessful breast feeding experiences can be prevented or solved through purposeful nursing action. Nurses need to accept the responsibility to help mothers gain knowledge and skill needed to successfully breast-feed their babies."[8]

Preparation of the mother *before* the actual breast feeding experience plays a large part in giving effective care. This should include instructions about "hand-washing," sterile technique procedures and other rituals associated with the feeding of the infant in the hospital. When the infant is brought to his mother for feeding, the delay from such tasks can be frustrating and stress-producing for both mother and baby.

Whenever it is indicated, the mother should be informed about the feeding reflexes of her infant (see p. 377). During the actual nursing period the nurse can reinforce this information (as necessary) and *show* the mother how to elicit these responses. It is essential that the mother be able to evoke these reflexes herself, since she ultimately must assume total responsibility. Too often the nurse takes over these aspects, and the mother does not get sufficient practice to acquire any skill during these first days in the hospital. It is not easy to "stand-by" and watch the inexperienced mother trying to breast-feed her baby without offering too much interference. But it is necessary to be careful not to disrupt the learning process.

Position. Assisting the mother to experiment with various positions which are comfortable during breast feeding is another important facet of care. The mother is sometimes asked whether she wants to nurse the baby sitting up or lying down. An inexperienced mother does not know this, although she may think she does, and she should be given an opportunity to try various positions, while help is available, and make her own choice.

A pediatrician (mother of four children, all breast-fed) suggests "while after a few days it may be more comfortable to nurse lying down, it

[7] Barnes, G. R., Jr., *et al.*: Management of breast feeding. J.A.M.A. 151:192-199, January 17, 1953.

[8] Iffrig, Sister M. C.: Nursing care and success in breast feeding. Nurs. Clin. N. Am. 3:353, June, 1968.

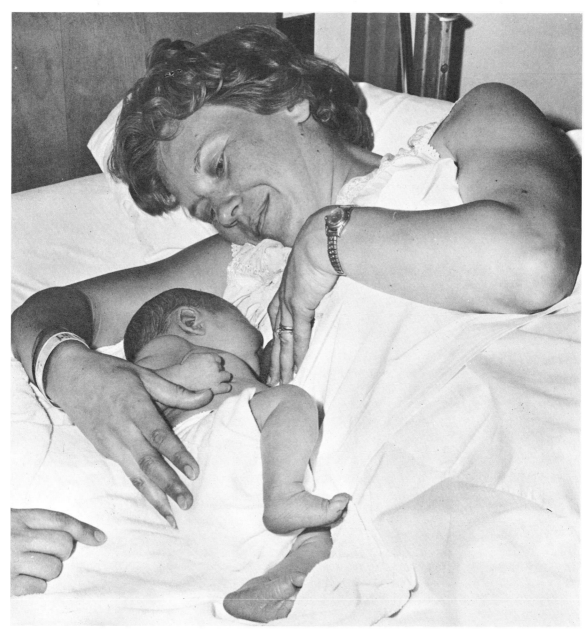

FIG. 15-9. Both the mother and baby should be comfortable during the nursing period. (MacDonald House, The University Hospitals of Cleveland, Cleveland, Ohio)

is just about impossible to get a newborn infant going at the nipple unless you sit up and use both hands for support of the baby."[9]

Another method, described by Sister Mary Charitas, is a technique called alternate massage.

---

[9] Streeter, B. N.: Suggestions to simplify breast feeding. J. Am. Med. Women's Assoc. 16:378, May, 1961.

. . . Alternate massage is a procedure of breast feeding that was developed to prevent common problems of early breast feeding. The nurse can teach it to any nursing mother. Alternate massage consists simply in alternating massage of the breast with the baby's nursing in order to complete each nursing period. It enables the baby to empty the breast, an achievement that insures the milk supply and at the same time prevents painful breasts and nipples. . .

How to Use Alternate Massage

. . . Put the baby to breast and observe how he nurses. Usually after the first minute or so the movements of the baby's mouth become long, slow and rhythmic. In this type of nursing the baby compresses the milk reservoirs with his gums and swallows milk. Such nursing avoids production of sustained negative pressure, which is responsible for injuring the nipple.

After a while you notice that the baby stops nursing, then he goes on as before. As the feeding proceeds, he rests more frequently and the character of the nursing changes from mouth movements that are long, slow and rhythmic to those that are rapid and shallow. Later there are still fewer slow rhythmic mouth movements and more of the sleepy rapid shallow type. It is the shallow kind of nursing that produces sustained negative pressure that hurts the nipple. The baby cannot extract milk from the breast when he nurses in this manner. Indeed he resorts to this kind of nursing only when the milk flows from the breast quite freely.

When the pattern of the baby's nursing changes from long, slow mouth movements to sleeping for the most part or to rapid shallow mouth movements, start alternating breast massage with the baby's nursing. Do not remove the baby from the breast; simply slip your hand to the back and middle portion of the breast near the armpit and gently massage the breast several times. While the breast is being moved the baby usually stops nursing, then responds by nursing with long, slow strokes. He may take only two or three strokes, however, because he can quickly pick up the milk that the massage has caused to move from the alveoli to the milk reservoirs. Then repeat the massage and permit the baby to nurse again. Often you will find the breast softening beneath your fingers. When one area softens, move your fingers to a new position and continue alternating breast massage with the baby's nursing until the entire breast has been softened.

It is important not to use breast massage until the character of the baby's nursing has changed from long, slow mouth movements to sleeping for the most part or to rapid shallow nursing. If massage is used before this time, the milk flows too fast for the baby to manage. . .[10]

If the infant is to nurse satisfactorily, he must be held properly by the mother; although some mothers seem to know how to support a baby at the breast, many are awkward, and definite instructions are helpful. Both the mother and the baby must be comfortable and in such a position that the baby can grasp the nipple *and the areola* without any undue effort. If the baby grasps only the nipple, he will not be able to draw out the

FIG. 15-10. Babies nurse better if the mother is relaxed and both the mother and the baby are comfortable.

milk; moreover, the mother's nipples are likely to be damaged. If the mother is lying down (Fig. 15-9), she should be on her side with her arm raised and her head comfortably supported. The baby should lie on his side, flat on the bed or so supported that he can grasp the breast easily. If the mother prefers to sit up to nurse, she should use a comfortable chair and a stool to support her feet, as necessary. It is often helpful to place a pillow under the arm that is supporting the infant (to reduce the tension on the muscles, Fig. 15-10); or to place a pillow under the baby to raise him to a sufficient height so that he may reach the breast easily. If the stitches of the episiotomy are bothersome, a rubber ring or a pillow under the mother's buttocks may be helpful. The nurse may have to work with the mother a bit to be sure that she is comfortable. Often mothers in their eagerness to get the baby on the breast become very tense and assume quite uncomfortable positions (although they assure the nurse

10 Iffrig: Op cit., pp. 347-349.

that they are "comfortable"). Patience and gentle reminding on the part of the nurse encourages these mothers to relax more readily.

Orientation of Infant. After the baby is placed beside the mother, he should be allowed a little time to accustom himself to the new environment and to hunt for the nipple himself. He should not be forced to nurse immediately, especially if he is hesitant or shows disinclination. If the rooting reflex is well developed (and as he smells the milk), he will turn toward the nipple or any object that brushes his cheek (see p. 350). Thus, if the mother or the nurse touches his cheek gently with the nipple, he will turn toward it, open his mouth and grasp it. Sucking usually follows closely thereafter. If the infant seems to have some difficulty in finding and grasping the nipple, although he seems to be eager, the mother or nurse can gently cup a hand around the baby's head and guide him to the nipple. Care should be taken, however, not to touch his cheek or to force his head, since he will only turn away and resist the pressure on his head. In addition, he may cry, and a crying baby tends not to grasp a nipple successfully even though he may be hungry.

Sucking Behavior of Infant. Babies will exhibit a wide variety of sucking behavior. Some, after finding the nipple, suck vigorously without stopping until they are satisfied. Others may suck vigorously for a time, appear to sleep or to rest

and then resume sucking. Still others mouth the nipple before actually sucking but eventually nurse well. Others seem rather disinterested in the whole thing and dawdle throughout the nursing period. When the milk comes in, however, a change usually is noted, and even these infants begin to nurse more in earnest.

The important point here is that individual differences do exist in infants, apparently from birth; hence care must be taken to allow for these differences. To try to force the infant into a style or speed that is not his will only result in screaming, resistance and refusal; the nursing period should be adapted to the infant and not the infant to the nursing period. Mothers, especially, are appreciative of learning about this; often they think there is "*a* way to nurse" and do not realize the differences in eating behavior that infants have. Giving mothers anticipatory guidance and instruction in this aspect of nursing a baby is a very important component in nursing care.

If the infant is to suck effectively, he must place the nipple well back in his mouth, close his lips tightly around the areola, and squeeze the nipple against his palate with his tongue. He then can compress the lactiferous sinuses behind the areola and draw the milk into his mouth by sucking. He empties the breast through a combination of compression and suction. As he nurses, he moves his jaws up and down to compress and empty the sinuses; his tongue, as it draws the nipple back against the palate, suctions the milk from the nipple. Swallowing occurs when enough milk has been obtained to induce the reflex. This activity is carried on rhythmically, interspaced with periods of rest, until the infant is satisfied.

When the nurse assists the mother, she should be sure that the baby has the nipple on top of his tongue and that enough of the areola is in his mouth to prevent damage to the nipple. If he has a good grasp, his jaws will move up and down regularly, and sucking and swallowing movements can be seen in his cheeks and throat. If his grasp is poor, sucking and swallowing may be infrequent and/or absent, although his jaws may continue to move. If the nurse notes that the breast tissue seems to press against the infant's nose and thus obstructs his breathing, she can instruct the mother to take her forefinger and gently compress the tissue so that it no longer impinges on the infant's nose. Care should be taken not to pull the nipple away from the infant in this maneuver.

Usually, getting the nipple in his mouth and tasting the milk seem to increase the baby's interest

Fig. 15-11. Nursing shield. In the treatment of sore or cracked nipples this soft, natural rubber shield may be used for their protection during the nursing periods. (The Pyramid Rubber Company, Ravenna, Ohio)

and ability to nurse. If the infant does not seem too interested or adept, moistening the nipple by expressing a few drops of colostrum or milk often encourages sucking.

Occasionally, a breast shield (Fig. 15-11) may be used to start the infant nursing if for some reason he cannot grasp the nipple. Continued use of this appliance is unwise, since the breasts cannot be emptied because the lacteal sinuses are not compressed during the nursing. The shield can be useful during the first few minutes of nursing to draw the nipples out if they are flattened by engorgement or inversion. Usually, however, even inverted nipples become prominent if the alveolar area is compressed gently by the fingers before nursing; they generally evert more when the infant sucks. The shield may be used also for a short period if the mother's nipples become sore; some nipple pain is experienced by most women during the first days of nursing, but generally it subsides as milk secretion begins, and the baby becomes satisfied. Mothers often state that the pain disappears when the let-down reflex occurs. The care of sore nipples is discussed below.

Giving Support and Supervision. If the infant has taken the nipple without difficulty and has been sucking well for several minutes, the nurse can feel fairly assured that no further assistance is necessary *at this time.* If she leaves the mother and infant, however, she should place the bell cord within reach and instruct the mother to ring if she feels that she needs further help. Moreover, she should make a point of looking in occasionally to observe the progress of the two. Letting the mother have reasonable periods of managing the nursing process by herself will instill confidence in her, but she never should be left without adequate instruction and reassurance. Often, the presence of the nurse is all that is necessary to give the mother the necessary encouragement.

Both the mother and the nurse must realize that many infants do not nurse too well during the first week of life. Unfortunately, the shortened hospital stay only diminishes the time that professional assistance can be given. Therefore, a referral to a public health agency may be indicated, and this possibility should be explored with the mother before she leaves the hospital. If the infant does not seem to respond satisfactorily to the nursing situation during the time that he is in the hospital, he should not be forced. As previously stated, a crying, upset baby will not take a nipple well; rather, he should be cuddled and

soothed until he becomes quiet. If the baby still refuses or cannot nurse after about 10 or 15 minutes of effort on the part of the nurse and mother, it is better to stop and to try again when the baby seems to be more ready. If the infant does not appear to be hungry, it is permissible to omit a feeding. If he is evidencing hunger, some physicians advise giving a bottle but still offering the breast at the next feeding. Often, after a few days and with bottle feedings, an infant who has been disinterested and resistant to the breast suddenly takes hold and begins to nurse with vigor. Since the mother can become very discouraged, when her baby is nursing poorly, it is important that the nurse support the mother in her attempts to continue nursing. Patience, reassurance and adequate guidance are key factors in helping the mother over this initial adjustment.

Care of the Nipples

Too much emphasis cannot be placed on the care of the nipples to facilitate breast-feeding. Cleanliness is a cardinal principle. Thus, keeping the nipples clean and dry is basic to keeping them in good condition (see p. 155).

Sore nipples are a frequent "complaint" during the mother's early breast-feeding experience, and so she should be instructed to report any discomfort in order that corrective measures may be instituted at once.

The nipples are best treated after each nursing period with the application of a bland cream or ointment, such as lanolin or a commercially prepared compound (e.g., Massé Nipple Cream or Vitamin A and D Ointment). Painting the nipples with tincture of benzoin or alcohol has long been used to toughen tender nipples, but this has a tendency to dry the skin; in fact, alcohol has been demonstrated to be destructive to the nipple during lactation. Many hospitals are now advocating the use of a thermalite (therapeutic) lamp for tender or cracked nipples; the affected breast is exposed for 20 to 30 minutes twice a day. The mother should be advised that even the exposure of the breast to fresh air for similar periods is beneficial, because this is a measure she may resort to after she returns home.

When a sore nipple is examined, it may be found to be fissured (cracked) or to have a small erosion (raw area). The primary treatment for either condition is rest, in order to avoid further irritation and to allow time for healing. In the majority of cases a nipple shield (Fig. 15-11) may be used for protection so that the infant may continue to

Fig. 15-12. First position in the expression of breast milk from a large, pendant breast, showing the thumb and fingers properly placed and pressing backward.

Fig. 15-13. Second position, showing the thumb and finger pressed deeply into the breast, at the same time compressing the breast well behind the nipple. This deeper pressure is necessary in a round, virginal-shaped breast.

Fig. 15-14. Second position, showing compression of the breast between the thumb and fingers, well behind the nipple, and the milk coming in a stream. Care is exercised to avoid pinching or bruising the breast tissue.

nurse. If there is any bleeding from the fissure or erosion, nursing usually is discontinued. Under such conditions, manual expression should be instituted to empty the breast, not only to continue to stimulate lactation, but also to relieve engorgement. The nurse should make every effort to recognize the early symptoms of "cracked nipples" so that further problems can be avoided. These raw areas afford an easy portal of entry for pathogenic bacteria to gain access to the breast and to cause mastitis. Abscess of the breast is very painful and often disastrous. Not only does it result in the immediate suspension of breast-feeding but it also may prevent the

suckling of future babies (see Chap. 21, Complications of the Puerperium).

Length of Nursing Time

The infant will begin nursing, from 1 to 5 minutes, from one or both breasts. Gradually, the time is increased according to the tolerance of the mother's nipples. When lactation is well established, the nursing period is approximately 20 minutes, although there may be a wide variation, depending on the infant's sucking pattern. When the breasts are full, and the milk flow is easily ejected, the breast usually is emptied in the first 5 minutes or so of nursing. The baby may continue to suck, or he may fall asleep. If the infant continues to suck for an inordinately long time (30 to 45 minutes), this may be an indication that there is not enough milk present, and that he is still hungry, or it may be an indication that he sucks intermittently and therefore takes longer to get the milk. Again, he may wish merely to suck, even though he is not hungry. If secretion of milk is not the problem, it is wiser to let him proceed at his own pace than to attempt to hurry him, so long as nipple irritation does not occur. Sometimes the let-down reflex is so active that the milk literally streams, and the baby not only does not have to suck very hard but may have difficulty in swallowing fast enough to keep up with the stream. Placing the baby in a more upright position is sometimes helpful in preventing choking in these cases. He may have to nurse a bit, stop, and then continue as he learns to cope with the increased stream.

Bubbling. The mother should be instructed in the technique of bubbling her infant (see Chap. 15). This may be done when she changes breasts, or midway and at the end of the feeding period. If the infant has had difficulty in beginning to nurse, it is usually better to bubble him at the end of the feeding. Breast-fed babies tend not to swallow as much air as bottle-fed infants; hence the need for bubbling usually does not present much of a problem.

Schedule. A self-regulatory or self-demand schedule is the usual accepted practice today, especially for breast-fed babies; that is, the baby is fed when he indicates hunger by crying and body posture. The infant cries when he is hungry because actual contractions in his stomach cause him pain. If he is fed when he cries and is experiencing pain, he learns to associate food with the relief of pain. Thus food (and mother who supplies it) become pleasant factors in his life. If, on the other hand, he is made to wait until "time" for feeding, he may not nurse well because he is exhausted from crying or has lost his feeling of hunger. Similarly, if a baby is "sleepy" and not allowed to wake up sufficiently by himself, he also will not nurse well and will soon resent efforts made to wake him up. Slapping the soles of his feet, spanking his bottom and the like generally are not effective. These infants may want to nurse only every 6 to 8 hours for the first few days; later they enjoy more frequent nursing periods.

Most average-sized babies regulate themselves on an *approximate* 4-hour schedule. Smaller infants may prefer 3 hours. However, the nurse and the mother must remember that a wide variation will exist; the interval at times may be from 2 to 6 hours and sometimes as long as 8 hours. Usually, however, there will be 6 to 8 feedings in 24 hours. Each infant also will vary his own schedule. For instance, after a few days the mother may notice that the infant wants to eat every 2 hours or so. She usually can meet the demand, since frequent nursing stimulates the milk production. Care must be taken that her nipples do not become sore because of the frequent sucking, or that she does not become fatigued. The nurse will want to be particularly careful in observing mother and baby during this time. If the mother does evidence the above signs, then the nurse, after checking with the doctor, may suggest that a bottle be given for one feeding so that the mother may rest.

Complemental Feedings. This subject has long been controversial. Some physicians (and mothers) feel that giving the infant any artificial feedings diminishes the success of breast-feeding and is extremely detrimental to establishing and maintaining lactation (see Suggested Reading). Others feel that there are legitimate indications for an occasional artificial feeding. A variety of feedings may be used (i.e., plain water, glucose water, dilute formula, full-strength formula). If the mother is to use complemental feedings when she gets home, the nurse will want to be sure that she understands their preparation, the kind and the amount of feedings, and the indications for their use.

Expression of Milk

There are some instances in which the mother is desirous of breast-feeding, but for certain reasons the infant cannot be "put to breast." There are also situations in which the breast-fed infant is not able to empty the breast completely. At such times it becomes necessary to utilize artificial means to empty the breasts of milk; otherwise, if this condition is allowed to persist for several days, lacteal secretion is inhibited, and the future milk supply may be jeopardized.

The hands of the person expressing the milk should be washed thoroughly with warm water and soap and dried on a clean towel. Since the daily care of the breast is designed to maintain cleanliness, the same cleansing ritual required before putting the baby to breast would be utilized here.

Manual Expression. This can be done by nurse, but it is preferable to teach the mother how to

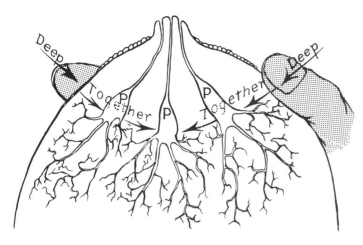

FIG. 15-15. Illustrating the movements needed to force milk out of the little pockets "P" in which it collects. Place a finger and a thumb on opposite sides of the nipple at "Deep." Press deeply into the breast in the direction of the black arrows. Then compress the breast together in direction of the arrows toward center point "P." This will force the milk out of the ducts in streams. "Deep" and "together" express in two words the motions required. (After U. C. Moore, Nutrition of Mother and Child)

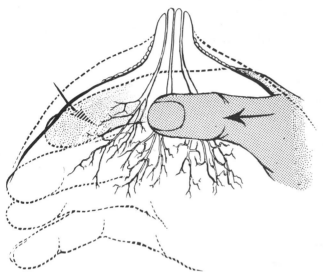

FIG. 15-16. Diagram showing the method of expressing the milk from the breast, as the mother would view it from above, by compressing the milk pockets between the thumb and forefinger. The 3 unused fingers are used to support the breast. This represents the second or "together" motion. (After U. C. Moore, Nutrition of Mother and Child)

carry out this procedure while she is in the hospital. In this way she can have guided practice under the supervision of the hospital nurse, so that when she has to do it after she returns home, her confidence and ability will be increased.

A sterile glass or wide-mouthed container should be in readiness before beginning, and if the milk is to be fed to the infant, a sterile bottle and cap also will be needed. It may be desirable first to massage the breast for a few seconds to stimulate the flow of milk, and in such instance it is helpful to lubricate the hands with a drop of mineral oil. Breast massage should be done with a gliding movement of the hands. The pressure exerted should be firm, even, and, above all, gentle. First, place one hand on top of the other above the breast, then as they are drawn apart turn the

fingers downward and encircle the breast. As the hands sweep forward toward the areola, they should cup the breast, drawing it forward and upward, and glide off without ever touching the areola or the nipple. If the breast is pendulous, care should be taken to allow it to fall gently.

One hand is used to support the breast and to express the milk; the other, to hold the container which will receive the milk. Although some authorities advocate that the right hand be used to milk the left breast, the decision as to which hand is used should depend on how the mother can accomplish this with the greatest of ease. The forefinger is placed below and the thumb above the outer edge of the areola. The forefinger should be kept straight so that pressure can be exerted between the middle of this finger and the

FIG. 15-17. Electric breast-pump. Suction system provides vacuum up to 15″ of mercury. Control allows patient to regulate degree of suction to her requirements and comfort. (Gomco Surgical Manufacturing Corp., Buffalo, N. Y.)

ball of the thumb. As they are alternately compressed and released, with the area of the collecting sinuses between them, milk is forced out in a stream (Figs. 15-12 to 16). It is of paramount importance here to avoid pinching and possibly bruising the breast tissue. The fingers should not slide forward on the areola or the nipple during the milking process. However, they must be moved in clockwise fashion around the areola, each time compressing and releasing the fingers on that area, so that all the collecting sinuses may be emptied.

Many obstetricians advocate this method of emptying the breasts rather than using the breast pump, because the action more nearly simulates the action of the infant's jaws as it nurses. Furthermore, since no mechanical equipment is required, it is a method which can be readily used when necessary after discharge from the hospital.

Electric-Pump Expression. Several types of electric breast pumps employing the principle of intermittent negative pressure are used in hospitals (Fig. 15-17). The physician may prescribe their use to empty the breasts of milk, as in some cases to reduce engorgement, or to draw out inverted nipples.

The nurse should be familiar with the instructions pertaining to the particular electric pump that she is using. If she is teaching the mother how to pump her breasts, it is wise to make sure that she understands how to use it, and especially how to control the vacuum.

Low suction will express the milk without discomfort or injury. For whatever purpose the electric breast pump is used, the suction should be increased gradually to prevent irritation to the nipple and needless pain which, in turn, might cause anxiety in the mother and retard the flow of milk. Suction should be intermittent to simulate the sucking of the infant. It takes approximately 5 to 12 minutes to empty a breast completely, depending on the stage of lactation, but pumping should be stopped as soon as milk ceases to flow. If it is used solely to draw out inverted nipples, it should be used only until the nipple becomes erect. A breast should never be pumped longer than 15 minutes at any one time. However, if the mother experiences back or chest pain, an indication that the breast is dry, the pumping should be stopped immediately.

The breast milk obtained should be measured and the amount recorded. When only one breast is pumped at a time, the record should indicate whether it was the right or the left, so that the next time the other breast can be pumped. If the milk is to be fed to the infant, it should be poured into a sterile nursing bottle, labeled with the infant's name, the time and the date and refrigerated immediately. To ensure further safety in the hospital, milk that is saved for an infant in this way should be sterilized before it is fed to him.

The electric breast-pump machine may be used for more than one mother and thus should be washed with soap or detergent each time that it is used. In addition, certain removable parts, such as the breast-pump bottle and cap, the breast funnel and the rubber connection tubing, must be washed thoroughly, wrapped and autoclaved immediately after use.

Hand-Pump Expression. At times a hand breast-pump may be used. Suction is obtained by alternately collapsing and releasing the rubber bulb. The principles of use and action are the same as those for the electric pump. Since this appliance is used also for more than one mother, it should be washed thoroughly in soap or detergent, rinsed and autoclaved.

Hygiene of the Mother

Rest and Adequate Nutrition. Perhaps these two are the most important considerations for the lactating mother. The detrimental effects of fatigue and worry already have been discussed. In the hospital the nurse is able to act as a buffer between the mother and some of these problems. In addition, the mother is relieved of household responsibilities and is able to have meals served to her. When she leaves the hospital, she no longer has this somewhat protected environment. Thus, it is important that the nurse make sure that the parents understand the importance of rest and adequate nutrition, and that the parents have made adequate plans to provide for them. If it is at all possible, the mother should have help at home. Her main energies then can be directed to the care of the infant and giving attention to her husband and other children. Housekeeping chores will have to be simplified and the mother's activity restricted so that she will get sufficient rest. Since her sleep will be broken at night, naps during the day become particularly *essential*—they should not be considered a luxury. Without adequate rest, the milk supply soon will be reduced to a dribble. If heretofore the woman has been very active, she may need special help to realize the importance of naps and rest periods. It is helpful, also, if visitors (including relatives) are restricted; they can become fatiguing to the mother, and they may be a source of potential infection to the newborn.

Diet. The daily diet of the lactating mother

should be similar to that taken during pregnancy, with the addition of about 700 calories and amounts of the various nutrients (protein, calcium, iron, vitamin A, thiamine, riboflavin, niacin, vitamin B_6, vitamin B_{12}, and ascorbic acid) as recommended by the Food and Nutrition Board of the National Research Council[11] (see Chap. 8, Antepartal Care). These increased demands in the diet during lactation can be supplied with the addition of a pint of milk, one serving of vegetable and one of citrus fruit, an egg and one large serving of meat. Foods which the mother knows from experience disagree with her should be avoided; but the old belief that certain foods eaten by the mother will cause colic in her infant is now discredited. However, as previously stated in Chapter 14, certain drugs may be excreted in the mother's milk in sufficient quantity to affect the breast-fed infant.

Caloric allowances must be adjusted for the variation in energy requirements which result from differences in the body size of women. Another important consideration in determining additional energy requirements for lactation is that they be proportional to the quantity of breast milk produced, and compatible with maintenance of the mother's weight. Since the quantity of breast milk produced varies from woman to woman, the caloric intake should be adjusted in relation to the mother's actual milk production. The basic diet should be supplemented by approximately 120 calories for each 100 cc. of breast milk that is produced. Let us assume that a mother has an average yield of breast milk of 850 cc. per day. In this instance an additional allowance of up to 1000 calories might be utilized.

The National Research Council recommends an additional 20 Gm. of protein per day in the mother's diet. This allowance should be estimated according to the quantity of breast milk secreted and the protein content of this milk.

The vitamin and mineral intake should be adjusted also to supply the needed amounts for lactation. The average riboflavin content, for example, is approximately 40 mg./100 cc. of human milk. The World Health Organization Expert Committee on Nutrition in Pregnancy and Lactation assumes the average daily human milk secretion to be 850 cc., with an upper limit of 1200 cc.

---

[11] Recommended Dietary Allowances. 7th revised edition, Publication No. 1694, National Academy of Sciences National Research Council, Washington, D.C., 1968.

Vitamins B_6 and B_{12} have been added to the list of recommended daily dietary allowances in the 1968 revision. The increased need of vitamin B_6 for lactation is indicated by the amount of vitamin B_{12} in human milk (approximately 0.1 mg./liter). During lactation 2.5 mg. of vitamin B_6 is required in the mother's diet.[12]

The value of a high protein diet to the mother cannot be stressed enough. The mechanism by which food is converted into milk protein is not very efficient; therefore, approximately 2 Gm. of food protein is needed to produce 1 Gm. of milk protein. The greater part of this protein intake (98 Gm. daily) should be in the form of animal protein, since this type supplies all the essential amino acids.

A high fluid intake also is necessary for milk production. Between 2,500 and 3,000 cc. is recommended for the mother engaged in usual activity under pleasant environmental conditions. More may be required in hot weather or with physical exertion. This fluid intake should include a good deal of water as well as other beverages. Many mothers find that taking a beverage prior to nursing facilitates the let-down reflex.

If the mother's diet was adequate in pregnancy, then additions rather than changes are all that will be necessary. It is important that the nurse ascertain that the mother is aware of these additions. If she is not, then guidance must be given. Often nursing mothers do not realize that their nutritional needs increase even over the needs of pregnancy, and they try to go back to their pre-pregnant diet. Increasing the milk intake to at least 1½ quarts daily will meet the additional protein, thiamin, riboflavin, calcium, phosphorus and niacin needs. Supplementing the citrus fruit recommendations in pregnancy with generous servings of other fruits and vegetables will meet the vitamin C requirements. An adequate vitamin D intake can be obtained by supplementing the vitamin-D-rich foods recommended during pregnancy. To further ensure optimum vitamin and mineral intake, many physicians will prescribe that the vitamin supplement capsules taken during pregnancy be continued.

The mother's weight is one of the best criteria in determining adequate caloric intake. It should remain stationary; wide fluctuations will necessitate adjustment of her diet, usually in carbohydrate and fat intake (this statement is based on the assumption that she has an adequate protein intake). The mother may take all foods in moderation as long as they agree with her. The old notion that certain foods (chocolate, the "strong" vegetables such as cabbage, onions, garlic) were excreted through the milk and would upset the baby is no longer universally held.

DEBATABLE ITEMS. Some physicians feel that certain foods, such as berries and chocolate, may produce an allergic reaction in the baby. If the mother has any question regarding these matters, she should consult her physician. Alcohol may be taken in moderation; many mothers find that a glass of sherry or beer before nursing relaxes them considerably and facilitates the let-down reflex. Smoking does not directly influence the lactation process when it is done in moderation, but it should be avoided for the reasons stated in Chapter 8.

Drugs. Many drugs are excreted in the milk, as was explained in Chapter 14, and it is particularly important for the mother to consult her physician before she attempts any self-medication, *even though she has taken the drug before*. Small doses of aspirin, milk of magnesia, mineral oil and some of the bulk-producing laxatives usually may be taken without passing harmful effects to the infant; however, it is well to advise the mother to inform her doctor if she feels she must continue to use any of them.

Weaning

Occasionally, it becomes necessary to wean the baby suddenly. In these cases the physician will follow the regimen for "drying up the breasts" as described on pages 312 to 313. Most often, weaning is done gradually. There does not appear to be any "best" time for this procedure. Sometimes, with the introduction of solid foods the infant tends to take the breast less, and the milk supply consequently will diminish. However, many infants appear to relish solids and still continue to nurse well. It is essential to good health that the baby have solid foods by the age of 6 months at the latest. By this time his iron reserve has been depleted, and foods rich in protein and iron are particularly important. Provided that the baby receives a varied diet that includes meat, eggs, fruits and vegetables, there is no indication for weaning other than the natural inclinations of the mother and the baby. The process can be done gradually, with a cup and/or bottle offered in place of the breast. As the stimulation decreases, so does the milk supply, and lactation gradually

---

[12] Ibid., p. 19.

FIG. 15-18. Breast exercise. After breast-feeding has been discontinued the breasts seem to be soft and flabby. These simple exercises may help to restore firmness of tissues because they involve the pectoral muscles which lend secondary support to the breasts. Stand with feet apart, toes turned in slightly, abdomen in and up, buttocks tucked under and head held high. Hold fingertips together, with arms at shoulder level. Press fingers together sharply and firmly. Relax and repeat 10 times.

ceases. Usually no engorgement ensues; if any should occur, the mother should be instructed to consult her physician.

Breast Exercises

Mothers are sometimes concerned about the temporary increase in the size of the breasts during lactation. When breast-feeding has been discontinued, the breasts soon approximate their previous size and firmness, particularly if needed support has been maintained. There are exercises which, if done regularly, may be helpful. The breast itself is made up of glandular tissue and fat (see Fig. 2-35), and since there is an absence of elastic tissue, exercises cannot directly hasten the return of the breasts to their former state. However, exercises that involve the pectoral muscles may be helpful, because these muscles lend secondary support to the breasts (Figs 15-18, 19). These exercises may be started when the mother is no longer breast-feeding, should be limited at first and increased only as the mother can tolerate them without fatigue.

PARENTAL GUIDANCE AND INSTRUCTION

A considerable amount of health supervision throughout the mother's pregnancy is devoted to anticipatory guidance, not only to provide for her immediate care, but also to help her plan and prepare for the time when she takes her new infant home from the hospital. A good foundation to facilitate this transition has been laid in this way, but it may lose some of its effectiveness unless certain aspects are reinforced in the immediate puerperium.

Each mother's understanding and ability will vary, depending largely on her background and previous experiences. Undoubtedly, the primipara who has not been accustomed to infants will have much to learn about the care and handling of her new baby. On the other hand, the multipara may feel uncertain about the response of an older child to the new baby and thus require guidance in understanding and dealing with sibling rivalry. Many mothers need to know more about their own care; others need to know how to facilitate certain adjustments within the home or the family group. If the mother knows what she can expect and what to do, she usually can handle simple problems which might otherwise cause fear or apprehension.

Proper care for the mother during the puerperium emphasizes the need for rest, nourishing food and protection from worry. Parents, as a rule, seem to be under the impression that once the delivery is over, normality is restored and they can resume their usual activities immediately. however, it is agreed that it may be weeks before the generative organs have returned to normal size and position, and the emotional and endocrine adjustments may be even more delayed.

Since the nurse is in close and continuous contact with the mother, she should assume the responsibility of giving this anticipatory guidance and/or reinforcing or delegating that part which might be done more suitably by others. One of the most important points to be emphasized is that the mother should proceed *as slowly as possible* in the postpartal period at home. The general feeling of well-being and the excitement of having the baby, together with the emotions

FIG. 15-19. Breast exercise. Lie flat on back with knees and thighs flexed to place spine firmly on the floor. Abdomen is kept flat. Breathe naturally and do exercises slowly. (1) Holding a small book in each hand, stretch arms out level with shoulders. (2) Raise arms forward from body to bring books together, keeping arms straight. Lower arms to outstretched position. (3) Raise arms forward as in No. 2; then carry them, held straight together, to floor behind head. Return arms to outstretched position. Repeat. Stop all exercises before feeling tired.

aroused in the "taking-hold" phase, all too often provide so great a stimulus that the mother has a tendency to overdo. If there are other children in the household, especially toddlers, the demands on the mother may be considerable.

If it is at all possible, the major responsibilities of housekeeping should be taken over by a "helper," so that the mother can be more relaxed and devote herself primarily to caring for her new infant and spending more time with the immediate family. At this time family relationships can be strengthened if the mother is not overwhelmed with apprehension and fatigue. The subject of household assistance needs to be explored thoroughly with the mother (and if necessary, the father). The parents may need help in realizing what possibilities and alternatives they have in this matter. Some parents, for instance, manage very nicely when the husband takes some vacationtime and assumes management of the household. However, it must be remembered that not all husbands are able (or willing) to shoulder this considerable task. Other parents can rely on parents, in-laws or relatives for a time. Still others must hire

outside help; in these cases the expense and consequent budgeting may have to be discussed. If outside help is employed, then the mother may have some question as to whether a housekeeper or a "nurse" (to take care of the baby) would be more desirable. This, of course, will depend on many factors. Most mothers find that when they are relieved of the heavy housekeeping chores, the "care" of the baby is relatively easy and provides an opportunity to get thoroughly acquainted with the new addition to the household.

The nurse should not "recommend" one type of helper over another. Rather, she should explore the subject with the mother, point out the alternatives that the parents have, and let them make the final decision. This approach would be appropriate for any other aspect of guidance.

By the time that the mother leaves the hospital she should have at least a basic understanding of her own condition and status, and she should know what physical and emotional changes to expect. In addition, she should be familiar with the daily care of her baby and know what to expect of him, together with any other important

FIG. 15-20. Setup used for baby bath demonstration in the mothers' classroom. Note paper bag for discarded cotton balls, pillowcase for a laundry hamper and step on can for diaper pail. (MacDonald House, The University Hospitals of Cleveland, Cleveland, Ohio)

FIG. 15-21. Luncheon "round table" for small group of mothers to learn about their own care and their baby's through guided group discussions. (MacDonald House, University Hospitals of Cleveland, Cleveland, Ohio)

Fig. 15-22. Individual teaching.

details related to his care. Parents should know how and where to contact the physician if before the next scheduled visit there should arise any medical problem pertaining to either the mother or the infant.

Since the present-day maternity stay is rather short, some type of follow-up service often is desirable and necessary. Therefore, parents should be offered information about the services of the public health nursing agency in their community, and how they may use these services. In cases of obvious need a referral to an agency should be instituted before the patient leaves the hospital.

Husbands who have accompanied their wives to parents' classes are usually much more conscious of this period and prepared for it. Often they plan their time at home so that they can help to assume some of the responsibilities. It is not so much physical help that is needed as it is the satisfactions gained by the mutual "sharing" engendered by the partnership. If the mother takes special care to express her appreciation of her husband's awareness and consideration, then this initial readjustment period becomes less tedious and truly gratifying to both.

Individual Teaching

Regardless of the fact that a mother may attend all the group classes offered in the maternity hospital, each mother should be given individual help to learn how to handle and care for her infant while she is in the hospital, particularly if this is her first baby. Many new mothers are timid at first because they do not know what to expect of their infants, or they are afraid of what they will do to them because of their own feelings of inadequacy. A mother who has had no previous experience with infants will need some guided practice in changing diapers, dressing her baby and handling the infant in general (Fig. 15-22). Rooming-

FIG. 15-23. Knee-chest position may be advised by the physician if the uterus has not returned to its almost normal position.

CORRECT — Chest resting on bed, thighs perpendicular to surface.

INCORRECT—Chest on pillow, thighs slant away from body.

INCORRECT — Resting on elbows, thighs slant inward toward body.

in units provide an environment in which the mother can have such an experience over an extended period of time. However, even in situations where the infants are kept in a central nursery, the nurse should plan to spend some time with the mother, in addition to the regular feeding periods, to help her learn to care for her baby. If hospital staffing permits the time, it may be desirable for some mothers to bathe their own infants at the bedside, under the nurse's guidance, before leaving the hospital. There is no reason that such practices should violate the "clean nursery technique" if they have been properly planned. A rooming-in experience is undoubtedly beneficial for mother, father and baby. But when this is not possible because of hospital facilities or policies, a daily extended visiting period can be extremely helpful. In this way the parents and the baby can become better acquainted in the security of the maternity division, where experienced personnel are near at hand to answer the mother's questions and to offer advice.

Postpartal Exercises

Certain exercises are advantageous to the mother during the postpartal period to strengthen the abdominal muscles, to promote involution and a general sense of well-being (see page 203).

Discharge Instructions

Before the mother is discharged from the hospital, the physician will give her instructions about her care and the rate at which it is prudent for her to resume normal activities in the following weeks at home. She is told to avoid any heavy work and to get as much rest as possible during the next 3 weeks (see p. 307). Her schedule should be planned to include morning and afternoon rest periods and adequate sleep at night. Stair climbing should be limited until the 2nd week at home. If the mother is advised to take exercises to strengthen abdominal and perineal muscles, the physician will specify when they may be started and the frequency with which they are to be done. The hair may be washed at any time, and tub baths or showers are permissible. The mother usually is advised not to have intercourse or to take a vaginal douche until after the "6-week check-up" to prevent infection and trauma to the newly healing organs and structures. Instructions concerning eating habits and regulation of the bowels are discussed.

If the medical care of the infant is being supervised by a pediatrician, he may give the mother home-going instructions concerning her baby; otherwise this is taken care of by the obstetrician. The mother should be given specific information about feeding, skin care, clothing, sleep, bowel habits, behavior and the early growth and development of her infant.

Many hospitals provide printed home-going instructions for maternity patients. When these are used, it is the responsibility of the nurse to make sure that the mother understands them before she leaves the hospital.

The maternity programs of most public health agencies include home visits by the nurse. When a referral has not been made by the hospital nurse, the mother should be informed that such services are available in the community and told how to secure them if she should need help with the care of the baby.

The importance of follow-up care for both mother and baby should be stressed. The mother is instructed that it is essential for her to keep the appointment for her "6-week check-up." The infant should be checked in 4 weeks and regularly thereafter by a private physician or in one of the well-baby clinics sponsored by the department of health.

Family Planning

Brutally high death rates approximated so closely the high birth rates for vast aeons that the population of the world remained stationary or almost so. The human female, a relatively slow breeder even among mammals, had to reproduce close to her physiologic maximum if the family, the tribe and the nation were to survive. It took the human population from the beginning of time to about 1850 to reach its first billion. It reached 2 billion in approximately another 80 years. The third billion was added in about 30 years; and at the present rate of growth the prospects are that the next 30 years will add not just 1 billion inhabitants to the globe, but a number that may approximate 3 billion. Dr. Irene Taeuber, one of our most conservative demographers, forecasts another 391 million people for Africa by the end of the century (only 30 years hence), 421 million more for Latin America, and 2 billion, 350 million additional for Asia.

The reasons for these soaring figures are plain enough. As the result of worldwide and highly efficacious public health measures, the death rates, especially in developing countries, have fallen precipitously. But in these very countries the same high birth rates prevail as obtained decades ago. This imbalance between births and deaths leads inevitably to such figures as those just cited. Since it would be unthinkable to suggest any measures to increase death rates, the only solution to the problem, short of the Four Horsemen of the Apocalypse, is reduction in the number of births.

Even at present population levels, the majority of the world's populace subsists on near-starvation diets. Malnutrition is the inevitable forerunner of anemia and increased vulnerability to infectious diseases. Infants and children are the hardest hit. Overcrowding abets the dissemination of infectious diseases and vitiates any attempts at hygienic living. Excessive population is therefore an all-important health problem. For this reason the American Public Health Association, the American Medical Association and other pertinent organizations have long since endorsed family planning as an urgent health need.

The important role that the nurse, both the maternity and the public health nurse, can play in the extensive movement to control excessive fertility is reflected in the numerous articles in nursing journals on this subject, as indicated by the bibliography of this chapter. For example, the Editor of *Nursing Outlook,* Alice M. Robinson, wrote in an editorial:

There is no need to advocate any particular concept or belief or method; but it is the nurses' grave and imminent responsibility to give the widest possible help and hope and understanding to the end that guidance in family planning is made unequivocally and universally available to parents, regardless of their socioeconomic status.[13]

She properly points out, moreover, that "*all* major religious groups—Jewish, Catholic and Protestant—agree on the necessity for *responsible, planned* parenthood." It might be added in this connection that at least one method of contraception has the approval of all religions. Certainly, in this modern changing age it is incumbent on every nurse to be aware of all of the available methods of birth control. The nurse should be conversant with the advantages and disadvantages of each method, both at the mechanical and psychological levels, as they relate to the individual patient and her husband. The choice of a suitable contraceptive depends on many factors and will vary even from year to year in any couple's contra-

---

13 Robinson, A. M.: The principle, not the method. Nurs. Outlook 12:27, September, 1964.

ceptive life span. These factors include expense, bathroom facilities, frequency of intercourse, number of children, the risk the couple wishes to take, illness, physical problems, and individual variations with each couple.

The nurse should also be acquainted with the increasing availability of vasectomy and tubal ligation in any hospital or area in which she is working. Studies have shown that one fourth to one third of all couples at the present time are looking toward this permanent method of contraception when their families are completed.

Those who are in conscience committed to the moral teachings of the Roman Catholic Church may find that only two of these methods are ethically acceptable to them; we have asterisked both. The nurse who in conscience finds that she cannot give general contraceptice advice should state this to her patients. This will allow patients to go elsewhere for the information which they wish to have.

Oral Progestins. Oral contraceptives ("The Pill") have been publicized so extensively in the lay press that their existence is common knowledge. They owe their effect to the suppression of ovulation caused by the administration of certain hormones, and they constitute the most efficacious contraceptive method known. The program involves setting up a "controlled menstrual cycle" by administering one of these pills daily for 20 days, beginning with the 5th day of the menstrual cycle. Because these compounds have estrogenic as well as progestational effects, they provoke endometrial withdrawal bleeding 3 or 4 days after discontinuance. Since it is possible to control the menstrual cycle by these agents, they are also used extensively as therapeutic measures in women with menstrual abnormalities. Their secondary effects are decreased menstrual flow and decreased menstrual cramping. As contraceptive agents they are superb, if taken correctly. There is some suggestive evidence of an increased incidence of thrombophlebitis with the pill. In your discussions with patients this fact should be mentioned, but it should also be pointed out that the medical risks of pregnancy are greater. The couple should use the best available contraceptive that does not make them fearful of consequences or emotionally uncomfortable. This choice is often a compromise. Upon stopping the pill, some women will have an immediate return of ovulation and menstrual periods, and some may not have menstrual periods for three to six months. Ovarian damage due to pill usage has not been demonstrated. Future pregnancies are not affected.

Intra-uterine Devices (IUD). This technique (actually an ancient practice but only recently validated scientifically) involves the insertion into the uterine cavity of a small, usually flexible appliance, the length or diameter of which is approximately three quarters of an inch. This foreign object is allowed to remain in the uterus as long as contraception is desired. These devices have been made in various shapes (spirals, loops, rings) and of various materials (plastic tubing, nylon thread, stainless steel). Although the mechanism by which these appliances prevent conception is obscure, they are about 97 per cent effective (three pregnancies in 100 users with the IUD in place). They rank second only to the oral progestins and are probably equal to the properly used diaphragm in the protection they afford. The advantages of intra-uterine devices are that they are inexpensive and, once inserted, require no further attention, provided that they remain in place. This brings us to the main drawback of these appliances: they frequently are expelled. Moreover, some of the appliances have to be removed because of bleeding or cramps. Spontaneous expulsion or necessary removal by the physician occurs in 15 to 20 per cent of all cases with the devices now being used.

Many of the commonly used IUD's have a nylon string attached which serves two purposes: (1) it aids in removal, and (2) it allows the patient to check for its presence by palpating the strings at the level of the cervix. You should emphasize to your patients that it is important to check for the presence of the IUD before each sexual exposure in the first 6 to 9 months. After this time, the chance of spontaneous expulsion without the patient's knowledge is low, and it is at this time that the quoted 97 per cent rate of effectiveness is valid. Also, the rate of expulsion and physician removal is greater than 20 per cent in the patients who have never been pregnant, and many physicians reserve this method for the multiparous patient. There are probably two factors operating here: 1) the irritability of the nulliparous uterus, and (2) the lack of sufficient motivation on the part of the girl or woman who has never been pregnant to tolerate the initial 2 to 3 months of cramping and spotting. The severity of these latter symptoms with the IUD may vary from none to quite severe or intolerable. These devices are being widely used throughout the world, especially in developing countries, where their low cost and lack of any need for continuing motivation constitute particular advantages.

The Diaphragm. The diaphragm is a dome-shaped rubber cup, which may range in diameter from 7 to 10 cm. and is inserted into the vagina and over the cervix prior to intercourse and then removed, no sooner than 6 hours after intercourse. The use of the diaphragm insures the placement of spermicidal jelly over the cervix. The diaphragm, by itself, is not a contraceptive device; it must be used with a spermicidal jelly or cream which is placed in the diaphragm between it and the cervix.

A common objection to the diaphragm is the vaginal manipulation necessary to insert it, a procedure which is repugnant to some women. This problem is easily solved if the patient is fitted with a flat or coil spring diaphragm (in contrast to the arc flex diaphragm). These diaphragms may be used with an "inserter" which allows the patient to insert it like a tampon, without touching the genital area. The arc flex diaphragm cannot be used with an inserter, as they now exist. It was designed for ease of manual insertion, and may, in some cases, give a better fit in the presence of a mild cystocele. Some women, after one or more pregnancies cannot be fitted with a diaphragm. You may assure your patient that neither she nor her husband will be aware of the presence of a well-fitted diaphragm. Although its efficacy is good, the diaphragm has lost favor in view of the greater efficacy and acceptability of the oral contraceptives and intrauterine devices (foregoing paragraphs).

The Condom. The condom is one of the more effective contraceptive devices, if used properly. The patient will probably tell you that she knows this but there is really a decrease in "sensation" or that her husband will not use one for the same reason. You might point out that no method of contraception is perfect (i.e., all of them have some disadvantages for one or both partners or have some anxiety-producing aspects). You should reassure the patient that they are safe if used before any penetration, and seldom, if ever, break. This information will help those couples who are anxious about other forms of contraception. The fear of pregnancy and of some contraceptives can lead to abstinence and a difficult marriage relationship, unless you can help with alternatives.

*The Safe Period or Rhythm. The rationale of the safe period or the rhythm method is that when there are regular periods, ovulation occurs at approximately the same time in each cycle (i.e., 14 days *prior to the beginning* of the next cycle). The ovum is capable of being fertilized only for a period of 48 hours, at the most, after ovulation. Theoretically, therefore, abstinence from sexual intercourse on that day and for the two days before and after (a total of five days) should forestall conception.

In actual experience, however, even normal regular periods are often 1 to 2 days in either direction (e.g., 28 ∓ 2 days). This puts the day of ovulation in the same four day range ∓ 2 days, and the period of abstinence must then be, realistically, about eight days. For more accuracy the basal body temperature should be used.

The most important point about the rhythm method and its repeated failures, really has more to do with the longevity of the sperm than with the day of ovulation. Sperm are found in the cervical mucus as soon as 20 seconds after ejaculation and as late as five days after ejaculation. These are active sperm and any active sperm must be regarded as capable of fertilizing an egg. There are many "day 6 and day 7" pregnancies that attest to this fact (i.e., that intercourse on day 6 or 7 of a 28 day cycle resulted in pregnancy).

If rhythm is to work, there must be regular periods, and abstinence for at least fourteen days out of each 28 day cycle. Intercourse during the first five days of a cycle (menses) is not contraindicated, except on an aesthetic basis by some couples nor is it contraindicated during the last five or six days of a cycle, if these can be determined accurately.

*Basal Body Temperature. This method is a more accurate variation of the rhythm method, but it entails an effort that few women are willing to make. If the periods are regular, she can take her oral temperature each day for three cycles and record it and submit it to her physician for analysis (see Fig. 3-4 and Chap. 3). Special thermometers are sold at most drugstores for this purpose. The rise in temperature indicates the day of ovulation, but if periods are regular an estimate is just as accurate (by subtracting 14 from the first day of the period).

If there are irregular periods, theoretically the woman could take her temperature every morning and record it; when she sees the degree rise sustained for a three day period, she can assume that ovulation has occurred and that intercourse is safe, in terms of contraception. Only the most motivated patients will do this for much more than three or four months and the method still requires long periods of abstinence prior to the rise in temperature.

Couples are much more motivated to use this method for detecting ovulation (if there is an infertility problem) than for contraception.

Douches. Not a method of contraception.

Jellies, Creams, Suppositories, Foams. These contraceptives are cheap and available without consulting a physician, but they are relatively ineffective because the woman cannot be sure of the placement or the retention of the spermicidal agent. These are especially useful for the patient who is contemplating another pregnancy and has been on the pill. She could stop the pill a few months earlier than the time she planned for conception and use a contraceptive (foams, jellies, creams, etc.) that is less effective until her periods are reestablished (see oral progestins). A contraceptive failure at this time is not the catastrophe that it might have been a few months earlier.

Withdrawal. Withdrawal or coitus interruptus is an extensively used method of contraception and appears to be satisfactory to a large proportion of couples. However, withdrawal, as a method of contraception is a compromise at best. It requires a tremendous amount of concentration and will-power on the part of the husband and trust on the part of the wife. This trust is not always well founded and creates anxiety. Neither of these factors are really conducive to relaxation and pleasure and leave the couple with a very distorted idea of what sexual pleasure is or can be. Also, there is a pre-ejaculatory secretion ranging in quantity from a few drops to as much as 1 cc. of seminal fluid. This is especially true when there has been prolonged erection. This fluid frequently has motile sperm in it, and we must assume that they have the capability of fertilizing an egg.

Lactation. Menstruation may occur at any time during lactation though it is frequently delayed until nursing is stopped. The absence of menstrual periods during lactation should not be taken as evidence that ovulation has not occurred. Ovulation may occur, as evidenced by conceptions during this period, and it will occur *prior* to the onset of any menstruation. Even if the mother uses breast-feeding as the sole means to feed her newborn infant, after the third month she should not depend upon lactation to control fertility. The nursing mother should use some method of contraception if she does not wish to become pregnant.

Contraceptive Advice for the Postpartal Patient

Patients may be reluctant to discuss methods of contraception with their doctor for the six-week postpartal period because he has usually told them to abstain until the six week visit. Patients are more realistic, especially the multiparous patient, and she will discuss this with the nurse if she is given the opportunity. Of all the methods available, the condom is the only method that should be used during this period. The insertion of the IUD and the use of the diaphragm or foams and other spermicidal agents should be postponed until involution of the uterus is complete. Withdrawal might be suggested if the couple has used this method previously. Some doctors will put their patients on the pill immediately after delivery, whether or not the mother is nursing. Some doctors will not prescribe the pill for use during the nursing period.

SUGGESTED READING

Adels, M. J., and Rogers, S. F.: Use of a new non-narcotic analgesic for postpartum pain. Am. J. Obstet. Gynec. 84:952-955, October 1, 1962.

American Public Health Association: Policy statement on population. Am. J. Public Health 104:2102, December, 1964.

Ayd, F. J.: The teenager and contraception. Pediat. Clin. N. Am. 16:355-361, May, 1969.

Bristol, W. M.: Comparative effectiveness of compressional and supporting breast binders in suppressing lactation. Nurs. Res. 15:203-206, Summer, 1966.

Brodsky, J. D., and Greenstein, C.: Air embolism associated with pregnancy and the puerperium. Illinois Med. J. 112:5, 1957.

Cahill, I.: Child-Rearing Practices in the Culture of Poverty. NLN Convention Papers, 1967.

Calderone, M. S.: Manual of Family Planning and Contraceptive Practice. Baltimore, Williams & Wilkins, 1970.

Eppink, H.: An experiment to determine a basis for nursing decisions in regard to time of initiation of breastfeeding. Nurs. Res. 18:292-299, July, 1969.

Evans, R.: Needs identified among breastfeeding mothers. ANA Clinical Sessions, 1968 Dallas, pp. 162-171, New York, Appleton-Century, 1968.

Evans, R. T., et al.: Exploration of factors involved in maternal physiological adaptation to breastfeeding. Nurs. Res. 18:28-33, January-February, 1969.

Goodwin, B.: What is maternity nursing?, in Jeffries, J. E. (ed.): Can Maternity Nursing Meet Today's Challenge?, Ross Round Table on Maternal and Child Nursing, pp. 45-51, Ross Lab., 1967.

Gorden, R. E., and Gorden, K. K.: Social factors in prevention of postpartum emotional problems. Obstet. Gynec. 15:433-438, April, 1960.

Henning, E., et al.: A dynamic nursing appraisal of the puerperium, in Lytle, N. (ed.): Material Health Nursing, pp. 153-163, Dubuque, Iowa, Wm. C. Brown, 1967.

Hilliard, M. E.: New horizons in maternity nursing. Nurs. Outlook 15:33-36, July, 1967.

Hutcheson, H.: Patient education for low-income women in a family planning program. ANA Clinical Sessions, pp. 20-24, New York, Appleton-Century-Crofts, 1968.

Iffrig, Sister M. C.: Nursing care and success in breast-feeding: effectiveness of alternate massage. Nurs. Clin. N. Am. 3:345-354, June, 1968.

Joint Committee on Family and Child Welfare and Committee on Health: The Right to Birth Control Information in Family Planning, New York, Community Service Society of New York, June, 1964.

Josselyn, I. M.: Cultural forces—motherliness and fatherliness. Am. J. Orthopsychiat. 26:264-271, April, 1956.

Kallaus, J.: The mother in the maternity unit. Am. J. Nurs. 65:120-127, April, 1965.

Larsen, V. L.: Stresses of the childbearing year. Am. J. Public Health. 56:32-36, January, 1966.

Lesser, M. S., and Keane, V. R.: Nurse-Patient Relationships in a Hospital Maternity Service. St. Louis, C. V. Mosby, 1956.

Manisoff, M. T.: Family Planning; A Teaching Guide for Nurses. New York, Planned Parenthood—World Population, 1969.

Maternity Center Association: Preparation for Childbearing. ed. 2, New York, Maternity Center Association, 1969.

Meir, G.: The role of hospital nurses in family planning. Am. J. Nurs. 65:86-91, July, 1965.

Menczer, J., and Eskin, B.: Evaluation of postpartum breast engorgement by thermography. Obstet. Gynec. 33:260-263, January, 1969.

Newton, N. and Newton, M.: Psychologic Aspects of Lactation. New Eng. J. Med. 277:1179-1188, November 30, 1967.

————: Mother's Reactions to their Newborn Babies. J.A.M.A. 181:206-210, July 21, 1962.

Pierson, E. C.: Sex is Never an Emergency. Philadelphia, Lippincott, 1971.

Recommended Dietary Allowances, rev. ed., Publication No. 1694, Washington, D.C., National Academy of Sciences, National Research Council, 1968.

Reeder, S.: Becoming a mother—nursing implications in a problem of role transistion. ANA Regional Clinical Conferences, pp. 204-210, 1967.

Rich, O. J.: Hospital routines as rites of passage in developing maternal identity. Nurs. Clin. N. Am. 4:101-109, March, 1969.

————: The Initial Feeding Experience as Maternal Role Enactment, Maternal Child Nursing Conference, School of Nursing, University of Pittsburgh, pp. 37-41, June, 1966.

Rubin, R.: Basic maternal behavior. Nurs. Outlook 9:683-686, November, 1961.

————: Puerperal change. Nurs. Outlook 9:753-755, December, 1961.

————: Maternal touch. Nurs. Outlook 11:828-831, November, 1963.

————: The family-child relationship. Nurs. Outlook 12:36-39, September, 1964.

————: Food and feeding—a matrix of relationships. Nursing Forum 6:195-205, Spring, 1967.

Smith, R. R., and Hodgson, J. S.: Study affirms benefits of postpartum tub baths? Hosp. Topics 44:101-102, October, 1966.

Streeter, B. N.: Suggestions to simplify breastfeeding. J. Am. Med. Women's Assoc. 16:377-378, May, 1961.

Williams, B.: Sleep needs during the maternity cycle. Nurs. Outlook 15:53-55, February, 1967.

Yunek, M. J.: Postpartum care is more than a routine. Nurs. Outlook 17:50-52, January, 1969.

Zacha, M. C.: Nursing goals in working with families under multiple stress. Nurs. Clin. N. Am. 4:69-75, March, 1969.

The Womanly Art of Breastfeeding. Franklin Park, Illinois, LaLeche International, 1963.

CONFERENCE MATERIAL

1. The patient's husband is severely injured the day after her infant is born. What provision can be made by the hospital to keep the patient informed about conditions at home and the care of her three other children?

2. What instructions should be given to the primipara and her husband concerning her care following delivery and discharge from the hospital? How can the public health nurse participate most effectively in this family's care?

3. What approach would you use to help a mother who was undecided about whether or not to breast-feed her infant?

4. Why is the postpartal examination important? What is the nurse's role in relation to the examination?

5. A mother tells the nurse that she wants to breast-feed her baby for 6 to 8 months because she knows that she cannot become pregnant so long as she is nursing. How can the nurse reply?

6. What are the pros and the cons of early ambulation of the maternity patient?

7. How can the nurse help a nursing mother so that she can make her limited food budget provide well-balanced meals for the family? The family consists of the mother, the father (employed as a factory worker) and two small children.

8. A young mother is concerned that her 2-year-old child will be jealous of the new baby. How can this problem be handled?

9. What health teaching would you consider necessary to include as you give a bath to a primipara the first morning after delivery? A multipara?

Study Questions

Unit Four: Nursing in the Normal Puerperium

Read through the entire question and place your answer on the line to the right.

1. Soon after the mother was normally delivered, she complained of feeling chilly. The nurse observed that she was having a chill. In addition to reporting this to the physician, which of the following measures would the nurse carry out?
   A. Provide external warmth to the mother with blankets.
   B. Give a heart stimulant.
   C. Prepare to give oxygen.
   D. Give a hot drink.
   E. Place the mother in shock position.

   Select the number corresponding to the correct letter or letters.
   1. A only
   2. A and C
   3. A and D
   4. B and E
   _____

2. If a mother making satisfactory progress has a pulse rate of 90 immediately before delivery, what average rate or rates would be considered to be favorable soon after delivery?
   A. 60
   B. 70
   C. 80
   D. 90
   E. 100

   Select the number corresponding to the correct letter or letters.
   1. C only
   2. A, B and C
   3. C, D and E
   4. All of them
   _____

3. The appearance of the lochial discharge normally changes during the process of involution. In the space provided after the descriptive phrase in Column 2, place the letter of the period of time in Column 1 that corresponds to it.

Column 1	Column 2	
A. First day	1. Clotted blood with strings of membrane	_____
B. From 1 to 2 days	2. Brownish color; thin, scanty	_____
C. From 4 to 7 days		
D. From 8 to 14 days	3. Blood mixed with small amounts of mucus	_____
E. Third week	4. Pinkish color; moderate amount	_____
F. Seventh week	5. Yellow, creamish color	_____
G. Not at all	6. Dark-brown with occasional bright-red	_____
	7. Characteristic stale odor	_____
	8. Characteristic foul odor	_____

4. A good understanding of the physiologic changes taking place in the mother during the puerperium is a basis for good nursing. Which of the following processes are believed to accomplish involution of the uterus?

A. The contraction of stretched muscle fibers
B. The elimination of endometrium along with blood and serous discharge
C. The casting off of a portion of the spongy layer of the decidua
D. The generation of new endometrial lining from the layer of decidua attached to the muscular wall
E. The formation of new endometrium

Select the number corresponding to the correct letters.
1. A, B and D
2. A, C and D
3. C and E
4. All of them   _____

5. The nurse should be able to evaluate the observations she makes of her patient's condition. Which of the following changes in the height of the fundus would you consider to be indicative of normal progress of involution?

A. Twelve hours after delivery—1 cm. above umbilicus
B. Second day after delivery—6 in. above pubis
C. Fourth day after delivery—3 in. above pubis
D. Eighth day after delivery—2 in. above pubis
E. Tenth day after delivery—1 in. above pubis

Select the number corresponding to the correct letter or letters.
1. A only
2. A and C
3. B, D and E
4. All of them   _____

6. Which of the following seem to be the advantages gained from early ambulation after delivery?

A. Improves bowel and bladder function
B. Mothers seem to regain their strength more readily
C. Minimizes the chances of hemorrhage
D. Hastens involution of the uterus
E. Eliminates incidence of thrombophlebitis

Select the number corresponding to the correct letters.
1. A and B
2. A, C and D
3. B, C and E
4. All of them   _____

7. Although the procedures for perineal care vary from hospital to hospital, in what respects do they all agree?

A. Requiring the nurse to carry out surgical aseptic technic
B. Endeavoring to protect the patient against infection from external sources
C. Using forceps to handle sponges in cleansing vulva
D. Requiring that each sponge be used for one stroke only
E. Requiring that perineal pads be sterile when applied

Select the number corresponding to the correct letters.
1. A and E
2. A, B and C
3. B, D and E
4. All of them   _____

8. To keep the nipples in good condition for breast feeding, which of the following should be included in their daily care?
   A. Keep the nipples clean and dry.
   B. Wash with warm water once a day.
   C. Wash with mild antiseptic solution prior to each feeding period.
   D. Cover the nipples and areola with clean plastic breast squares to prevent contamination.
   E. If nipple is sore, discontinue breast-feeding until tenderness subsides.

   Select the number corresponding to the correct letters.
   1. A and B
   2. A, C and D
   3. B, D and E
   4. All of them   _____ _____

Note: The key to the correct answers to these questions is given on page 613.

UNIT FIVE
Nursing the Normal Newborn

Care of the Newborn Infant
Care of Low Birth Weight and Premature Infants

Care of the
Newborn Infant

16

Physiology of the Newborn • Characteristics of the Newborn
The Environment of the Newborn • Nursing Care of the Newborn • Infant Feeding
The Mother and Her Newborn

INTRODUCTION

From the standpoint of maternity care, the infant will be considered through the neonatal period (the first 4 weeks of life).

During pregnancy the unborn infant has been protected and nourished by his mother, but at birth he suddenly becomes an "independent" individual and undergoes the most profound physiologic changes that are encountered at any period of life. Some of these alterations are immediate, but they are all permanent and therefore significant.

Since these first days and weeks are so critical, the nurse is called on to give expert nursing care when she assumes care of the newborn. She must use the utmost care in handling the baby, keeping him warm and protecting him from exposure and injury. She must also make accurate observations and record and report them. Her communication and teaching skills are utilized, since she must ensure the infant's future well-being by helping the parents to develop an understanding of their baby's needs and to acquire skill in his care. In this way she reinforces their concept of themselves as adequate parents. The nurse also must be aware that some parents need assistance in developing healthy attitudes regarding child-rearing practices, so that the infant can make a satisfactory emotional and social adjustment. A close parent-infant relationship must be fostered (and provision made for this in the hospital environment), and communication must be maintained between the nurse and the parents. Thus, the care of the newborn infant presents an interesting challenge to those in maternity nursing.

PHYSIOLOGY OF THE NEWBORN

Recent research[1] has indicated that the infant must pass through approximately 6 overlapping stages before he becomes entirely adapted to extra-uterine life. During these stages he is in a "transition" period which he must negotiate successfully if he is to survive and to develop normally. The 1st step or stage begins with labor, when the fetus receives the stimulation from the uterine contractions and the changes in pressure as the membranes rupture. As he passes through the 2nd step, he encounters a variety of foreign stimuli—light, sound, heat, cold, gravitation, etc. In the 3rd stage, he must begin breathing. Stages 4 and 5 require profound changes and reorganization in the functioning of the organ systems and metabolic processes. Here he must initiate respiration, change from fetal to neonatal circulation, alter hepatic and renal function and pass meconium. Stage 6 demands further reorganization of the metabolic processes to achieve a viable, steady state. This includes changes in blood oxygen saturation, reduction of enzymes, diminution in postnatal acidosis and recovery of the neurologic

---

[1] Arnold, H. W., *et al.*: Transition to extra-uterine life. Am. J. Nurs. 65:77-80, October, 1965; Desmond, M. M., *et al.*: The clinical behavior of the newly born: Part I, The term baby. J. Pediat. 62:307-325, March, 1963.

FIG. 16-1. A healthy newborn infant 4 hours after birth. MacDonald House, The University Hospitals of Cleveland, Cleveland, Ohio)

tissues from the trauma of labor and delivery. Since these changes take time, it is no wonder that the infant's natal day is so crucial to his life and future well-being.

Respiratory Changes

During the 4th month of pregnancy the infant apparently attempts respiratorylike movements. Some authorities feel that amniotic fluid is aspirated during this activity; others feel that the lungs actually manufacture amniotic fluid. At any rate, amniotic fluid seems to pass in and out of the lungs. Yet during gestation the lungs perform no other function.

Initiation of Respiration. With birth, however, profound changes occur. Now the lungs must exchange the oxygen and the carbon dioxide in the blood, work hitherto performed by the placenta. Exactly what initiates respiration is as yet unclear. It is believed to be a combination of physical, sensory and chemical factors, but precisely how each of these influences the other and to what degree is not known exactly. There is some evidence to indicate that the sudden change from intra-uterine to extra-uterine life produces enough physical stimulation to prompt respiration. It may be that the passive motion of the joints and the squeezing of the infant's thorax during delivery, as well as his spontaneous movements after birth, also contribute to minute ventilation and influence the other physical and sensory factors. It is worth noting in this regard that mothers of the various mammalian species, as they vigorously lick and cleanse their offspring after delivery, do, in fact, seem to apply a deliberate mechanical sensory stimulation to their young.

The chemical changes that occur in the blood as a result of the transitory asphyxia that occurs during delivery seem to be of paramount importance. These include a lowered oxygen level, an increased carbon dioxide level, and a lowered pH. If the asphyxia is prolonged, then depression of the respiratory center ensues rather than stimulation, and resuscitation is usually necessary (see Chap. 23). A vigorous infant often breathes seconds after birth and certainly within 1 minute of delivery.

A great effort is required to expand the lungs and to fill the collapsed alveoli. Surface tension in the respiratory tract as well as resistance in the lung tissue itself, the thorax, the diaphragm, and the respiratory muscles must be overcome. Moreover, any obstruction (i.e., mucus, etc.) in the air passages has to be cleared. The first active inspiration comes from a powerful contraction of the diaphragm, which creates a high negative intrathoracic pressure, causing a marked retraction of the ribs because of the pliability of the baby's thorax. This first inspiration distends the alveolar spaces which heretofore have been filled with fluid. Any remaining fluid that is left is reabsorbed rapidly if the pulmonary capillary blood flow is adequate, since it is hypotonic and passes easily into the capillaries. After several minutes of breathing, lung expansion should be complete.

Respiration in First and Second Periods of Reactivity. A healthy infant begins life with intense activity. This phase has been designated by some authorities as the 1st period of reactivity (see Suggested Reading). In this phase the infant exhibits outbursts of diffuse, purposeless movements which alternate with periods of relative immobility. At this time respiration is rapid (reaching as high as 80 breaths per minute), and there may be *transient* flaring of the alae nasi; retraction of the chest and grunting are not uncommon. Tachycardia also is present, at times reaching 180 beats per minute in the first minutes of life and thereafter falling to an average of 120 to 140 beats per minute.

After this initial response the baby becomes relatively quiet and does not respond intensely to either internal or external stimuli. He relaxes and may fall asleep. His first sleep occurs on an average of 2 hours after birth and may last anywhere from a few minutes to 2 to 4 hours.

When he awakes, he is again hyperresponsive to stimuli, and he begins his 2nd period of reactivity. His color may change rapidly (from pink to moderately cyanotic), and his heart rate responds to stimulation, becoming rapid. Oral mucus may be a major problem in respiration during this period. Choking, gagging and regurgitation alert the nurse to the presence of mucus, and appropriate intervention must be taken (see Chap. 23). Since the length of the 2nd period of reactivity is variable, the nurse must be particularly alert for the first 12 to 18 hours of the infant's life.

Character of Normal Respiration. As the infant adapts successfully to extra-uterine life, his respiration usually ranges from 35 to 50 breaths per minute. They are easily altered by internal and external stimuli. Normally, his respiration is quiet and shallow. This can be observed most accurately by watching the movement of the abdomen, since his respiratory activity is carried out largely by the diaphragm and the abdominal muscles. Periods of dyspnea and cyanosis may occur suddenly in an infant who is breathing normally (even after the transition period and after several days). This *may* indicate some anomaly or other pathologic condition and should be reported promptly. Therefore, the nurse should notify the physician if the respiration drops below 35 or increases beyond 50 when the infant is at rest, or if dyspnea or cyanosis occur.

Circulatory Changes

The anatomic changes that occur with birth have been discussed previously in Chapter 4. The nurse will recall that a rapid change takes place, with oxygenated blood being distributed in a manner similar to that of circulation in an adult.

Total Blood Volume. The amount of time between birth and the clamping of the umbilical cord is an important factor in determining the amount of the infant's total blood volume. For instance, the baby receives an additional 50 to 100 cc. of blood if the cord is clamped and cut after pulsations have ceased. This is due to the fact that as the uterus contracts, it pumps blood from the placenta into the baby's circulation. The increased blood volume is quickly readjusted through the elimination of excess fluid.

The peripheral circulation of the newborn is somewhat sluggish. It is felt that this accounts for the residual cyanosis of the infant's hands, feet and circumoral area. The nurse will note that these areas often remain mildly cyanotic for 1 or 2 hours after delivery. The general circulatory lability probably accounts for the mottled appearance of the baby's skin when it is exposed to air and for the "chilliness" of the infant's hands and feet.

The pulse rate, like the rate of respiration, also is labile and generally follows a pattern similar to that of the respiration. When the respiration is rapid, the pulse tends to be rapid; similarly, when the respiration slows down, so does the pulse. As previously stated, the pulse is affected by both internal and external stimuli, and thus the nurse can be more accurate if she counts the *apical* pulse rate while the baby is quiet. The normal rate is usually 120 to 150 beats per minute, but it may rise to 180 with crying and other intense activity. When the infant is asleep, the rate may range from 70 to 90 beats per minute.

The blood pressure is characteristically low, being around 80/46 at birth and rising to 100/50 by the 10th day. Since the extremities of the newborn are so small, accurate auscultation is difficult. If any accuracy is to be obtained, proper equipment is essential. A cuff 1 inch wide should be used and should cover two thirds of the upper arm or thigh.

Erythrocyte Count and Hemoglobin Concentration. The newborn infant has a much higher erythrocyte and hemoglobin level than an adult. The erythrocyte level ranges between 5,000,000 and 7,000,000 per microliter, and the hemoglobin level is usually 15 to 20 Gm. per 100 ml. of blood. These higher rates are needed by the baby in utero for adequate oxygenation. After birth the need no longer exists, since the lungs are functioning, and a gradual decrease takes place, particularly during the 2nd and the 3rd weeks of life. There is usually a slight *increase* in these concentrations on the 1st and the 2nd postnatal days; this is due in part to the extra amount of blood received through delayed clamping of the cord and to the subsequent readjustment of the blood volume. The gradual decrease in the erythrocyte count and the hemoglobin concentration results in a "physiologic" neonatal anemia, which disappears spontaneously. Clinical symptoms usually do not appear (except in cases of nutritional problems and/or infection), and no therapy is needed. The lowest counts are reached when the infant is 3 months old, when the hemoglobin level ranges between 11 and 12 Gm. per 100 ml. of blood, and the erythrocyte count between 4,000,000 and 4,300,000 per microliter; after that there is a gradual increase.

PHYSIOLOGIC JAUNDICE. Another effect of the destruction of the red blood cells is the so-called physiologic jaundice which usually is seen on the 2nd or the 3rd day of life. It is thought that an increase in serum bilirubin results from the breakdown of the red blood cells, and this, together with a temporary inability to remove the bilirubin, results in the jaundice. The condition usually begins to subside on the 6th or the 7th day, and it should disappear by the 2nd week of life. A bilirubin concentration of 13 mg. per 100 ml. of blood is beyond the physiologic limit and a total serum bilirubin above 18 to 20 mg. per 100 ml. is termed hyperbilirubinemia (see Chap. 23). Since the physiologic jaundice does not usually manifest itself until the infant is 2 or 3 days old, the nurse must be alert for any signs of jaundice before that time, especially in the first 24 hours of the baby's life. This latter type of jaundice is generally pathologic and should be reported immediately so that treatment can be instituted.

Blood Coagulation. Immediately after birth the intestinal tract of the infant does not harbor the bacteria necessary to help to synthesize the very important substance, vitamin K. Other substances important in blood coagulation are manufactured in the liver and are under the influence of vitamin K; these substances are temporarily diminished. Thus the infant suffers from a transitory deficiency in blood coagulation. This condition occurs between the 2nd and the 5th postnatal days and returns to normal spontaneously in several more days. Some physicians feel that this deficiency can be minimized or prevented by the administration of a small dose of vitamin K_1 at the time of birth (see Chaps. 13 and 23).

White Blood Cells. The normal newborn has a wide range in the total number of white blood cells. A leukocytosis (15,000 to 45,000 cells per microliter) is present at birth, with polymorphonuclear cells accounting for a large percentage of the total count. During the first few days after delivery there is a considerable decrease in the total count, as well as a shift in the type of predominating cell. The polymorphonuclear neutrophils decrease, and the lymphocytes increase, so that by the end of the 1st week the lymphocytes predominate.

Temperature Regulation and Metabolic Changes

The temperature-regulating mechanism of the newborn infant is not fully developed at birth; thus his heat production is somewhat low, and he responds readily to environmental heat and cold stimuli. At birth his body temperature is assumedly the same or higher than that of his mother; however, at birth it may drop 1 or 2 degrees in spite of the application of external heat and blankets. With chilling the drop is even more precipitous and dangerous for the baby. If the infant is given adequate covering and protection, the temperature soon begins to rise, and it returns to normal in about 8 hours. The nurse should keep in mind how easily the infant responds to environmental cold and heat and avoid subjecting the baby to wide variations in temperature.

Basal Metabolism. Since the surface area of the newborn is large in comparison with his weight, his basal metabolism per Kg. of body weight is higher than that of an adult.

Thus his CALORIC REQUIREMENTS are high during infancy. About 50 to 55 calories per pound of body weight per day suffice in the beginning. However, because of the increase in activity during the neonatal period and the energy requirements needed for the baby's rapid growth at this time, an increase in the caloric requirements may be needed after several days. Caloric needs will vary a good deal, even for infants of the same age and weight. Activity seems to be a determining factor. An infant who moves about a good deal, cries, etc., will need more calories than his more phlegmatic counterpart. The infant's caloric needs usually are based on weight-gain, well-being and satiety. A caloric intake of about 110 to 120 calories per Kg. of body weight per day (50 to 55 calories per pound per day) is usual after the first few days.

The infant's FLUID REQUIREMENT also is greater per Kg. of body weight than that of an adult. This is due to his increased muscular activity, caloric intake and basal metabolism.

Transitory Fever of the Newborn. This condition sometimes occurs between the 2nd and the 4th day of life. It is caused by a low fluid intake and the usual fluid loss that occurs in the immediate postnatal period. The temperature may rise as high as 38.9° to 40° C. (102° to 104° F.), the skin is dry, the fontanels may be depressed, the urinary output may be decreased, and a weight loss may occur. This condition is found most often in infants who do not take their feedings well (or who do not suck well) or in those who take only small, infrequent feedings. Both the fever and the subsequent side-effects can be remedied by increasing oral feedings (i.e., giving the baby water between milk feedings or administering parenteral fluids).

Neurologic Changes

The nervous system of the newborn is immature; that is, it is neither anatomically nor physiologically fully developed. Although all neurons are present, many remain immature for several months, and some, for years. Thus, the infant is uncoordinated in his movements, is labile in his temperature regulation, and has poor control over his musculature: he "startles" easily, is subject to tremors of the extremities, etc. However, during the neonatal period, development is rapid, and as the various nerve pathways controlling the muscles are used, the nerve fibers connect with one another. Gradually, more complex patterns of behavior emerge, and the higher cerebral levels begin to function.

Reflexes are important indices of the baby's normal development, for their presence or absence at certain times reflects the extent of normality in the functioning of the central nervous system.

The *Moro* or *startle reflex* (Fig. 16-2) indicates an awareness of equilibrium in the newborn. This reflex should be elicited when the baby is lying quiet. A sudden stimulus such as a change in position, a jarring of the crib, a jerking of the blanket or clothes, or even a loud noise (which jars his position) causes the baby to draw up his legs, to bring his arms forward in an embracing motion, and usually to cry. The movements should be symmetrical. If they are not, injury to the part that lags should be suspected. The Moro reflex should be present at birth; normally it disappears by 3 months of age. If it cannot be elicited at birth, edema of the brain may be present and/or injury to the brain. As the edema subsides, the reflex returns, and it should be demonstrable on the day following delivery. If frank brain damage has occurred, the reflex will be absent for several days; if the damage is not

FIG. 16-2. Moro reflex.

FIG. 16-3. Tonic neck reflex.

too severe, the reflex will return in 3 or 4 days. Occasionally, the reflex is present at birth but disappears over the first days. Increasing cerebral edema or slow intracranial hemorrhage then are suspected.

When the *tonic neck reflex* is elicited, the infant assumes a "fencing" position; that is, he lies on his back with his head rotated to one side. The arm and the leg on the side to which he is facing are partially or completely extended, and the opposite arm and leg are flexed (Fig. 16-3). This reflex also disappears in a few months, since it is another manifestation of the immaturity of the newborn's nervous system.

Several reflexes are involved in feeding. The *rooting reflex* causes the baby to turn his head toward anything that touches his cheek. This is helpful when he is searching for food. Brushing his cheek with the mother's breast, for example, enables him to find the nipple for nursing. The *sucking reflex* (Fig. 16-4) stimulates sucking movements whenever anything brushes the infant's lips. Normally, this reflex is present at birth and accompanies the *swallowing reflex*, absence of which indicates immaturity, narcosis, brain injury or retardation. Moreover, if it is not stimulated, it ceases to exist. The *gag reflex* operates when the infant takes more into his mouth than he can swallow. He can cough or hiccup a little if fluid does go "down the wrong way."

Since the infant is not well coordinated, he may have difficulty in bringing several of these reflexes into play at the proper moment, and he will need help from his mother or nurse. For instance, he may succeed in finding the nipple when he attempts to nurse, but if he gets the nipple under his tongue, successful sucking and swallowing are inhibited. It is important that the mother understand these feeding reflexes, so that she can help her infant. Often the inexperienced mother, in her anxiety to assist the infant to nurse, attempts to turn his head toward the breast by pushing on his cheek. The rooting reflex therefore is elicited, and the infant promptly turns his head in the opposite direction. This causes no end of consternation for both mother and baby.

The *grasp reflex* (Fig. 16-5) is present at birth in both the hands and the feet. The infant will grasp any object placed in his hands, cling briefly,

FIG. 16-4. Sucking reflex.

and then let go. Even at birth he may be able to hold onto an adult's forefinger so securely that he can be lifted to a standing position. Although the baby cannot actually grasp with his feet, stroking the soles causes the toes to turn downward as though trying to grasp. The grasping movements are a reflex action at birth, but with practice and experience they soon become voluntary and purposeful.

The *stepping* or *dancing reflex* is another action that is present at birth but soon disappears. This reflex causes the infant to make little stepping or prancing movements when he is held upright with his feet touching a surface. After this reflex diminishes, the infant will not attempt stepping motions until he is ready to stand and to walk. However, he does exercise the leg muscles a great deal and seems to derive a great deal of enjoyment from waving and kicking his legs about.

The next group of reflexes might be termed protective since they are necessary and at times essential to the preservation of the newborn's safety. The *blinking reflex* occurs when the infant is subjected to a bright light. The *cough and the sneeze reflexes* clear his respiratory passages. The *yawn reflex* draws in additional oxygen. These, together with the infant's ability to cry when uncomfortable, to withdraw from painful stimuli, to resist restraint, etc., are all defensive measures. As the baby grows and develops, these together with the other reflexes mentioned either diminish or become more highly developed according to the need. Thus, the infant's behavior patterns become more complex and highly developed.

Gastrointestinal Changes

It is well for the nurse to remember that the newborn, to be able to swallow, must have his food placed well back on his tongue, since he does not have the ability to transfer food from his lips to his pharynx. This means that the nipple should be placed well inside the infant's mouth. Sucking is facilitated by strong sucking muscles and ridges or corrugations in the anterior portion of the mouth. In addition, the *sucking pads* (deposits of fatty tissue in each cheek) prevent the collapse of the cheeks during nursing and further make sucking effective. This fatty tissue remains (even when fat is lost from the rest of the body) until sucking is no longer essential to the baby's getting food. The salivary glands are immature at birth and manufacture little saliva until the infant is about the age of 3 months.

Stomach, Intestines, Digestion. The capacity of the newborn's stomach is rather difficult to measure, since the feedings may empty easily

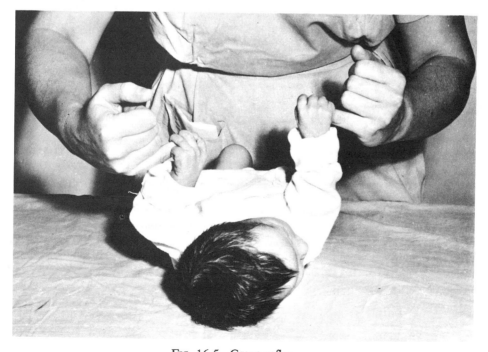

Fig. 16-5. Grasp reflex.

into the duodenum even before the feeding is completed. The capacity has been estimated to be approximately 50 to 60 cc. The cardiac sphincter is not as well developed as the pyloric sphincter, and hence the baby should be "bubbled" several times during the feeding so that any swallowed air can be eructed.

The newborn's intestinal tract is proportionately longer than that of an adult. Although it contains a large amount of secretory glands and a large surface for absorption, its elastic tissue and musculature are poor and not fully developed. Furthermore, nervous control is variable and inadequate. Nevertheless, the infant digests and absorbs a tremendous amount of food in proportion to his body weight.

Most of the digestive enzymes seem to be present and adequate, with the exception of pancreatic amylase and lipase. These last are somewhat deficient for several months but eventually reach a normal amount. The infant can digest simple foods more easily, but has a difficult time with the more complex starches. Protein and carbohydrates are easily absorbed, but fat absorption is poor.

REGURGITATION; VOMITING. The nurse and the mother will note that often the baby regurgitates (spits up) soon after a feeding. Sometimes regurgitation happens as long as 60 minutes after a feeding. This occurs because of the imperfect control of the cardiac sphincter and the immaturity of the nervous control. Activity also seems to be implicated, since the more active infant tends to spit up more often and for longer periods than the more quiet infant. The condition can be minimized by bubbling the infant well during and after feedings and by avoiding overfeeding. Handling the infant gently (and as little as possible) after feedings and placing him on his right side with his head and trunk elevated slightly also are helpful measures.

Occasionally, actual vomiting occurs during the first several days after birth. It is felt that this may be due to the secretions and material that were swallowed by the infant during delivery. Another cause is the swallowing of air by the infant during a feeding. This condition should subside within 2 or 3 days (with proper feeding, bubbling and positioning) and requires no special treatment. If the condition persists, however, or if the vomiting is of a projectile nature, then the physician should be notified immediately (see Chap. 23).

Stools. The baby's stools change daily during the first week of life, and their changes and amount should be recorded accurately (see p. 375-376)

Kidney Function and Urinary Excretion

The kidneys of the newborn function quite efficiently at birth. During fetal life, even though the placenta takes care of waste excretion, they become functional, and urine can be found in the bladder of the fetus as early as the 4th month of gestation. Excretion begins during the 9th week of gestation. Since the baby has urine in his bladder at birth, he may void at delivery; but sometimes urination is delayed for as long as 12 to 24 hours. Voidings during the first days after birth may be scanty and somewhat infrequent (unless edema is present) until feeding increases the fluid intake and consequent output. The number and the amount of voidings gradually increase until the infant is urinating as many as 30 times a day after the immediate postnatal period (see p. 376). With the development of bladder control, the frequency again decreases. The urine of the newborn (after the first voiding) has a high specific gravity and may appear to be quite cloudy due to the mucus and urate content as well as its high concentration. As the infant takes an increasing amount of fluid, the specific gravity gradually drops, and the cloudiness disappears, leaving the urine the usual straw color and almost odorless. Uric acid excretion is high in the newborn period, and this substance, when excreted on the diaper, may appear as reddish or "brick-dust" stains. Since the material looks like blood, it is sometimes thought that the infant is suffering from hematuria (see p. 376).

Changes in Hepatic Function

During fetal life the liver performs an important role in blood formation, and it is thought that it continues this function to some degree after birth. Later in the neonatal period it produces substances that are essential in the coagulation of the blood (see p. 348). If the mother's iron intake has been adequate during pregnancy, enough iron will be stored in the infant's liver to carry him over the first months of life when his diet (primarily milk) is iron-deficient. About the 5th month, however, the baby's iron reserve is depleted, and unless foods containing iron are given, a deficiency will ensue.

CHARACTERISTICS OF THE NEWBORN

Immediately after birth or within the next few hours the physician will give the infant a complete physical examination. This usually includes: head (fontanels, overriding of skull bones), eyes, mouth (palate, gums, tongue), heart, lungs, abdomen, extremities, genitalia and anus. The measurements of the infant are noted, such as the circumference of the head and the shoulders, and the weight and the length. The average full-term boy baby weighs from 7 to 7½ pounds (about 3,300 Gm.) at birth; girl babies weigh a little less. The average length of a full-term infant at birth is about 20 inches (51 cm.).

The physician will scrutinize the infant carefully for any deformity (e.g., cleft palate, clubfoot), injury (e.g., cephalhematoma, fracture of the clavicle) or abnormality (e.g., tonguetie, phimosis). If a malformation or an injury is found, the physician will advise concerning the infant's care and will assume the responsibility for telling the parents about their baby.

General Appearance

The nurse should be familiar with the characteristics of the normal newborn so that she can distinguish them from the abnormal. For example, certain symptoms which might be cause for concern in an older child (e.g., rapid rate and rhythm of respiration), when observed in a newborn infant, may merely represent normal neonatal physiology. Also, it is well for the nurse to take a look at him from the standpoint of how he appears to his mother. The healthy newborn infant has many characteristics which momentarily may look unusual to her. The nurse should be ready to talk with the mother about her baby and to answer her questions. A daily inspection sponge bath affords the nurse an excellent opportunity to observe the infant's anatomy and behavior, and thus to become familiar with the infant (see p. 372).

Position and Movements. The newborn infant usually lies with his arms and legs flexed, or tending to imitate the position that he has been accustomed to in utero. When the infant is awake, he sucks, yawns, sneezes, blinks and stretches. His movements for the most part are purposeless. For the first day or two he sleeps most of the time, but even while he is relaxed and quiet, he occasionally may exhibit some coarse, jerky movements. During the first few weeks of life he may lie with his head turned to one side

Fig. 16-6. Molding of the head.

and the arm and leg on that side extended, while the other arm and leg are drawn up (tonic neck reflex). If he is awakened suddenly or startled by jarring or a loud noise, he will thrust his arms out in an "embracing motion" (Moro reflex).

Head. The infant's head is large, comprising about one quarter of his size, and with cephalic presentations may initially appear to be asymmetrical because of the molding of the skull bones during labor. The suture lines between the skull bones and the anterior and the posterior fontanels can be palpated easily (Fig. 5-1). When the nurse's hand is passed over the fontanels, the areas should feel soft but neither bulged nor depressed. The anterior fontanel, the diamond-shaped and larger of the two (normally 2 to 3 cm. wide and 3 to 4 cm. long), may feel smaller for the first several days when there is marked overriding of the skull bones. The posterior fontanel is triangular in shape and is located between the occipital and the parietal bones. It is smaller than the anterior fontanel and may be almost closed at birth. Occasionally, the scalp is covered with a thick growth of hair which sheds for the most part before the permanent hair appears.

The face is small and round, and the lower jaw appears to recede.

Eyes and Visual Perception. The eyes are closed much of the time but will open spontaneously if the infant's head is lifted (a valuable point to remember when one wants to inspect

Fig. 16-7. Erythema toxicum. This "newborn rash" develops more frequently on the back, the shoulders and the buttocks. (MacDonald House, The University Hospitals of Cleveland, Cleveland, Ohio)

the eyes). Recent research[2] has indicated that the infant from birth can see and discriminate

[2] Fantz, R. L.: Pattern discrimination and selective attention as determinants of perceptual development from birth *in* Kidd, A. H., and Rivoire, J. L. (eds.): Perceptual Development in Children, New York, International Universities Press, 1965.

patterns as the basis for form perception. This capacity is rather limited by imperfect oculomotor coordination and inability to accommodate for varying distances. Moreover, the eye, the usual pathways and the visual part of the brain are poorly developed at birth. Nevertheless, although the baby's vision is much less acute than an

Fig. 16-8. Preparation of the infant, restrained for circumcision. (*Left*) Board, padded and covered with plastic, as used in many hospitals for circumcision. (*Right*) The infant, restrained on the board with towels, ready for circumcision.

Fig. 16-9. Technique of circumcision, using hemostat, scalpel and sutures. After cleansing penis and surrounding area, the prepuce is stripped back with the help of a partial dorsal slit (A to D). The prepuce is now clamped and excessive prepuce cut off (E). The suture material used is plain 00 or 000 catgut in a very small needle (F and G), but some physicians prefer silk.

adult's, a good deal of visual experience is possible for him. Visual patterning seems to be particularly stimulating or interesting to him, more so than color or brightness alone. For instance, he will show a preference for a face or a solid object rather than a blob of light or a bright color. Thus, even the newborn sees a patterned and organized world which he explores discriminatingly (albeit with his limited means). When and how his visual contact with environment makes a lasting impression on his behavior remain topics for future research. Most mothers do not realize that their infant can see as well as he does, and they appreciate being informed of this fact. In addition, some mothers become exceedingly anxious when they observe strabismus or nystagmus in their infants, but they should be reassured that

this lack of coordination is normal during the first few months of life.

All babies' eyes are blue or a slatey gray color at birth. By the time that the infant is 3 months old, they have achieved their permanent color, although complete pigmentation of the iris does not occur until the infant is about 1 year of age. Since the lacrimal glands are not functioning at birth, the baby does not shed tears when he cries. Tears do not appear for several weeks and sometimes for several months. There may be some edema of the lids and/or purulent discharge caused by the silver nitrate (see p. 367). The changes in the vascular tension of the eyes during delivery sometimes cause small areas of subconjunctival hemorrhage. These areas disappear spontaneously in 1 or 2 weeks and are not significant.

Ears and Hearing. The ear and the nerve tracts for hearing are anatomically mature at birth, and the newborn can hear after his first cry. Hearing apparently becomes acute within several days as the eustachian tubes become aerated, and the mucus in the middle ear disappears.

Lips, Mouth, Cheeks. The lips are sensitive to touch, and any stimulation of this nature usually elicits the sucking reflex. Moreover, the rooting reflex is well developed, so that when the cheek is stroked on one side the infant will turn his head in that direction. In conjunction with sucking, a labial tubercle may be present on the center of the upper lip, as well as the sucking pads (fat) in the cheeks. At this time the tongue does not extend far beyond the margin of the gums because the frenum is normally short. A mother's concern that her baby is tonguetied is usually unwarranted.

It is well known that during the first 2 months of life the newborn infant has a great need to suck and will usually suck on anything that comes

-in contact with his lips. Newborn infants can suck while sleeping and nonnutritive sucking can have a quieting effect on excited babies. One study revealed, when infants sucking on pacifiers were tested during ordinary restful sleep, that sucking renders the sleeping infant unresponsive to external stimuli.[3]

Body; Skin. The infant's neck is short. His chest is round and slightly smaller in circumference than his head. The breasts may be engorged initially and may even secrete "witch's milk." This condition, like menstruation, a vaginal tag or enlarged labia in girl babies, is due to a hormonal factor and without interference will disappear spontaneously. In boy babies the scrotum appears to be relatively large, and the prepuce is long and adherent to the glans penis (this separates in several months). The abdomen is round and protruding due to the relative size of

---

[3] Wolff, P. H., and Simmons, M. A.: Nonnutritive sucking and response thresholds in young infants. Child Develop. 38:631-638, 1967.

FIG. 16-10. Technique of circumcision with Yellen clamp. After cleansing area and stripping back prepuce as shown in Figure 15-9, the cone of the Yellen clamp is placed over the glans and the prepuce put on a stretch with sutures (A). The prepuce is now drawn through the beveled hole of platform (B). Screwing down clamp crushes prepuce, producing hemostasis. Three to 5 minutes of such pressure is necessary to prevent subsequent bleeding. The excess of the prepuce is then cut away (C) and the clamp removed (D). (Yellen, H. S.: Am. J. Obst. & Gynec. 30:146)

Fig. 16-11. Postcircumcision inspection for bleeding.

the abdominal organs and weak muscular structures. The respiratory movements are largely diaphragmatic, and breathing is rapid, shallow and irregular.

The infant's skin appears to be thin and delicate and is often dry and peeling. The baby's color may be pink, reddish or pale, becoming very ruddy when he cries. Initially, the hands and the feet are quite blue, due to the sluggish peripheral vascular circulation, but this cyanosis of the extremities soon disappears, often within a few hours. Vernix caseosa, a white cheesy material which has been a protection to the skin while the fetus is floating in amniotic fluid in the uterus, may be apparent, particularly in the creases of the body. Also, on the body there may be large areas of fine downy hair called lanugo. Milia may be present on the nose and the forehead, and small flat hemangiomas may be apparent on the nape of the neck, the eyelids or over the bridge of the nose. These so-called "stork bites," clusters of small capillaries, usually disappear spontaneously during infancy.

In nonwhite infants, dark bluish areas are usually apparent on the buttocks or the lower back. These "mongolian spots" have no relationship to mongolism and will disappear spontaneously during late infancy. A pilonidal "dimple"

resulting from an irregular fold of skin sometimes is seen in the midline over the sacrococcygeal area.

Miscellaneous Conditions

At times the following conditions are seen in the normal newborn infant. Although they are not serious, they do represent some deviation from what is "usual." Moreover, they often cause concern in the parents; thus the nurse should be familiar with them so that she can answer any questions that the parents may have and give appropriate reassurance.

Icterus Neonatorum. This is an exceedingly common condition during the 1st week of life and, as the name implies, is characterized by jaundice. Physiologic jaundice is dependent on the normal neonatal rise in the serum bilirubin level (see p. 348). It makes its appearance, as a rule, on the 2nd or the 3rd day of life and disappears without treatment about the 6th or the 7th day. Almost 1 baby in 3 shows icterus, which often is due to physiologic jaundice. Most authorities attribute it to inadequate liver function and the destruction of red cells which takes place during the 1st week of life. The mother may be assured that the condition is due to a normal process and will clear up within a few days.

Erythema Toxicum. Sometimes referred to as the newborn rash, erythema toxicum is a blotchy

Fig. 16-12. Hypertrophy of breast in infant developing in the neonatal period.

erythematous rash which may appear in the first few days of life (Fig. 16-7). The erythematous areas, which develop more frequently on the back, the shoulders and the buttocks, have a small blanched wheal in the center. The cause of this skin disturbance is obscure, and no treatment is necessary. The rash is transient and likely to change appreciably within a few hours, and it may disappear entirely within a day or so.

Milia are pinpoint-sized pearly white spots which occur commonly on the nose and the forehead of the newborn infant. When touched gently with the tip of the finger, these spots feel like tiny, firm seeds. They are due to retention of sebaceous material within the sebaceous glands, and if they are left alone, will usually disappear spontaneously during the neonatal period. Mothers often mistake milia for "whiteheads" and may attempt to squeeze them if the nurse or the physician has not warned them against such practice.

Phimosis. In many male infants the orifice in the foreskin of the penis is so small that the foreskin cannot be pushed back over the glans. This condition is known as phimosis. Although it is rarely of sufficient degree to obstruct the outflow of urine or to cause any immediate symptoms, it is undesirable because it prevents proper cleanliness. Phimosis may be corrected either by stretching the orifice of the foreskin with a hemostat, or by circumcision. Both of these procedures are carried out by the physician, but sometimes the nurse is asked to stretch the foreskin gently every

day after having first received detailed instructions from the physician. Preparation of an infant for circumcision, two common methods of performing the operation, and also postcircumcision inspection are depicted in Figures 16-8 to 11.

Breast Engorgement. Engorgement of the breasts is common during the neonatal period in both male and female infants (Fig. 16-12). It is due to the same causes that bring about mammary engorgement in the mother—that is, endocrine influence. In the case of the infant, its breasts have been acted on throughout pregnancy by the estrogenic hormone which passes to it through the placenta from the mother. This is the same hormone which prepares the mother's breasts for lactation. When it is withdrawn after birth, changes in the infant's breasts take place similar to those in the mother.

Mammary engorgement in the newborn subsides without treatment, but sometimes it persists for 2 or 3 weeks.

Menstruation occasionally occurs in newborn girls and is due to estrogenic hormone, as just described. It usually amounts only to slight spotting and need cause no special concern.

THE ENVIRONMENT OF THE NEWBORN

Prevention of Infection

The prevention of infection is of paramount importance in caring for the newborn. Everyone who is in contact with infants must assume this

Fig. 16-13. The central nursery. (MacDonald House, The University Hospitals of Cleveland, Cleveland, Ohio)

responsibility; this includes parents as well as personnel. Staff should take special care to instruct parents so that their activities conform to the prevention of infection. The basis of "good" technique in handling the infant is thorough hand washing with an antiseptic detergent or a soap (or detergent) containing hexachlorophene. Some institutions require scrubbing with a brush; others feel that detergent, water and friction are sufficient. Whichever the procedure, meticulous hand washing is essential, whether the infant is cared for in the central or regular nursery or in a rooming-in situation. The parents and the staff should be especially careful to wash their hands before a feeding and after a diaper change. The parents will need instruction about the importance (and technique) of proper hand washing, and reinforcement should be given as necessary during the hospital stay.

As with personnel in the delivery room (see Chap. 13), all nursery staff should have a pre-employment physical examination and a yearly physical examination thereafter to minimize the possibility of spreading infection from the staff among the newborn. In addition, any staff member who contracts *any* infection (i.e., respiratory, gastrointestinal, skin lesions, etc.) should remain away from the nursery and contact with the newborn until the infection is gone *completely*.

If the mother manifests signs of infection and has been in contact with her infant, the infant will be isolated from the other babies (usually in the isolation or observation nursery) and will be removed from the mother's presence until her disorder is treated and cleared. Since the mother may be concerned about being separated from her baby and miss him, the importance of the precautions should be explained thoroughly. If the mother is concerned about continuing breastfeeding (and her condition permits), her breasts can be pumped to ensure stimulation and a continued supply of milk. Her milk is discarded, how-

FIG. 16-14. Rooming-in 2-bed unit.

ever, as an added precaution, until her infection subsides. The mother who has not had contact with her infant before she evidences signs of infection, also will be separated from her infant, and the foregoing explanation and management of feeding is applicable to her also.

Babies who are delivered outside a hospital environment are not admitted to the regular newborn nursery. They usually are cared for in the observation nursery or with the mother in a rooming-in situation.

To further reduce the hazards of infection from outside sources, the number of visitors may be restricted in the maternity area, and no visitors are allowed in the nursery proper. Children also are excluded from the maternity unit, since various infections and particularly communicable diseases are so prevalent among them. To further ensure cleanliness, members of the staff wear special gowns when they care for infants. These gowns should be short-sleeved so that a thorough scrub or wash may be given the hands, the forearms and the elbows, and the gowns should be changed for each "shift" and more frequently if soiled.

Masks are no longer worn, since they must be changed every 20 to 30 minutes to be effective, and, in fact, they can become a reservoir of bacteria when not applied and changed properly. Occasionally, the mother will be instructed to wear a mask in tending the baby if she has had a recent cold, or if she develops a cold when she goes home. The nurse should make certain that she understands the principles underlying the application and the wearing of the mask and especially that she be aware of how her hands can be contaminated in adjusting and tying it. Even at home a clean mask should be worn each time the need arises, and the mother should be instructed to wash her hands each time after she adjusts it.

Types of Care for the Newborn

The Central Nursery System. The central or general newborn nursery on the postpartal division is designed for the care of a variable number of healthy newborn infants (Fig. 16-13). In this system the infants are brought to their mothers at certain specified times during the day—generally for feeding and/or visiting. The staff assumes the responsibility for all the care of the babies. Some authorities feel that the separation of mother and child (and husband) in this manner results in an unnatural fragmentation of the family at a momentous time for building family unity (see Suggested Reading). Also with the emergence of the many drug-resistant organisms that abound in the hospital environment, the danger of epidemics (whenever a large aggregate of persons collect) is enhanced. Certainly, in a central nursery system the contact among the mother, the infant and the father is not as extensive as it would be in a rooming-in plan. However, the hospital's physical plant may make a central nursery arrangement the only type feasible. Moreover, some mothers prefer the type of care that is given under a central nursery system for a variety of reasons. At any rate, some type of central nursery usually is found in most hospitals. Control of the physical facilities and stringent personnel policies accomplish a good deal of protection of the newborn so managed. For instance, cribs should be placed at least 2 feet apart with 3-feet-wide aisles between the cribs. Limiting the number of infants in a nursery from 8 to 12 also is helpful. Requiring all personnel to put on clean gowns before entering the nursery, limiting the number of individuals who may enter the nursery, and requiring strict adherence to nursery aseptic technique on the part of nursery personnel, all aid in protecting the infants. Washing the hands and arms to the elbows and scrubbing the fingernails thoroughly before entering the nursery, as well as washing the hands carefully before and after handling each baby, afford additional protection.

The central nursery is a so-called "clean" nursery. But it must be understood that there is a difference in nursery technique between what is considered to be "nursery clean" and what is considered to be "baby clean" (i.e., what is clean for an individual baby). There should be no common equipment, such as a common bath table, used in providing care for the babies. There should be provisions in the nursery so that individual technique can be followed. Each infant should have his own crib and general supplies, so that he can be given such care as his daily inspection bath or be diapered or dressed in his own bed. Most cribs are constructed with a built-in cabinet for the infant's own supplies (clean diapers, shirts and linens) and a drawer to hold the containers for cotton balls, safety pins, thermometer, etc. When such cribs are not available, improvised units for the infant's crib

should be obtained so that individual-care technique can be carried out.

If there is any evidence of a questionable infection at the time of delivery, if the infant is born on the way to the hospital, or if the infant is suspected of having an infection of the eyes, the skin, the mouth or the gastrointestinal tract, the infant should not be admitted to the central nursery.

Observation Nursery. Maternity hospitals should have an observation nursery where infants suspected of developing an infectious condition may be kept until the presence or absence of infection is determined. When a definite diagnosis of infection is made, the infant must be transferred immediately to an isolation nursery away from the maternity division.

Aside from the fact that infants in the "suspect" or observation nursery must be segregated from others, and naturally require closer supervision and care because of suspected infection, their nursing care otherwise should be like that given a healthy newborn infant.

Rooming-in. This term has been applied to the plan of having the new infant share his mother's hospital unit so that they may be cared for together. This type of arrangement has come to mean much more than caring for the mother and the infant in the same unit of space. Rather, it implies an attitude in maternal and infant care that supports parental education and is based on recognition and understanding of the needs of each mother, infant and family. Rooming-in often is discussed as if it were a modern innovation. Historically, however, all mothers back to paleolithic times "roomed-in" until the central nursery was instituted during the first 2 decades of the 20th century (see Suggested Reading). Nevertheless, rooming-in as it is practiced today does represent a departure from the concept of the "traditional" central nursery.

Attitudes in maternal and infant care have changed, in part because of increased insight into the needs of the mother, her baby and the family as a unit. Rooming-in plays an important part in the family-centered approach to maternity care, for it not only provides an environment which fosters a wholesome, natural mother-child relationship from the very beginning, but it also affords unlimited opportunities for the parents to learn about the care of their baby.

To have a rooming-in program function successfully requires administrative planning and sound preparation of the entire hospital staff and

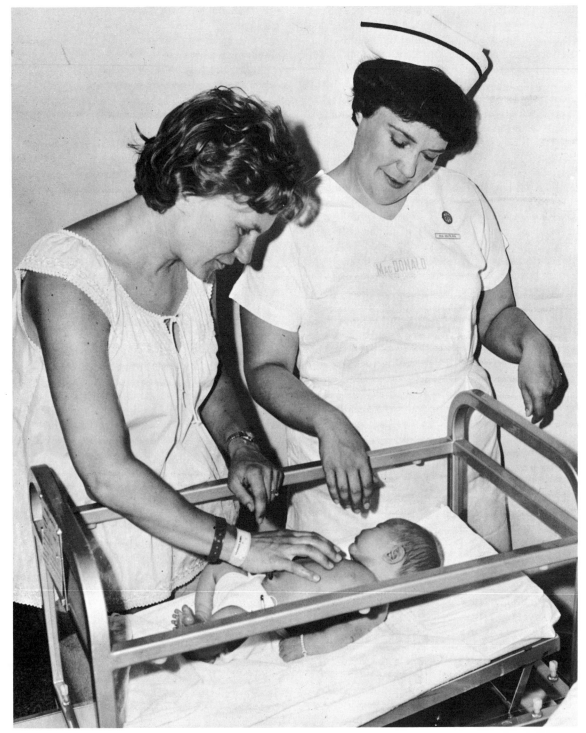

FIG. 16-15. Rooming-in arrangement. Mother has opportunity to learn about her new baby. (Mac-Donald House, The University Hospitals of Cleveland, Cleveland, Ohio)

the parents who use it. Generally, it demands a different architectural arrangement. Adequate space must be allowed for the mother's unit to accommodate the regular equipment needed for her, as well as that needed for the infant's care. Different physical plans for rooming-in arrangements have been developed, some units to accommodate one mother, others for as many as four of them. Each rooming-in unit should have an adjoining nursery and its own workroom. Where it has not been feasible to make major changes in the physical plan of a maternity hospital to provide for continuous rooming-in, some hospitals have adopted a modified rooming-in program, providing extended time for the mother and her baby to be together during the day but otherwise utilizing the central nursery.

The newborn infant must be protected from sources of infection regardless of where he is cared for. The same basic principles for asepsis employed in the nursery must be followed in infant care in the rooming-in unit. Some years ago Dr. Edith Jackson said that it was possible to provide "the essential psychological satisfactions" which the mother and baby derive from a rooming-in experience "without losing the hard-won safeguards to physical health."[4] This has been demonstrated, for epidemic infections, such as diarrhea and skin infections, which sometimes occur in large hospital nurseries have not been observed in rooming-in programs.

Individual mothers must be taken into consideration as to whether or not they should have rooming-in. Some mothers will want to have their babies with them most of the time so that they can get to know them and learn to care for them under the guidance of the nurses and the physicians. Other mothers may not want rooming-in, particularly multiparas, because they feel that this is an opportunity for rest and freedom from responsibility. Many mothers feel that they would enjoy rooming-in but hesitate because they do not feel sufficiently able to assume the care or the responsibility for the baby at this time. These mothers need help, of course, to understand that the nurse is there to help them, and that they do not have to take over any more of the infant's care than they feel able or want to do. It is interesting to note that research[5] has indicated

Fig. 16-16. Maternal touch in an initial contact of mother with her newborn. (MacDonald House, The University Hospitals of Cleveland, Cleveland, Ohio)

that these negative feelings and qualifications are not as significant or widespread as one might think.

Nurses with understanding and interest often can anticipate the mother's needs and desires and can be of invaluable help to her. Much of the practical care of the new baby must be learned by the new mother during her brief hospital stay to supplement the theoretical knowledge she has gained during the antepartal period. At this time the mother usually needs close supervision and guidance from the nurse so that she may develop confidence in her own ability to handle and care for her baby. The father, also, may share in some of these experiences and learn much about his baby and his baby's care. With this kind of preparation, parents of first babies in particular do not feel so helpless when they return home. These shared experiences undoubtedly contribute to an excellent foundation for stable and secure family relationships.

[4] Jackson, E. B.: Should mother and baby room together? Am. J. Nurs. 46:17, 1946.

[5] Ringholz, S., and Morris, M.: A test of some assumptions about rooming-in. Nurs. Res. 10:196-199, Fall, 1961.

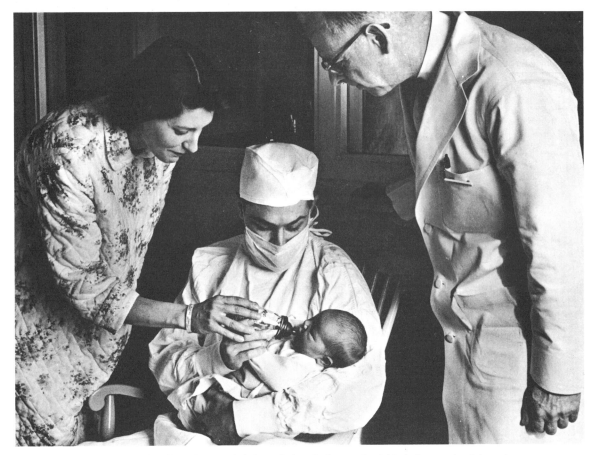

Fig. 16-17. Rooming-in unit. Mother is assisting father to feed his baby as physician observes.

NURSING CARE OF THE NEWBORN

Initial Care

In the delivery room the initial care has been given to the infant's eyes and the cord, and appropriate identification has been added. The baby should be watched to see that he is kept warm (a most important detail), that respiration is normal, that color is good and that there is no bleeding from the cord (see Chap. 13).

It is customary in many maternity hospitals today to provide a "receiving" nursery on the labor and delivery division so that closer supervision and care for the infant may be assured immediately following the delivery.

Observations

The infant's natal day, as previously stated, is the most hazardous during the postnatal period. Therefore, it is important that the nurse take particular care with her observations during the first 24 hours of the baby's life. The receiving or transition nursery in the labor or the nursery sections affords an excellent physical environment (similar to that of recovery room care for adults) for the extensive observations that are necessary (see Suggested Reading). "High-risk" babies (infants who have been exposed to or have experienced a prolonged labor, difficult labor, fetal distress, maternal complications during pregnancy and/or labor, respiratory distress, etc.) especially need intensive observation and often special equipment for their care, such as incubators, suction equipment, etc.

Behavior and Physiologic Responses. Because these are indicative of normal reactions in the newborn, they should be observed and recorded, as well as any abnormal signs. For instance, the frequency and the type of cry are important, since the infant aerates his lungs in this way. Moreover, the type of cry may be indicative of cerebral damage (see Chap. 23). In a vigorous, normal infant the cry should be lusty and should

Fig. 16-18. Rooming-in arrangement. Mother cares for her newborn. (MacDonald House, The University Hospitals of Cleveland, Cleveland, Ohio)

occur especially when the baby is handled or moved. If this does not happen, and the infant seems "sleepy" or depressed, it may be necessary to stimulate him to cry every hour or more frequently, depending on the degree of depression. This response may be aroused by changing his position or rubbing his back, head or feet. Occasionally, with a drowsy infant it becomes necessary to slap or rub the soles of the feet *gently* to elicit the necessary cry. The time of the baby's first stool and voiding should be noted, for this will give an indication of proper excretory function. It is sometimes necessary for the nurse to check with the delivery room records to see

whether the infant voided or defecated at delivery. Finally, the newborn's general activity, muscle tone and reflexes (especially the Moro and the sucking reflexes) should be observed. A healthy infant will be active, evidence good muscle tone and respond with behavior appropriate to the various reflexes (see pp. 349-351).

Respiration and Color. These should be given close attention, for they are good indices of whether or not the newborn is experiencing respiratory insufficiency. Dyspnea, rapid respiration exceeding 50 breaths per minute, and persistent cyanosis should be reported to the physician. Since mucus in the nasopharynx often

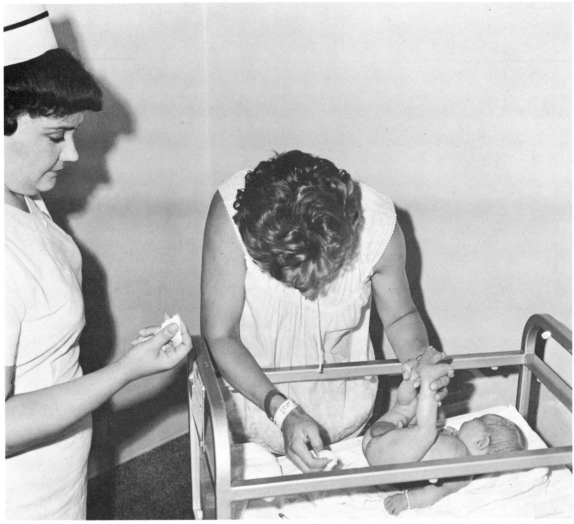

FIG. 16-19. Rooming-in arrangement. Nurse provides guided learning experiences for mother caring for her newborn. (MacDonald House, The University Hospitals of Cleveland, Cleveland, Ohio)

causes respiratory distress, the nurse should be particularly watchful for its presence. Gagging, vomiting, breath holding, retraction of the head, choking and cyanosis are all signs of the presence of mucus. It is particularly prone to develop in the 2nd period of reactivity following the first sleep. Postural drainage and the technique for aspirating mucus are explained in Chapter 23.

Condition of the Cord. This should be noted; any oozing or hemorrhage should be reported immediately, and the cord should be reclamped or retied as indicated. Oozing more often occurs between the 2nd and the 6th hours of life and frequently is associated with crying or the passage of meconium.

The baby's skin should be observed also for pallor and jaundice as well as cyanosis. Pressing the skin with a finger often enables clearer visualization of jaundice. The blanching that occurs with the maneuver provides a contrast that shows up the icteric color more clearly. The significance of pallor and jaundice in the first 24 hours is explained in Chapter 23.

The infant's temperature should be checked frequently (every hour), and particularly if external heat is being applied. Even though the infant's temperature may have been quite low at first, he responds readily to external changes in temperature. Therefore, care must be taken that he does not become overheated.

Continuing Care

Cleansing. The daily cleansing of the infant affords the nurse an excellent opportunity for making the observations that are necessary during the immediate postnatal period. The materials used for the bath, its frequency, etc., may vary from institution to institution. Several decades ago the daily soap and water and oil baths were replaced with merely wiping off excess vernix with dry or slightly moist cotton balls. The diaper area was cleansed as necessary. However, in view of the increase in staphylococcal infections in newborn nurseries, the American Academy of Pediatrics recommends a sponge bath with a liquid detergent containing 3 per cent hexachlorophene after birth and every other day thereafter. A sponge bath is necessary until the cord drops off. In most institutions the suggestions of the Academy of Pediatrics are adhered to. On alternate days the diaper area and other soiled areas are cleansed with warm water as necessary. Thus some cleansing of the infant occurs daily, and the nurse should utilize the opportunity to inspect the baby thoroughly.

Assessing the Mother's Understanding. In the verbal exchanges with the mother during the daily care of the baby it is important that the nurse assess the mother's understanding and her skill in caring for her infant. Any basic principles or procedures related to infant care that the mother finds necessary and useful should be part of the nurse's teaching plan for the mother during her hospital stay. A referral to a public health agency may be necessary to ensure appropriate follow-up, particularly if the mother is inexperienced. The following principles of care can be conveyed easily to the mother (and the father when he is present).

Eyes. In the daily care of the baby no special treatment other than necessary cleansing with sterile water is given the baby's eyes unless there is a discharge. Any redness, swelling or discharge should be reported and recorded on the chart. There may be some reaction from the medication used for prophylaxis against ophthalmia neonatorum, but the physician will prescribe treatment if necessary.

Cord. Babies do not receive a tub bath until the cord has separated, and the umbilicus has healed. A cord dressing is considered to be unnecessary in most hospitals since exposure to the air enhances drying of the cord; nevertheless, it is still used in some institutions. If a cord dressing is used, it is removed when it becomes soiled, or when the baby is taken to the nursery for its initial bath. If the cord is left exposed to the air, some physicians prefer that the base be wiped with alcohol daily to encourage drying further and to discourage the possibility of infection.

No attempt should be made to dislodge the cord before it separates completely. If there is a red inflamed area around the stump or any discharge with an odor, this condition should be recorded and brought to the physician's attention immediately. The cord usually becomes detached from the body between the 5th and the 8th days after birth, but its detachment may be delayed until the 12th or the 14th day without causing any concern (Fig. 16-20). When the cord drops off,

Fig. 16-20. The umbilical cord drying.

the umbilicus is depressed somewhat and usually free from any evidence of inflammation. No further treatment is necessary, except to keep the part clean and dry. When inflammation is present, the physician will give specific orders for care.

Adherent Foreskin. In a male infant, adhesions between the prepuce and the glans penis are very common. The foreskin may be extended beyond the glans. Reduction to a very small opening is spoken of as phimosis (see p. 358). A curdy secretion, called smegma, may form in considerable amount and collect under the prepuce behind the glans. Also, small amounts of urine may be retained. Any of these conditions favor irritation and, if found, should be reported to the obstetrician. He may perform the delicate operations of separating the adhesions, stretching the prepuce or circumcising the baby.

The manipulation following dilation and retraction is difficult at first, and should be done gently. The foreskin must be replaced immediately; if not, edema may result, rendering the replacing difficult.

Care Following Circumcision. When the newborn infant is circumcised, the main principles of postoperative care are to keep the wound clean and to observe it closely for bleeding (Fig. 16-11). For the first 24 hours the area is covered with a sterile gauze dressing to which a liberal amount of sterile petrolatum has been added.

Mothers are naturally anxious about their babies at this time, so, as soon as it is feasible after the circumcision has been done, the nurse should take the baby to his mother for a brief visit. She can be reassured that the procedure has not been very painful for her child. The infant will cry during the operation, but this is due as much to the necessary restraints as to the discomfort. Occasionally, a local anesthetic will be used, but generally the procedure is performed without it. Thus, the infant may be fed immediately after the circumcision, and both mother and baby seem to enjoy the comfort that the feeding and cuddling bring. It is unwise, however, to keep the baby away too long from the careful observation of the nurse.

FIG. 16-21. Inspection of cord stump.

Fig. 16-22. Retracting foreskin for cleansing penis (uncircumcised). (MacDonald House, The University Hospitals of Cleveland, Cleveland, Ohio)

The infant's diaper should be applied so that only one layer of the material covers the penis. This lessens the danger of masking any bleeding that might occur. In changing the infant's diaper the nurse should hold his ankles with one hand so that he cannot kick against the operative area. Unless the physician orders otherwise, the circumcision dressing can be removed postoperatively when the infant voids for the first time. If a length of petrolatum gauze was applied firmly to the site of operation, the physician may wish it to be left in place for 24 hours. Cleansing must be done gently but can be accomplished as necessary with cotton balls moistened with warm tap water. A fresh sterile petrolatum dressing usually is applied to the penis each time the diaper is changed for the first day. The penis must be observed closely for bleeding, and during the first 12 hours should be inspected every hour. It is advisable to place the infant's crib where he can be watched conveniently. Moreover, to keep all the nursing personnel alerted, some signal, such as a red tag, can be attached to the identification card on the crib. If bleeding occurs, usually it can be controlled with gentle pressure. Some physicians leave a p.r.n. order for local application of

Adrenalin 1:1,000 solution to the bleeding point; but if bleeding persists, the physician should be notified immediately.

Since the length of the maternity stay has been considerably shortened, circumcision may be done on the 2nd or the 3rd postnatal day or even before the baby leaves the delivery room. To overcome the transitory coagulation deficiency, some physicians administer vitamin K_1 at birth. Sometimes the operation is performed on the day preceding discharge; therefore the nurse should ascertain the physician's wishes for aftercare and make certain that the mother knows how to care for her newly circumcised infant. Generally, the care will be the same as that described.

Care of Girl Babies. Similar adhesions sometimes are found about the clitoris in female infants and, when observed, should be reported to the obstetrician. The smegma which may accumulate between the folds of the labia should be gently and carefully cleansed with moistened cotton balls, using the front-to-back direction and a clean cotton ball for each stroke. Occasionally, a slight bloody discharge may come from the vagina (see p. 358). This usually is due to a hormonal reaction and rarely reappears; cleanliness is the only treatment necessary. Very infrequently, the discharge may be caused by injury; if the discharge persists, it should be reported to the doctor.

Weight. The baby should be weighed on the birth date and every day or every other day thereafter. If the infant remains in the hospital longer than 5 days, he should be weighed at intervals prescribed by the medical staff. His weight should be recorded accurately.

During the first few days after birth the infant may lose 5 to 10 per cent of his birth weight. This is due partly to the minimal intake of nutrients and fluid and partly to the loss of excess fluid. About the time the meconium begins to disappear from his stools, the weight begins to increase, and in normal cases does so regularly until about the 10th day of life, when it may equal the birth weight. Then the baby should begin to gain from 4 to 6 ounces per week during the first 5 months. After this time the gain is from 2 to 4 ounces weekly. At 6 months of age the baby should be double his birth weight, and he should triple it when a year old. This is one way to note the baby's condition and progress; when the baby is not gaining, that fact should be reported to the physician. Besides gaining regularly in weight and strength, the baby should be happy and good-natured when awake and inclined to sleep a good part of the time between feedings.

Pulse and Temperature. The clinical record of a normal baby should show a variation in pulse of 120 to 150. Only experience can teach a nurse to count an infant's pulse rate accurately (see p. 347). Touching his wrist will generally startle him and noticeably accelerate the heart beat. The pulse can always be felt at the temporal artery to best advantage, particularly during sleep. The rectal temperature may normally vary a whole degree (see p. 348). A premature baby, who may have a temperature below that of a normal baby, will stabilize his temperature within 24 to 72 hours somewhere between 96° and 98° F., depending on his weight—the smaller the baby, the lower the temperature will be.

Crying. After the baby is born and has cried lustily, he becomes quiet and usually sleeps. After the eyes, the cord and the skin have received the necessary care, he is dressed and placed in a warm crib and usually does not cry unless he is wet, hungry, ill or is moved. A nurse soon will learn to distinguish an infant's condition and needs from the character of his cry, which may be described as follows. A loud, insistent cry with drawing up and kicking of the legs usually denotes colicky pain; a fretful cry, if due to indigestion, will be accompanied by green stools and passing of gas; a whining cry is noticeable when the baby is ill, premature or very frail; a fretful, hungry cry, with fingers in the mouth and flexed, tense extremities, is easily recognized; and there is a peculiar, shrill, sharp-sounding cry which suggests injury. A nurse should make every effort to recognize any deviation from the usual manner in which a baby announces his normal requirements. Moreover, she should convey this information to the mother, since it is essential that the mother learn to interpret her infant's cues. The

FIG. 16-23. Taking axillary temperature.

FIG. 16-24. I.M. injection for infant.

newborn has only his posture and his voice at this time to inform others of his needs.

"HYPERTONIC" BABIES. Occasionally, the nurse will find that an infant seems to be fussy from birth. He appears very active, startles easily, cries readily and more frequently (and apparently for no reason), is alert and awake much of the time and in general does not fit the usual pattern of activity, feeding and sleeping described. Some physicians term these babies "hypertonic", that is, they do not seem to be able to relax as well as other infants. The parents, particularly, may find their adjustment to their new baby difficult and anxiety-provoking until they are informed (or learn by trial and error) that this is "normal behavior" for this child. Too often they assume they must be doing something "wrong" since in spite of their efforts their baby remains fussy, tense and crying. The nurse can be very helpful to the parents in giving them anticipatory guidance about their baby's behavior and helpful ways in which he can be soothed. She should inform the physician of her observations so that he may advise the parents appropriately. These infants usually respond favorably to being held securely. Thus, wrapping them snugly with a receiving blanket, cuddling them securely, changing their position slowly and surely rather than quickly, all help to allay undue tenseness. Of course, rocking the baby and walking with him are particularly successful measures, but no parent can or should do this over protracted periods of time.

Any new activity or procedures should be introduced to this kind of infant slowly. For instance, when he is given a tub bath for the first time, he should be placed in a small amount of water very slowly and each lower extremity immersed gradually. This will help him to be less frightened and startled. The parents should not consider an occasional evening out a luxury; rather it should be considered a necessary item in the care of their baby. These infants do place greater demands on their parents than do infants of a more placid nature, and a short time away from the baby does wonders in restoring the perspective and good humor of the parents.

Care of the Skin. The skin is thin, delicate, extremely tender and very easily irritated. Since the skin is a protective covering, breaks in its surface may initiate troublesome infection; hence skin disturbances constitute an actual threat to the baby's well-being.

The new baby does not perspire, usually, until after the 1st month, and he does not react to cold by having "goose flesh." In warm weather, or if the baby is dressed too warmly, he may develop prickly heat, a closely grouped pinhead-size rash of papules and vesicles, on the face, the neck and wherever skin surfaces touch. Fewer clothes and some control over the room temperature will help to relieve the discomfort.

BATHING. In the majority of hospitals today, elaborate procedures for bathing the infant have been discarded. It is recommended, as previously stated, that the skin be cleansed every other day with sterile cotton or a soft washcloth, warm water and a hexachlorophene detergent (see p. 367). Blood is removed from the skin after the delivery, but no attempt is made to remove the vernix caseosa thoroughly unless it is stained with blood or meconium. The vernix caseosa serves to protect the skin and disappears spontaneously in about 24 hours. If it remains in the creases and folds of the skin longer than 2 days, it is apt to cause irritation. In this case gentle wiping usually removes it sufficiently. On the alternate days that the hexachlorophene bath is given, an inspection bath should be given, at which time the infant can be "spot cleansed" as needed with the moistened cotton balls. The use of strong soap, oil and baby powder is discouraged by many pediatricians because of the sensitivity of the newborn's skin. The nurse should pay particular attention to cleansing (and drying) the scalp and all creases at the neck, behind the ears, under the arms, the palms of the hands and between the fingers and the toes, under the knees, the soles of the feet, and in the groins, the buttocks and the genitals.

Basic Principles. Each nurse will develop her own manner of bathing the newborn according to her manual dexterity, the size and the activity of the infant, and the facilities available. Several basic principles should be observed.

First, all equipment, clothing and supplies should be assembled so that the infant never is left alone or exposed unduly. Safety pins should be closed and placed out of the reach of the baby. Receptacles for soiled clothing, cotton balls, etc., should be available.

FIG. 16-25. Exposing buttocks to air.

Second, care should be taken so that the environment is free from drafts and warm enough (i.e., 75° to 80° F.). The nurse should not have to interrupt the bath to close a door or a window. The water for the bath should be about 98° to 100° F. Water that feels warm to the elbow is approximately that temperature.

Third, in giving the bath the nurse should proceed from the "cleanest" areas to those that are "most soiled." Thus, the eyes are bathed first, then the face, ears, scalp, neck, upper extremities, trunk, lower extremities, and finally the buttocks and the genitals. Each of these in turn is washed, *rinsed well* and dried. To prevent undue exposure, a portion of the infant can be undressed at one time, bathed and then redressed.

Finally, *the infant never should be left alone,* even on a large work area; one hand should be kept on him at all times.

Demonstration and Practice. Each mother should have an opportunity to observe a demonstration of a sponge bath and, if at all possible, to give a bath to her infant. The various principles enumerated above can be conveyed to the mother readily. In addition, the nurse should explore with the mother what facilities are available in the home so that the necessities can be met and undue expense and difficulty avoided. For instance, a large drainboard which can be washed and padded adequately (and is a comfortable height for handling the infant) can be utilized for the bath area. A large pan or basin does very well for the bathtub in the early weeks; it should be kept only for the baby's use. Thus, the extra expense of special equipment can be minimized.

THE CORD TIE should be left in place until the cord drops off; the clamp is removed in 24 hours, provided that the umbilical stump has dried sufficiently. The nurse should observe whether the skin is clear, pink, cyanotic, blotchy or jaundiced and if there is dryness present.

BUTTOCKS. Sometimes, despite good nursing

FIG. 16-26. The new baby comes home to his family.

Fig. 16-27. The children wanted to hold their new brother. Sitting in the armchair and holding the baby are Kathy, age 2½ years, and Flip, age 4½ years.

care, the infant's buttocks become reddened and sore. A diaper rash may occur which is caused by the reaction of bacteria with the urea in the urine. This in turn causes an ammonia dermatitis. The most important prophylaxis lies in keeping the diaper area clean and dry. Sometimes, petroleum jelly, baby oil or a bland protective ointment, such as vitamin A and D ointment, is prescribed by the doctor. Pastes may not be advised, because they are much more adhesive than ointments and thus create cleansing problems.

A simple treatment which is often effective is merely to expose the infant's reddened buttocks to air (Fig. 16-25) and light several times a day, using care to keep the infant covered otherwise. Warm daylight may be all that is necessary, although the use of a "lamp" treatment is more effective and at the same time provides a measure of warmth. An ordinary gooseneck lamp with a screened bulb (no stronger than 40 watts) can be placed on the table so that it is a foot or more away from the infant's exposed buttocks. The light may be used for 30 minutes at a time. Because the skin is already irritated, the nurse should exercise care not to burn it further by using too strong a bulb or placing the light too close.

If the condition occurs at home, the treatment described above also is appropriate, and the mother can be so instructed. Boiling the diapers is another effective measure, since this destroys the bacteria. However, many of the detergents and conditioners nowadays have antibacterial agents in them; these may be effective in washing the diapers. Care should be taken to rinse the diapers thoroughly, since the residue of the detergent, etc., in itself can be irritating. In this respect the modern diaper services have very effective

FIG. 16-28. Father gives the baby his bottle as Kathy and Flip help.

facilities; many sterilize diapers and entire layettes as part of the service.

Sleeping. The baby will need rest and sleep with as little handling as possible. If he is well and comfortable, he usually sleeps much of the time and wakes and cries when he is hungry or uncomfortable. He may sleep as much as 20 hours out of 24 (although this varies considerably from infant to infant). It is not the sound sleep of the adult; rather he moves a good deal, stretches, and at intervals awakens momentarily. Since he responds so readily to external stimuli (and this may make him restless), his clothing and coverings are important. They should be light in weight, warm but not too warm, and free from wrinkles and "bunches." His position should be changed frequently when he is awake. He can be placed on either side or on his abdomen, especially when he is ready for sleep. If he is positioned on his back, then someone should be present, for if the baby regurgitates, he is more likely to aspirate in this position. As he gets older and learns to roll over, he will assume the position that he likes most for sleep.

Intestinal Elimination. During fetal life the content of the intestines is made up of brownish-green tarlike material called meconium. It is composed of epithelial and epidermal cells and lanugo hair that probably were swallowed with the amniotic fluid. The dark greenish-brown color of the meconium is due to the bile pigment. During fetal life and for the first few hours after birth the intestinal contents are sterile. Apparently, there is no peristalsis until after birth, because normally there is no discoloration of the amniotic fluid.

STOOLS. For the first 5 or 6 days, the stools gradually change from meconium to transitional stools (after which they become the regular milk stools). During this time the color of the stools changes from tarry black to a greenish black, to greenish brown, to brownish yellow and thence to greenish yellow. The transitional stools are composed of both meconium and milk stools; hence their variation in color. After the transitional stools the color gradually changes to a soft yellow of a smooth pasty consistency with a characteristic foul odor if the infant is formula-

FIG. 16-29. Bath time for the baby. Kathy and Flip are allowed to help.

fed. Stools of breast-fed infants tend to be golden yellow and of mushy consistency. Most newborns pass the first stool within 12 hours of birth—nearly all have a stool in 24 hours. If an infant has not passed a stool by this time, intestinal obstruction must be considered as a possible reason for the delay, and the baby must be observed closely. The number of daily stools on about the 5th day of life is usually 4 to 6. As the infant grows, this number decreases to 1 or 2 each day. The type of stool may be influenced by the mother's diet. However, there may be slight variations from the normal, which may have little significance if the baby appears to be comfortable and sleeps and nurses well. If the baby's stools have a watery consistency, are of a green color, contain much mucus, and flatus is being passed, the condition may be evidence of some digestive or intestinal irritation and should be reported to the physician. The number, color and consistency of stools should be recorded daily on the baby's record.

Urinary Elimination. Urinary activity of the fetus is evidenced by the presence of urine in the amniotic fluid. The baby usually voids during delivery or immediately after birth, but the function may be suppressed for several hours. However, if the baby does not void within 24 hours, the condition should be reported to the physician, as retention of the urine may be due to an imperforate meatus. After the first 2 or 3 days the baby voids from 10 to 15 times a day. When the urine is concentrated, red or rusty stains on the wet diaper may be due to uric-acid crystals in the urine.

INFANT FEEDING
The Newborn's Ability to Handle Food

One of the major physiologic adaptations which the infant must make in the transition from intrauterine to extra-uterine life concerns the source of his nourishment and the ability to take food into his body, to digest it and to assimilate it. During prenatal life the nutritive substances for growth and handling of waste products are provided for by means of the placental circulation (see Chap. 4). Thus, prior to birth the gastro-intestinal tract has not been required to utilize muscle, chemical or absorptive activity in handling food. Clement Smith makes the analogy that the digestion and the absorption of food is, like the respiration of air, a function that the infant has had no opportunity of practicing during its fetal career.[6] Following delivery not only must the gastrointestinal tract begin abruptly to process a rather large amount of food, but the infant must begin to suck and swallow to take the food into his stomach. The infant's capacity to take the food in and digest it is adequate when the food is appropriate (i.e., breast milk or milk formula) and when it is appropriately given.

Certain important considerations in relation to the development of the infant's digestive apparatus and infant feeding will be recalled here, because they have a direct bearing on feeding practices. The student is urged to utilize the appropriate references in the Suggested Reading at the end of the chapter for more thorough study, as well as to build on content in normal nutrition, physiologic chemistry, etc., covered in background courses.

SUCKING AND SWALLOWING REFLEXES. The infant's ability to take in food through his own efforts demands the ability to suck and to swallow. At birth the sucking and swallowing reflexes are already present, and normally they are quite strong. It is known that the swallowing reflex, as well as peristaltic movements in the stomach, become active during the last 2 months of fetal development, because bits of vernix caseosa and lanugo are found with other debris in the meconium stool. The nurse who has witnessed the birth of babies can easily recall how the infant is able to swallow mucus, and how sometimes, even while the initial care is being given in the delivery room, the infant will begin to suck on anything that gets near his mouth.

STOMACH AND INTESTINES. At the time of birth the infant's stomach is small, its capacity is approximately 50 to 60 cc., but it is capable of considerable dilatation. During feeding the infant's stomach is able to stretch to at least 3 or 4 times its approximate capacity. It is not merely distended by the amount of food taken in (i.e., milk), but also by the amount of air the infant swallows as he sucks the milk or cries. In the act of crying the infant tends to gulp in air.

The gastric musculature is somewhat deficient at birth. In contrast, the glandular structures in the mucosa are present, although shallow in contrast with those of the adult. The relatively greater length of the intestinal tract and the weakness of the abdominal musculature to serve as a supporting structure explain in part the reason that considerable distention of the stomach is possible.

Although gastric digestion is not considered to be a factor of primary importance to the nutrition of the newborn infant, many of the findings reported by Clement Smith in his textbook could be useful in the consideration of infant feeding schedules. For example, the stomach empties more slowly in the newborn period than any other time in life. However, the distended stomach is able to adjust its content by promptly emptying some or all of its content into the duodenum. A number of the studies on gastric motility have demonstrated wide individual differences in emptying time. The major portion of the feeding usually leaves the stomach in less than 3 or 4 hours, although the greater portion of this occurred 1½ to 2 hours after the meal. In some instances the emptying time of the infants' stomachs took more than 8 hours. It was found also that the introduction of a second feeding before the stomach was empty caused portions of the first feeding to remain somewhat longer in the stomach than if the stomach was emptied from the last feeding before the next was offered. Another important finding is that human milk leaves the stomach somewhat more rapidly than cow's milk, although a formula made of cow's milk which has been boiled leaves the stomach more rapidly than that which is fed without this additional preparation.

Infant Nutrition. In the last several decades progress in scientific developments has made artificial feeding (formulas) so much like human breast milk in chemical composition that they are, in fact, almost identical. Although it is generally considered that the best food for the baby is that designed by nature—human breast milk—the individual differences in mothers and babies must be considered in the practical situation. It is the mother who makes the decision of how she wants to feed her baby, and the nurse should support her in this decision.

[6] Smith, C. A.: The Physiology of the Newborn Infant. ed. 3, p. 228, Springfield, Charles C Thomas, 1959.

Some advantages of feeding breast milk are: it is exactly the correct chemical composition for babies, is constantly available (and no preparation is necessary), is at an even temperature, is free from bacteria, and causes a lower incidence of allergy.

In artificial feeding the differences in caloric allowances required for various infants will depend on: (1) the individual nutritional needs and (2) the infant's rate of growth. All of the infant's nutritional needs, except that for growth, can be met by providing 33 calories per pound per day. When the component necessary for growth is added, approximately 42 calories per pound per day will be required. One might anticipate that by the time some infants are 10 to 14 days old, they may consume 55 calories per pound per day, but this should not be followed rigidly.

Self-regulatory Feedings. A permissive feeding regimen for newborns means that babies should be offered as much formula or feeding as they seem to want and should not be forced to take the amount prescribed unless forcing has been specifically ordered by the responsible physician.

The variation in baby readiness and the desirability of individualizing the time of starting feedings needs to be stressed. The time of initiating feedings will depend on evidence of the infant's hunger and the readiness of the baby. Once the first feeding has been offered, the routine or prescribed schedule for offering feedings should be followed.

The permissive feeding regimen for breast-fed newborns may require even more flexibility. A mother who is breast-feeding may desire to begin breast-feeding her baby before the time specified by hospital routine for the first water feeding, as sometimes happens when the nursery requires that the first feeding be water and given by the nurse prior to other feedings. Unless there is a maternal complication or contraindication, every baby should visit his mother at each feeding time, starting with the first feeding of "breast" or "bottle," but excluding the 2 A.M. feeding period for the first visit unless the mother wants to see her baby at this time.

Composition of Human Milk. Breast milk, as it leaves the mother's breast, is a sterile fluid. It should have an alkaline or possibly a neutral reaction, but never an acid reaction. Colostrum cells should be absent after the 12th day, and the fat globules should be small, numerous and of uniform size.

Milk is a natural emulsion and consists of about 10 per cent of solids and 90 per cent of water. The solid substances are fat, sugar, proteins and salts. The fat of milk is the cream, the sugar is the kind known as "lactose," or "milk-sugar," and the protein makes up the bulk of the curd.

Artificial Feeding

Formula feeding has become the predominant mode of nurture for infants born in American hospitals today. In survey findings reported by Meyer involving 2,928 U.S. hospitals with more than 2½ million births in 1966, 73 per cent of infants discharged from the nurseries were receiving only bottle feeding.[7]

The most significant change to come into the hospital newborn nursery in more than 50 years (i.e., since the advent of the central nursery system) is the use of disposables and unit packaging. This includes ready-to-feed formulas in disposable containers.

Prepared milk mixtures in throw-away containers with sterile nipple units attached represent the newest development in infant feeding in the hospital. The prepared milk mixtures are said to have features which improve on evaporated milk or whole milk formulas.[8]

In artificial feeding it is necessary to modify the milk to approximate as nearly as possible the chemical and the physical characteristics of human milk. When human milk and cow's milk are compared, the difference in fat and protein content needs to be considered. Cow's milk is diluted, and therefore carbohydrate is added to the newborn infant's formula. It is generally accepted that even normal fat in milk (3.5%) is poorly tolerated. Thus, cow's milk is diluted essentially to lessen the fat component of the formula. In addition, when whole milk is diluted, the casein curd is more flocculent in the infant stomach and thus aids in the digestion of milk. In diluting the formula the carbohydrate of milk also is diluted inadvertently and should be restored to the original amount (4.5%) or more to furnish additional calories for optimal nutrition and weight gain. The added carbohydrate may be in the form of granulated sugar, corn syrup or a commercially prepared carbohydrate modifier. Added carbohydrate permits normal metabolism of fats, allows protein to be used to build new tissues instead of serving to provide calories, and encourages normal water balance.

---

[7] Meyer, H. F.: Current feeding practices in hospital maternity nurseries. Clin. Pediat. 8:69, February, 1969.

[8] *Ibid.,* p. 72.

TABLE 16-1. COMPARATIVE DATA ON RELATIVE COMPONENTS IN HUMAN MILK, COW'S MILK AND EVAPORATED COW'S MILK IN NORMAL DILUTION (ACCORDING TO NELSON)*

	NORMAL DILUTION		APPROXIMATE PERCENTAGE COMPOSITION IN NORMAL DILUTION (GRAMS PER 100 ML.)			
TYPE OF MILK	RATIO	CALS./OZ.	PROTEIN	FAT	CARBO-HYDRATE	MINERALS
Human milk, average	undiluted	20	1.1	4.5	6.8	0.2
Cow's milk, market average	undiluted	20	3.3	3.5	4.8	0.72
Cow's milk, evaporated (Standard brands)	1:1	22	3.6	4.2	5.3	0.75
Commercial premodified milks:						
Modified milk, Baker†	1:1	20	2.2	3.3	7.0	0.6
Bremil, Borden	1:1	20	1.5	3.5	7.0	0.5
Carnalac, new formula, Carnation	1:1	20	2.28	2.69	8.23	0.5
Modilac, Gerber	1:1	20	2.15	2.6	7.6	0.37
Enfamil, Mead†	1:1	20	1.5	3.7	7.0	0.35
Similac, Ross†	1:1	20	1.7	3.4	6.6	0.38

* Nelson, W. E. (ed.): Textbook of Pediatrics, ed. 8, p. 139, Philadelphia, Saunders, 1964.

† Also available in powdered form.

The physician will prescribe the formula for the infant and give specific directions concerning its use. Various milk formulas are used today: diluted pasteurized milk with added carbohydrate, diluted evaporated milk with or without carbohydrates added, fresh skimmed milk, powdered skim milk, or one of the brands of prepared milk preparations (see Table 16-1). Of these milk formulas, the most widely used formula is diluted evaporated milk with added carbohydrate. It should be noted that evaporated milk has several advantages: It is safe because it is sterilized in an unopened can, it is convenient to store, the cost is relatively low, and the formula is simple to prepare. An evaporated milk formula for the newborn infant is usually made up of one part evaporated milk diluted with two parts of water and carbohydrate in sufficient amount to meet the required calories.

Essential nutritional requirements are a basic consideration in the computation of a formula for the newborn infant. Certain "rules of thumb" concerning nutrients and formula computation are as follows:

1. *Proteins.* One and one half ounces of cow's milk per pound of body weight equals 1.5 Gm. of protein per pound, which equals one tenth of body weight.

2. *Carbohydrates.* One tenth ounce per pound of body weight equals 1 ounce per 10 ounces of milk prescribed, which also equals 1 per cent of

the body weight. One third of the carbohydrate should be derived from the milk of the mixture, and the remainder added in the form of starch or sugar. Later in the first year the carbohydrate is given in the form of a starch cereal, and the carbohydrate in the milk formula may be reduced at that time.

3. *Fats.* Anywhere from 3 to 5 per cent is included, no specific amount being stipulated. If the fats are restricted, a larger amount of protein or sugar, or both, is required for energy sources. The suitable quantity of fat is supplied in amounts of milk which furnish the required amounts of protein. An excess of fat is not to be desired.

4. *Minerals.* An adequate mineral-salt intake is supplied to any infant when 1½ ounces of milk per pound of body weight are given. Enough iron is stored in the liver of the normal infant (from the hemoglobin breakdown after birth) to suffice until about the 4th or 5th month. This deficiency is usually made up by the addition of the solid food supplements (egg yolk, fortified cereals, vegetables and fruit) which are usually added before this time, except in the completely milk-fed infant who refuses or is not offered these iron-containing foods in the first year.

5. *Water.* The requirement for water varies from 10 to 15 per cent of the body weight, or may be expressed as 1½ to 2½ ounces per pound of body weight. This is supplied in the milk itself, in the diluent of the milk mixture, and supple-

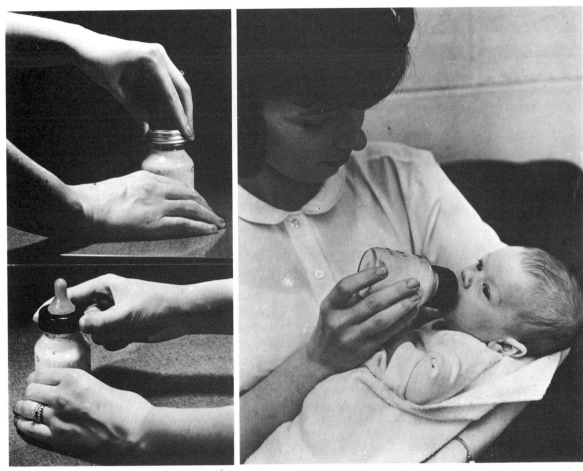

FIG. 16-30. The ready-to-use commercially prepackaged sterilized formula provides a safe, simple 3-step feeding for the convenience of the mother at home. At feeding time, (*left, top*) remove lid, (*left, bottom*) apply sterilized nipple, and (*right*) feed the baby. (Ross Laboratories, Columbus, Ohio)

mented to instinctive demands by offerings of water and fruit juices between feedings.

6. *Calories.* The average requirement for growth in the first year is 50 calories per pound of expected weight, two thirds of this caloric need being supplied by the milk and one third by the added carbohydrate.[9]

---

[9] Meyer, H. F.: Infant Foods and Feeding Practice. p. 72, Springfield, Charles C Thomas, 1960.

Formula Computation. A simple problem with which to apply the basic rules of formula computation would be the food needs of an infant weighing 10 pounds at 2 months of age, having weighed 6 pounds at birth. This infant would probably take 3 oz. more than his age in months (2) which would be (2 months plus 3 equals 5) 5 oz. per feeding. In 24 hours he probably would be satisfied with five feedings; hence, he would need 25 oz. in a total 24-hour period.

EXAMPLE—WHOLE MILK MIXTURE

1½ oz. whole milk per lb. of body weight (10 lb.) ....Milk, 15 (fluid) oz. = 300 cal.

1 oz. CHO [carbohydrate] per 10 oz. milk used ....Cane sugar, 1½ oz. = 180 cal.

Diluent to make up total 24-hour amount ....Water, 10 (fluid) oz.

5 feedings of 5 oz. each ....25 (fluid) oz. = 480 cal.

Calorically, this should effect normal growth since it provides 48 calories per pound. Should it not provide normal weight increase of about 5 to 7 oz. per week, or should the infant fail to be satisfied by evidencing signs of hunger, the milk proportion could be increased, or the total amount be enlarged, or additional CHO added, or all of these could be changed to fit the infant's needs.

In calculating a formula with evaporated milk and a corn syrup for the same hypothetical infant, the construction would be as follows:

EXAMPLE—EVAPORATED MILK MIXTURE

1 oz. evaporated milk per lb. body weight ....Evap. milk, 10 (fluid) oz. = 440 cal.
1/10 oz. CHO per lb. body weight ....Corn syrup, 1 (fluid) oz. = 120 cal.
Diluent to make up total 24-hour amount ....Water, 14 (fluid) oz.
5 feedings of 5 oz. each ....25 (fluid) oz. = 560 cal.

With this mixture the calories are increased to 56 per pound, which might easily be tolerated by said infant, especially if he were active and hungry and needed more food.[10]

Directions for Making Formula. The hands should be washed before assembling the equipment. All equipment used for the preparation of the formula should be kept separate (Fig. 16-31). If bottled milk is used, the outside of the bottle should be washed with soap and cool water as soon as received, and the bottle should be placed in the refrigerator. If canned milk is used, the top of the can should be washed with soap and water, using friction, and then thoroughly rinsed. Hot water should be poured over the top just before it is opened. All equipment should be washed thoroughly in warm soapy water and

rinsed well so that no milk film remains to hold bacteria.

Bottles and Nipples. The 8-ounce bottle is a good size to use and should be graduated in ounces and half ounces so that it will be possible at all times to know exactly how much food the baby has taken. A sufficient number of bottles and nipples should be sterilized to supply the feedings for the 24-hour period. It is always safer to have 1 or 2 extra bottles and nipples in reserve in case of breakage.

The shape of the bottle should be such that every part of the inner surface can be reached with a brush to facilitate cleaning.

The holes in the nipple are usually small, but they may be made the required size by heating a fine sewing needle with its eye fixed in a cork (used as a handle). The point is held in the flame until red hot, then accurately plunged into

---

[10] Meyer, *op. cit.*, p. 75.

FIG. 16-31. Formula equipment. Sterilizer with bottle rack and tight-fitting lid; six 8-ounce nursers (for formula) and two 4-ounce nursers (for water and orange juice) complete with nipples, caps and sealing disks; quart-size formula pitcher with clearly marked graduations; nipple jar with perforated (for sterilizing) and solid lids; long-handled tongs; table knife; long-handled mixing spoon; can opener; set of measuring spoons and a funnel-strainer. (Pyramid Rubber Company, Ravenna, Ohio)

Fig. 16-32. Mother feeds formula to her newborn baby. Note the correct angle to hold the baby's bottle. (MacDonald House, The University Hospitals of Cleveland, Cleveland, Ohio)

one of the three holes and withdrawn quickly. The procedure needs practice before holes of proper size can be made. Some nipples have crucial incisions instead of punctured holes to prevent them from clogging.

The test of proper hole size is made by holding the bottle, filled with milk and with the nipple attached, upside down. The milk should escape drop by drop, and if it runs in a stream, the hole is too large. The objection to the large hole is that the baby nurses too rapidly, which causes indigestion, colic and other disorders. If the stream is very rapid, the baby may have difficulty in swallowing.

Aseptic Method. In this method the bottles, nipples, nipple caps and equipment used in making the formula are sterilized before the formula is prepared. The mother will need a glass or enamel pitcher in which to mix the formula, a measuring cup, measuring spoons, tablespoon (to mix the formula), funnel (depending on the size of the bottle mouth), can opener (if canned milk is used) and some kind of tongs that can be sterilized. The tongs will be used as a forceps to handle the equipment. These items, together with the bottles, caps, and nipples are placed in a large pan or sterilizer half full of water and boiled vigorously for 10 minutes. The equipment and the bottles, nipples, etc., may be done separately if the sterilizer cannot accommodate such a large load. Care should be taken to place the forceps in such a way that the handles can be reached easily after sterilization. If the mother must reach into the water for them, then she contaminates the water and hence the materials being sterilized. After sterilization the formula is made according to directions. A specific amount of the formula is put into each bottle. The bottles are then nippled, capped and refrigerated.

Terminal Sterilization. In this method the formula is prepared under a clean but not aseptic technique. The equipment, bottles, nipples and nipple caps are washed thoroughly but are not sterilized. The formula is prepared and poured into the bottles, and the nipples and the caps are applied loosely. They then are placed in the sterilizer, covered with a tight-fitting lid and sterilized by having the water boil rapidly in the bottom of the sterilizer for 25 minutes. In this method, formula, bottles, nipples and protectors are all sterilized in one operation. Before the formula is refrigerated, the screw collar should be made secure. The majority of hospitals use the autoclaving method, but in the home the procedure immediately above is used. In each method the formula must remain sterile and the nipple untouched and sterile until it reaches the baby's mouth.

There is a variety of bottles and nipples on the market, many of them sold as "units" (bottle, nipple and nipple protector).

Hunger. If the baby is not getting enough food, he will wake before his regular nursing time and be obviously hungry. He will cry and fret, refuse water with apparent disgust, and when a feeding is offered, seize the nipple ravenously and nurse with great vigor. Often for the very young infant, increasing the amount of feeding

Fig. 16-33. Bubbling the baby. (MacDonald House, The University Hospitals of Cleveland, Cleveland, Ohio)

is all that is necessary. For an older infant, increasing the concentration of the formula and/or its amount may be necessary. Solids sometimes are introduced at this time to help allay the hunger. Occasionally, a baby appears to be hungry between feedings when in reality he is only thirsty. He may be given a small amount of tepid boiled water to satisfy his thirst.

Bubbling. After 5 minutes or so, or in the middle and at the end of each feeding, the infant should be held in an upright position and his back *gently* patted or stroked (Fig. 16-33). Pounding the baby on the back vigorously is neither effective for bubbling him nor conducive to his well-being. The change in position (from semireclining to upright) is the important factor in eliciting a bubble. Often holding the infant upright and pressing him against the breast is all that is necessary. Because the new infant's gastrointestinal tract is labile, milk may be eructated with gas bubbles. Care should be taken to ensure adequate "bubbling" before the infant is placed back into the crib, thus preventing milk regurgitation.

Regurgitation. Regurgitation, which is merely an overflow and often occurs after nursing, should not be confused with vomiting, which may occur at any time and is accompanied by other symptoms. This regurgitation is the means of relieving the distended stomach and usually indicates that the baby either has taken too much food or has taken it too rapidly.

Assisting the Mother Feeding Her Infant

The feeding of the baby is one of the first tasks which must be achieved in the mothering role. The young inexperienced mother undoubtedly will need guidance, assistance and emotional support in feeding her new baby whether she feeds him by breast or by bottle. The help given by the nurse in the first feeding experiences not only helps the mother to deal with her anxiety in handling the new baby and in coping with the manipulative problems related to feeding him, but it lends her the emotional support that she so desperately needs in surmounting her own stress in the situation. The mother who has never handled a small infant before, being confronted with a sleepy or a squirmy infant, can feel all the more inadequate as she realizes that the responsibility to nourish this "bundle of joy" is hers.

The environmental climate surrounding the feeding of the baby should be peaceful and unhurried (Figs. 15-9, 10). The mother should be rested and ready. She should not have been rushed through a previous task, such as the morning bath or other daily care routine procedures, to meet a deadline imposed by the baby's feeding schedule. The nurse who brings the baby to his mother should avoid hurrying him to his mother's bedside, pushing the crib into the room, and leaving at once with the remark, "I'll be back to give you your baby as soon as I get the other babies out." Meanwhile, the mother looks at her hungry fretful baby in his crib, and often she is afraid to pick him up lest she be reprimanded for failing to wait for the return of the harassed nurse.

Expanding Contacts With the Baby. When babies are kept on a routine feeding schedule in the conventional maternity hospital, the mother's contacts with her baby are sometimes limited to the feeding period. It is unfortunate when the mother feels she must begin to feed her baby the moment she takes him into her arms. Feeding often takes up most of the time mothers and infants are together in the hospital, leaving little

opportunity for their getting acquainted otherwise. Smith has described a plan whereby the demand feeding regimen to meet the needs of the individual baby was successfully achieved in a maternity hospital.[11] To provide some flexibility in the routine schedule, babies easily could be brought to their mothers at least 15 minutes before the feeding time and left with them for a similar period of time afterward, if the mothers so desired, without disrupting hospital routine. This plan would relieve some of the mother's stress at the beginning of the feeding period by allowing her more freedom to hold the baby leisurely, look at him or fondle him as she chooses. For mothers who are breast-feeding, this contact would have a positive effect on the let-down factor.

Getting Insight into the Mother's Goals and Problems. One must always bear in mind that each mother has her own goals in each new maternity experience. The astute nurse will utilize opportunities to assist the mother in achieving the mother's goals in accordance with the mother's individual capacity. Some time spent in purposeful conversation with the mother in addition to the time when her baby is with her may help the nurse to gain further insight into the mother's concerns. Even when hospital staffing is limited, the nurse who organizes her activities thoughtfully usually can find the "extra" time to accomplish what she considers to be the most important components of patient care.

One of the most obvious ways for the nurse to support the mother in the feeding experience is to stay with the mother until both mother and baby are settled, and then, in leaving the bedside to let the mother know that she is immediately available. The nurse who takes time to listen to what the mother is saying and to observe the interaction between the mother and baby often can identify problems that the mother is experiencing.

For example, the nurse left Mrs. Bee comfortably feeding her 2-day-old son. When she returned to the room 10 minutes later, Mrs. Bee looked up and said, "He only sucked for 2 minutes and now he's asleep. Look at him. Is his skin a little yellow? I can't make him take any more." Most mothers will verbalize their concerns, though they may not ask directly for help. In this instance the nurse responded with concern, "You wonder if he's had enough to eat?" The mother responded as she looked down at the baby, "Yes," and then went on to talk about her

11 Smith, C. S.: Demand feeding in the newborn nursery. Nurs. Outlook 6:514-515, September, 1958.

Fig. 16-34. Maternal identification processes are active. (See Figs. 16-34 to 16-43) Observe the mother's use of touch and visual perception as she looks at her sleeping baby on her lap. (MacDonald House, The University Hospitals of Cleveland, Cleveland, Ohio)

awkwardness in handling the baby and the bottle at the same time. She said, "I wonder whether perhaps I have tired the baby."

The nurse meets the mother's concern half way by her inquiry. At the same time, she must use judgment not to create concerns that do not exist. Responding to the mother's remarks in a way that leaves the conversation open and encourages the mother to express her concerns is not only helpful to the mother but also likely to give the

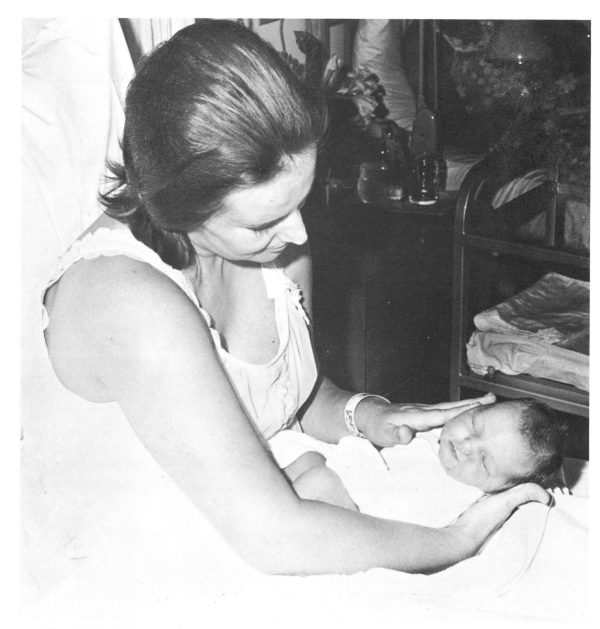

Fig. 16-35. Mother uses her fingers to stroke cheek of her sleeping baby. (MacDonald House, The University Hospitals of Cleveland, Cleveland, Ohio)

nurse important clues about what the mother at the moment feels are "problems." The words that the nurse uses to speak with the patient are important, but even more important is the feeling communicated in this interaction between two people.

THE MOTHER AND HER NEWBORN

With the birth of her baby the mother must assume a new role, along with all its concomitant tasks and responsibilities. Moreover, these adjustments must be undertaken before physical and psychological restoration from pregnancy and labor is complete. Since the adaptation to motherhood usually evolves as a slow, often unconscious modification of the individual's attitudes and activities, the professionals who provide for the mother's and the infant's care in the hospital are not always cognizant of what mother and baby experience in the early days of homecoming.

Fig. 16-36. Mother holds sleeping baby on her forearm to look at him. (MacDonald House, The University Hospitals of Cleveland, Cleveland, Ohio)

The literature on the development of maternal behavior (see Suggested Reading) tends to support the fact that primigravidas are generally more awkward and anxious and have more early concerns about their abilities to care for their newborn than do multiparas. One cannot assume that because the newly delivered mother seemingly makes a "good adjustment" during the first days after birth in the hospital that the adaptation will be smooth and uncomplicated after she returns home. This early period of adjustment—particularly during the first week of the infant's life—is a crucial one. Thoughtful nursing intervention at this time can make a significant contribution to the welfare of the family. Therefore it becomes important to ask what the nurse in the hospital might do to prepare the mother more adequately for coping with problems that she may encounter on going home with her new baby.

Carpenter interviewed mothers of first-born infants to determine the kinds of help they needed for themselves and their babies in the first months at home following delivery.[12] She reported that mothers in the lower socioeconomic groups not only have more difficulties than their more affluent

[12] Carpenter, H. M.: The Need for Assistance of Mothers With First Babies During the Three-Month Period Following the Baby's Birth. New York, Columbia University, 1965.

FIG. 16-37. Mother brings baby closer to her body. Observe the mother's use of maternal touch. (MacDonald House, The University Hospitals of Cleveland, Cleveland, Ohio)

FIG. 16-38. Mother cradles baby in her arm. (MacDonald House, The University Hospitals of Cleveland, Cleveland, Ohio)

neighbors but are also less likely to have assistance from relatives or friends, or the services of a private physician. In relation to their own health, concerns most frequently mentioned were about the condition of the perineum and breasts, fatigue and depression. The mothers expressed needs in relation to feeding and other care-taking activities for their babies. In addition, they felt they needed better understanding of the baby's behavior, especially the normal ranges of infant behavior.

Presently, more seems to be known about maternal attitudes and practices in general than about the specifics of maternal behavior—at least that assumption can be made from what appears in the literature. How do mothers interact with their babies? What clues can be observed of mother and baby in a reciprocal relationship that inform us about the nature of the identification processes? (See Figs. 16-34 to 16-43) In order to provide appropriate nursing care it becomes important to know, for example, how mothers behave when they feed their babies. Escalona discusses differences in social experiences of young infants.[13] Some mothers care for their babies as if they are very fragile things. These mothers are task-oriented and approach routine care of their babies completely separate from social interaction. Their interaction, for example, does not evoke the baby's smiles or vocal responses.

Maternal touch (see writings of Rubin and Bowers in Suggested Reading) has reciprocal value for both mother and infant. The mother uses her fingers, hands and arms to explore and fondle her baby as she begins to establish a relationship with the baby. As she caresses the baby she is going through identification processes with him which assist her in "claiming" him as her baby. This is significant for the infant in his growth and learning. For the maternity nurse these understandings should make the difference in the quality of her care. Mothers should not only be given the opportunity to look at and learn to care for their babies in an unhurried fashion

[13] Escalona, S. K.: The Roots of Individuality. p. 47, Chicago, Aldine, 1968.

FIG. 16-40. Mother relaxes body, leans back against pillows as she takes baby's hand between her fingers. (MacDonald House, The University Hospitals of Cleveland, Cleveland, Ohio)

FIG. 16-39. Mother encircles baby with both arms, enfolds him to her breast. (MacDonald House, The University Hospitals of Cleveland, Cleveland, Ohio)

while they are in the hospital but they should have planned opportunities for social experiences with their babies. In many maternity hospitals mothers must wait until the nurse, or her assistant, hands the baby to his mother to be fed, and then relinquish him to the nursery personnel when he has hardly finished feeding because this is the "routine."

Mothers' Concerns About Their Babies

Every new mother experiences concerns to some degree about caring for her newborn infant. The mother who has had other babies may feel quite confident in performing the mothering tasks for the baby, but at the same time she may wonder how on returning home she ever will be able to manage her time and energy to give all the children and her husband what they need and what she would like to give them. On the other hand, the mother with her first baby may have many early concerns about fulfilling the infant care

activities, such as feeding and bathing the baby, if she has had little or no experience.

Feeding the Baby. This is a major area of concern during the first weeks.[14] Adams found that the mother's questions usually were related to the amount and the frequency of feeding. The first days after delivery the mothers were asking how to prepare formula, but by the end of the week they were more interested in getting answers to questions about how to feed the baby, how often to feed and the amount of feeding. Mothers who were breast-feeding wanted to know about the adequacy of their milk supply. "Is he getting enough?" was a frequent question.

Bathing the baby is another task that mothers must learn to carry out, one that often causes concern. At first the task itself seems most important, thus, how to bathe the baby (i.e., the procedure, seems most urgent). But after new mothers have had some experience in handling their infants, they are more interested, as home-going approaches, in learning how they are going

[14] Adams, Martha: Early concerns of primigravida mothers regarding infant care activities. Nurs. Res. 12:72, Spring, 1963.

FIG. 16-41. Baby awakens on mother's lap. Observe mother's interaction with crying baby. (MacDonald House, The University Hospitals of Cleveland, Cleveland, Ohio)

FIG. 16-42. Mother comforts her crying baby. (MacDonald House, The University Hospitals of Cleveland, Cleveland, Ohio)

to hold a squirming, soapy baby during his bath, and how to bathe him in a tub.

The baby's crying is of greater concern to mothers after the first week of life. When the baby spends most of his time in the hospital nursery, the mother may not get a chance to hear him cry, and she may wonder whether he can. One mother was ready to go home from the hospital (on her 5th postpartal day) and had never heard her baby cry. As the nurse wheeled his crib into the room that morning, the baby was crying lustily from hunger. The mother's face lighted up with great satisfaction as she said, "Now I *know* he can cry!" Mothers want to know why the baby is crying. With appropriate anticipatory guidance in the hospital, they can be helped to learn about the infant's communication through crying and how to interpret various kinds of crying.

Other Areas of Concern. "Concerns," according to Adams, "are areas of special interest or worry to mothers as indicated by questions pertaining to particular areas of care." Other questions they ask are related to care of the navel and/or circumcision, sleeping, taking the baby outdoors for the first time, hiccups, weight gain, rashes. Fathers, too, have concerns about tasks they must learn, particularly how to hold and to handle the new baby.

The Relation of Teaching to Areas of Concern. An understanding of how new parents view their problems with infant care activities must underlie any preparation for teaching mothers and helping them to learn about their babies and their care. The small group demonstrations of the infant bath and formula preparation are rather basic, but they need to include time for mothers' questions to be answered. There is a real need to have small group discussion conferences for new mothers, where they can initiate the conversation in the presence of a professional nurse who can act as a discussion leader or resource person.

Clinical Study: A Nurse and a New Mother

A clinical study in maternity nursing was carried out for the purpose of studying the nurse-patient interaction and nursing intervention with a young primigravida during the early puerperium.* There was conscious evaluation of the

---

* Part of a pilot project supported by Grant STIMH 7988-03 from the National Institute of Mental Health, United States Public Health Service.

Fig. 16-43. The baby continues to cry. Observe the mother-infant interaction in this relationship. (MacDonald House, The University Hospitals of Cleveland, Cleveland, Ohio)

nurse-patient interaction by the nurse during the relationship. Also, there was an attempt to apply psychosocial concepts to this situation by reflecting on the psychodynamics of behavior. Because Olive Rich's writings have particular significance for maternity nurses, she has graciously consented to share them with the authors for use in this textbook (see Suggested Reading).

The Clinical Experience

The patient selected, a 24-year-old primigravida, had no major complications during pregnancy, labor or delivery. The nurse had daily contacts with the patient for 7 days, beginning with the day of delivery and extending through the day of discharge. The nature of the contacts varied. At times the contact was solely for verbal and nonverbal interaction; at other times other facets of nursing care were included (e.g., assisting the mother with breast-feeding and teaching her how to carry out manual expression of breast milk). After the discharge of the mother from the hospital the nurse had three significant contacts with the patient in her home and three significant contacts by telephone. In the course of this experience there was only one direct interaction of the nurse with the patient alone. The patient had the same roommate throughout her hospital stay, and at home her mother and mother-in-law were both present—the latter intermittently—during the first two contacts with the nurse.

This clinical nursing study is directed to an examination of the possible dynamics involved when a patient who has made a good adjustment in the hospital suddenly encounters major problems on arriving home with her new baby. During the early postpartal days the patient's behavior was assessed by several staff members in the hospital setting as confident, mature, "doing just fine," and physically able and calm. In contrast, after the first 52 hours at home the young mother found herself fatigued and depressed. As she summarized it: "I just wasn't prepared for all this."

So that the student can understand and evaluate the nursing intervention, a fairly detailed description of the patient in the hospital and on the nurse's first visit to the home will be presented. As a further basis of understanding, concepts of the psychodynamics of pregnancy and childbearing as presented by selected authors will be discussed. Application will be made to this unique patient situation in the areas in which data are available. Finally, there will be some evaluation of the means of nursing intervention that were utilized and some reflective questioning about what other measures might have been of further help in preparing this mother for being at home with her baby.

The First Seven Days

The nurse's first contact with Mrs. X was on the afternoon of her day of delivery. Although Mrs. X had been in labor for more than 24 hours and had not slept for about 36 hours, she was sitting up in bed, making preparations to have her baby for a visit. She had seen her baby briefly on two previous occasions but had not held him. The nurse brought the baby from the nursery, placed him in his mother's arms, and waited for her comments. At first she looked and looked, not touching the baby's face but holding him quite securely.

PATIENT: "I don't know why, I expected him to be a towhead. I was when I was born. (*After a pause*) I don't see any forceps marks. They've trimmed his fingernails. Are his eyes blue?"

NURSE: "Most babies' eyes tend to be more blue than brown at first. What color would you say your eyes are? Your husband's eyes?"

PATIENT: "Mine are hazel. His are brown."

NURSE: "It is possible that you could each have the characteristic of blue eyes to pass on to a child."

PATIENT: "He looks like his daddy."

NURSE: "What part of him? Can you tell?"

PATIENT: "No, not really. His nose maybe."

NURSE: "You can unwrap him if you'd like."

PATIENT: "He has big feet. Look at his long toes."

Mrs. X continued for about the next 30 minutes to hold the baby quite comfortably and to comment about him in a similar vein. Little pauses threaded her observations as she went on: "He was a very active baby when I was carrying him. What's he doing? Is he hiccupping? What can he really see? He has a nice pink color. Does he have a bridge in his nose? I was born without one. Has he been given water yet? His ears are so big! At least they seem to be, in relation to his head."

The questions and comments were stated rather matter-of-factly with a certain objectivity and a seeming lack of involvement, as though she were commenting on any baby in the nursery. Mrs. X did not speak to the baby, kiss him or show much change in voice or face during the first prolonged encounter with her baby. The nurse remained with the mother the entire time and offered once to take the baby back to the nursery, assuming that she might be tired, but she wanted to keep him longer. In this one contact with the baby, the mother displayed facets of maternal behavior as described by Rubin.[15]

These observations of the mother's first holding of the baby are presented in considerable detail because they introduce Mrs. X's continued relationship with her baby as the nurse saw it in the hospital. Mrs. X, of course, gained skill in handling the baby but continued to relate to him in a matter-of-fact manner. No spontaneous expression of delight in her child was observed.

Mrs. X made an apparently rapid physical recovery from childbirth. Even on the day of delivery she was able to sit on her episiotomy and did not complain of perineal pain. The gastrointestinal and urinary systems readily assumed normal functioning. The mother made no complaint of afterpains, even when nursing the baby. She had only minimal engorgement of the breast tissue and only occasional nipple tenderness during her 7 days in the hospital. Mrs. X's perception of her postpartal status was similar to this. On the day after delivery she was sitting on the side of her bed, with her legs hanging down. The nurse attempted to intervene.

NURSE: "Some mothers like to sit that way for feeding their babies. But they don't think about the

---

[15] Rubin, R.: Basic maternal behavior. Nurs. Outlook 9:683-685, November, 1961.

fact that they've no backrest and no support for their arms, and that their feet hang down without support. They don't understand why they're tired until after it happens. Wouldn't you like to lie down in your bed or sit in the arm chair for feeding the baby?"

PATIENT: "No, I'm just fine. I feel good. I felt just fine all during pregnancy. You know, I worked until the 7th month."

On another occasion:

NURSE: "I see you have skimmed milk."

PATIENT: "That was my only problem during pregnancy—weight gain. I must have gained 30 to 35 pounds."

Other persons commented about Mrs. X's well-being. Her mother said, "I'm proud of how well she's done." The obstetrician spent a minimal amount of time with her during his hospital rounds. She had few questions and had "no problems." The pediatrician commented, "That's the kind of mother it takes to be successful with breast-feeding—one who's calm and doesn't get all flustered." Her roommate, who had a 16-month-old child whom she had breast-fed for several months, commented, "She's *so* mature." Whenever other nurses were asked about Mrs. X, they would report, "Oh, she's doing real well. She's just fine."

Mrs. X appeared to adjust with minimal difficulty to her first mothering task, that of feeding the baby. The baby nursed the first time the breast was offered and at fairly frequent intervals during the prelactation period. Mrs. X didn't appear to be upset about some of the baby's sleepy times during this period. She would hold the baby but not overstimulate him or urge him to nurse. There were no problems concerning the configuration of the breast or nipple for breast-feeding. About the 3rd postpartal day Mrs. X had some engorgement, and by the next day she had milk enough to affect a gain in the baby's weight. He continued to gain, and she was kept informed about his daily gain in weight until they were discharged from the hospital.

Although the nurse observed that Mrs. X did not express much spontaneous delight in her baby, the following interaction should be noted:

PATIENT: "Will the baby be coming to me at 2 o'clock this morning?"

NURSE: "You don't have milk yet, do you? There's no reason to disturb your rest until you have milk for the baby. Do you want to tell the nursery nurse, or should I?"

PATIENT: "I think I would like to have him—just to hold him."

NURSE: "Are you sure you don't need the rest? The purpose for bringing him at 2 A.M. is for his feeding and your comfort in relieving the milk, once it comes in. You may have him, if this is what you wish."

PATIENT: "I would like to have him."

Mrs. X said that she could use the signal system to call for anyone or to ask for anything during her hospital stay, but that it wasn't necessary; she had whatever she needed. From observation and discussion it seemed that Mrs. X was offered the "usual" guidance given to a new mother by the nurses. She had some assistance the first few days during the feeding periods, and she was included in a demonstration class for mothers on bathing the baby. She was presented with the possibility of her baby's being in her room for 2 to 3 hours in the afternoon for an "extended visit." (During this time the mother has the opportunity to observe her baby, to diaper and dress him, and to feed him if she desires.) Mrs. X took advantage of the extended visit during the last 2 afternoons she was in the hospital.

There were several instances of cues which verbally portrayed some of Mrs. X's need for instruction and guidance. The following exchange occurred in the first meeting:

NURSE: "I would like to help you with getting acquainted with your baby and with being a new mother."

PATIENT: "Sure. I don't know very much."

Several days later:

PATIENT: "I don't know just what I'm supposed to eat when I'm breast-feeding."

Then, several days later:

PATIENT: "They're going to bring him in to be with me from 1 to 4 tomorrow afternoon. I can diaper him and dress him. I need this kind of opportunity."

And still later:

NURSE: "Some doctors have printed instructions about their views of baby care."

PATIENT: "I hope mine does. There's so much I need to know."

On the second day of the extended visit experience the nurse came into the room and found the babies of both mothers asleep.

PATIENT: "I've had a busy time changing diapers and shirts."

NURSE: "What went on?"

PATIENT: "Well, he was messy before the feeding, so I changed him. Then I nursed him for 5 to 6 minutes, and he needed changing again. I had his clean diaper partly on him, and he voided all over his shirt and diaper. So I changed his shirt for the first time. There are three dirty diapers and a dirty shirt in the paper sack. They should have brought me a shopping bag!"

This was stated with a bit of humor accompanied by a moderate degree of frustration in the voice. (The nurse did not attribute any particular significance to these comments at this time.)

The patient expressed some concern and frustration about the length of her labor.

PATIENT: "Just how do you tell how long labor is? I had my first contraction at 3 A.M. on Sunday, and the baby wasn't born until 5 A.M. on Monday."

NURSE: "It's hard to judge when labor begins. Some

of the early contractions are helping to thin and soften the cervix—and are useful. We call that prelabor. They don't accomplish anything very dramatic, though."

PATIENT: "I had a lot of back pain. I finally called the doctor, and he said to come into the hospital. But they slowed down when I got here. It would have been easier to stay at home longer. I had hardly dilated at all when I got here. If I'd been home, I could have been up and around. I was lucky, though. I was able to be up to the bathroom. There's no place to walk. I guess they don't like you walking up and down the corridors up there. The doctor had to give me something to stimulate labor, but then it wasn't too long—about 3 or 4 hours."

NURSE: "I don't know how one prepares a first-time mother for labor. Was it anything like you expected?"

PATIENT: "You can read a lot, and people can tell you. But you don't really know what to expect until you experience it yourself. I'm glad it's over, though, because I didn't know what it would be like."

NURSE: "I think mothers have two kinds of feelings about labor. They're eager to have it begin—"

PATIENT: "They're anxious to have the baby here."

NURSE: "They're tired of carrying that heavy uterus around. It's awkward."

PATIENT: "That never bothered me. I always felt fine."

NURSE: "Was that your main impression, that labor was long, and there was a lot of back pain?"

PATIENT: "Yes. I had no pains in the front, only pain in the back. I don't remember too clearly, because they gave me some medication to sleep. Dr. O said it would be a long time."

On another occasion (following the attendance of both patients in the room at the baby bath demonstration on Mrs. X's 4th postpartal day):

PATIENT: "They used the baby of another one of Dr. O's patients, one who delivered just 50 minutes after I did. There was a sort of race to see who'd get to the delivery room first."

NURSE: "You made it."

PATIENT: "Yes, but she'd come in only a few hours before."

NURSE: "And you'd been at work for at least 20 hours."

PATIENT: "Yes, and then some. I hope it won't be so long the next time. It shouldn't, should it?"

NURSE: (*To patient's roommate*) "Is it, Mrs. A? Was it as long this time?"

PATIENT'S ROOMMATE: "No, but I have rather short labors. My first was only 8½ hours, and this one was 5 hours."

NURSE: "That's right. You're the one who has babies quite easily."

PATIENT: "You're lucky!"

Further discussion about labor continued (not all included here).

NURSE: "At least you're ready to have one more."

PATIENT: "Yes."

PATIENT'S ROOMMATE: "When I had my first baby, I said on the delivery table, 'Well, I'm ready to have another.'"

PATIENT: "I don't think I'd have said that."

NURSE: "But by the fourth day you are ready."

PATIENT: "Maybe even two days ago I'd have said it."

In summary, the nurse's evaluation of the patient at the time of homegoing was as follows:

1. She experienced a minimal amount of (physical) discomfort, less than what the nurse had observed in the immediate puerperium of a primipara in a long time.

2. She was concerned about her baby's welfare, although she related to him with some degree of objectivity and distance. She proceeded with the mothering skills of feeding, dressing and handling him with considerable naturalness and lack of apparent frustration. She didn't request much assistance from the nursing or medical staff in relation to her care or the baby's.

3. She seemed to have realistic plans for managing when she went home. Her mother-in-law lived with them and could assist with cooking, cleaning and answering the telephone. Her mother would come at intervals to assist with the laundry and heavier duties. Her husband would be there evenings and nights, and she would take care of herself and the baby.

The more dominant themes would lead one to assume that she would manage at home in a similar manner with maturity, calmness and matter-of-factness. The nurse herself would always have assumed so, had she not been privileged to see Mrs. X at home on the 9th postpartal day.

After First 52 Hours at Home

The nurse called the X residence about 6:15 P.M. on the day after the mother's discharge from the hospital. This time was selected to fit into the family's usual 5:15 P.M. dinner hour, as described by Mrs. X during her hospital stay. The purpose of the nurse's call was to determine whether this would be a suitable time to visit the family at home. Mrs. X's mother-in-law answered the telephone but soon called her son, because Mrs. X was feeding the baby.

PATIENT'S HUSBAND: "Hello."

NURSE: "Good evening. How's the new father?"

HUSBAND: "Pretty good."

NURSE: "I had mentioned to your wife that I might stop today, but that I would call first to see how things were going."

HUSBAND: "She's running a little behind schedule. We're going to have our dinner as soon as she's finished feeding the baby."

NURSE: "Perhaps I should wait and come tomorrow—or another time."

HUSBAND: "The baby was kind of fussy around 2."

NURSE: "2 P.M.?"

HUSBAND: "No, 2 A.M. this morning. I guess she was up most of the night with him."

NURSE: "Has she had any rest today?"

HUSBAND: "Not too much. Her mother said she would come over for a while this evening."

The conversation continued a short while. The nurse indicated that she would call again the next day to ascertain an appropriate visiting time. The nurse telephoned about 1:30 P.M. the following day.

PATIENT: "How are you?"

NURSE: "How are *you* is the question."

PATIENT: "I guess I'll survive."

NURSE: "You guess you'll survive?"

PATIENT: "I've just finished feeding him. He seemed hungry. He nursed for about 20 minutes. I'm getting him settled now."

NURSE: "How did it go last night?"

PATIENT: "He slept real well from about 11 P.M. to 2:15 A.M."

NURSE: "That was over 3 hours."

PATIENT: "Then he had a fussy period after I fed him. He didn't go back to sleep until about 4:30. I gave him some water. He took about 2 ounces. Then I had to wake him about a quarter to 8."

NURSE: "That was pretty good. He slept more than 3 hours *that* time."

PATIENT: "My husband was up with me, too."

There was further telephone discussion about feeding, and the nurse made arrangements to come for a visit within the next few hours.

Mrs. X was seated in an armchair. The front of her dress was open, but the brassière was in place. The baby was dressed in a kimona and wrapped in a receiving blanket. Mrs. X looked pale and tired. She didn't look up right away. The nurse sat down on a hassock near the mother's chair.

NURSE: "How are things going by now?"

PATIENT: "I just wasn't prepared for all this. I felt so good in the hospital."

PATIENT'S MOTHER: (*Rubbing lotion on creases of infant's arms and legs*) "I told Mary when she was pregnant that she ought to go to some classes, and she said, 'What do I want to go to classes for?'"

NURSE: "I don't really know *how* parents can be prepared for these early days. Classes help some, but perhaps one needs to experience them. I don't know if you can really get prepared!"

PATIENT'S MOTHER: "I think he's growing. I think I can see him growing."

NURSE: "You think you can see him change each day?"

PATIENT'S MOTHER: "Yes, I think I'm enjoying the baby more than Mary. She's so tired—and she has the responsibility."

Mrs. X excused herself. While she was gone, her mother commented:

PATIENT'S MOTHER: "She hasn't had much sleep. She's very tired. Everything's so new to her. I came

over Monday night a while so she could get some rest. Now I helped with the laundry and bathed the baby just before his feeding."

Mrs. X returned with her mother-in-law and introduced her to the nurse. She sat down in the living room now, where the four adults were seated, and where the baby was asleep in his bassinet.

NURSE: (*To patient*) "I see you have something here to drink."

PATIENT'S MOTHER: "She's not eating very well. Says she's not hungry. I made her a steak sandwich for lunch. She only ate half of it—and some salad and some milk."

NURSE: "When you're so tired, it's hard to be interested in food."

PATIENT: "I just have to force myself. I'm not hungry."

NURSE: "What about fluids? Are you drinking plenty?"

PATIENT: "I'm drinking quite a bit. Milk, fruit juices, water."

NURSE: "How has today gone in comparison with yesterday?"

PATIENT: "Everything's so new. Things all seem to come at once. I don't know where to start. I've never been around babies much. Some people have younger brothers and sisters; others have baby sat. I never did much of that, at least not with such a small baby. Not even with my niece and nephew. My sister-in-law was so protective that even my mother couldn't get close to the baby."

NURSE: "There are a lot of young women who haven't had the benefit of caring for small babies."

PATIENT: "Everything's so new. I just want to do the right thing." (With this statement her eyes became watery and red, and the tears nearly spilled over.)

MOTHER-IN-LAW: "Mary's doing a fine job."

NURSE: "You had some question last night about how long the baby was nursing, and how to keep him awake. How has this been today?"

The discussion continued with details for feeding and other events surrounding the baby.

PATIENT: "Last night my husband said, 'You're never going to breast-feed another baby!'"

NURSE: "Why do you think he said that?"

PATIENT: "He compares our baby with my brother's child, who takes 8 ounces from the bottle and sleeps all night. He forgets that he's a 2-month-old baby!"

The discussion focused for a while on bathing the baby.

PATIENT: "I haven't done that yet. I'll need to take hold. There's so much I don't know about. It's different seeing it done than doing it."

NURSE: "Perhaps right now, if you're tired, it's just as well to let someone else bathe him. *You're* the only one who can feed him. Others can do some of the other things."

PATIENT: "I'm used to work. It's not that. I

worked in an office for 6 years. I began to work even when I was in high school, when I was 15. You grow up fast under those circumstances."

NURSE: "You probably needed to have things pretty carefully scheduled, to work full time and to manage a house and take care of your husband."

PATIENT: "You can say that again."

NURSE: "Now you have a squirming, crying bundle that doesn't fit into any schedule. Remember, Dr. M said he's not even sophisticated enough to know he shouldn't have his fussy periods at night."

PATIENT: "If you only knew when it would *end*, you know—not even on the day, but which *week*."

NURSE: "If there were only some limits which you could count on, you mean, knowing that sleeping through the night would happen by such and such a time."

PATIENT: "It's not knowing that's hard."

Further conversation revealed that Mrs. X had expressed some of her feelings by crying, and that her husband had found her weeping when she'd gotten up to be with the baby during a fussy time at night. The nurse gave some guidance about scheduling, feeding, placement of the baby's crib, and she answered questions of Mrs. X and her mother. It was near the dinner hour, and the nurse made plans to visit again in a few days.

Just by chance Mrs. X's mother met the nurse in a distant part of the hospital. The following remarks are excerpts from the mother's comments: "My daughter was so sure of herself during pregnancy. I wanted her to go to prenatal classes to learn about babies, but she didn't want to. . . . She feels so inadequate. I wasn't prepared for her depression. She seems to feel so inadequate about the bath."

The expressed concerns of Mrs. X's mother added weight to the previous question of what was happening to cause such a marked change in Mrs. X's behavior and performance in her new role. What facets of nursing care in the hospital could have been utilized to prepare Mrs. X more adequately for coping with problems on her return home?

At the beginning of the third day, 52 hours after she returned home, Mrs. X seemed to experience the low point of her "depression." The following day the baby began to sleep longer between feedings. Mrs. X began to get more rest, her appetite improved, she felt stronger, and she bathed her baby. There were still frustrations and problems to be handled, but they seemed to be more manageable. For instance, on Monday of her 2nd week at home, the nurse telephoned at 3:30 in the afternoon to see whether she might stop for a visit. Mrs. X said that everything was topsy-turvy, and that she was still trying to get herself dressed. However, she had bathed the baby, and she was preparing dinner. The following week the nurse made her third visit to the home. It was her first contact with the patient alone. Although the nurse was aware that the "right moment" had

probably passed for helping Mrs. X with the distress she expressed by nearly crying, she did introduce the subject. The following interaction occurred with some expression of feeling, but there was no weeping or overt manifestation of anxiety as the "first 52 hours" were discussed.

NURSE: "You've been home a little more than a week now. Is it what you expected? Anything like what you envisioned it would be?"

PATIENT: "I had *no* idea what to expect. I was never with small babies. I just didn't know how much time and work a baby would take. It's a 24-hour responsibility."

NURSE: "Those first days must have been pretty difficult. You must have felt a bit helpless at not knowing what to do when the baby cried."

PATIENT: "Yes, they were. Sunday wasn't so bad. I'd just come home, and people were around. My mother was here. But then Monday mother had to work, and my husband went to work, I was alone with the baby except for my mother-in-law. I knew how to change a diaper, but that was about all. I wanted to do the right thing for the baby."

NURSE: "I'm sure a mother wants to respond to her baby's needs, but deciding what is the right thing is hard. It is a lot of responsibility, to be a mother, a parent."

PATIENT: "I think we're getting acquainted. I can tell his cry when he's hungry; I can tell when he has gas by the way he draws up his legs."

NURSE: "You are more certain about making decisions as to what to do for him? You can decide when he needs milk—or water?"

PATIENT: "Yes. This week is so much better than last."

NURSE: "Did other things bother you those first days—beside not knowing what to do with the baby? The house?"

PATIENT: "Well, yes. I do have certain ways of doing things, and when other people help, they can't know how you do them. I've always been very healthy."

NURSE: "So you're not accustomed to having people help you?"

PATIENT: "No, I've always been quite independent. I've worked since I was 15. I worked until my 7th month of pregnancy. I felt so well in the hospital."

NURSE: "Yes, we kept talking about that, and kept looking for some problems, but—"

PATIENT: "There weren't any. Not even my stitches hurt after the 2nd day."

NURSE: "When you came home, you hit a low point."

PATIENT: "I wasn't prepared for being so depressed. I guess it's called the 'baby blues.' "

NURSE: "Some people have this experience in the hospital. Did it happen to you there?"

PATIENT: "Not really—maybe only once. One evening my husband didn't come to see me because he wasn't feeling well, but he didn't tell me until later. That upset me, because I wish he'd tell me. Maybe I could do something to help him."

NURSE: "You probably haven't felt so helpless in a long time as you did those first several days."

PATIENT: "No, I haven't. If we have another baby, I'd know more what to expect. . . ."

It may be helpful to have further information about Mrs. X and the significant people in her environment. Mrs. X is the younger of two children born to parents of different religious faiths. Although her father is in the family picture, Mrs. X did not once refer to him. Mrs. X's mother, on the other hand, has played an active role. She visited her daughter in the hospital and assisted her daughter with household tasks on the days in which she was not working. The mother commented that her daughter has always been a "good girl," and that she never had to worry about her when she was out on a date. If she were going to be late, she'd always call. Some of the interactions previously shared might provide some clues about her opinion of her daughter's adequacy as a mother.

There is little information about Mrs. X's brother except that he has been to college, is married, is the father of two children, and lives with his family in a nearby suburb. On the other hand, Mrs. X mentioned twice that she had gone to work when she was 15 (there are gaps in information here as to the reason for working and the nature of her work). On graduation from high school Mrs. X went to work as a bookkeeper and continued to work in that position through the 7th month of her pregnancy.

Mr. and Mrs. X have been married for several years. Mr. X, who is 9 years older than his wife, has been employed as a craftsman with the same company for the past 13 years. Mrs. X spoke with delight in her voice and her face when she told that her husband was thinking of painting a banner with the words "Welcome home, Mary and Johnny." On the day of discharge from the hospital, when the nurse first saw them together, they seemed to relate with warmth but with a certain self-consciousness and reserve. He was attentive in helping her into the car.

The nurse observed the new parents together briefly on two occasions in their home. On the day Mrs. X was so depressed, she eagerly listened for sounds of the car as the time for her husband's homecoming drew near. When he did come into the living room, she immediately offered to get his slippers. On another occasion he slipped his arm around her waist as she was in the kitchen warming a bottle of water for the baby. The X's are not in financial distress; they have two cars, hospitalization insurance, more than adequate equipment for the baby, and are buying a new suburban home.

They are eager to move into their new home. The advent of the baby has crowded them, since Mr. X's mother also lives with them in their 2-bedroom house. This necessitates placement of the baby's equipment in their bedroom and the baby in the living room. Mr. X's mother is an elderly woman who has a serious chronic illness. Mrs. X expressed her desire to contribute toward making a home for her mother-in-law and making her life as pleasant as possible. She commented several times on how well she and her mother-in-law got along. When the nurse was in the home, Mrs. X's mother-in-law was friendly and courteous, but she kept busy with her household tasks instead of joining in the conversation.

Comments and Conclusions

The concept that pregnancy is a period of disequilibrium and maturational crisis needs to be reiterated to professionals working with women during the childbearing cycle. This may need special emphasis in relation to the woman who has an uncomplicated pregnancy and childbirth experience, since it is usually the woman with problems and complications who occupies the major portion of the nurse's attention. Pregnancy involves profound physiologic and psychological changes. An intensive longitudinal study of 15 women during pregnancy and the 1st year after delivery was conducted by Bibring et al. in Boston. The theoretical framework on which the study is based is as follows:

Pregnancy is a crisis that affects all expectant mothers, no matter what their state of psychic health. Crises, as we see it, are turning points in the life of the individual, leading to acute disequilibria which under favorable conditions result in specific maturational steps toward new functions. We find them as developmental phenomena at points of no return between one phase and the next when decisive changes deprive former central needs and modes of living of their significance, forcing the acceptance of highly charged new goals and functions. Pregnancy as a major turning point in the life of a woman represents one of these normal crises, especially for the primigravida who faces the impact of this event for the first time. We believe that all women show what looks like remarkable, far-reaching psychological changes when they are pregnant. The outcome of this crisis, then, has profound effects on the early mother-child relationships.[16]

The final results of the study have not been published, but they may contribute significantly to understanding the nature of the crisis and the maturation expected.

Bibring states that the crisis does not end with

_____

[16] Bibring, Grete, et al.: A study of the psychological processes in pregnancy and of the earliest mother-child relationships. Psychoanal. Stud. Child 14:25-26, 1959.

the birth of the baby but continues into the puerperium and perhaps beyond:

The findings that crisis continues, more or less so, beyond parturition offer strong support in favor of the proposition that the frequent problems in the early mother-child relationship are partly due to an as yet incomplete reorganization of the mother's psychic equilibrium at the time of delivery.[17]

Deutsch agrees that the crisis period extends beyond the delivery of the baby.[18]

Pregnancy and childbirth could be discussed much more extensively as a general crisis, but it may be more helpful to investigate some of the possible components of the crisis and to reflect on those which may be applicable to Mrs. X's situation. The first several posthospital days illustrate an obvious crisis period for Mrs. X.

Components of the Crisis Situation

A very complex component of the crisis and disequilibrium has to do with the relationship of psychosexual development and maternal feelings.

Deutsch[19] writes extensively about motherhood, pregnancy, confinement and lactation in relation to Freud's concepts of psychosexual development. For example, breast-feeding the baby may arouse the erogenous area of the nipple and create sexual sensations. The nursing mother may be confused by the aroused sexual feelings and the feelings of love and responsiveness as she nurses her baby.

There is limited data from which to assess Mrs. X's situation in regard to the psychosexual component. Mrs. X appeared to be rather matter-of-fact about the process of breast-feeding. She would prepare the nipple for feeding in the presence of her roommate and the nurse, and she allowed the nurse to touch her breast to assist the baby in obtaining proper grasp of the areola. She practiced the technique of manual expression of breast milk at the same time her roommate was practicing, although a certain degree of privacy was planned during this teaching-learning experience.

Mrs. X did not ask questions of the nurse or the obstetrician concerning the appropriate time for renewing sexual intercourse in relation to the process of vaginal and perineal healing. The nurse introduced the subject, and Mrs. X seemed to appreciate the guidance offered, since the obstetrician had not included this in his homegoing instructions.

On three different occasions the subject of subsequent pregnancies and child spacing was indirectly introduced by giving information in relation to breast-feeding and ovulation. Mrs. X did not pursue the topic with further discussion or questions. She seemed to remain somewhat guarded and reserved in all of the relationships, and thus one would expect that she would maintain this reserve in the area of psychosexual material.

Closely aligned with the psychosexual component of the crisis is Caplan's description of the change in equilibrium between the ego and the id. He likens the usual relationship of id and ego to an iceberg, the portion above the surface being the ego and the portion below the surface being the id. During pregnancy the iceberg turns upside down and allows id material to come to the surface rather easily. Fantasies and wishes are consciously expressed with a relatively minimal production of anxiety.[20]

Caplan describes the pregnant woman as a kind of battery that needs to be charged. If those significant to her are not able to meet her needs for being nurtured, she may have more difficulty in extending herself to her child during those early months when the child has many needs but gives little to the mother in response to the fulfillment of those needs.

Rubin analyzes the passive and the dependent phases of the puerperium. These were discussed in Chapter 14.

There is very little data about Mrs. X's period of pregnancy except that she felt fine and continued to work until the third trimester of pregnancy. One would, however, question the degree to which she was allowed to be dependent and to receive care during the early puerperium in the hospital. She did "take in" rest and food, but on the day after delivery she was already taking her own bath in the shower. She had no obvious or particular reasons to request or demand nursing or medical care. One could question whether she might have been better fortified to cope with the baby at home if there had been more attention to the "battery-charging" process.

There are clues that Mrs. X is a "giving" person who does not ask much for herself. She was accustomed to giving herself to a job and to her family. She invested herself in her mother-in-law to provide "pleasant moments" for a woman with a serious illness. She invested herself in her husband in proper feeding ("He's not been served a TV dinner since we were married!") and in caring ("Would you like your

---

[17] Ibid., p. 20.

[18] Deutsch, Helene: Psychology of Women. p. 261, New York, Grune & Stratton, 1945.

[19] Ibid.

[20] Caplan, Gerald: Concepts of Mental Health and Consultation. Children's Bureau Publication No. 373, p. 51, Washington, D.C., 1959.

slippers?"). She might well have had some conflicting feelings about the reversal in role with these significant people. It might have been easier for her to receive care from hospital personnel, because helping is an expected part of their function; but to receive care from those to whom she usually extended herself was quite a different situation.

Another component of the crisis of child-bearing is the inescapable revival of feelings about the woman's relationship with her own mother. This relationship is always influenced by guilt feelings. The degree to which further independence from her mother is sought is somewhat in direct proportion to the extent of her guilt feelings. She is caught between two poles: that of needing her mother or a mother substitute in providing care and guidance in the new role of motherhood, and that of asserting that she is now the mother.

The fate of the identification with the mother is another factor that determines the course of pregnancy. In every instance the capacity for motherhood is related to this identification. The ego of the pregnant woman must find a harmonious compromise between her deeply unconscious identification with the child, which is directed toward the future, and her identification with her own mother, which is directed toward the past. Wherever one of these identifications is rejected, difficulties arise. In the first case the fetus becomes a hostile parasite, in the second the pregnant woman's capacity for motherhood is weakened by her unwillingness to accept her identification with her own mother.[21]

Many questions could be raised about Mrs. X's mother's advice that she attend some classes during pregnancy and her daughter's expressed lack of need and interest in attending prenatal classes. The question of why Mrs. X refused to attend classes has many facets. It is interesting to note the mother's response on the "52nd hour," the day of frustration and depression: "I told her when she was pregnant she ought to go to some classes." Perhaps Mrs. X did not need to depend on her mother too much during pregnancy or in the hospital period. She did indeed need her mother in the early-days at home. She needed her mother to do the laundry, to bathe the baby, and to give guidance in understanding the needs of her child. How could Mrs. X work through becoming a "coequal" with her own mother in terms of motherhood when she felt so helpless and inadequate in meeting her baby's needs?

Mrs. X's responses in "I just wasn't prepared for this. . . . I just want to do the *right* thing," may communicate something of ego inadequacy in relation to motherhood. She once commented ironically, "They call babies a bundle of joy!"

---

[21] Deutsch, *loc. cit.,* p. 145.

She was afraid to do certain things for the baby. The day after she had bathed the baby for the first time:

PATIENT: "It wasn't so bad once I did it. I just was afraid to be by myself to bathe him. I was afraid I wouldn't know what to do—like I couldn't get under one of his arms. So my sister-in-law says, 'Just skip it this time.' "

NURSE: "You were afraid you might hurt him."

PATIENT: "I had so much more confidence after I'd done it."

Something of the extent of her fear may be understood by the fact that it was *7 days* after she had given the first bath that she ventured to give the bath when she was alone. Similarly, she waited to give vitamins to the baby until her husband was at home with her. This is quite in contrast with her observation of the nurse's handling of the baby when he was regurgitating some mucus on his first day of life. When the nurse asked her if she'd know what to do, she said: "Just turn him on his side to get the mucus out—so it doesn't get in his throat."

Perhaps it is somewhat artificial to attempt to describe components of a crisis experience. Certainly in the actuality of a situation these components overlap and merge. However, for the purpose of attaining a closer understanding of the patient in order to help her to achieve her goals, there is value in investigating all aspects of the situation. For practical purposes it might be said that Mrs. X's crisis is a fairly predictable one. Therefore, the nurse's anticipatory guidance will be of immense benefit to the new mother during a necessarily critical period of her life.

SUGGESTED READING

General

American Academy of Pediatrics: Standards and Recommendations for Hospital Care of Newborn Infants, rev. ed., Evanston, The Academy, 1964.

Arnold, H. W. *et al.*: Transition to extra-uterine life. Am. J. Nurs. 65:77-80, October, 1965.

Blake, F., Wright, F. H., and Waechter, E. H.: Nursing Care of Children. ed. 8, Philadelphia, J. B. Lippincott, 1970.

Battaglia, F. C., and Lubchenco, L. O.: A practical classification of newborn infants by weight and gestational age. J. Pediat. 71:159-163, August, 1967.

Brackbill, Y., and Thompson, G. G.: Behavior in Infancy and Early Childhood, New York, Free Press, 1967.

Buchanan-Davidson, D. J.: What we can learn from meconium. Am. J. Nurs. 63:112-113, July, 1963.

Buetow, K. C., *et al.*: Effect of maintenance of "normal" skin temperature on survival of infants of low birth weight. Pediatrics 34:163-170, August, 1964.

DeLamerens, S., *et al.*: Neonatal bilirubin levels after use of phenothiazine derivations for obstetrical analgesia. J. Pediat. 65:925-928, December, 1964.

Escalona, S. K.: The Roots of Individuality. Chicago: Aldine Publishing Co., 1968.

Eisenberg, R. B., *et al.*: Auditory behavior in the human neonate: Preliminary report. J. Speech Hearing Res. 7:245-269, September, 1964.

Fantz, R. L.: Pattern discrimination and selective attention as determinants of perceptual development from birth *in* Kidd, Aline H., and Rivoire, J. L. (eds.): Perceptual Development in Children. New York, International Universities Press, 1965.

———: The origin of form perception. Sci. Am. 204:66-72, May, 1961.

———: Visual experience in infants: decreased attention to familiar patterns relative to novel ones. Science 146:668-670, October 30, 1964.

Gryboski, J. D.: The swallowing mechanism of the neonate: I. Esophageal and gastric motility. Pediatrics 35:445-452, March, 1965.

Haynes, U.: A Developmental Approach to Case-finding. Children's Bureau Publication #449, Washington: Government Printing Office, 1967.

Hervoda, A.: Nursery evaluation of the newborn, Am. J. Nurs. 67:1669-1671, August, 1967.

Keitel, H. G.: Preventing neonatal diaper rash. Am. J. Nurs. 65:124-126, May, 1965.

James, L. S., *et al.*: Respiratory physiology of the fetus and newborn infant. New Eng. J. Med. 271:1403-1409, December 31, 1964.

Levin, S.: Baby habits, genesis and ontogenesis. Speculation on prehistory, biblical history and some phenomena of babyhood. Clin. Pediat. 3:741-742, December, 1964.

MacCready, Jean: A Feeding Room for Babies. Am. J. Nurs. 64:117, July, 1964.

Marlow, D. R.: Textbook of Pediatric Nursing. ed. 3, Philadelphia, W. B. Saunders, 1969.

Meyer, H. F.: Current feeding practices in hospital maternity nurseries. Clin. Pediat. 8:69-72, February, 1969.

———: Infant Foods and Feeding Practice. ed. 2, Philadelphia, W. B. Saunders, 1965.

Nelson, W. E. (ed.): Textbook of Pediatrics. ed. 8, Philadelphia, W. B. Saunders, 1964.

Parmalee, A. H., Jr., *et al.*: Infant sleep patterns from birth to 16 weeks of age. J. Pediat. 65:576-582, October, 1964.

Polgar, G.: The first breath: A turbulent period of physiologic adjustment. Clin. Pediat. 2:562-571, October, 1963.

Pryor, K.: Nursing Your Baby. New York: Harper and Row, 1963.

Riker, A. P.: Breastfeeding. Public Affairs Pamphlet No. 353S, New York, Public Affairs Pamphlets, 1964.

Ringholz, S., and Morris, M.: A test of some assumptions about rooming-in. Nurs. Res. 10:196-199, Fall, 1961.

Shipley, T., *et al.*: The human electroretinogram in the first day of life. J. Pediat. 65:733-739, November, 1964.

Silverman, W. A., and Parke, P. C.: Keep him warm. Am. J. Nurs. 65:81-84, October, 1965.

Smith, C. A.: The first breath. Sci. Am. 109:27-35, October, 1963.

Stembera, Z. K.: Umbilical blood flow in healthy newborn infants during the first minutes after birth, Am. J. Obstet. Gynec. 91:568-574, February 15, 1965.

Stern, E., *et al.*: Sleep cycle characteristics in infants. Pediatrics 43:65, January, 1969.

Wolff, P. H., and Simmons, M. A.: Nonnutritive sucking and response thresholds in young infants. Child Develop. 38:631-638, 1967.

The Mother and Her Newborn Infant

Adams, M.: Early concerns of primigravida mothers regarding infant care activities. Nurs. Res. 12:72-77, Spring, 1963.

Anthony, E. J., and Benedek, T.: Parenthood: Its Psychology and Psychopathology. Boston: Little, Brown, 1970.

Barnes, G. R., Jr., *et al.*: Management of breast feeding. J.A.M.A. 151:192-199, January 17, 1953.

Benson, L. G.: Fatherhood: A Sociological Perspective. New York: Random House, 1968.

Bibring, G. L., *et al.*: A study of the psychological processes in pregnancy and of the earliest mother-child relationship. Psychoanal. Stud. Child 16:9-72, 1961.

Bowers, R.: Touch—A Pilot Study in Clinical Teaching. Maternal Child Nursing Conference, pp. 31-33, University of Pittsburgh School of Nursing, June, 1966.

Bowlby, J.: Maternal Care and Mental Health. Geneva, World Health Organization, 1952.

Brody, S.: Patterns of Mothering. New York, Internat. Univ. Press, 1956.

Caplan, G.: An Approach to Community Mental Health. New York, Grune & Stratton, 1961.

Carpenter, H. M.: The Need for Assistance of Mothers With First Babies During the Three Month Period Following the Baby's Birth. New York, Teachers College, Columbia University, 1965.

Clark, A.: The beginning family. Am. J. Nurs. 66:802, April, 1966.

———: The adaptation problems and patterns of the expanding family, the neonatal period. Nurs. Forum 5:92-109, 1966.

Deutsch, H.: Psychology of Women, vol. 2, Motherhood, New York, Grune & Stratton, 1945.

Disbrow, M. A.: Factors Involved in Successful Breast Feeding. U.S.P.H.S. Grant GN7901, unpublished, 1962.

Evans, R. T.: Needs Identified Among Breastfeeding Mothers, ANA Clinical Sessions, pp. 162-171, 1968.

Evans, R. T., et al.: Exploration of factors involved in maternal physiological adaptation to breastfeeding. Nurs. Res. 18:28-32, January-February, 1969.

Iffrig, Sister M. C.: Nursing care and success in breastfeeding. Nurs. Clin. N. Am. 3:345-354, June, 1968.

Keane, V. R.: Nursing care of the family after delivery. Bull. Am. Coll. Nurs. Midwifery 9:56-63, Fall, 1964.

Lesser, M. S., and Keane, V. R.: Nurse, Patient Relationships in a Hospital Maternity Service. St. Louis, C. V. Mosby, 1956.

McElin, T. W., et al.: The microbiological environment of a rooming-in maternity. Am. J. Obstet. Gynec. 83:907-917, April, 1964.

Mintern, Leigh, et al.: Mothers of Six Cultures. New York, John Wiley & Sons, 1964.

Moore, L., and White, G. D.: Comparisons of teaching methods in maternal and infant care. Nurs. Outlook 13:74-76, May, 1965.

Newton, M., and Newton, N.: The normal course and management of lactation. Clin. Obstet. Gynec. 5:44-63, March, 1962.

———: Psychologic aspects of lactation. New Eng. J. Med., November 30, 1967.

Parent-Child Relationships: The Role of the Nurse. New Brunswick, New Jersey: Rutgers University, May-June, 1968.

Rich, O. J.: Hospital routines as rites of passage. Nurs. Clin. N. Am. 4:101-109, March, 1969.

———: Personal communication to authors, 1965.

———: Clinical Study of a Primipara's Initial Adaptation to Mothering, U.S.P.H.S. Grant STIMH 7988-03, unpublished, 1965.

Richardson, S. A. (ed.): Childbearing: Its Social and Psychological Aspects. Baltimore: Williams & Wilkins, 1967.

Rossi, A. S.: Transition to parenthood. J. Marriage and the Family 30:26-39, February, 1968.

Rubin, R.: Basic maternal behavior. Nurs. Outlook 9:683-686, November, 1961.

———: Puerperal change. Nurs. Outlook 9:753-755, December, 1961.

———: Maternal touch. Nurs. Outlook 11:828-831, November, 1963.

———: The family-child relationship and nursing care. Nurs. Outlook 12:36-39, September, 1964.

Senn, M. J. E., and Hartford, C. (eds.): The Firstborn: Experiences of Eight American Families. Cambridge: Harvard University Press, 1968.

Simmons, J. E., et al.: Maternal variables and neonate behavior. J. Child Psychiat. 6:174-183, 1967.

VonRuden, J.: Relation Between Acceptance by the Nurse of the Feeding Method and Alleviation of Guilt Feelings in the Mother. ANA Regional Clinical Conferences, 1966.

Care of Low Birth Weight and Premature Infants

INTRODUCTION

The basic meaning of the word "prematurity" is underdevelopment. It refers to the inability of the infant who is born before the usual gestation period and/or who is under "normal" birth weight, to make an adaptation to extra-uterine existence to a degree comparable with the survival rates in mature infants. Thus, a premature infant has been defined arbitrarily as any infant of single or multiple birth that is born prematurely, at term or even past term with a weight of 2,500 Gm. (5½ lbs.) or less. Such an infant is usually less than 47 cm. (18 in.) in length and usually has been born prior to the 37th week of gestation. In recent years, the term low birth weight has been introduced as a supplement to "premature," since it is possible to have an infant born at term, who is immature and does not exceed the 2,500 Gm. minimum "mature" birth weight criterion. Although most authorities will agree that the definition of prematurity is still open to question, some progress has been made with the delineation of the "low birth weight" concept. However, there is still controversy over the definitions and the criteria to be applied. It has not been established, for example, when prematurity ought to be defined by weight or gestational age or both. Moreover, the two above mentioned terms continue to be used synonymously at times and differentially at other times. A *low birth weight* infant has been defined as any live born infant with a weight at birth of 2,500 Gm. (5½ lbs.) or less. A *premature* infant is a live born infant whose gestation period is less than 37 weeks regardless of weight.[1] Thus, a low birth weight infant may be premature, but a premature infant need not have a low birth weight. Moreover, two other criteria, development and body measurements, have been suggested. In the former some physicians regard the maturational level of enzyme systems, physiologic-anatomic functions, and neurologic behavior as indices of maturity and immaturity. Body measurements such as crown-heel length (47 cm. mature), crown-rump length (32 cm. mature) and head circumference (33 cm. mature) are used by some. However, as previously stated, there is no agreement as to the combinations which should be "standard" criteria. To be consistent with the literature (at the expense of some precision) we will use the term premature when referring to both types as a total condition or state of affairs. When referring specifically to either type as defined above, we will use the term low birth weight and qualify "premature" with early gestational age.

Prematurity ranks as the eighth cause of death in the United States and has become, in the eyes of many authorities, the largest single problem in contemporary obstetrics and pediatrics as well as public health. Despite the importance of this problem, little progress has been made in achieving

---

[1] Babson, S. G., and Benson, R.: Primer on Prematurity and High-Risk Pregnancy. P. 1, St. Louis, C. V. Mosby, 1966.

a desirable reduction in the rate. For instance, it still remains about 7 to 8 per cent in the white race and 12 per cent in the nonwhite races. These figures have held markedly constant for the last 75 years. Furthermore, little definitive knowledge has been obtained about the causes of this phenomenon. Many factors are known to be associated with it. Yet, no causal relationships have been demonstrated. Recently, investigators have found that some of the associations may be spurious and clouded by exogenous variables which are either undetermined or inaccurately measured. (For a thorough discussion of these considerations, see the Abramowicz and Kass articles in the Suggested Reading.) We do know, however, that the majority of deaths among newborns are associated with prematurity. The death rate of the low-weight neonate is forty times that of the full-sized infant born at term. Moreover, the incidence of cerebral palsy associated with prematurity may be as high as ten times, deficiency fivefold, and lethal malformations seven times over those in the nonpremature infant. Emotional disturbances, social maladjustments, visual and hearing defects are also multiplied. If this were not enough, medical and custodial costs for these individuals are incalculable. Without a doubt, this condition is truly one of the most urgent problems of modern medicine.

As the above figures indicate, nonwhites, the Negro race particularly, because they generally have smaller infants than whites, have a higher percentage of premature infants. Infants over the empirical weight, even though apparently born at full term, occasionally may be diagnosed by a physician as "premature" on the basis of other considerations, such as faulty maintenance of body temperature, particular feeding difficulties or certain physical characteristics. This may apply especially to infants born to diabetic or prediabetic mothers. Although the upper limit of weight has been established, the lower never has been accepted by any authoritative group, and the level at which a dividing line is drawn between abortions and premature infants remains a matter of personal or local preference. The lower limit will depend on the definition of abortion, but the 1,000 Gm. figure is the one most frequently used. If the baby is from 6 to 8 weeks or more premature, the diagnosis is comparatively easy because of weight, length and physical characteristics. The closer to full term the baby is, the greater are the chances for survival.

The nursing care that is required for prema-ture infants and their parents presents an interesting challenge for the nurse. The situation is a poignant one, for the life of the infant often hangs in the balance, and the postpartal course is complicated by concomitant psychological disorganization. The nurse is one of the key persons who is responsible for a successful outcome for both infant and parents.

FACTORS ASSOCIATED WITH PREMATURITY

Since more than half of the neonatal deaths in the United States are due to prematurity, and since these rates have remained constant for many years, the emphasis on preventive care must be stressed. If an amount equal to the money expended on premature care were applied to preventive care, it would be interesting to prognosticate the results. The causes of prematurity demand continued attention and research, since knowledge in this area is far behind the information now available about other aspects of obstetrics. Since there is little empirical evidence as to cause per se, it is perhaps wiser to speak of factors contributing to this condition.

Maternal factors contributing to prematurity usually can be demonstrated in only about one third of the cases. These include such obstetric problems as toxemia and premature separation of the placenta; those of fetal cause such as plural births, anomalies and hydramnios; and medicosurgical features such as intercurrent maternal disease (hypertension, venereal, thyroid, cardiac and diabetic disease) and operations. Other maternal factors are also of interest and have been shown to have some association (but again, no causal relationship) by various investigators. Some of the factors are: the age and parity of the mother, her marital status, overwork, cigarette smoking, small-heart syndrome, her history of previous pregnancy disaster, subfertility, her race, her nutritional status, her socioeconomic status, high altitude, and the quality of antepartal care. (For a more thorough discussion of these variables see the Babson and Benson book and the Abramowicz and Kass articles in the Suggested Reading.)

The *paternal role* in prematurity is largely theoretical and is yet to be clarified. Some investigators feel that older age, the transmission of Rh-positive genes to the offspring, chronic alcoholism, and diabetes mellitus may be factors that influence fetal development adversely.

TABLE 17-1. PREMATURE INFANT
Infants Classified by Weight and Gestational Age*

	5 LB. 8 OZ. (2,500 GM.) OR LESS			OVER 5 LB. 8 OZ. (2,500 GM.)	
	LESS THAN 37 WEEKS		37 WEEKS AND OVER GROUP III	LESS THAN 37 WEEKS GROUP IV	37 WEEKS AND OVER GROUP V
	LESS THAN 3 LB. 5 OZ. GROUP I	3 LB. 5 OZ. TO 5 LB. 8 OZ. GROUP II			
Percent of all deliveries	1	2	2 to 4	2 to 4	90 ± 3
Neonatal mortality (%)	65	10	3 to 4	2	Less than 0.5
Appellations	Immature premature	Premature	"Small for dates" Dysmature Postmature Pseudopremature Fetal malnutrition Intrauterine growth retardation Chronic fetal distress	"Pseudoterm"	Normal newborn infants
Characteristics	Weight loss, 20 percent ± 10 percent Translucent and edematous skin Decreased tone Erratic extremity movement Periodic breathing Moderate jaundice Physiologic immaturity in enzymatic and functional development	Weight loss, 10 percent ± 5 percent	Minimal weight loss, less than 5 percent Malnutrition Dry and scaly skin Increased tone Restricted Moro reflex Increased oxygen consumption Minimal jaundice Cries for and has increased capacity for food Anxious, open-eyed appearance	Same as for Group II but less marked	
Complications	Respiratory distress syndrome common Susceptible to infection Asphyxial injury to capillaries, with hemorrhage		Respiratory distress syndrome rare Hypoglycemia common Reduced skeletal growth Increase in congenital anomalies May have had chronic intrauterine asphyxia	Respiratory distress syndrome occasionally Often neglected because of the false reassurance of their size	
Special requirements	Incubator care		Early water, glucose, calories, and vitamins	Same as for Groups I and II	
Exceptions	Some immature infants who are also malnourished and undersized for their gestation, with some of the characteristics and nutritional requirements of Group III		Infants who are biologically small due to race, family pattern, or early growth arrest; usually not malnourished		Up to 10 percent of normal infants, who have had some degree of fetal malnutrition as in Group III, particularly when of postdate delivery

* Modified from Yerushalmy, J., van den Berg, Bea J., Erhardt, C. L., and Jacobziner, H.: Birth weight and gestation as indices of "immaturity," Amer. J. Dis. Child. 109:43, 1965.

From Babson, S. G., and Benson, R. C.: Primer on Prematurity and High-risk Pregnancy. St. Louis, C. V. Mosby, 1966. (Modified from Yerushalmy, J., van den Berg, B. J., Erhardt, C. L., and Jacobziner, H.: Birth weight and gestation as indices of "immaturity." Am. J. Dis. Child. 109:43, 1965.

Fetal conditions such as multiple birth, congenital anomalies, and certain specific diseases including rubella, malaria and chickenpox all can affect fetal development negatively. Finally, *placental factors,* such as placental insufficiency and abnormalities of the cord have been indicted. All in all, it becomes apparent that the condition of prematurity involves a variety of interrelated variables, some physiologic, some pathological, and some that defy such neat categorization.

CAUSES OF PREMATURE DEATHS

Perhaps one of the most discouraging findings has been the failure of survival rates among prematures to improve with time despite advances made in reducing maternal and infant mortality in general. Some earlier improvements were seen in the United States overall, from 1935 to 1948, as the neonatal mortality of these infants fell from 149 to 108 per 1000 premature live births. However, the situation leveled off, and now a slight but steady rising trend in mortality is now being recorded. One exception to this negligible improvement has occurred in infants weighing less than 1000 Gm.; their chance of survival has increased, probably due to the intensive attention and care required for these very small infants. At any rate, the overall mortality rate of prematures is still disproportionately high. By far the commonest cause of death among prematures is idiopathic respiratory distress syndrome (hyaline membrane disease). These terms are used to describe a syndrome of neonatal respiratory distress in which pulmonary hyaline membrane with atelectasis are the principal findings at autopsy. This condition is seen frequently also among infants who have been delivered by cesarean section and among babies of diabetic mothers. Other principal causes of death include anoxia, malformations, bronchopneumonia, septicemia and other infections and birth injuries (principally cerebral, for the blood vessels of the premature lack the supporting wall structure and are damaged very easily).

CHARACTERISTICS AND PHYSIOLOGY OF THE PREMATURE INFANT

General Description at Birth

As there are many degrees of prematurity, there are also various stages of anatomic and physiologic development. Many of the symptoms described below may vary in infants of approximately the same fetal age, depending on the factors associated with prematurity and the physical condition of the mother and the infant. At birth the premature baby lacks the subcutaneous fat which is deposited during the last 2 months of intra-uterine development. This gives the skin a transparent appearance with the blood vessels easily seen through the skin, which often is of a deep red color, sometimes with a cyanotic hue. These premature babies are prone likewise to develop icteric skin changes. Lanugo is usually abundant all over the skin surface but disappears within a few weeks.

The external ears and the nose are very soft, due to the underdeveloped cartilage. The ears lie very close to the head. The skull is round, in contrast with the long anteroposterior skull diameter of the full-term infant. The fontanels are large, and the sutures prominent. The fingernails and toenails may be immature, often not reaching the ends of the fingers and the toes.

The infant may be puny and small, or he may approximate full-term weight; yet the internal organs may be imperfectly developed, and these babies appear to be reluctant to assume the responsibility to live. The respiration is shallow and irregular, due to the lack of lung expansion and proper gaseous exchange. There are often periods of apnea. Due to the irregular respiration and the poorly developed function of swallowing, there is danger of aspiration of milk or vomitus, causing cyanosis and predisposing to pulmonary infections. The premature baby regurgitates his food readily, because the stomach is tubular in form, and the sphincters are poorly developed. The urine is usually scanty.

The walls of the blood vessels are weak, and the tendency to hemorrhage is great. Since the central nervous system is not fully developed, the premature infant is sluggish, must be wakened to be fed, and the muscular movements are feeble. The temperature is usually subnormal and fluctuating, due to the underdeveloped heat-regulating center. The cry is monotonous, whining, "kittenlike" and effortless, showing a lack of energy. All these symptoms are evidenced in varying degrees, according to the degree of immaturity.

Physiological Considerations

As we have seen in Chapter 16, the newly born infant must make certain adaptations to extra-uterine life. While the various stages or steps have not been delineated for the premature baby as they have for the normal newborn, it is apparent that his adaptations will be even greater and more difficult due to his anatomical and physiological deficits.

Respiratory System. The development of the lungs will depend upon the degree of maturity. For instance, the lungs of an infant weighing 2 pounds (900 Gm.) or less show small alveoli lined with cuboidal epithelium and surrounded by a meagre supply of capillaries (which prevent efficient gaseous exchange); the lungs of an infant weighing 6 pounds (2730 Gm.), on the other hand, show large alveoli, the walls of which are virtually formed by bare capillaries. There is a great increase in the capillary network between the 26th week and the 36th week of intrauterine life and for this reason, the ability of the lungs to sustain extrauterine life increases with each week of intrauterine existence. The more immature the infant, the less blood flow there is through the lungs; the remainder being shunted through the ductus arteriosus.

As we have seen with the mature newborn, the most critical event in the adjustment to extrauterine life is the establishment of ventilation by the previously unused lungs. The unexpanded lungs of any fetus are not just crumpled air sacs waiting to be filled; rather they are fluid filled organs requiring a great deal of negative intrapleural pressure (up to 60 cm. water has been used experimentally) for expansion. This great effort is necessary because of the viscosity of the fluid in the lungs, surface tension effects, and tissue resistance. The premature baby is often not capable of this enormous task because of the previously mentioned inadequacy in his capillary anatomy which impedes appropriate gaseous exchange, and because the respiratory centers of the brain which regulate depth and rate of respiration are not fully developed. In addition, these infants are hampered by weak respiratory muscles, a yielding thoracic cage, a decreased amount of pulmonary lipoprotein which reduces surface tension in the lungs and a deficient amount of fibrinolysins; hence primary and secondary atelectasis is common to these infants. The nasal passages are extremely narrow and the mucous membrane easily injured. The cough reflex is poorly developed or absent, making the danger of inhalation of regurgitated fluids very real.

In general then, an unstable respiratory system is a result of these deficits. Respiration tends to be irregular in rhythm and depth; there are periods of apnea during which cyanosis may develop. The infant utilizes his diaphragm more than his chest in his breathing, and if there is much atelectasis the thoracic cage is dragged down with each inspiration. In the severe cases, the sternum is sucked back towards the spine with inspiration, and expiration is accompanied by a short feeble grunt. It is important to remember that with these infants, respirations must be counted for at least a minute if any accurate respiratory rate is to be determined.

Cardiovascular System. *The heart* is relatively large at birth and often its action is slow and feeble. Extrasystoles occur and murmurs may be present at birth or soon after, which may later disappear as the fetal openings gradually close. As previously stated there is a decrease in the density of available capillaries in vital organs to take up sufficient oxygen in babies under about 1000 Gm. The extreme capillary fragility, especially of the intracranial vessels, together with the low plasma prothrombin level leads to a bleeding tendency in these infants. This tendency is evidenced by the frequency of ecchymosis of the skin as well as intraventricular hemorrhage and other internal bleeding.

The *systolic blood pressure* at birth is lower than that of the mature infant, and decreases with the birth weight. Infants weighing between 2 to 4 pounds (900 to 2,270 Gm.) generally have a systolic pressure of 45 to 60 mm. of mercury as compared with the 80 mm. of mercury for term infants. The level rises with the age of the child, being about 20 mm. by the end of the second week, and an additional 5 mm. by the age of two months.

The *pulse rate* ranges between 100 and 160, with the average around 140. Because of the tendency to arrhythmia, the pulse rate is most accurately obtained (as with the term infant) with a stethoscope counting the apical beat for a minute.

As with the mature infant, the premature has a relatively high *hemoglobin concentration* at birth which decreases to around 7 Gm./100 ml. of blood at 4 to 8 weeks of age. This is due to the premature's inadequacy in manufacturing hemoglobin, together with his relatively rapid rate of growth. After this time, the rate gradually increases until about 4 months when there is a second fall, characterized by hypochromia of the red cells. If a severe enough anemia develops in the first phase of hemoglobin decline, it may be treated with iron therapy. Some investigators have found for some unknown reason that *parenteral* (but not *oral*) administration of iron is

FIG. 17-1. Vital-signs wheel. Pulse rate, body temperature, respiratory rate, and respiratory performance are recorded on a data sheet at 6-hour intervals. To encourage the examiner to make each observation without knowledge of prior judgments, the preceding record is masked with the wheel. An index of respiratory distress is determined by grading each of five arbitrary criteria; grade 0 indicates no difficulty, grade 1 moderate difficulty, and grade 2 maximum respiratory difficulty. The "retraction score" is the sum of these values; a total score of 0 indicates no dyspnea, whereas a total score of ten denotes maximal respiratory distress. (Courtesy of Mead Johnson & Company, Evansville, Ind.) (Silverman, W. A.: Dunham's Premature Infants, p. 144, New York, Harper & Row, 1961)

FIG. 17-2. Posture of premature infant: (*Left*) Immediately after birth, (*center*) several hours later, and (*right*) after several days. (Redrawn from St. Anne Dargassies, Sr: La maturation neurologique du prématuré [The neurologic maturation of the premature infant]. *Neonatal Studies* 4:71, 1955.) (Silverman, W. A.: Dunham's Premature Infants, p. 125, New York, Harper & Row, 1961)

useful in prevention of the first phase of anemia. However, the later phase responds well to oral iron therapy and thus it has become customary to institute the oral form of therapy from the third week onward.

White Blood Cells. The white blood cell count at birth is lower than that usually found in the term infant (see Chap. 16). There is a predominance of polymorphonuclear cells, as with the mature infant, and the same decrease occurs in the total white cell count during the first week of life. However, the change to lymphocytic predominance may occur slightly later for the mature infant.

Jaundice in the Premature. The majority of premature infants become jaundiced around the second or third day of life. As is the case with term infants, the jaundice intensifies from the 4th to the 6th day and generally disappears by the second week. As far as we know, the mechanism responsible for this condition is approximately the same as that described for mature infants (see Chap. 16). Weight and degree of development appear to be related to the serum bilirubin value. The smaller the infant, the higher the peak of bilirubin value; 13 mg./100 ml. of blood is beyond the physiologic limit. In the very small premature, a value of 15 to 20 mg./100 ml. is often found, because of the inability of the premature's immature liver to dispose of the bilirubin which is liberated by the breakdown of the red blood cells.

When hyperbilirubinemia occurs (serum bilirubin in excess of 18 to 20 mg./100 ml. of blood), kernicterus may occur, and when the infant is particularly stressed (e.g., respiratory distress, difficult delivery) even less concentrations of bilirubin are required to produce kernicterus. Other conditions which predispose to this condition before the second day of life are (1) erythroblastosis, concomitant with the immature liver function and (2) an early gestational age of the infant.

Temperature Regulation. Even more so than the normal newborn, the premature infant's temperature regulating mechanism is poorly developed at birth. Since his peripheral circulation is also poor, his peripheral responses to heat and cold (i.e., sweating and shivering) are inadequate. Heat production is low and heat loss high because of the relatively greater body surface (in proportion to the weight) and the lack of subcutaneous fat.

Neurological System. The stage of development of the nervous system at birth will depend upon the degree of maturity. As with the normal newborn, all the premature's neurons are present, but they are not as fully developed and remain so for months and sometimes years. The least mature infants tend to lie quietly unless disturbed, waking only at intervals for feeding. External stimulation results in weak purposeless jerky movements and perhaps a feeble cry. As the infant matures, his movements tend to occur in little bursts of activity which can be quite vigorous, resulting in his wiggling from one end of the incubator to the other. At first the less mature infant will lie on his side in the "fetal position"; later he uncurls and after several days he lies on his back with his head rolled to one side, his hips flexed and abducted, and his knees and ankles flexed (frog position). The less mature the infant, the worse his muscle tone.

The vital centers controlling respiration and temperature are poorly developed, as are the centers controlling such important reflexes as coughing, swallowing and sucking. The Moro and tonic neck reflexes are present in normal infants of both low birth weight and early gestational age, as are the Chvostek and Babinski signs. Tendon reflexes are variable in all immature infants.

Gastrointestinal System. Larger prematures may have fairly good sucking and swallowing ability. The less mature infants, however, generally have feeble reflexes which, in the very immature, may be absent altogether. Because of the poorly developed mechanism for closure of the cardia and the relatively strong pyloric sphincter, regurgitation is common.

Again the powers of digestion depend upon the degree of prematurity, being rudimentary in infants of 26 to 28 weeks gestation but becoming more efficient as maturity increases. The stomach of a 2 pound (900 Gm.) infant at birth shows little folding of the mucosal surface (which reduces the surface area for absorption) and poor development of the secretory glands and muscle layers, as compared with that of a term baby with his deeply folded mucosal layer and relatively well-developed glands and muscle tissue. The premature infant appears to digest and absorb carbohydrates easily, proteins less well and fats badly, even though fat splitting enzymes are present at birth. This inability to manage fat leads to the often seen greasy and foul-smelling steatorrheic stools. When the newborn premature uses his glycogen stores he depends as usual on his body fat for energy; when food becomes available, he uses more calories from the carbohydrates and less from the fats than the term baby; thus, he resembles the fetus more in this respect since the fetus also depends on carbohydrates for its main source of energy.

The musculature of the bowel is weak and easily distended, so that there may be a tendency to constipation. Because of the thin abdominal wall, gastric peristalsis is seen; if distention is present, intestinal peristalsis also becomes visible.

Urinary System. In comparison to the normal newborn, the premature's renal function is impaired. Since the kidney tubules continue to be formed until term, the premature's kidneys are poorly developed. Thus, he cannot concentrate his urine well (which becomes important when he suffers from conditions involving an excessive water loss such as diarrhea or vomiting) and he is unable to excrete sodium and chloride well with resultant early water retention and edema. It is believed by many that the tendency to a more marked and prolonged acidosis in the newly born premature and his inability to excrete many drugs is probably due to the relatively poor development of the kidneys. Low pH levels (normal is 7.42) are regularly found in apparently healthy immature infants, and are not considered dangerous unless accompanied by conditions such as respiratory distress, vomiting or diarrhea.

Urination is scanty and infrequent for a few days after birth, due to the small amount of fluid that is usually administered. Urates are commonly present in some excess, thus giving a false positive for albumin by heat, acetic acid or trichloracetic acid tests.

Hepatic System. The liver is relatively large but its function is poorly developed in the smaller infants. This immaturity of the liver predisposes to jaundice (see p. 560) because of the inability of the liver to conjugate and excrete bilirubin. It has also been suggested that the low blood sugar found in the premature is hepatogenic, due to small liver glycogen stores. Lower serum protein levels, deficiency of blood clotting factors, and the deficient conjugation and detoxification of certain drugs are all attributed to liver immaturity.

NURSING MANAGEMENT

Since the life of the premature baby may depend on his nursing care, the nurse should realize the seriousness of this responsibility during this period of her nursing experience and make every effort to increase her knowledge and to develop her skill in caring for these infants.

Often, the first hours of the premature baby's life determine the outcome. He needs warmth, meticulous physical care, gentle handling, precise and careful feeding and protection from infection. It must be remembered always that the word "premature" means that this baby has arrived before he has had the opportunity to develop completely, and, if he is to live, this intricate development has to be completed against almost insurmountable odds—under conditions sometimes difficult even for the normal full-size baby.

Immediate Care

Since these infants come into the world "before their time," it is sometimes the nurse's duty to assist with the delivery and/or the care immediately after the delivery. Even if the delivery has been effected under aseptic conditions, the care given a premature infant may differ from that given to the full-size baby, depending on his condition. For the very small and feeble premature baby, the urgency of providing immediate warmth, humidity and oxygen as indicated may precede the care of the eyes and completion of the care of the cord. Moreover as we have seen, the premature is often one of a multiple birth; also his birth is often accompanied by premature separation of the placenta, hemorrhage and other disorders; thus his delivery complicates the mother's safety as well as his own. Teamwork is essential, that is, the combined efforts and skill of the obstetrician, pediatrician, anesthesiologist and nurse.

Whenever possible, the doctor will wait until the cord pulsation weakens before clamping it, so that the baby will benefit from the placental blood. The cord will be clamped or tied with special care because of the softness of the tissue, leaving space for a second ligature close to the body when a linen cord tie is used. The cord should be inspected at frequent intervals for bleeding, because of the increased tendency to bleeding and because prematurity is a predisposing cause of secondary hemorrhage. If a premature birth is anticipated, the pediatrician and anesthesiologist are usually notified to assist in their special areas. In almost all of these deliveries general anesthesia is contraindicated because prematures are so easily depressed by anesthetic and analgesic drugs. Therefore, the more specialized talents of the anesthesiologist are often required and he will also attend to any resuscita-

(A) A folded towel is placed under the shoulders. With the right hand the head is first lifted anteriorly and then rotated into partial extension ("sniffing position").

(B) A pencil-handle laryngoscope with a premature blade (Foregger & Co., New York) is held in the left hand and introduced through the right corner of the infant's mouth and swung to the midline; this moves the tongue to the left of the blade.

(C) Under direct vision through the slot in the right half of the blade the laryngoscope is dipped slightly and advanced so that the posterior surface of the epiglottis lies on the beak of the speculum. The tongue and epiglottis are lifted vertically, bringing the larynx into view.

(D) The right hand can now be released, and the infant's jaw is supported with the fifth finger of the left hand. An endotracheal catheter (Cole, size 10) is introduced at the right corner of the mouth and passed into the glottis through the vocal cords. The laryngoscope is then removed.

(E) A tube supplying oxygen is held in the operator's mouth. Inflation of the lungs is accomplished with short sharp puffs into the endotracheal tube, using only part of the volume of gas contained in the operator's mouth.

FIG. 17-3. Technique of mouth-to-tube resuscitation. (Silverman, W. A.: Dunham's Premature Infants, p. 97, New York, Harper & Row, 1961) tion needs of the infant, leaving the obstetrician free to attend the mother. Direct laryngoscopy, tracheal aspiration, intubation and mouth to tube insufflation have all been used. If there is any rule of thumb, it is "do only what has to be done" since the more manipulation, instruments, etc. that are introduced, the more danger there is with respect to injury and infection. In flaccid infants the tongue may lie against the pharyngeal wall and obstruct the airway. After the airway is cleared of foreign material, the head is extended and a small sized pharyngeal airway is inserted which often corrects the obstruction. If spontaneous respiration does not immediately occur, the lungs are inflated (see Fig. 17-3). If the mouth to tube technique has been used, then antibiotics are generally instituted to guard against infection. Care must be exerted to prevent injury of small premature infants during resuscitation. Injudicious squeezing of the chest and abdomen (see Chap. 23) may result in multiple rib fractures or subcapsular hemorrhage of the liver. Various types of drugs have been used to aid in establishing and/or maintaining respiration. The opiate antagonists (N-allylnormorphine) have been effective when given to mothers who have had large doses of opiates. There was a significant reduction in the time required to establish respiration and in the need for resuscitation in the babies. Some physicians inject N-allylnormorphine in an isotonic saline solution directly into the umbilical vein of the depressed infant with satisfactory results. It is stressed, however, that depression may be deepened if the apnea is due to other causes; therefore, great caution is used with these drugs. Various respiratory stimulants including nikethamide, alphalobeline, picrotoxin, and even caffeine sodium benzoate have been found to exert little or no significant effect on alleviating depression. Some physicians give sodium bicarbonate to depressed infants who have not responded to initial oxygen therapy. This is to alkalize the probable acidotic condition engendered by depression of respiration; heart action and blood flow through the lungs are thereby improved. The nurse will be responsible for collecting all materials and equipment and assisting the physicians in any manipulations of them (or the infant) that are required. She will also be responsible for notifying the various physicians and units of the premature's impending arrival. Her critical observation of the infant before, during and after any procedures is especially important at this time. The completion of necessary recording is to be accomplished quickly since early transfer of the infant is usually requested.

Since premature babies are more susceptible to infections, asepsis is imperative. However, if the infant's condition is very labile and/or critical, the installation of prophylactic eye drops may have to be deferred until his condition stabilizes; in these cases, the eyes can be wiped with moist sterile gauze. These infants are usually placed in the supine position with the shoulders elevated so that the abdomen is lower than the thorax. This is accomplished by placing a folded towel under the shoulders and back. It is thought that this position prevents the voluminous liver from being forced back by gravity to impinge upon the dome of the diaphragm, thus reducing respiratory capacity.

The maintenance of body temperature is essential. The premature's temperature tends to fall even more precipitously than the normal infant's at birth, because of his poor heat regulating ability. Therefore the baby should be wrapped in a warmed blanket and placed in a warm environment (90 to 92 degrees F.). This attention to warmth must be continued even while resuscitation is being performed. After any immediate resuscitation efforts are concluded, the infant is generally transferred as quickly as possible to the

FIG. 17-4. The position for premature infants recommended by Rossier. With the infant supine, a folded towel is placed under the back so that the abdomen is at a lower level than the thorax. In this position the neck is in slight hyperextension. (Redrawn from Rossier, A.: "Clinical Study of Respiration in Premature Infants." In *Anoxia of the Newborn Infant*. Oxford, England, Blackwell Scientific Publications, 1953.) (Silverman, W. A.: Dunham's Premature Infants, p. 119, New York, Harper & Row, 1961)

FIG. 17-5. Portable incubator, New York City Department of Health.

premature unit to insure a proper environment. The usual weighing, temperature taking, thorough physical examination, and eye prophylaxis are generally delayed until the infant is transferred to the nursery. Obvious congenital anomalies can be noted before the infant is transferred.

Continuing Care

Because of the magnitude of the premature problem, special nurseries and referral centers have developed for these infants in many urban areas. Space is usually allotted in the hospital separate from the term newborn nursery. In some cities, there is a large premature unit located in a medical center. When these infants must be moved from a hospital to a center or from a rural area to a hospital, effort is made whenever possible for safe transport to and from the hos-

pital (Fig. 17-5). It is strongly advised that the nurse who accompanies the infant be trained in resuscitative techniques.

As with initial care, continuing care revolves around maintaining temperature, preventing infection, maintaining respiration and nutrition of the infant.

Temperature Maintenance. Authorities vary as to the range of environmental temperature to which a premature should be subjected for best survival. Some suggest 90 to 97 degrees F.; some 90 to 92 degrees F. All agree, however, that the temperature is critical; it is generally accepted that the environmental temperature should support a *body* temperature of the infant of between 97 to 98 degrees F. In addition, it is advised that the premature's body temperature be brought up to this level, if necessary, and maintained *from birth* within this range, since significantly greater survival rates have resulted with this management. It is important to remember that these infants increase their heat production in cooler environments; this requires more oxygen, which places an added and at times an impossible burden on the already immature and often diseased lungs.

The premature's body temperature as well as his respiration is maintained in the artificial environment of the incubator, or as they are sometimes called, the isolette. The modern air-conditioned isolette is a miniature room in which the infant can live and be cared for under ideal conditions (i.e., desirable levels of heat, humidity and oxygen). As the infant matures, he will have less need for all three of the above in such exacting measured quantities; finally he will progress to a crib. There are several kinds of incubators currently in use, but the principle is the same, the differences being in the special construction details developed by various manufacturers. The nurse will want to familiarize herself with them since she will have a major responsibility in checking and maintaining the previously mentioned levels.

Modern incubators have controls on the outside of the unit to regulate the environment accurately and to adjust the bed from the hori-

FIG. 17-6. The Isolette incubator. (Air-Shields Inc., Hatboro, Pa.)

Bed temp. 80-90°F

115-125°F

FIG. 17-7. Homemade heated bed made from small canned goods box. The platform is 4 inches above the floor. The box is padded inside and outside with quilting. Three quarters of the bed is covered with a blanket. (Lundeen and Kunstadter: Care of the Premature Infant, Philadelphia, Lippincott)

zontal to the tilted positions (Trendelenburg and reverse-Trendelenburg positions) to facilitate treatments and care. Some have the "Servo-Control" to automatically adjust to needed temperature and humidity settings by means of an automatic sensing device (Thermistor) attached to the infant's skin. Special oxygen inlets provide adjustable oxygen concentrations (30 to 40 per cent is the usual recommended "maintenance" flow). Regardless of these built in sensors, the nurse will want to check and record the oxygen concentration with a reliable oximeter (oxygen analyser) placed at the level of the infant's nose; a similar device can be used to ascertain that humidity level. When oxygen therapy is no longer required, the incubator can be ventilated with fresh air from the room through a large, replaceable air filter or through an outside air attachment. Humidity can be controlled, and, by means of a nebulizer, supersaturated atmosphere can be created. Constant temperatures within the incubator can be regulated and maintained with a double-thermoswitch-controlled, sealed heating unit. Other features which are nonetheless important to the nurse are that these incubators are so designed that the infant can be observed from all sides through transparent windows. Moreover, hand holes with air-tight doors and self-adjusting "sleeves" permit the nurses and the physicians to care for the infant without disturbing the atmospheric conditions. The incubators are made of stainless steel and plastic and constructed for easy removal of all essential parts, without tools, to permit proper cleansing and sterilizing.

In an emergency situation—for example, when the infant is born prematurely at home in an outlying rural area—some means to protect the premature must be devised until an incubator can be brought from the local health agency. An incubator can be improvised from a box or a cardboard carton (Fig. 17-7). Such a specially prepared bed may be heated by electricity from a wire-screened 25- or 40-watt light bulb, or, if electricity is not available, by the use of hot-water bottles, or heated bricks or sandbags.

Prevention of Infection. Even though the isolette provides a more or less ideal environment, solicitous care must still be taken. The maintenance of asepsis in every detail must be maintained for these fragile babies. Scrupulous hand washing and gowning technique is to be observed. Personnel are also cautioned to avoid contact with sources of infection which might be transferred to the babies. There are usually special nursery gowns which will be worn when assuming care of these infants. The gowning procedure will vary from institution to institution but the underlying principle will be to keep as clean as possible anything that comes in contact with the premature. Masks are infrequently used in modern care as they have been found to harbor a rich source of contamination since moisture and bacteria from the nasopharynx collect in the mask folds, and even ordinary conversation distributes the infectious contents throughout the environment.

Rest is another important factor related to prevention of infection. These infants are to be shielded from excitement and disturbing influences, as these are tiring to the already weakened infants. Light can be curtailed, and loud or sudden noises should be avoided. As long as the infant requires humidity or oxygen therapy, all routine care, such as feeding, altering his position, necessary changing of linen or cleansing his skin, etc., is given in the premature bed.

The skin is extremely delicate and tender; and if diapers are used, they should be changed as soon as they become wet or soiled. Sometimes only a small pad is placed under the baby. Indeed, no clothing is really needed because of the controlled environment of the incubator. Most authorities recommend daily dilute hexachlorophene baths to curtail and prevent staphylococcus colonization of the skin and nasal passages. If an incubator is not available, the baby is dressed in a jacket of cotton and gauze or flannel.

The weight and temperature of the baby are both matters of importance and are carried out and recorded according to the hospital routine, as are the frequency and amount of voiding, and stools. Each institution will have its particular procedure, but the principles are the same as those when attending the normal newborn.

Maintaining Respiration. As previously stated, the establishment and maintenance of respiration is one of most critical import for these youngsters, and it is the nurse's responsibility to make careful, frequent observations and precise verbal and written recordings. It has been demonstrated that the first 5 minutes of life are crucial for the later successful outcome of the infant with respect to respiratory depression. Infants with unimproved respiratory function after these 5 minutes have a 4 times greater chance of dying in the first days than those infants whose condition improves or is good during this time. A majority of premature infants must receive oxygen initially because of respiratory depression or cyanosis or concurrent pathological conditions such as hemorrhage or erythroblastosis. Nevertheless, oxygen should not be used routinely and, except in an emergency, is to be prescribed by the physician. Oxygen therapy is often a life-saving measure for the infant, but it must be used judiciously and is to be administered at the lowest concentration compatible with life, since the oxygen requirements for these infants will vary according to weight, maturity and general condition of morbidity. If an incubator is not immediately available at birth (and respiratory difficulties are present) after necessary suctioning, the infant may be given oxygen by mask which is placed over the nose and mouth. This is to be considered a temporary emergency measure, and is to be removed promptly when the crisis is over and/or an incubator becomes available. The flow of oxygen can be set at a *maximum* of 3 liters when this method is used. When the premature infant is in an incubator, the lowest oxygen *concentration* to relieve the respiratory symptoms is to be employed; oxygen should not be ordered by liter flow when the incubator is utilized. Occasionally, higher concentrations (near 100%) may have to be employed to relieve general cyanosis or other conditions, but hourly reductions in the oxygen concentration must be carried out after these needs are met, to decrease any over oxygenation in the arterial blood of the infant.

One of the inherent dangers of this hyperoxia is the development of retrolental fibroplasia (see Chap. 23). It has been demonstrated that there is a relationship between the prolonged use of relatively high concentrations (40 per cent or more) of oxygen and the occurrence of this disease, which causes blindness in the premature (but not in the term infant). The high concentrations of oxygen causes arterial spasm of the fragile, still developing retinal vessels of the infant. The spasm is followed by obliteration and later by neovascularization, hemorrhage and retinal detachment. These processes produce the dense, fibrous tissue from which the disease takes its name. The reason that the premature (and not the term) infant is so susceptible to high oxygen concentrations is because of the immaturity of his retinal development. By 24 weeks gestational age, the retinal vessels have grown about 6 mm. from the optic nerve. Between 24 and 30 weeks no further growth occurs ("immature" fundus); after this time, however, growth again begins ("transitional" fundus). By about 34 weeks (weight 4 lbs. 6 oz. or 2,000 Gm.) the fundus is usually mature. During the "immature" and "transitional" developmental stages of the fundus, infants are liable to become victims of the disease, when injudicious concentrations of oxygen are employed which initiate the above pathological process; hence the preponderance of this disease among the very early gestational age and very low birth weight infants. Again, the nurse is responsible for seeing that the appropriate concentration is maintained.

Respiratory Patterns. The commonest respiratory rhythm of a quiet, larger healthy premature is the steady cogwheel type, with no pause between inspiration and expiration; the next commonest is the so-called adult rhythm with its inspiration, expiration pause. Other patterns such as inspiration-pause-expiration also occur. Sighs that interrupt the regular pattern are common and a sigh is often followed by an apneic pause. Periodic breathing, consisting of two or more periods of breathing per minute separated by an apneic pause of 3 seconds or more is more common among the small infants. Many authorities consider that anything that increases the minute volume of respiration reduces the incidence of this type of respiration.

TABLE 17-2. FEEDING GUIDE FOR PREMATURE INFANTS UNDER 2,000 GM. (4 LB. 8 OZ.)

FORMULA	AGE (IN DAYS)	VOLUME RANGES			
		ML./KG./DAY		ML./LB./DAY	
		IMMATURE*	UNDERGROWN*	IMMATURE	UNDERGROWN
10% glucose	0	20	30	9	14
Half, 10% glucose and half, full-strength	1	30	45	14	20
	2	40	60	18	26
	3	50	75	22	32
	4	60	90	26	40
	5	70	105	30	48
Full-strength formula (24 cal. per 30 ml.)	6	80	120	35	55
	7	90	135	40	60
	8	100	150	45	70
	9				
	10	110	160	50	75
	12	120	160	55	75
	15	130	160	60	75
	20	140	160	65	75

1. The volume ranges allow a choice of feeding amounts. Most premature infants are more safely fed in the lower ranges. *Supplemental parenteral fluids will be necessary if dehydration, lethargy, or excessive weight loss occurs.*

2. Multiply infant's weight (kg. or lb.) by volume to be given for that day and divide by twelve (number of feedings) for amount to be fed at 2-hour intervals.

3. Infants on reaching 1.5 kg. (3 lb. 5 oz.) should be placed gradually on a 3-hour feeding schedule (total volume given, divided by eight feedings).

4. Infants on the bottle and on reaching 1.8 to 2 kg. (4 to 4½ lb.) may be fed on a modified demand basis and at increased feeding intervals.
   Volume taken may range *above* 200 ml. per kg. (90 ml. per lb.).

Exceptions:

1. Infants in poor condition *for any reason* require a delay in oral feedings and the institution of parenteral fluids *from the first few hours of life.*

2. Any baby with distention, cyanotic or apneic attacks, or vomiting should have his feedings stopped and condition evaluated.

3. A stomach residual (at the time of the next gavage feeding) of over 1 ml. indicates a delay in emptying time. Feedings should be reduced and the event reported to physician for evaluation.

4. Malnourished infants require glucose and water soon after birth to support brain metabolism, due to deficient glycogen stores in liver.

* *Immature* refers to the very small, weak, and hypotonic premature infant. *Undergrown* infants are those who are small for their gestational age, with a greater need for calories.

From Babson, S. G., and Benson, R. C.: Primer on Prematurity and High-risk Pregnancy. St. Louis, C. V. Mosby, 1966.

"Normal" respiratory rates are difficult to determine since it is difficult to define the "normal" premature and the "normal" conditions under which they prevail. Two patterns have been associated with a low mortality rate and have thus been described as "normal." In the first pattern about 40 respirations per minute occur from birth onward without any significant fluctuations. In the second pattern rates over 60 respirations per minute occur in the first hour, with no significant increase, and subsequently decline. A significant increase is 15 or more respirations per minute above the average rate obtained in the first hour after birth.

The following patterns are always abnormal in the healthy term infant; so too in the premature but they are more expected because of the premature's developmental deficits. Simple retraction may be seen in which the chest and abdomen rise together, with a slight indentation over the sternal area. When this occurs, the nurse knows that observations must be increased and sharpened. This pattern is a warning sign and the physician may want to be alerted. Paradoxical breathing is considered a critical condition; the abdomen rises while the chest sinks. There is a marked chin lag and an audible respiratory grunt, indicating respiratory distress. The nurse will want to alert the physician, and keep him informed of any progress in the condition. This will mean exacting observation and frequent reporting.

Prolonged apnea (which is different from the periodic apnea discussed above) often occurs in cases of respiratory distress syndrome (see Chap. 23), as well as other pathological conditions such as infection, pneumonia and central nervous system injuries. Treatment usually consists of positive pressure oxygen therapy, and it goes without saying that these babies must have continuous observation since these spells are often repeated.

The nurse will also want to regulate other procedures such as bathing and weighing, to conserve the infant's strength and prevent apnea from sheer exhaustion. She will also want to position the infant in a lateral Sim's position or the supine position previously recommended to prevent mucus from reaching and remaining in the lungs. Changing position every 2 to 3 hours also aids in ventilating the lungs.

Maintaining Nutrition

In planning the feeding schedule for the premature infant, it is important to establish a food tolerance, since the intestinal tract (as well as other organs) is underdeveloped. The caloric needs of the premature baby are estimated according to the body weight. At first, the feeding should be in small amounts and then increased gradually to the amount that will produce a consistent gain, since vomiting, and consequent aspiration, distention and diarrhea may be due to over feeding. Early and more nearly optimal feeding in the case of the larger infant will contribute to lessened mortality and morbidity by preventing nutritive depletion and maintaining biochemical homeostasis. Hypoglycemia and hyperbilirubinemia, in particular, are reduced and growth and development at a critical period are supported. Prompt caloric supply for the undernourished infant is especially important.

Those infants in good condition (these are usually but not always the larger infants) with active

FIG. 17-8. Gavage feeding. When the premature infant does not require oxygen, the nurse can take him out of the incubator and hold him as she feeds him. (Babies and Childrens Hospital, The University Hospitals of Cleveland, Cleveland, Ohio)

peristalsis may be started on oral 5 to 10 per cent glucose water 6 to 12 hours after birth. For the infant in poor condition, no matter what the cause, oral feedings are usually withheld for several days if necessary and parenteral fluids instituted. If the infant is fed orally some physicians begin the infant on a trial of plain water, if it is retained, then glucose water or dilute modified cow's milk formula is instituted at 2-hour intervals. Some physicians begin with 5 to 10 per cent glucose water. Thus, there is a gradual replacement of water feedings by milk feedings, and a gradual increase in the amounts of milk and water at each feeding until caloric and fluid requirements are met. If an infant is taking about 180 cc. of full strength modified cow's milk formula per kilogram of body weight per day, then he is getting about 120 calories per kilogram per day which ensures an adequate weight gain.

Some physicians still prefer breast milk as the feeding of choice; unless the infant is vigorous, it is difficult to manage him on this type of feeding since there are very few mother's milk banks in this country, and it is often difficult for the mother to manually express enough milk for her baby's needs. A modified cow's milk formula has been found most effective as an all-around diet to supply nutritional requirements in the form and proportions that the premature can readily handle.

Prematures who weigh 3 pounds or less may be fed every 2 or 3 hours. Infants who weigh over 3½ pounds may be placed on a 4-hour feeding schedule. In addition to the feedings, the diets usually include vitamin and iron preparations. These additions are introduced when the feeding and schedule are fairly well established, and the infant is able to tolerate them. The stomach of the premature baby needs rest between feedings as much as that of the full-term baby; therefore, the interval should be regulated accordingly. The schedule should be as near that of a normal infant as is compatible with his progress.

When a very small and weak infant is on a 2 to 3 hour feeding schedule, gavage feeding (Fig. 17-8) is usually indicated. More recently, the indwelling catheters have not been recommended because mucus is produced which can block the airway in the weak premature, also purulent rhinitis and conjunctivitis may develop even with frequent tube changing; finally, the tube partially obstructs the airway. In addition, dropper feeding is not recommended because the swallowing reflex may be weak and easily fatigued, with a chance of overflow and aspiration.

Also considerable skill is required in controlling the volume and speed of release of feedings.

Feeding responsibilities are the nurse's and often she must pass the nasogastric tube as well. When gavage feeding is instituted, a French catheter no. 8 is introduced through the mouth; the distance is measured from the nose to the xiphoid process and is marked on the catheter. The infant is observed for any choking or gasping, which indicates the possibility of tracheal entry. The open end of the gavage tube can be inserted into a container of sterile water and if bubbles appear, then it is certain that the tube is in the trachea. The tube then must be removed and inserted properly. When the catheter is correctly placed, the tube is aspirated gently with a syringe; if a feeding residual of up to 1 ml. is returned, then the amount of the feeding is decreased by that amount. The residual need not be discarded; it can be fed as part of the new feeding. The nurse reports a residual of 1 ml. or more and skips that feeding. After checking the formula to determine correct temperature (tepid), the nurse will pour the formula through the barrel of the syringe; the milk is allowed to run slowly, with no pressure and minimal elevation of the syringe. During the feeding the infant is supported in a semi-reclining position. If the infant requires oxygen, he will be fed in the incubator. After the feeding, the infant is replaced in the incubator, and positioned with his head and shoulders slightly elevated, unless the physician prefers, and so specifies, another position. The larger infants may be placed on the abdomen or on the right side to facilitate emptying of the stomach. These positions guard against regurgitation and aspiration.

Bottle feeding requires that the infant have a good sucking and swallowing reflex which may take days or weeks to develop. The baby will indicate his readiness for the bottle by consistently sucking on the gavage tubing. When bottle feeding is instituted, the time of feeding is not to exceed 15 minutes as this will tire the youngster too much. A soft, average sized nipple with an adequate opening is used. The nurse can help the infant open his mouth to accept the nipple by applying gentle pressure on the infant's chin and touching his lips with the nipple. Again, the infant is held in the semi-erect position to facilitate "burping" and nursing. After the feeding he is positioned as described above. There are several precautions that the nurse will want to be aware of. The infant is not to be urged to accept more formula than is easily taken. Moreover, the bottle should be removed if he appears to be getting the milk too fast; in this case the infant will usually gasp, choke, or swallow so quickly as to interfere with his respirations. Any infant who shows reluctance to eat on two successive occasions will need critical reassessment. Feedings are to be discontinued if the baby vomits, becomes cyanotic, overdistends or develops frequent or diarrhea stools. Feedings should also be discontinued if there is 1 ml. or more of residual; again, the infant needs re-evaluation. Finally, the bottle of the premature is never to be propped. Any change of feeding habits in these infants is critical and *may be the first sign of illness*.

Currently in premature care, feeding by a medicine dropper usually is not used. When a medicine-dropper feeding is indicated for some specific reason, the glass tip should be protected by a small piece of rubber tubing which extends at least one quarter of an inch beyond the glass tip. When the infant is unable to suck, the swallowing reflex also is extremely weak. If a medicine dropper is to be used to feed such an infant, the procedure should be managed only by the most skilled practitioner, since aspiration can occur easily because of the poor swallowing reflex.

The other necessary care of the infant such as temperature taking, weighing, bathing, and dressing (if required) is usually done in conjunction with the feeding periods so that the infant may rest without interference at the other times. The nurse will want to gather any materials she needs and plan her care carefully so that she may implement her care as expeditiously as possible. Frequent entering the incubator is not in the interests of good aseptic technique and, of course, is very tiring to the infant. As previously stated, providing sufficient rest for these infants is an integral part of the therapeutic regimen.

PARENTAL REACTIONS

The birth of a premature infant, as was mentioned earlier, causes a certain amount of disorganization in the parents before they are able to master their feelings and come to accept the event. Since the baby may be born before term, parents often are deprived of the last 6 to 8 weeks in which the final psychological (and sometimes material) preparation for the birth is made. None of the physical and emotional signs of approaching labor (enumerated in Chap. 13) may happen. These are helpful to the mother in alerting her to the near approach of another new phase in the childbearing process, and this awareness in turn assists her in achieving a psychological preparation. The result, then, may be a rather abrupt arrival of the infant, and the event may be surrounded by several anxiety-provoking features: an unattended delivery, a longer hospital stay for her baby and perhaps herself, separation of the infant and herself, and most heartrending of all, a delicate infant who may be in danger of death.

Guilt feelings and a certain amount of grieving (see Chap. 23) in both parents are an invariable accompaniment. The parents ask themselves time and again such questions as: "What went wrong? What did we do? What made it happen? Can I really carry babies?" These guilt feelings and grief may be manifested in a variety of ways: general anger with the whole situation, self-deprecation, numerous complaints, blaming the spouse and/or attendants, insistent bids for reassurance and attention, profuse crying or extreme quiet and immobilization. Loneliness is also a problem, for the mother has no opportunity to see, hold, feed and examine her child as the other mothers have. We are all familiar with the wistful figure at the nursery window, gazing longingly through the glass, while the other mothers are occupied with feeding, changing and cuddling their infants. The loneliness continues when the parents go home without their infant, and because of the continued separation, the task of integrating the new member into the household is delayed. In addition, most mothers are concerned about whether they will be able to take adequate care of their babies when they do bring them home. The mother may still carry a picture of the frail infant surrounded by all the nursery paraphernalia and not realize that her baby will be reasonably mature when he is discharged from the hospital.

To cope with this concern, she may ask considerable questions while she is in the hospital and demand reassurance about the baby's condition; on the other hand, she may be quiet and uncommunicative, quite overwhelmed with the anticipated enormous responsibility. The economic drain on the finances cannot be overlooked, either; with medical and hospitalization expenses what they are today, the cost is considerable. Even for those who have adequate medical insurance, the maternity benefits are usually distressingly low. This, of course, adds to the general anxiety and strain of the situation.

Supportive Care. Although there is much that is specialized in the physical care activities for the premature infant, the mother's physical care remains generally the same as that for any normal postpartal course. Thus, the emphasis on care for these mothers is 2-fold. (1) They need help to facilitate their emotional adjustment (this holds true for the father as well) and (2) they need help in preparing for the care of the infant when they bring him home. The nurse will find Caplan's delineation of the mental hygiene activities of the nurse during pregnancy and the puerperium helpful in implementing these foci: (1) ego strengthening and general support, (2) mobilization of environmental resources of love and support, (3) anticipatory guidance, and (4) help in specific crises.[2]

The nurse can do much to strengthen the mother's ego by helping her work through her guilt feelings and grief and thus reinforce her concept of herself as an adequate, worthy person. To do this, the nurse must provide opportunities for the mother to ventilate her feelings and to question the situation. It is often difficult for the nurse to answer all the questions the mother and father ask her, especially if the prognosis for the baby is guarded. Yet, to avoid the questions or problems is to deprive the parents of a valuable avenue of coping with the problem. The fears and the fantasies engendered by not knowing are often worse than the facts, even though the facts are unfortunate. As the nurse listens to the mother and the father and reflects their concerns, she helps them to arrive at a clearer notion of the reality of the situation; thus they are able to separate fact from fancy and to work through to a more positive acceptance of their situation. The nurse can expect some negative feelings to be expressed, and the patient may go through a period of self-pity. An accepting, nonjudgmental attitude will help the patient to move to a more positive frame of mind.

Keeping the lines of communication open between the nursery staff and the patient is another useful supportive measure; the nurse on the postpartal unit can prepare herself with the latest reports regarding the baby's condition, so that she will have the information to give to the parents. Especially when the mother cannot be taken to see her baby in the premature nursery, it is very helpful if the nurse in the premature unit can make regular visits to the mother on the ward

---

[2] Caplan, Gerald: The mental hygiene role of the nurse in maternal and child care. Nurs. Outlook 2:14-19, January, 1954.

to inform her of her infant's progress. If circumstances within the unit prevent this, contact with the mother by telephone may be substituted. This two-way communication between the floor and the nursery helps the patient to feel that everyone is "tuned in" on her situation and concerned about her. It also gives her the opportunity to know the personnel who are responsible for the care of her baby, and this is reassuring in itself.

When the mother is able, she can be allowed to visit the nursery at least to observe her baby for a time. Some mothers find this difficult at first, especially if the infant is very small and/or ill. It is a wise nurse who allows the mother to indicate her readiness for such visits and gives appropriate encouragement as the mother is able to face the situation and take more responsibility.

Since the mother will be grieving to a certain extent and will be lonely, any environmental resources available that will convey love and support should be utilized. Certainly, her husband and available relatives are possible resources, as well as interested and empathic professional personnel. Often the latter, because they can be objective, are very helpful. Nurses must remember that the husband and wife must work through this mutual crisis, and even though they are both upset, they can gain strength and support from each other if they are helped to utilize positive coping mechanisms. If the family has a religious affiliation, their clergyman can lend valuable assistance also during this time.

All avenues of support are to be explored with the parents. If the mother seems to benefit from visitors or visiting with the other patients, then there need be no restriction of visiting privileges. There is no reason to isolate a mother in a room by herself (even if there has been a fetal demise) without ascertaining whether the mother needs to be alone for a time. If possible, the same nurse should be assigned to her care, for if the mother is to work through her feelings, she must have time to build a trust relationship, and this takes at least several encounters. Other personnel, such as the social worker, may be helpful if aid is needed financially, or strict budgeting is necessary. Another source of help that can prove invaluable is the public health or visiting nurse. The need for a referral for these patients and their infants never should be overlooked. Most patients are delighted to have someone to rely on during the first difficult days when they bring the baby home. Furthermore, some patients cannot make much progress during their short hospital stay in expressing their feelings and in working through the problem. Thus, they need a competent person when they return home to help them in this, as well as in making necessary arrangements in preparation for the baby's homecoming.

In making a referral, it is well to keep in mind the criteria for an appropriate referral, as stated by Wolff: it has merit; it is practical; it fits the patient's individuality; the right of the patient to say no is preserved.[3] The nurse should be particularly cognizant of the last point and present the referral as something that would be useful (describing its advantages), but allow the patient the option of making the decision. If there is refusal on the first try, the nurse always can reintroduce the topic later after the mother has had time to reconsider and is more aware of the factors involved in the home care of her baby. Although a nurse may know, as a professional, that follow-up is necessary, far more cooperation will be elicited from the parents if they have a choice in the matter.

Several hospitals are allowing the mothers to come into a portion of the premature unit to visit and feed their babies when the condition of the baby permits. At the same time they institute a counseling program on feeding and psychological aspects of care, which incorporates anticipatory guidance concerning the condition and the needs of the infants on arrival home. Coping with sibling rivalry also may be included. Appropriate reading material is given, and follow-up is done to see that the material is understood. This approach is very helpful, for it alleviates some of the separation and loneliness between mother and child and later fosters self-reliance and confidence in the mother at home.

In implementing the final mental hygiene activity, the nurse will want to remember that the advent of a premature birth is a crisis in itself; however, the parents may have to adjust to various related crises (e.g., a sudden, downward turn in the baby's condition, financial embarrassment, unexpected developments regarding other children and relatives, etc.). Thus, she should be prepared to help the parents to deal with these as they arise, and to seek appropriate resources for them if the matter lies beyond her competence. Her knowledge of the principles of communication and supportive care will be utilized here as they would be in any other crisis situation. Her willingness and ability to allow the parents to ventilate and work through their feelings about the situation is of prime importance. The nurse is one of the key persons in the care of the premature infant and his parents.

GROWTH AND DEVELOPMENT

Growth and development of the premature is primarily dependent upon the degree of immaturity at birth. Much will depend on the ability of the infant to meet the conditions attendant at birth and to adjust to the changes in his new environment. The majority (about 65 per cent) of prematures weigh between 2,000 and 2,500 Gms. Outcomes for these infants are good barring complications. An additional 20 per cent weigh between 1,500 to 2,000 Gms. and if prompt good care is provided, they also have a chance of a good outcome. As birth weight decreases, chances of satisfactory growth and development also decrease, even though "survival" rates may be good. In general, infants who react well to prompt treatment and care make their adjustment usually by the end of the first year. Others may require several years to match the "normal" child at that age, and some, unfortunately, really never "catch up" in various respects. Nearly all longitudinal studies indicate a continued difference in height and weight as compared with standard populations. Caution must be used in interpreting these findings, since these data may be confounded by the inclusion of children who show reduced growth as a result of central nervous system damage or deficiency, poor nutrition, or low birth weight with intrauterine growth retardation. When these children are excluded, few significant differences are found.

The nurse is often asked by the parents if their premature baby will ever develop as well and become as strong and sturdy as one born at term. As we have seen, depending upon birth weight, the little one has a good chance of doing so. Although he may be slower in regaining his birth weight, he is likely to gain approximately the same amount of weight (i.e., an average gain of 13 to 15 pounds) as the full term infant during the 1st year. Evidences of progress in his development are temperature stability, the increased vigor of his cry, stronger muscular activity, evidence of appetite and hunger, more normal periods of sleep, changes in the appearance and the character of his skin due to the addition of the

---

[3] Wolff, I. S.: Referral—a process and a skill. Nurs. Outlook 10:253-256, April, 1962.

subcutaneous fat, the development of reflexes and general signs of health. Individual variations occur, of course, but the developmental level achieved by the small premature infant during his 1st year generally will be lower than that expected for his chronologic age. Authorities differ in opinion concerning the length of time these infants may require to attain the physical and the intellectual developmental status of a full-size infant of comparable age. The World Health Organization's Expert Committee on Maternal and Child Health states:

It has been shown, for instance, that premature children may grow less quickly, have lower intelligence scores and more mental and physical handicaps than children of heavier birth weight. Again, the mechanism is by no means obvious and the specific influence of low birth weight is as yet unclear. Poor growth and development may merely be a reflection of an unfavorable environment.

The current definition of prematurity is based on the criterion of birth weight and there is no reason to suppose that children comparable in birth weight will also be comparable in viability or development.[4]

Parents of prematurely born infants invariably need special guidance and support to help them develop confidence in their ability to care for their baby, particularly in anticipation of taking him home from the hospital. The nurse has a real responsibility to help them so that they are adequately prepared for the baby's homecoming.

SUGGESTED READING

Abernathy, J. R., et al.: Birth weight, gestation and crown-heel length as response variables in multivariate analyses. Am. J. Public Health 56:1281-1286, August, 1966.

Abramowicz, M., and Kass, E. H.: Pathogenesis and prognosis of prematurity. New Eng. J. Med. 275:878-885, October 20, 1966.

———: Pathogenesis and prognosis of prematurity. New Eng. J. Med. 275:938-943, October 27, 1966.

———: Pathogenesis and prognosis of prematurity. New Eng. J. Med. 275:1001-1006, November 3, 1966.

———: Pathogenesis and prognosis of prematurity. New Eng. J. Med. 275:1053-1059, November 10, 1966.

Babson, S. G., and Benson, R. C.: Primer on Prematurity and High-Risk Pregnancy. St. Louis: C. V. Mosby, 1966.

Blake, F. G., Wright, F. H., and Waechter, E. H.: Nursing Care of Children. ed. 8, Philadelphia, J. B. Lippincott, 1970.

Canice, Sister M.: Mothers in the nursery. Am. J. Nurs. 64:101, November, 1964.

Caplan, G.: The mental hygiene role of the nurse in maternal and child care. Nurs. Outlook 2:14-19, January, 1954.

Committee on the Fetus and Newborn, American Academy of Pediatrics: Standards and Recommendations for Hospital Care of Newborn Infants, rev. ed., Evanston, Illinois, 1964.

Cornblath, M., et al.: Research and nursing care in the premature nursery. Am. J. Nurs. 62:92-96, July, 1962.

Crosse, M. V.: The Premature Baby. London, Churchill, 1966.

Drillien, C. M.: The Growth and Development of the Prematurely Born Infant. Edinburg, Livingstone, 1964.

Early feeding of the premature infant. Nutrition Reviews 24:295-297, October, 1966.

Eastman, N. J.: The great deterrent: Prematurity. Bull. Sloane Hosp. Wom. Winter, 1964.

Eastman, N. J., and Hellman, L. M.: Williams Obstetrics. ed. 13, New York, Appleton, 1966.

Follow-up of prematures in the journals. Children 12:35, January-February, 1965.

Gunter, L.: Psychopathology and stress in the life experience of mothers of premature infants. Am. J. Obstet. Gynec. 86:333-340, June, 1963.

Hasselmeyer, E. G.: Behavior Patterns of Premature Infants. Washington, D.C., U.S. Department of Health, Education, and Welfare, 1961.

Holt, L. E., Jr., and Snyderman, S. E.: The feeding of premature and newborn infants. Pediat. Clinics North America 13:1103-1115, November, 1966.

Ingles, T.: Maria, the hungry baby. Nurs. Forum 5, No. 2:36-47, 1966.

Jonxis, J. H. P., et al.: The Adaption of the Newborn Infant to Extra-uterine Life. Illinois, Charles C Thomas, 1964.

Kaplan, D. M., and Mason, E. A.: Maternal reactions to premature births viewed as an acute emotional disorder. Am. J. Orthopsychiat. 30:539, July, 1960.

Lees, M. H., et al.: Thermal requirements of undergrown human neonates. Biologia Neonatorum 10, No. 5-6:288-301, 1966.

McCann, M., and Thomas, T.: Milk solute-induced nephropathy in the premature infant: an hypothesis. Current Therapeutic Research 9:174-178, March, 1967.

Marlow, D. R.: Textbook of Pediatric Nursing, ed. 2, Philadelphia, W. B. Saunders, 1965.

Neal, M. V., and Nauen, C. M.: Ability of premature infant to maintain his own body temperature. Nurs. Research 17:396-402, September-October, 1968.

---

[4] World Health Organization, WHO Expert Committee on Maternal and Child Health: Social Aspect in the Teaching of Obstetrics and Gynaecology, Technical Report Series, No. 266, p. 9, Geneva, 1963.

Nelson, W. E.: Textbook of Pediatrics. ed. 8, Philadelphia, W. B. Saunders, 1964.

Owens, C.: Parents' response to premature birth. Am. J. Nurs. 60:1113-1118, August, 1960.

Peeples, E. H., and Francis, G. M.: Social-psychological obstacles to effective health team practice. Nurs. Forum 7, No. 1:28-37, 1968.

Petruska, R.: A one page record for prematures. Am. J. Nurs. 63:67-68, March, 1963.

Samsudin, M. D., and Williams, M. L.: Rational use of skim milk in a complete infant formula. Am. J. Clinical Nutrition 20:1308-1311, December, 1967.

Silverman, W. A.: Dunham's Premature Infants. ed. 3, New York, Hoeber, 1961.

————: Diagnosis and treatment: Use and misuse of temperature and humidity in care of the newborn infant. Pediatrics 33:276-277, February, 1964.

Tarumoto, Shoso: A clinical study on the growth and development of low birth weight infants. Hiroshima J. Med. Sciences 15:239-270, September, 1966.

Thaler, O. F.: Grief and depression. Nurs. Forum 5, No. 2:8-22, 1966.

The newborn monitor. Hosp. Progress 49:26-27, June, 1968.

Ujhely, G. B.: Grief and depression—implications for preventive and therapeutic nursing care. Nurs. Forum 5, No. 2:23-35, 1966.

Vulliamy, D. G.: The Newborn Child. London, Churchill, 1967.

Wallace, W. M.: Problems and progress in infant nutrition—a long view. Current Therapeutic Research 9:133-135, March, 1967.

Wolff, I. S.: Referral—a process and a skill. Nurs. Outlook 10:253-256, April, 1962.

Wortis, H., et al.: Development of lower-class premature children born in and out of wedlock. Social Work 9, No. 4:42-49, 1964.

CONFERENCE MATERIAL

1. What is the responsibility of the hospital and the nurse in preparing the mother to care for her baby after they leave the hospital?

2. What advice and help could you give the mother to help her to adjust the new baby in the home and to prevent (or deal with) sibling rivalry when there is a 2-year-old brother who is accustomed to having the undivided love and attention of his parents?

3. Compare the physiologic development of the premature infant with that of the normal full-term infant.

4. What are some other means which could be employed to supply external heat for the premature infant who requires it when a mechanical incubator is not available?

5. What information can you give parents about the "well-baby clinic" in your community?

Study Questions

Unit Five: Nursing the Normal Newborn

Read through the entire question and place your answer on the line to the right.

1. The neonatal period constitutes one of the most important periods of life because of the profound physiologic changes which occur. Which of the following statements concerning these alterations are correct?
   A. Certain of these physiologic changes are immediate; some are delayed.
   B. All of these physiologic changes are immediate.
   C. All of these physiologic changes are permanent.
   D. Certain of these physiologic changes are temporary.

   Select the number corresponding to the correct letters.
   1. A and C
   2. A and D
   3. B and C
   4. B and D

2. Which of the following reasons best explain why the maternity hospital should adopt the rooming-in plan for the mother and her newborn?
   A. All mothers need the experience gained thereby.
   B. Selected mothers and babies may profit where the plan could be adopted.
   C. All mothers want this type of service.
   D. Most infants cry too much in a central nursery.
   E. All infants need this added attention.

   Select the number corresponding to the correct letter or letters.
   1. A only
   2. B only
   3. A, C and D
   4. B, C and E

3. What type of initial bath usually is given the newborn infant?
   A. Tub bath.
   B. Spray bath.
   C. Oil bath.
   D. Sponge bath with a 3 per cent hexachlorophene solution and warm water.
   E. Cleansing of the genitals with warm water and sterilized cotton.

4. What is the reason for selecting this method of skin care in the above question?
   A. The infant's skin must be washed thoroughly to prevent irritation.
   B. It stimulates circulation.
   C. Special oils provide nourishment to the tissues.
   D. It prevents infection.
   E. It lessens the amount of staphylococcus colonization of the infant's skin and nasopharynx.

5. What is the usual procedure for the daily care of the genitals of the male infant who is not in need of circumcision?
   A. Wash externally with soap and water; otherwise let alone.

B. Retract and cleanse under the foreskin with cotton ball moistened with warm water. Replace foreskin over glans after cleansing.

C. Retract and cleanse under the foreskin with alcohol.

D. After cleansing, apply sterile petrolatum under the foreskin.

E. Stretch the prepuce and lubricate with mineral oil.

B

6. What is the principle underlying the concept of demand feedings for the newborn infant?

A. Maintaining a regular 4-hour schedule to establish eating habits.

B. Feeding the infant every 2 to 3 hours to stimulate digestion.

C. Fitting individual feedings to individual needs.

D. Permissive feeding schedule causes less conflict with the mother's household activities.

E. More frequent feedings assure an adequate nutritional intake.

C

7. The young mother asks how she will know when her baby is hungry. Which of the following responses would be most appropriate for the nurse to reply?

A. "All crying indicates hunger."

B. "Feed the baby whenever he is awake."

C. "He will cry, fret and suck on anything in contact with his lips."

D. "Offer him water first; if he refuses the water, then feed him."

C

8. What is the established birth weight below which the infant is considered to need special premature care, regardless of whether or not he is born prematurely according to dates?

A. 4 pounds

B. 4½ pounds

C. 5 pounds

D. 5½ pounds

E. 6 pounds

D

9. The appearance of a healthy newborn infant's stools normally will change during the neonatal period. Which of the following types of stools, in sequence of appearance, would the nurse observe in the healthy infant?

A. Dark, tarlike

B. Clay-colored, soft

C. Mottled greenish-brown, soft

D. Smooth, yellow

E. Green, curdy

Select the number corresponding to the correct letters.

1. A and D

2. A, C and D

3. B, C and E

4. All of them

2

10. How does the composition of mother's milk compare with cow's milk?

A. Human milk contains more protein.

B. Human milk contains less protein.

C. Human milk contains more carbohydrate.

D. Human milk contains larger fat globules.

E. Human milk contains less iron.

Select the number corresponding to the correct letters.

1. A and C

2. A, C and E

3. B, C and D

4. B, D and E

3

11. Which of the following features are characteristic of the premature infant and distinguish him from the full-size infant?
   A. The infant is usually puny and weighs less than 2,000 Gm.
   B. The infant's head is proportionately large, his skull is round or ovoid in shape, and his facial features are small and angular.
   C. The skin is soft, transparent and may be covered with lanugo.
   D. These infants whimper and cry rather constantly, although the cry is weak.
   E. The body temperature is unstable and thus responds rather readily to changes in the temperature of the environment.

   Select the number corresponding to the correct letters.
   1. A and B
   2. B, C and D
   3. B, C and E
   4. All of them   3
   _____

12. When the mother learned that her premature infant was receiving gavage feedings she asked the nurse why this was being done. Which of the following reasons may be correct for the nurse to reply?
   A. "This method of feeding your baby was indicated because he became exhausted when he tried to swallow."
   B. "Feeding your baby this way prevents him from vomiting and thus eliminates the danger of his aspirating formula into his lungs."
   C. "Feeding your baby this way conserves his strength and permits him to receive food into his stomach when sucking or swallowing may be difficult."
   D. "He can be given his formula quickly this way and so he does not have to be handled as much."
   E. "A tiny baby's resistance to infection is poor, so gavage feeding is really a protective measure against such infections as thrush, which he might acquire if he were bottle-fed."

   Select the number corresponding to the correct letter or letters.
   1. A only
   2. C only
   3. B, C and D
   4. B, D and E   C
   _____

13. In caring for premature infants, which of the following precautions should be taken against retrolental fibroplasia?
   A. The administration of oxygen should be discontinued as soon as feasible.
   B. The concentration of oxygen in the incubator housing the infant should be tested periodically and kept at less than 40 per cent.
   C. Daily determinations of the serum bilirubin level should be done when there is any indication of proliferation of the retinal capillaries.
   D. High humidity should be maintained in the incubator constantly.
   E. The infant's eyes should be protected from bright lights.

   Select the number corresponding to the correct letters.
   1. A and B
   2. A, C and D
   3. B, D and E
   4. All of them   1
   _____

14. How can the public health nurse assist the family in the care and the supervision of the premature infant?
   A. Visit the home before the infant leaves the hospital to evaluate the home situation and give anticipatory guidance to the parents as necessary.
   B. Help the family to understand that the infant is still premature and must have the same kind of skillful, protective care in a sheltered environment similar to that in the hospital premature nursery.

C. Make daily visits to the home to bathe the infant, prepare the formula and, in general, give suggestions and guidance to the mother about her infant's care.
D. Visit the home again after the infant is discharged from the hospital to give the family guidance and assistance as necessary.
E. Help the family to understand that this infant requires a great amount of undisturbed rest and thus should not be held or cuddled as much as the full-size infant.

Select the number corresponding to the correct letters.

1. A and D
2. A, C and E
3. B, C and E
4. All of them

15. The premature infant has difficulty in regulating his body temperature because heat regulation is one of the least developed functions of his body. Which of the following conditions are responsible for this?

A. The surface area of the premature infant is relatively smaller than that of a normal full-term infant in proportion to body size.
B. Lack of subcutaneous fat which would furnish a measure of insulation
C. Limited ability to produce body proteins
D. Poor reflex control of skin capillaries
E. Frequent episodes of diaphoresis causing loss of body heat

Select the number corresponding to the correct letters.

1. A and C
2. B and D
3. B, C and E
4. All of them

Note: The key to the correct answers to these questions is given on page 613.

UNIT SIX
Operative Procedures in Obstetrics

Operative Obstetrics

Operative Obstetrics

18

Episiotomy and Repair of Lacerations • *Forceps* • *Version* • *Cesarean Section*
Destructive Operations • *Induction of Labor*

A number of special procedures which the physician may use to assist the mother in labor and delivery come under the heading of operative obstetrics. These include episiotomy and repair of lacerations, the application of forceps or vacuum extractor, destructive operations on the fetus, version, cesarean section, and induction of labor.

EPISIOTOMY AND REPAIR OF LACERATIONS

Except for clamping and cutting the umbilical cord, episiotomy is the most common operative procedure performed in obstetrics. In view of the fact that this incision of the perineum, made to facilitate delivery, is employed almost routinely in primigravidas, the procedure has been discussed in the section on the conduct of normal labor (see Chap. 13).

Lacerations of the perineum and the vagina which occur in the process of delivery (see Fig. 13-35) have also been covered earlier in the text, because some tears are unavoidable even in the most skilled hands. The suturing of spontaneous perineal lacerations is similar to that employed for the repair of an episiotomy incision but may be more difficult because such tears often are irregular in shape with ragged, bruised edges.

FORCEPS

Some of the common types of obstetric forceps are illustrated in Figures 18-1 to 4. The instrument consists of two steel parts which cross each other like a pair of scissors and lock at the intersection. The lock may be of a sliding type, as in the first three types shown, or a screw type, as in the Tarnier instrument. Each part consists of a handle, a lock, a shank and a blade; the blade is the curved portion designed for application to the sides of the baby's head. The blades of most forceps (the Tucker McLane is an exception) have a large opening or window (fenestrum) in them to give a better grip on the baby's head, and usually they have two curves: a cephalic curve, which conforms to the shape of the baby's head, and a pelvic curve, to follow the curve of the birth canal. Axis-traction forceps, such as the Tarnier, have a mechanism attached below which permits the pulling to be done more directly in the axis of the birth canal. An axis-traction handle is also available for use on standard forceps.

The two blades of the forceps are designated as right and left. The left blade is the one which is introduced into the vagina on the patient's left side; the right blade goes into the right side. If the nurse is assisting the obstetrician, she should articulate and disarticulate the forceps and make sure that she knows which blade is which.

It may become necessary to deliver the baby by forceps for reasons related to the mother's welfare (maternal indications), or because of conditions associated with the baby's condition (fetal indications). Among the more common maternal indications are: Malposition of the fetal head, toxemia of pregnancy, threatened rupture of the uterus and inability of the mother to push after full dilatation of the cervix, because of conduction anesthesia, exhaustion, or heart disease. The chief fetal indication for forceps delivery is fetal distress, as suggested by a slow, irregular fetal heart. Many obstetricians, however, deem it desirable to deliver almost all primigravidas with forceps electively, in the belief that the operation spares the mother many minutes of exhausting bearing-down efforts and relieves pressure on the baby's head. This is usually referred to as "elective forceps."

Forceps operations never are attempted unless the cervix is completely dilated. Forceps delivery is contraindicated unless the vertex is engaged (i.e., the greatest biparietal diameter of the fetal head is at, or has already traversed, the pelvic inlet). Usually, but not always, when engagement has occurred, the vertex is at or below the ischial spines. In the vast majority of cases today, the forceps delivery is carried out at a time when the baby's head is on the perineal floor (visible or almost so) and internal rotation may already have occurred, so that the baby's head lies in a direct antero-posterior position.

FIG. 18-1. Simpson forceps.

FIG. 18-2. Tucker McLane forceps.

FIG. 18-3. Kielland forceps. (A) Front view; (B) side view.

FIG. 18-4. Tarnier axis-traction forceps.

This is called *low forceps,* or "outlet forceps." When the head is higher in the pelvis but engaged, its greatest diameter having passed the inlet, the operation is called *midforceps.* If the head has not yet engaged, the procedure is known as *high forceps.* High-forceps delivery is an exceedingly difficult and dangerous operation for both mother and baby and is rarely done. The obstetrician will inform the nurse of the type of instrument he wishes to use. Autoclaving is the usual type of sterilization employed, and several pairs of the generally approved forceps, each encased in suitable wrappings, are autoclaved and kept in the delivery room for immediate use. The other instruments needed for a forceps delivery are the same as those required for a spontaneous delivery, plus those necessary for repair work (see Chap. 13).

Anesthesia is recommended, but in low-forceps deliveries it may be light, and in many institutions this type of operation is performed successfully under pudendal block anesthesia. The patient is placed in the lithotomy position and prepared and draped in the usual fashion. After checking the exact position of the baby's head by vaginal examination, he will introduce two or more fingers of his right hand into the left side of the vagina; these fingers will guide the left blade into place and at the same time protect the maternal soft parts (vagina, cervix) from injury. Taking the left blade of the forceps in his left hand, he introduces it into the left side of the vagina, gently insinuating it between the baby's head and the fingers of his right hand (Fig. 18-5). The same procedure is carried out on the right side, and then the blades are articu-

direction
of
insertion

FIG. 18-5. Insertion of forceps blade.

lated. Traction is not continuous but intermittent (Fig. 18-6); and between traction, the obstetrician will partially disarticulate the blades in order to release pressure on the baby's head. Episiotomy is almost routine nowadays in these cases.

Vacuum Extractor

Occasionally, the nurse may see an instrument known as the vacuum extractor used in place of the forceps. The vacuum extractor consists of a metal cup that is applied to the fetal head and tightly affixed there by creating a vacuum in the cup through withdrawal of the air by a pump (Fig. 18-7). Cups are supplied in various sizes. The largest cup which can be applied with ease is selected for use. Vacuum is created slowly, and the suction creates an artificial caput within the cup, providing a firm attachment to the fetal scalp. Traction then can be exerted by means of a short chain attached to the cup, with a handle at its far end.

VERSION

Version consists of turning the baby in the uterus from an undesirable to a desirable position. There are three types of version: external, internal and Braxton Hicks.

External Version. This is an operation designed to change a breech presentation into a vertex presentation by external manipulation of the fetus through the abdominal and the uterine walls. It is attempted in the hope of averting the difficulties of a subsequent breech delivery. Obstetricians find the procedure most successful when done about a month before full term; it often fails, however, either because it proves to be impossible to turn the fetus around, or because the fetus returns to its original position within a few hours. Some obstetricians disapprove of it altogether.

Internal Version. Sometimes called internal podalic version, this is an operation designed to change whatever presentation may exist into a breech presentation (see Fig. 18-8). With cervical dilatation complete, the whole hand of the operator is introduced high into the uterus, one or both feet are grasped and pulled downward in the direction of the birth canal. With his external hand the obstetrician may expedite the turning by pushing the head upward. The version usually is followed by breech extraction (p. 481). Internal version finds its greatest usefulness in cases of multiple pregnancy in which the birth of the second twin is delayed, or when the second twin is in a transverse lie. It is now almost never used in other circumstances.

Braxton Hicks Version. In this procedure, two fingers are introduced into a partially dilated

Fig. 18-6. Applied forceps and direction of traction.

Fig. 18-7. Application of the vacuum extractor and delivery of the fetal head.

cervix and, after manipulating the fetus to effect turning, one leg is drawn through the cervix. The operation is not designed to bring about immediate delivery and never is followed at once by extraction. Its purposes are either to compress the lower uterine segment with the infant's buttock (see placenta previa, p. 466), or, more rarely, to stretch the cervix with the infant's thigh so that labor may be initiated. It is rarely used in modern obstetrics.

CESAREAN SECTION

Cesarean section is the removal of the infant from the uterus through an incision made in the abdominal wall and the uterus. The main indications for cesarean section fall into five groups: (1) disproportion between the size of the fetus and that of the bony birth canal, that is, contracted pelvis (p. 484), tumor blocking birth canal, etc.; (2) certain cases in which the patient has had a previous cesarean section, the operation being done because of fear that the uterus will rupture in labor; (3) certain cases of very severe toxemia of pregnancy, but rarely in eclampsia; (4) certain cases of placenta previa and premature separation of the normally implanted placenta; (5) fetal distress, actual or impending. When a cesarean section is done prior to the onset of labor, as the result of a pre-arranged plan, it is referred to as "elective" cesarean section (as with "elective low forceps," the obstetrician is not forced to perform the operation immediately but elects to do it as the best procedure for mother and baby).

Main Types of Cesarean Section

Although there are four types of cesarean section, the lower segment section is usually the operation of choice. In this operation, the uterus is entered through an incision in the lower segment. Other types of cesarean section include the classical cesarean section, in which the incision is made directly into the wall of the body of the uterus; the extraperitoneal cesarean section, in which the operation is arranged anatomically, such that the incision is made into the uterus without entering the peritoneal cavity; and cesarean-hysterectomy, which involves a cesarean

FIG. 18-8. Internal podalic version. Elbow length gloves are usually worn for this operation.

FIG. 18-9. Classic cesarean section. (*Left*) Uterus packed off with warm, moist gauze pads. Start of incision with knife. (*Right*) Continuation of incision with bandage scissors.

section of any variety followed by removal of the uterus.

The Low Segment Cesarean Section. This procedure is usually the operation of choice for a number of important reasons. Since the incision is made in the lower segment of the uterus, which is its thinnest portion, the operation is associated with minimal blood loss, and the incision is easy to repair. The lower segment is also the area of least uterine activity, and thus the possibility of rupture of the scar in a subsequent pregnancy is lessened. Since the incision can be properly peritonealized, the operation is associated with a lower incidence of postoperative infection. The initial incision (the abdominal cavity having been opened) is made transversely across the uterine peritoneum, where it is attached loosely just above the bladder. The lower peritoneal flap and the bladder are now dissected from the uterus, and the uterine muscle is incised either vertically or transversely. The membranes are ruptured, and the baby is delivered. After the placenta has been extracted and the uterine incision sutured, the lower flap is imbricated over the uterine incision (Fig. 18-9, 10). This two-flap arrangement seals off the uterine incision and is believed to prevent the egress of infectious lochia into the peritoneal cavity.

Classical Cesarean Section. A vertical incision is made directly into the wall of the body of the uterus; the baby and the placenta are extracted, and the incision is closed by three layers of catgut sutures (Figs. 18-11, 12). Thus, this approach requires traversing the full thickness of the uterine corpus. It is still recommended in certain circumstances. It is particularly useful when the bladder and lower segment are involved in extensive adhesions resulting from a previous cesarean section, and occasionally is selected when the fetus is in a transverse lie or when there is an anterior placenta previa.

Extraperitoneal Cesarean Section. By appropriate dissection of the tissues around the bladder, access to the lower uterine segment is secured without entering the peritoneal cavity. The baby is delivered through an incision in the lower uterine segment. Since the entire operation is done outside the peritoneal cavity, neither spill

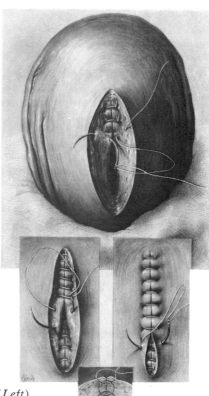

FIG. 18-10. Classic cesarean section. (*Left*) Delivery of infant. (*Right*) Method of suturing uterus.

Fig. 18-11. Low cervical cesarean section. (*Left*) High Trendelenburg position, bladder empty, with catheter in place. The peritoneum over lower portion of uterus is picked up with tissue forceps to determine how far up it is loosely attached to uterus. A transverse incision of the peritoneum, slightly concave downward, is to be made about 1 inch below the point where the peritoneum is firmly attached to the uterus.

(*Right, top*) The lower edge of the incised peritoneum is picked up by the tissue forceps and gently

stripped off the underlying uterine segment by finger dissection.

(*Right, bottom*) The upper flap of loose peritoneum has been stripped from the underlying muscle by finger dissection and is held back by a retractor. A small incision with a scalpel is made at the upper end of the lower uterine segment and carried downward with bandage scissors.

of infected amniotic fluid nor subsequent seepage of pus from the uterus can reach the peritoneal surfaces. This approach was used extensively in the pre-antibiotic era, but is rarely employed today.

Cesarean Section—Hysterectomy. (Synonym: Porro's operation). This operation comprises cesarean section followed by removal of the uterus. It may be necessary in certain cases of *premature separation of the placenta,* in patients with multiple *fibroid tumors of the uterus,* and in some circumstances is done electively for sterilization purposes.

Preparation

Preparations for cesarean sections are similar to those for any other abdominal operation, except that in these cases it includes preparations for the care of the infant. An elective cesarean section allows ample time for a physical examination, routine laboratory studies, typing and crossmatching blood and other customary procedures. However, if there is an emergency, or if labor has started, then such preparations must be made with

expediency. In any event, the usual hospital procedure should be followed.

Nursing Care

When the patient is admitted for an elective cesarean section, nursing care which is routine for any waiting mother (e.g., checking fetal heart tones and being alert to prodromal signs of labor) is employed. A short time before the operation the skin should be shaved to remove all hair from the abdomen. The abdomen is shaved, beginning at the level of the xiphoid cartilage and extending out to the far sides and down to the pubic area. A retention catheter is inserted to ensure that the bladder remains empty during the operation and attached to a constant drainage system. One should make certain it is draining properly before the procedure. The preoperative medication usually ordered is atropine. The use of narcotic drugs prior to delivery is avoided because of their depressant effect on the infant, but these medications should be readily available. Oxytocic drugs (e.g., oxytocin and ergonovine) should be ready in the operating room so that they can be administered promptly on the verbal order of the obstetrician when the infant is born.

In addition to the preparation of the operating room for the surgical procedure, preparation for the care of the infant must be accomplished. There must be a warm crib and equipment for the resuscitation of the infant. An infant resuscitator, such as the Kreiselman, is an efficient mechanical device, because it is equipped with heat, suction, oxygen (open mask and positive-pressure) and an adjustable frame to permit the proper positioning of the infant. Furthermore, such a resuscitator provides a convenient place to give initial care to the newborn. A competent

person should be present at cesarean section to give the infant initial care and to resuscitate it, if necessary. This person may be a professional nurse, but in many hospitals today it is customary to have a pediatrician present so that he may "take over" the care of the infant as soon as it is born and thus free the obstetrician to devote all of his attention to the mother.

Usually postoperative care is the same as that following any abdominal surgery. It is well to remember that the patient who has had a cesarean section has had both an abdominal operation and a delivery. The patient must be watched for hemorrhage, as after any delivery. The

FIG. 18-12. Low cervical cesarean section. (*Left, top*) Extraction of baby with forceps. Oxytocin (1 cc.) intramuscularly is usually given as soon as the head is delivered. (*Right, top*) After delivery of baby and placenta, edges of the lower segment incision are grasped with ring forceps and sutured. (*Right, bottom*) After upper peritoneal flap is pulled down over the uterine wound and sutured, the lower flap is pulled upward and sutured with running suture.

perineal pad must be inspected frequently. If the abdominal dressings are bulky, it may be difficult to palpate the fundus to see if the uterus is well contracted, but if the dressings are not massive, and do not extend above the level of the umbilicus, the nurse may feel the consistency of the fundus. Oxytocics may be ordered to keep the uterus contracted and to control bleeding. The vital signs should be checked regularly until they have stabilized, and if there is any indication of shock or hemorrhage, it should be reported promptly. Although there may be no visible signs of external hemorrhage, one would suspect internal hemorrhage if the pulse rate becomes accelerated, the respiration increases in rate, or the blood pressure falls, bearing in mind, of course, that the drop in blood pressure could be due to the effects of some types of anesthetic drugs.

If the retention catheter is to remain in place until the following morning, it should remain attached to "constant drainage" and should be watched to see that it drains freely. Intravenous fluids are usually administered during the first 24 hours, although small amounts of fluids may be given by mouth after nausea has subsided. A record of the mother's intake and elimination is kept for the first several days or until the need is no longer indicated.

Sedative drugs should be used to keep the mother comfortable and encourage her to rest. Her position in bed during the early postoperative hours may be dictated by the type of anesthesia that she received. She should be encouraged to turn from side to side every hour. Deep breathing and coughing should also be encouraged to promote good ventilation. Today most mothers delivered by cesarean section are allowed early ambulation. It is felt that this contributes considerably to maintaining good bladder and intestinal function.

The patient's husband should be permitted to visit his wife as soon as it is feasible. The mother will be anxious to see her infant, too, and it should be brought to her as soon as she is able to see it. The nurse should remain with the mother while she has her infant with her.

The general care of the mother will be similar to that given any postoperative or postpartal patient. Daily breast care and perineal care are carried out per routine. The mother may have the afterpains, engorgement of the breasts and the emotional reactions which often accompany a normal delivery.

DESTRUCTIVE OPERATIONS

Destructive operations (designed for the most part to reduce the size of the baby's head and thus to expedite delivery) are rarely done in modern obstetrics. Even in large maternity hospitals many years may pass without a single destructive operation. This salutary state of affairs is attributable in part to the widespread extension of prenatal care, in part to better management of women in labor, and in part to the availability of cesarean section, which makes it safe to effect abdominal delivery even in neglected cases. In the event that a destructive operation is necessary, the obstetrician will choose the necessary instruments.

INDUCTION OF LABOR

By the induction of labor is meant the artificial bringing on of labor after the period of viability. Induction of labor is indicated when continuation of pregnancy would affect maternal health, or when there are conditions in the mother which would affect fetal well-being. Complications of pregnancy which may require induction include toxemia, diabetes, hemolytic disease, and postmaturity (see Complications of Pregnancy). In some centers, labor is induced electively at term for convenience.

Medicinal Induction. Since it was believed that the intestinal peristalsis produced by a cathartic is somehow transferred to the uterus, with the consequent initiation of uterine contractions, castor oil has long been employed to induce labor. It was often followed by the administration of a hot soapsuds enema. While this is a harmless approach, it usually fails.

An efficient and safe method for the induction of labor is the administration of oxytocin by intravenous drip. The properties of this oxytocic agent and its use in the third stage of labor have already been discussed on page 270. Since oxytocin has dangerous potentialities when administered to a pregnant woman, the dosage used is always extremely small. Administration by intravenous drip assures a uniform, although infinitesimal, concentration of the agent in the blood stream. The amount of oxytocin being administered can be readily controlled and is governed by the response of the uterus. Oxytocin has also been administered intramuscularly, but this approach is no longer recommended. Since the response of a given patient is not predictable, there is no way to select an appropriate intramuscular dose.

FIG. 18-13. Nurse checks rate of flow of intravenous oxytocin solution. (MacDonald House, University Hospitals of Cleveland)

For the intravenous administration of oxytocin the physician will usually ask for a flask containing 500 cc. of 5 per cent glucose, to which he will add the quantity of oxytocin which he wishes to use. The intravenous equipment is set up as usual so that the number of drops flowing per minute can be closely observed in the observation tube. This is extremely important, and the physician will specify the precise number of drops per minute which he wishes employed. Initially, the drip should be run very slowly—4 to 5 drops/minute. The rate of administration should be increased gradually thereafter, always being governed by the response of the patient (Fig. 18-13).

The administration of oxytocin to a gravida carries certain hazards, and it is obligatory for her safety and that of the baby that a physician or a nurse be in constant bedside attendance to make certain that the number of drops flowing per minute does not change and to watch for certain untoward effects. The observer must check the rate of flow of the oxytocin solution at frequent intervals to make certain that it remains constant. The duration and the intensity of each uterine contraction must be watched closely and recorded. Any contraction lasting over 90 seconds indicates that the quantity of solution is too great, and the rate of flow should either be decreased or tentatively discontinued altogether. Furthermore, the fetal heart rate should be counted and recorded. It will be recalled that the fetal heart tones should return to their normal rate and rhythm within 15 seconds or so after the termination of a contraction, and any persistence of fetal bradycardia is another indication for discontinuation of the oxytocin drip. In the event that the nurse should be left alone with the patient while the intravenous-drip oxytocin technique is being employed, and she observes any abnormalities in the uterine contractions or the fetal heart tones, she should turn off the solution *immediately* and report her findings to the physician. The major advantage of the oxytocin drip is that it may be discontinued immediately in the event that untoward effects should be observed—an obvious safety factor.

Artificial Rupture of the Membranes. Amniotomy, or artificial rupture of the membranes is a common method of enhancing labor. Amniotomy has also been used to induce labor. When the patient is near term and the cervix is favorable, it is almost always followed by labor within a few hours. The membranes serve as a barrier against bacterial invasion. For this reason, once this barrier has been eliminated by amniotomy, delivery should be accomplished expeditiously. Many obstetricians now feel that the primary use of amniotomy for labor induction is tantamount to burning one's bridges, and that the procedure should be delayed until after the initiation of good contractions with intravenous pitocin.

Amniotomy is accomplished after placing the patient in the lithotomy position and carrying out antiseptic preparation of the vulva. The first two fingers of one hand are inserted into the cervix until the membranes are encountered. A long hook, similar to one blade of a disarticulated vulsellum tenaculum, or an Allis clamp, is inserted into the vagina, and the membranes are simply hooked and torn by the tip of the sharp instrument. As much fluid as possible is allowed to drain. The quality of the fluid should be noted. Normally, it is watery-clear. Fetal heart tones should be checked immediately after amniotomy, extra care should be exercised, as there is an increased possibility of cord prolapse.

So far as the nurse is concerned, these obstetric operations do not differ greatly from any other surgical procedures. The direction of these operations is entirely the responsibility of the physician, and the nurse's share consists of these three responsibilities: (1) having everything in readiness beforehand, (2) giving reassuring advice to the patient and her family and (3) making sure that no opportunity is lost in rendering all possible assistance to the physician.

CONFERENCE MATERIAL

1. A mother, Para 2, is admitted to the hospital at 42 weeks' gestation for induction of labor. Her membranes have been artificially ruptured and intravenous oxytocin has been started. Discuss the nursing care of this mother from this time until she is in active labor.

2. What specific nursing care would you give to a mother who sustained a third-degree perineal laceration as the result of a precipitous labor?

3. A 38-year-old gravida 5 had an uneventful pregnancy until the last trimester, when she developed pre-eclampsia. Now, at term, she is admitted to the hospital because of suspected abruptio placenta and, after consultation, is to have an emergency cesarean section. Discuss the nursing care of this mother from time of admission until she is taken to the operating room for surgery.

4. A primigravida, who has 3-year-old adopted twins, is delivered by low cervical cesarean section because of pelvic injuries received in an auto accident 6 years earlier. Discuss the nursing care of this mother following cesarean section.

SUGGESTED READING

Eastman, N. J., and Hellman, L. M.: Williams Obstetrics, ed. 13, New York, Appleton, 1966.

Fields, H., Smith, K., and Green, J.: Induction of Labor. New York, The Macmillan Company, 1965.

Wulff, G. J. L., Jr. (ed.): Symposium of forceps delivery. Clin. Obstet. Gynec., 8:811-918, 1965.

Study Questions

Unit Six: Operative Procedures in Obstetrics

Read through the entire question and place your answer on the line to the right.

1. Which of the following structures are involved when an episiotomy is performed?
   A. The vaginal mucosa
   B. The levator ani muscle
   C. The glans clitoris
   D. The cardinal ligament
   E. The fourchet

   Select the number corresponding to the correct letter or letters.
   1. A only
   2. A and B
   3. A, B and E
   4. All of them   3

2. Obstetric forceps are frequently used to facilitate delivery. In which of the following conditions would it be indicated to deliver the infant by forceps?
   A. The cervix fails to dilate completely.
   B. The mother has heart disease.
   C. The mother has a contracted pelvis.
   D. Prolapse of the umbilical cord
   E. Passage of meconium-stained amniotic fluid in vertex presentation

   Select the number corresponding to the correct letters.
   1. A and B
   2. B, D and E
   3. C and E
   4. All of them   2

3. Which of the following principles should be observed in the use of intravenous oxytocin to stimulate labor?
   A. The condition of the fetus must be satisfactory.
   B. It should be used only in cases of secondary uterine inertia.
   C. It should not be given to a multipara who has had 4 or more full-term pregnancies.
   D. It should be used in cases of borderline pelvis.
   E. A responsible person should be in constant attendance while the mother is receiving intravenous oxytocin.

   Select the number corresponding to the correct letters.
   1. A and B
   2. A, C and E
   3. B, D and E
   4. All of them   2

4. What specific treatment should be included in the care given a mother who has had a repair of a second-degree laceration of the perineum?
   A. Give daily routine perineal care.

B. Serve a soft diet until the 5th postpartal day.
C. Omit enemas until the 5th postpartal day.
D. Limit activities in regard to early ambulation.
E. Encourage the mother not to sit erect until wound has healed.

Select the number corresponding to the correct letter or letters.
1. A only
2. A, D and E
3. B, C and D
4. All of them   1

5. After a cesarean section, which of the following symptoms might indicate that the patient is having excessive bleeding?
A. Accelerated pulse and respiration and drop in blood pressure
B. Pain and tenderness in operative area
C. Abdominal distention
D. Sanguineous drainage from the abdominal wound and the vagina
E. Apprehension and restlessness

Select the number corresponding to the correct letters.
1. A and B
2. A, C and D
3. A, D and E
4. All of them   3

6. In caring for a mother who has been delivered by cesarean section, which of the following are usually employed to keep the uterus contracted and control bleeding?
A. Oxytocic drugs
B. Gentle massage of the fundus if it becomes relaxed
C. Icebag to the operative area
D. Pressure dressings and tight abdominal binder
E. Keep the patient flat in bed for the first 6 hours postoperatively.

Select the number corresponding to the correct letter or letters.
1. A only
2. A, C and D
3. B, C and E
4. All of them   1

Note: The key to the correct answers to these questions is given on page 613.

UNIT SEVEN
Maternal Disorders Associated With the Childbearing Cycle

Complications of Pregnancy
Complications of Labor
Complications of the Puerperium

Complications of Pregnancy

19

Toxemias of Pregnancy • *Hemorrhagic Complications* • *Hyperemesis Gravidarum*
Coincidental Diseases and Pregnancy

INTRODUCTION

Regardless of the fact that from a biologic point of view childbearing is considered to be a normal reproductive process, the borderline between health and illness is less distinctly marked during this time because of the numerous physiologic changes that occur in the mother's body during the course of parturition. The importance of early and continued health supervision during pregnancy is paramount for the total well-being of the mother and her infant, for such preventive care makes possible the early detection of warning signals of potential pathologic conditions, so that serious problems can be averted or controlled by prompt treatment (see Chap. 8).

Certain "common complaints" are experienced by most expectant mothers to some degree; these are the so-called minor discomforts of pregnancy, which are not serious in themselves but nevertheless detract from the mother's feeling of comfort and well-being. Since these discomforts are usually related to normal physiologic changes occurring within the mother's body and are not in themselves pathologic, they have been included in the chapter on antepartal care (see Chap. 8). However, minor discomforts, if neglected, may lead to a major complication.

The maternal disorders associated with pregnancy may be considered from the standpoint of the complications of the pregnancy itself and from the standpoint of the complications that are related to the coincidental diseases which occur during pregnancy. There are only a few major complications of pregnancy, but they present a serious health problem (e.g., the toxemias of pregnancy). The coincidental diseases which may occur during pregnancy are those which might occur at any other time as well, because the pregnant woman is subject to any disorder or disease which might affect a nonpregnant person. However, when these illnesses arise coincident to pregnancy, the disorder is likely to complicate the pregnancy, the disorder itself may be aggravated by the pregnancy, or both effects may result.

Certain complications of pregnancy may seriously jeopardize the health of both the mother and her unborn infant. The complications which primarily affect the mother and the maternal aspects of those having dual implications will be discussed in this chapter. Although dramatic progress has been made in reducing maternal as well as perinatal morbidity and mortality, some problems remain unsolved. Despite expanding social programs, a great many underprivileged women receive inadequate or no prenatal care. In contrast to those women with optimal care, these have an increased rate of complications, morbidity, and mortality, both maternal and perinatal.

A review of the most recent statistics indicates that there were, in 1967, 987 maternal deaths. The overall maternal mortality rate is 28 per 100,000 live births, 19.5 for the white population and 69.5 for nonwhites. Of the 987 deaths, 127 (12.8%) were due to sepsis, 189 (19.2%) to toxemia, 142 (14.4%) to hemorrhage, and 104 (10.6%) to abortion with sepsis. The remaining 425 (43%) were the result of various causes, including accidents and coincidental disease. In addition, maternal complications during pregnancy have a significant influence on perinatal morbidity and mortality, as demonstrated in Table 19-1.

TABLE 19-1. INFANT DEATHS CAUSED BY NEONATAL DISORDERS ARISING FROM CERTAIN DISEASES OF THE MOTHER DURING PREGNANCY, UNITED STATES, 1963*

CAUSE OF DEATH†	NUMBER OF DEATHS		
	TOTAL	WITH IMMATURITY	WITHOUT MENTION OF IMMATURITY
Certain Disease of Early Infancy:			
Neonatal disorders arising from certain diseases of the mother during pregnancy; attributed to:	741	466	275
Toxemias of pregnancy	245	157	88
Maternal diabetes	223	131	92
Maternal rubella	4	1	3
Toxoplasmosis	25	2	23
Other or unspecified diseases of mother during pregnancy	244	175	69

* Department of Health, Education, and Welfare: Vital Statistics of the United States 1963, vol. II, Part A, Table 1-20, Washington, D.C., U.S. Government Printing Office, 1965.

† Classified according to the Seventh Revision of International Lists, 1955.

TOXEMIAS OF PREGNANCY

"The toxemias of pregnancy are disorders encountered during gestation, or early in the puerperium, which are characterized by one or more of the following signs: hypertension, edema, albuminuria, and in severe cases, convulsions and coma."[1] Despite decades of intensive research, the cause of toxemia is still unknown. The name itself would give rise to the supposition that these conditions are due to circulating toxins in the blood, derived presumably from the products of conception; but this is probably not correct. Whether toxemia represents an exaggeration of the various physical changes which normally accompany pregnancy, or whether it depends on some entirely new deviation from the normal course of pregnancy is still one of the most important unsolved problems in the whole field of human reproduction.

The toxemias of pregnancy are a very common complication of gestation, being seen in 6 or 7 per cent of all gravidae. They rank among the three major complications (hemorrhage, puerperal infections and the toxemias of pregnancy) responsible for the vast majority of maternal deaths and account for some 1,000 maternal deaths in the United States each year. As a cause of fetal death they are even more important. It can be estimated conservatively that at least 30,000 stillbirths and neonatal deaths each year in this

country are the result of toxemias of pregnancy. The great majority of these deaths are due to prematurity of the infant.

The huge toll of maternal and infant lives taken by the toxemias of pregnancy is in large measure preventable. Proper antepartal supervision, particularly the early detection of signs and symptoms of oncoming toxemia and appropriate treatment, will arrest many cases and so ameliorate others that the outcome for baby and mother is usually satisfactory. The nurse is often the first to encounter the early signs and symptoms, not only in the hospital outpatient department but also on home visits, and it is of utmost importance that she be constantly on the lookout for them so that treatment may be instituted at the earliest possible moment.

Classification

The toxemias of pregnancy have heretofore been classified in many forms. In 1952 The American Committee on Maternal Welfare revised its classification as follows:

1. Acute toxemia of pregnancy
   A. Preeclampsia
      1. Mild
      2. Severe
   B. Eclampsia
2. Chronic hypertensive (vascular disease with pregnancy)
   A. Chronic hypertensive vascular disease without superimposed acute toxemia

---

[1] Definition established by The American Committee on Maternal Welfare, April 1, 1952.

1. Those cases in which hypertension was definitely known to exist before the onset of pregnancy
2. Cases of early hypertension before the 24th week

B. Chronic hypertensive vascular disease with superimposed toxemia

3. Unclassified toxemias

Acute toxemia of pregnancy is divided into two stages: *preeclampsia* (the nonconvulsive stage) and *eclampsia* (the convulsive stage). The condition is classified as *preeclampsia* when, after the 24th week of pregnancy, a gravida who previously has been normal in the following respects develops sudden elevation of blood pressure, albuminuria or edema (one or more of the symptoms). Certain criteria have been established to divide preeclampsia into two groups: "preeclampsia mild" and "preeclampsia severe," depending on the symptoms. In *preeclampsia mild,* the systolic blood pressure is found to be 140 mm. Hg or more, or is elevated 30 mm. or more above the usual level; the diastolic pressure will be 90 mm. Hg or more, or is elevated 15 mm. or more above the usual level. Abnormal blood pressures must be observed on two occasions or more at least 6 hours apart, because a single reading may be misleading. The albumin in the urine is small in amount but must be of sufficient degree on 2 or more successive days. Persistent edema involving the hands and the face is present. The condition is classified as *preeclampsia severe* if any one of the following signs or symptoms is present: (1) a systolic blood pressure of 160 mm. Hg or more, or a diastolic pressure of 110 mm. or more; (2) marked albuminuria; (3) oliguria; (4) cerebral or visual disturbances; (5) pulmonary edema or cyanosis. Once the preeclamptic patient has a convulsion, she passes into the stage called *eclampsia.*

Chronic hypertensive vascular disease, sometimes called essential hypertension, is a disease which is not peculiar to pregnancy. When pregnancy aggravates the already existing hypertension so that the gravida with this chronic process develops an acute elevation of blood pressure and a significant degree of albuminuria, the condition is called *chronic hypertensive vascular disease with superimposed acute toxemia.* This disease is seen in all stages of gestation but is prone to occur between the 24th and 30th weeks. Furthermore, the symptoms may increase in severity to the stage of eclampsia.

Preeclampsia

As has been stated in the previous classification of the toxemias of pregnancy, preeclampsia is characterized by a sudden elevation in blood pressure, albuminuria and edema in a gravida who previously has been normal in these respects. It is the forerunner or prodromal stage of eclampsia; in other words, unless the preeclamptic process is checked by treatment or by delivery, it is more or less likely that eclampsia (convulsions and coma) will ensue. Characteristically, preeclampsia is a disease of the last 2 or 3 months of pregnancy and is particularly prone to occur in young primigravidae. The underlying disease processes of preeclampsia and eclampsia are probably identical, the chief difference being that the latter goes on to convulsions and coma, whereas the former does not.

Signs and Symptoms. The earliest warning signal of preeclampsia is sudden development of hypertension. Accordingly, the importance of frequent and regular blood pressure estimations during pregnancy cannot be emphasized too strongly. The absolute blood pressure reading is probably of less significance than the relationship it bears to previous determinations and to the age of the patient. For example, a rise from 110/70 to 135/85 in a young woman is a more urgent danger signal than a rise from 135/85 to 150/90 in a patient at 35.

The next most constant sign of preeclampsia is sudden, excessive weight gain. If cases of preeclampsia are studied from the viewpoint of fluid intake and output, it is at once apparent that these sudden gains in weight are due entirely to an accumulation of water in the tissues. Such weight gains, in other words, represent latent edema and almost always precede the visible face and finger edema which is so characteristic of the advanced stages of the disease. From what has been said, it is apparent that scales are essential equipment for good antepartal care. Weight gain of 1 pound a week or so may be regarded as being normal. Sudden gains of more than 2 pounds a week should be viewed with suspicion; gains of more than 3 pounds, with alarm. Weight increases of the latter magnitude call for more frequent blood pressure determinations, and if these latter are also abnormal, hospitalization with intensive treatment is indicated. In investigating suspected edema, it is well to ask the patient if her wedding ring is becoming tight, since finger and facial edema is a more valuable sign of preeclampsia than is swelling of the ankles. In the

FIG. 19-1. (*Left*) Facies in preeclampsia. Note edema of eyelids and facial skin and general coarsening of features. (*Right*) Same patient 10 days after delivery.

facies of a patient with outspoken preeclampsia, the eyelids are swollen, and, associated with the edema, marked coarseness of the features develops (Fig. 19-1).

The sudden appearance of *albumin in the urine,* with or without other findings, always should be regarded as a sign of preeclampsia. A complete urinalysis, including a microscopic examination, will help to exclude infection as a cause of proteinuria. Usually it develops later than the hypertension and the gain in weight and for this very reason must be regarded as being of serious omen when superimposed on these other two findings.

But the very essence of preeclampsia is the lightninglike fulminance with which it strikes. Although the above physical signs of preeclampsia usually give the physician ample time to institute preventive treatment, it sometimes happens that these derangements develop between visits to the office or the clinic, even though they be only a week apart. For this reason it is imperative that all expectant mothers be informed, both verbally and by some form of printed slip or booklet, in regard to certain danger signals which they themselves may recognize. Insofar as the toxemias of pregnancy are concerned, the following symptoms demand immediate report to the doctor: (1) severe, continuous headache; (2) swelling of the face or the fingers; (3) dimness or blurring of vision; (4) persistent vomiting; (5) decrease in the amount of urine excreted; and (6) epigastric pain (a late symptom).

It should be emphasized that the three early and important signs of preeclampsia, namely, hypertension, weight gain and albuminuria, are changes of which the patient is usually unaware. All three may be present in substantial degree, and yet she may feel quite well. Only by regular and careful antepartal examination can these warning signs be detected. By the time the preeclamptic patient has developed symptoms and signs which she herself can detect (such as headache, blurred vision, puffiness of the eyelids and the fingers), she is usually in an advanced stage of the disease, and much valuable time has been lost. Headache is rarely observed in the milder cases but is encountered with increasing frequency as the most severe grades are met. In general, patients who actually develop eclampsia often have a severe headache as a forerunner of the first convulsion. The visual disturbances range from a slight blurring of vision to various degrees of temporary blindness. Although convulsions are less likely to occur in cases of mild preeclampsia, the possibility cannot be entirely eliminated. Patients with severe preeclampsia should always be considered as being on the verge of having a convulsion.

Treatment. Prophylaxis is most important in the prevention and the control of preeclampsia. Since in its early stages preeclampsia rarely gives rise to signs or symptoms which the patient herself will notice, the early detection of this disease demands meticulous antepartal supervision. Rapid weight gain or an upward trend in blood pressure, although still in the "normal" range, are danger signals. Every pregnant woman should be examined by her obstetrician every week during the last month of pregnancy and every 2 weeks during the 2 previous months. The most promising prophylaxis of the disease lies in reduction of sodium intake and curtailing weight gain in all pregnant women. Finger edema is a frequent forerunner of preeclampsia, which may precede the hypertension by several weeks and is a valuable warning sign.

AMBULATORY PATIENT. When the patient's symptoms are mild (i.e., there is minor elevation of blood pressure with minimal or no signs of edema and proteinuria), treatment may be instituted at home in the hope that symptoms will abate. During this period the patient should be examined by the physician at least twice a week, and she should be given a strict regimen to follow, as well as careful instructions in regard to symptoms to report promptly. The patient's activities should be restricted, and she should understand that bed rest during the greater part of the day is most desirable. Sedative drugs, such as phenobarbital, may be prescribed to encourage rest and relaxation, the dosage being dependent on the severity of the condition. Of major importance is a salt-poor diet. Therefore, the patient should be instructed so that she understands which foods have appreciable sodium content and therefore must be excluded from her diet, in addition to the fact that no salt may be added to her food in the kitchen or at the table. The diet should be well balanced but restricted in caloric content if the patient's weight gain indicates the need. It should contain ample protein, particularly lean meat, eggs and a quart of milk daily. Fluid intake should be maintained at 2,500 cc. daily; in hot weather, at 3,000 cc. Carbonated beverages should be avoided because of their sodium content.

The restriction of sodium in the diet of the preeclamptic patient is directed at reducing the edema. Even in normal nonpregnant persons an increased intake of sodium chloride causes water retention. Pregnant women, particularly gravidae suffering from preeclampsia, show a marked tendency to retain sodium, and there is reason to believe that this tendency of the tissues to retain sodium is closely correlated with their tendency to hold water. To superimpose still more sodium in the diet on this already existing sodium and water retention is obviously unwise. Since the accumulation of sodium and water precedes the development of hypertension and proteinuria in preeclampsia, the control of such retention is sufficiently important that diuretic therapy is indicated on an ambulatory basis if dietary measures fail. Such diuretic regimens are described subsequently. Some workers have even suggested the routine use of a low salt diet and diuretics in all patients who are "toxemia prone," such as young primigravidae and diabetics. Although it is difficult to determine whether diuretics alone can prevent toxemia, certainly in combination with diet and careful prenatal care they can.

HOSPITAL PATIENT. In the event that the patient's condition does not respond promptly to ambulatory treatment, she should be hospitalized without delay. A systematic method of study should be instituted upon admission to the hospital. A general physical examination and history should be obtained promptly, followed by constant vigilance for the development of such symptoms as headache, visual disturbances and edema of the fingers and the eyelids. Body weight should be obtained on admission and every other morning thereafter. Blood pressure readings should be taken every 4 hours except between midnight and morning, unless the midnight blood pressure has risen. Daily fluid intake and output records should be kept, and urine specimens sent to the laboratory daily for analysis for albumin and casts. Retinal examination is always included as part of the admission physical examination and is done every 2 to 3 days thereafter, depending on the findings. Blood chemical determinations are also included. Once the patient is admitted to the hospital, complete bed rest is essential.

DRUGS AND DIET. Even in milder cases, minimal doses of sedative drugs are helpful. Phenobarbital, 32 mg. (½ grain), may be given 4 times a day, or twice this dosage in cases of moderate severity. The dietary regimen previously described should be adhered to, or it may be indicated to restrict the sodium chloride to less than 3 Gm. daily. In such cases it may become necessary to substitute one of the commercial sodium-free milk powders in place of regular milk, since a quart of milk itself contains about 1.25 Gm. of sodium chloride. The most commonly used diuretics today are the thiazides, such as chlorothiazide (Diuril), 0.5 to 1.0 Gm. daily, or hydrochlorothiazide (Esidrix), 50 mg. daily. These drugs increase the excretion of both sodium and water without producing acidosis, but at the same time, when given in adequate doses, cause a marked loss of potassium. If not recognized, potassium depletion may become symptomatic, causing fatigue and muscular weakness. This problem can be avoided by administering supplemental potassium, or with dietary measures such as an increased intake of citrus fruit and juices. Some physicians avoid the problem by administering the drugs intermittently (3 days out of 5, or 5 out of 7). Occasionally, a patient may become refractory to the thiazides, in which case there are even more potent drugs available, such as ethycrynic acid or lasix. It is important to be sure that the problem is only one of refractoriness to the diuretic and not a true worsening of the toxemia, which would certainly require more drastic measures than a change in diuretics.

When severe preeclampsia develops, immediate and intensive therapy is imperative. Sedation is of major importance to forestall convulsions. The dosage of drugs employed should be regulated so that they produce drowsiness and sleep, from which the patient can be easily awakened, and also suppress the hyperactive reflexes of the patient. The drug most often used as a sedative and an anticonvulsant under these circumstances is magnesium sulfate. In addition to being an excellent anticonvulsant, magnesium causes vasodilation and, therefore, is also effective in lowering blood pressure. For rapid action, an I.V. dose of 20 to 30 ml. of a 10 per cent solution (2 to 3 Gm.) is used. Very often the drug is given intramuscularly in doses of 10 to 20 ml. of a 50 per cent solution (5 to 10 mg.). The dose is divided, half given into each buttock, and often 1 to 2 ml. of 1 per cent procaine is added to the injection to minimize discomfort. A repeat dose of magnesium sulfate should not be given unless the reflexes and respiratory rate have been checked, since it depresses both. The antidote is calcium, and an ampule of calcium gluconate should always be readily available when magnesium is being administered.

The barbiturates can also be used, the dose being larger (60 to 120 mg. every 4 to 6 hours) than for mild cases and the route of administration parenteral. If the patient is in labor, it is well to avoid barbiturates because of their depressant effect on the fetus. Although many use morphine in the management of severe preeclampsia, it would seem best reserved for the patient who has the added stimulus of pain (i.e., labor). Minimizing this stimulus will certainly reduce the likelihood of a seizure. In addition, there are an increasing number of favorable reports on the use of Diazepam (Valium) in such cases.

DELIVERY. Despite all efforts, the condition may persist to a marked degree, and in that event induction of labor may become necessary for the welfare of mother and infant (see Chap. 22. Fetal Diagnosis and Treatment). In occasional instances when the preeclampsia is severe and fulminating and conditions for induction of labor are not favorable, cesarean section may be the procedure of choice.

Postpartum. The signs and symptoms of preeclampsia usually abate rapidly after delivery, but the danger of convulsions does not pass until 48 hours have elapsed postpartum. Therefore, continuation of sedation throughout this interval is indicated. In the majority of cases the elevated blood pressure as well as the other derangements have returned to normal within 10 days or 2 weeks. In about 30 per cent of cases, however, the hypertension shows a tendency either to persist indefinitely or to recur in subsequent pregnancies. For this reason the prolonged follow-up of these patients is highly important.

Nursing Care. The nurse's responsibility in the detection and care of cases of preeclampsia is manifold. Since this complication of pregnancy is common and may occur antepartally, intrapartally or postpartally, it is important for the nurse to observe all maternity patients closely for the first indication of early symptoms, as well as to be quick to recognize and report any evidence pointing to an aggravation of the process. The early symptoms and the manifestations related to more severe preeclampsia, such as persistent headache, blurred vision, spots or flashes of light before the eyes, epigastric pain, vomiting, torpor or muscular twitchings, are all vastly important. Data collected in relation to these symptoms in addition to an accurate record of weight gain, fluid intake and elimination, diet and attitudes and behavior, when it is accurately recorded, can assist the physician in evaluating the symptoms and planning his course of therapy.

In setting the therapeutic atmosphere, the nurse should see that the environment is as comfortable and pleasant as possible. The patient should be in a single room, free from the stimuli of noise, strong lights and the presence of unnecessary equipment which might frighten her. To the best of her ability, the nurse must protect the patient from needless traffic into the room; otherwise, the coming and going of personnel to the bedside may be so constant that it could interfere with the efficacy of the treatment being carried out. Every effort should be exerted to relieve the patient's anxiety, which sometimes is brought about by apprehension regarding her illness or may be due to concern for the welfare of her family at home.

Regardless of the severity of the toxemia, certain responsibilities are carried out by the nurse. Medications ordered must be administered promptly, the prescribed diet should be supervised, a careful record of intake and elimination kept, blood pressure readings and basal weights taken, specimens collected and labeled accurately, and observations of slight symptoms or change in condition should be reported immediately, both verbally and on the patient's record. Since rest is a major consideration in the care of this patient, the nurse should plan a schedule of activities so that the patient is disturbed as little as possible. Medications, treatments and nursing procedures should be administered at the same time as far as the physician's orders will permit, but always with the thought in mind that only as much as will not overtire the patient should be planned for any one time. When any treatment is ordered, the procedure is best carried out after sedation has been administered. Before heavy sedation is initiated, any removable dentures or eyeglasses should be removed and stored in a secure place. If the patient is not in labor, the nurse must be alert to watch for signs of labor, particularly after sedation has been given. Any time an intravenous fluid is administered, if the physician has not specified the rate at which the fluid is to flow, it should be given slowly.

The nurse should see that the equipment necessary for the safe and efficient care of the patient is immediately available and in good working order. A padded mouth gag should always be ready for use at the bedside to prevent the patient from biting her tongue in the event that a convulsion develops. Trays for catheterization equipment and for the administration of special medications constitute part of the necessary equipment. Since water retention plays such a large role in the disease, and urinary output is likely to be diminished, an indwelling bladder catheter may be ordered to ensure accuracy in obtaining output from the kidneys. Since the urinary output must be watched carefully, it is imperative to see that the retention catheter is draining properly at all times. In severe cases suction apparatus should be readily available for aspirating mucus, as well as equipment for the administration of oxygen, should symptoms such as cyanosis or depressed respiration indicate the need.

Eclampsia

Clinical Picture. As indicated, the development of eclampsia is almost always preceded by the signs and symptoms of preeclampsia. A preeclamptic patient, who may have been conversing with you a moment before, is seen to roll her eyes to one side and stare fixedly into space. Immediately, twitching of the facial muscles ensues. This is the *stage of invasion* of the convulsion and lasts only a few seconds.

The whole body then becomes rigid in a generalized muscular contraction; the face is distorted, the eyes protrude, the arms are flexed, the hands are clenched and the legs are inverted. Since all the muscles of the body are now in a state of tonic contraction, this phase may be regarded as the *stage of contraction*; it lasts 15 or 20 seconds.

Suddenly the jaws begin to open and close violently, and forthwith the eyelids also. The other facial muscles and then all the muscles of the body alternately contract and relax in rapid succession. So forceful are the muscular movements that the patient may throw herself out of bed, and almost invariably, unless protected, the tongue is bitten by the violent jaw action. Foam, often blood-tinged, exudes from the mouth; the face is congested and purple, and the eyes are bloodshot. Few pictures which the nurse is called upon to witness are so horrible. This phase in which the muscles alternately contract and relax is called the *stage of convulsion*; it may last a minute or so. Gradually the muscular movements become milder and farther apart, and finally the patient lies motionless.

Throughout the seizure the diaphragm has been fixed with respiration halted. Still no breathing occurs. For a few seconds the woman appears to be dying from respiratory arrest, but just when this outcome seems almost inevitable, she takes a long, deep, stertorous inhalation, and breathing is resumed. Then coma ensues. The patient will remember nothing whatsoever of the convulsion or, in all probability, events immediately before and afterward.

The coma may last from a few minutes to several hours, and the patient may then become conscious; or the coma may be succeeded by another convulsion. The convulsions may recur during coma, or they may recur only after an interval of consciousness, or they may never recur at all. In the average case, from 5 to 10 convulsions occur at longer or shorter intervals, but as many as 20 are not uncommon. Convulsions may start before the onset of labor (antepartum), during labor (intrapartum) or anytime within the first 48 hours after delivery (postpartum). About a fifth of the cases develop postpartally.

Upon physical examination, the findings of eclampsia are similar to those in preeclampsia, but exaggerated. Thus, the systolic blood pressure usually ranges around 180 mm. Hg and sometimes exceeds 200 mm. Hg. Albuminuria is frequently extreme, from 10 to 20 Gm. per liter. Edema may be marked but sometimes is absent. Oliguria, or suppression of urinary excretion, is common and may amount to complete anuria. Fever is present in about half the cases.

In favorable cases the convulsions cease, the coma lessens, and urinary output increases. However, it sometimes requires 1 or 2 days for clear consciousness to be regained. During this period eclamptic patients are often in an obstreperous, resistant mood and may be exceedingly difficult to manage. A few develop actual psychoses. In unfavorable cases the coma deepens, urinary excretion diminishes, the pulse becomes more rapid, the temperature rises, and edema of the lungs develops. The last is a serious symptom and usually is interpreted as a sign of cardiovascular failure. Edema of the lungs is readily recognizable by the noisy, gurgling respiration and by the large quantity of frothy mucus which exudes from the mouth and the nose. Toward the end, convulsions cease altogether, and the final picture is one of vascular collapse, with falling blood pressure and overwhelming edema of the lungs.

Like preeclampsia, eclampsia is a disease of young primigravidae, the majority of cases occurring in first pregnancies. It is more likely to occur as full term approaches and is rarely seen prior to the last 3 months. Eclampsia is particularly prone to develop in twin gestations, the likelihood being about 4 times that in single pregnancies.

Prognosis. Eclampsia is one of the gravest complications of pregnancy; the maternal mortality ranges, in different localities and in different hospitals, from 5 to 15 per cent of such cases. The outlook for the baby is particularly grave, the fetal mortality being about 20 per cent. Although it is difficult in a given case to forecast the outcome, the following are unfavorable signs: oliguria; prolonged coma; a sustained pulse rate over 120; temperature over 103° F.; more than 10 convulsions; 10 or more Gm. of albumin per liter in the urine; systolic blood pressure of more than 200; edema of lungs. If none of these signs is present, the outlook for recovery is good; if two or more are present, the prognosis is definitely serious.

Even though the patient survives, she may not escape unscathed from the attack but sometimes continues to have high blood pressure indefinitely. This statement applies both to preeclampsia and eclampsia. Indeed, about 10 per cent of all preeclamptic and 5 per cent of all eclamptic patients are left with chronic, permanent hypertension. It is of even more importance to note that a still larger percentage of these women (about 50 per cent of preeclamptics and 30 per cent of eclamptics) again develop hypertensive toxemia in any subsequent pregnancies. This is known as "recurrent" or "repeat" toxemia. These facts make it plain that careful, prolonged follow-up of these mothers who have suffered from preeclampsia or eclampsia is imperative. Moreover, the prognosis for future pregnancies must be guarded, although, as the figures indicate, such patients stand at least an even chance of going through subsequent pregnancies satisfactorily.

Principles of Treatment. Since the cause of eclampsia is not known, there can be no "specific" therapy, and treatment must necessarily be empirical. By "empirical" treatment is meant the utilization of those therapeutic measures which have yielded the best results in other cases. It is thus based on experience. Since the experience of different doctors and different hospitals varies considerably, the type of therapy employed from clinic to clinic differs somewhat in respect to the drugs used and in other details. However, the general principles followed are almost identical everywhere. For the nurse to memorize some particular regimen of therapy, as given in this textbook or as used in this or that hospital, will serve little purpose in her later career and conduces to an undesirable rigidity of attitude. However, she should grasp thoroughly the general principles involved. These are enumerated as follows:

1. PREVENTION. Let it be emphasized again that eclampsia is largely (but not entirely) a preventable disease. Vigilant antepartal care and the early detection and treatment of preeclampsia will do more to reduce deaths from eclampsia than the most intensive treatment after convulsions have once started.

2. CONSERVATIVE TREATMENT. Since eclamp-

sia never occurs in nonpregnant women, nor in men, it is reasonable to believe that it must be due in some way to the pregnant condition. By the same token it might be concluded that the best way to treat eclampsia would be to terminate the pregnancy at once, that is empty the uterus. This was the therapy employed in the early years of the century and is known as the "radical treatment" of eclampsia; either the cervix was forcibly dilated and the baby extracted, or cesarean section was employed. The results were disastrous. A quarter to a third of the mothers died, often on the operating table from shock.

Dissatisfied with the poor results yielded by the radical treatment of eclampsia, about 1910, physicians began treating the convulsions with sedative drugs, ignored the pregnancy and allowed labor to start whenever it would. The most famous method of therapy of this sort is the Stroganoff regimen, based on sedation by means of morphine and chloral hydrate. The results were dramatic: the maternal mortality fell to 10 per cent, and the fetal mortality was no worse than before. Other physicians tried other sedative drugs and other means of combating the convulsions, but as long as they refrained from interfering with the pregnancy, the results were as good as Stroganoff's, that is, only 1 woman in 10 was lost. This program, whereby the eclamptic convulsions are treated by sedation or otherwise, the pregnancy ignored, and labor allowed to start when it will, is known as the "conservative treatment" of eclampsia.

This totally conservative approach, although bringing about an improvement over "radical" treatment, is no longer advocated in most cases. "Ignoring" the pregnancy results in an undue number of fetal deaths as well as unnecessarily prolonged maternal jeopardy. In the patient with eclampsia, efforts to effect delivery are instituted 12 to 24 hours after the seizure, when adequate sedation has been established and as much diuresis as possible accomplished. Delivery should be accomplished by the most expeditious means. Only in exceptional cases, with very small (immature) fetuses, is conservatism attempted. Most often in these cases the results are poor (i.e., the fetus dies in utero, the maternal status worsens, or spontaneous labor ensues). It is interesting to note that labor frequently begins spontaneously within 24 hours after an eclamptic seizure, even though the cervix is unripe at the time of the convulsion. The reasons for this are unknown;

however, it is an efficient protective measure for both mother and fetus.

3. SEDATION. The purpose of administering sedative drugs is to depress the activity of the brain cells and thereby stop convulsions. The drugs most commonly employed are described below.

Magnesium Sulfate. This drug is an excellent central nervous system depressant, and therefore anticonvulsant, and also a smooth muscle relaxant which causes dilatation of peripheral blood vessels and thereby reduces blood pressure. For these reasons it is probably the most common drug used in eclamptic patients. The routes of administration, doses and precautions have already been discussed. Since the situation with the eclamptic patient is so urgent, the drug is most often given intravenously, at least initially.

Barbiturates. Rapid-acting drugs, such as intravenous Amytal Sodium (0.3 to 0.6 Gm.), are often used to control the seizure, while subcutaneous doses of Luminal Sodium (0.1 to 0.3 Gm.) may be used subsequently.

Morphine. Although large doses (15 to 30 mg.) of morphine have been used commonly in the past as a first line of defense, it has become apparent that there are other more effective anticonvulsants which cause less respiratory depression.

Paraldehyde and Chloral Hydrate. These drugs are now largely of historic interest.

Other Drugs. Valium, previously described, and other drugs are now coming into use and may with further study serve to replace those agents presently used. The nurse should bear in mind that this is a changing field with new drugs continually coming to the fore. Those approaches which are standard in one hospital may seem foreign in another. The important principle concerning sedation is that it be adequate to control the initial convulsion, sufficient to prevent further seizures, and yet cause as little respiratory depression as possible. If the patient happens also to be in labor, with delivery proximate, fetal depression also becomes a consideration.

4. PROTECTION OF PATIENT FROM SELF-INJURY. The eclamptic patient must never be left alone for a second. When in the throes of a convulsion, she may crash her head against a bedpost or throw herself onto the floor; or she may bite her tongue violently. To prevent the latter injury, some device should be kept within easy reach which can be inserted between the jaws at the

Fig. 19-2. Improvised mouth gag inserted between jaws of eclamptic patient to prevent tongue injury. (Putnam, Tracy J.: Convulsive Seizures, Philadelphia, Lippincott)

very onset of a convulsion. A piece of heavy rubber tubing, a rolled towel or a padded clothespin is often employed (Fig. 19-2). The nurse must take care in inserting it not to injure the patient (lips, gums, teeth) and not to allow her own finger to be bitten.

Eclamptic patients must never be given fluids by mouth unless thoroughly conscious. Failure to adhere to this rule may result in aspiration of the fluid and consequent pneumonia.

5. PROTECTION OF PATIENT FROM EXTRANEOUS STIMULI. A loud noise, a bright light, a jarring of the bed, a draft—indeed, the slightest irritation—may be enough to precipitate a convulsion.

6. PROMOTION OF DIURESIS. When an eclamptic patient begins to excrete substantial quantities of urine, the outlook is encouraging. Accordingly, efforts are generally made to stimulate renal activity. This is most often done by the intravenous administration of hypertonic glucose solution, usually about a 20 per cent solution in amounts ranging from 200 to 500 cc.

Often now Mannitol (25 to 50 Gm.) by intravenous "push" dose is used to promote diuresis. Efforts to induce a diuresis are safer if the patient's central venous pressure is being monitored. Should the CVP be high (above 12 cm. H_2O), the use of osmotic diuretics such as 20 per cent glucose of Mannitol, or indeed large volumes of fluid, is risky and could well result in cardiac overload and pulmonary edema.

Nurse's Responsibilities in Eclampsia. The nurse's responsibilities in the management of a case of eclampsia are serious. Some of them have already been mentioned in the discussion of treatment. Although eclampsia usually is regarded as the climax to a mounting preeclamptic toxemia which has been present, the nurse must remember that it is occasionally observed as a fulminating case in an apparently normal woman who may develop severe symptoms in the span of 24 hours. In the event that eclampsia occurs, the best quality of nursing care is necessary. The attack may come on at any time, even when the patient is sleeping. During the seizure it is necessary to protect the patient from self-injury. Never leave the patient for an instant unless someone is actually at the bedside to relieve you. Gentle restraint should be used to guide the patient's movements whenever necessary to prevent her from throwing herself against the head of the bed or out of it. Canvas sides, as well as pads at the head and the foot of the bed, are helpful. The padded mouth gag should be inserted between the upper and lower teeth at the onset of a convulsion to prevent the tongle from being bitten. Regardless of the fact that the nurse is exceedingly "busy" with the patient when a seizure occurs, she should make careful and complete observations of the duration and the character of each convulsion, the depth and duration of coma, the quality and the rate of pulse and respiration and the degree of cyanosis. A careful record should be kept so that this information can be used by the physician in treating the patient. During the coma which follows, care must be taken to see that the patient does not aspirate. It is understood, of course, that one never gives an eclamptic patient fluids by mouth unless it is certain she is fully conscious. The position of the patient in bed should be such that it promotes drainage of secretions and the maintenance of a clear airway. It may be necessary to raise the foot of the bed of the comatose patient a few inches to promote drainage of secretions from the respiratory passage. When this measure must be resorted to, it is particularly important to watch for signs of pulmonary edema, which would be aggravated by this position. The head of the bed may need to be elevated to relieve dyspnea. Even though the patient should be disturbed as little as possible, her position should be changed at hourly intervals.

The patient should be protected from extraneous stimuli. Light in the room should be eliminated except for a small lamp, so shaded that none of the light falls on the patient. Although the room should be darkened, the light should be sufficient to permit observations of changes in condition, such as cyanosis or twitchings. A flashlight, directed well away from the patient's face, may be used during catheterization and rectal installations and during the physician's examinations. Sudden noises, such as the slamming of a door or the clatter of a tray as it is placed on a table, and jarring of the bed must be avoided, because they are often sufficient stimuli to send the patient into convulsions. Only absolutely necessary conversation should be carried on in the room, and this should be in the lowest tones possible.

The fetal heart tones should be checked as often as time will permit. Also, the nurse must watch for signs of labor. In eclampsia this may proceed with few external signs, and occasionally such a patient gives birth beneath the sheets before anyone knows that the process is under way. Be suspicious when the patient grunts or groans or moves about at regular intervals, every 5 minutes or so. If this occurs, feel the consistency of the uterus, watch for "show" and bulging and report your observations to the physician. Convulsions which occur during labor may speed up this process, and more rapid preparation for delivery should be made. During the delivery, the same atmosphere of quiet should be maintained, and glaring lights should be kept away from the patient's face.

Throughout the care of the eclamptic patient a careful account of fluid intake and output should be recorded, along with all the other observations and pertinent data. And, since further complications of pregnancy may occur in eclampsia, the patient should be observed for signs and symptoms of cerebral hemorrhage, abruptio placentae, pulmonary edema and cardiac failure.

Preeclampsia and eclampsia have been discussed in some detail because the nurse's role in the management of these conditions is extremely important.

Chronic Hypertensive Vascular Disease

As the name implies, this is a process in which high blood pressure is present before pregnancy. Difficulty is encountered in establishing such a diagnosis, because many women are not seen between pregnancies and blood pressures are, therefore, not recorded. Also, there is normally a decrease in blood pressure during the second trimester which could mask a preexisting hypertension, if the patient does not report for care until the 4th or 5th month of gestation. The diagnosis is justified if hypertension is detected prior to the 24th week of gestation. Most often patients with chronic hypertension are multiparae and commonly over the age of 30.

At least 75 per cent of such patients are able to successfully complete their pregnancies, with no significant change in the status of their hypertension. Fifteen per cent develop superimposed preeclampsia, an occurrence which carries an ominous fetal prognosis (20 per cent mortality), and even an increase in maternal mortality (1 to 2 per cent).

The treatment, then, for the majority of these patients with benign chronic essential hypertension is no different than for the non-pregnant patient. It includes salt restriction, diuretics, restricted activities, sedation and antihypertensives. The pregnancy is allowed to run its normal course under such circumstances. In the case of superimposed preeclampsia, after 24 to 48 hours of intensive medical therapy, pregnancy termination is generally indicated. Even though the baby may be premature, its chances for survival under these circumstances are generally better outside the uterus. In a small number of patients the hypertension will be so severe, with evidence of kidney involvement, severe retinal changes, or cardiac involvement, that therapeutic abortion might be considered if the patient comes to medical attention in the first trimester. It is also well to consider the advisability of postpartum tubal ligation in this group of patients who are generally older, with established families, and for whom additional pregnancies may represent a serious health hazard. This, of course, can only be a recommendation, the final decision resting with the patient and her husband.

HEMORRHAGIC COMPLICATIONS

The causes of bleeding in pregnancy are usually considered in relation to the stage of gestation in which they are most likely to cause complications. Frequent causes of bleeding during the first half of pregnancy are abortion, ectopic pregnancy and hydatidiform mole. Although hydatidiform mole is a less common cause (it occurs once in about 2,000 pregnancies), it is nevertheless important, because uterine bleeding is its outstanding symptom. The two most common causes of hemorrhage in the latter half of pregnancy are placenta previa and abruptio placentae.

Abortion

Definitions. Abortion is the termination of pregnancy at any time before the fetus has attained a stage of viability, that is, before it is capable of extrauterine existence.

It is customary to use the weight of the fetus as an important criterion in abortion. Infants weighing 1,000 Gm. (2 lbs., 3 oz.) or less at birth possess little chance for survival, whereas those above this weight have a substantial chance

of living. Thus, many authorities regard a pregnancy which terminates when the fetus weighs 1,000 Gm. (about 28 weeks of gestation) or less as an abortion. On the other hand, a small percentage of infants weighing 1,000 Gm. or less do survive. Modern advances in the management and care of premature infants have made it possible for smaller and smaller infants to survive, so fetuses weighing only 800 to 900 Gm. (1 lb., 13 oz. to 2 lbs.) may live. For this reason many authorities now maintain that fetal weight of 1,000 Gm. or less but more than 400 Gm. is classified as immature, and that fetal weight of 400 Gm. (about 20 weeks of gestation) or less constitutes an abortion. It is obvious, therefore, that how the termination of pregnancy is classified in different hospitals will depend wholly on the interpretation to which they subscribe. In summary, the following definitions are generally used. The termination of pregnancy at any time when the fetus weighs 400 Gm. or less is defined as an *abortion*. Infants weighing between 401 and 1,000 Gm. are called *immature*.

A premature infant is one born after the stage of viability has been reached but before it has the same chance for survival as a full-term infant. By general consensus, an infant which weighs 2,500

Threatened

Inevitable

Incomplete

Complete

Fig. 19-3. Stages of abortion. (Cooke, Willard R.: Essentials of Gynecology, Philadelphia, Lippincott)

Gm. or less at birth is termed *premature;* one which weighs 2,501 Gm. (5½ lbs.) or more is regarded as *full term.*

It is well to remember that premature labor does not refer to abortion. *Premature labor* is the termination of pregnancy after the fetus is viable but before it has attained full term. Although the cause of many premature labors cannot be explained, the condition can be brought on by maternal diseases, such as chronic hypertensive vascular disease, abruptio placentae, placenta previa, untreated syphilis or a mechanical defect in the cervix.

As a measure to bring about greater uniformity in the interpretation of the terms "abortion," "miscarriage" and "viability," the World Health Organization, in 1950, introduced certain new definitions which, in effect, would substitute the term "early fetal death" for "abortion" and would tabulate all live births and fetal deaths in 4 groups, according to length of gestation.

Terminology of Abortion. The term "abortion" includes many varieties of termination of pregnancy prior to viability but may be subdivided into two main groups, namely, spontaneous and induced. *Spontaneous abortion* is one in which through natural causes the process starts of its own accord. *Induced abortion* is one which is artificially induced whether for therapeutic or other reasons. The laity often employ the word "miscarriage" to designate spontaneous abortion, and the nurse will do well, in discussing the matter with patients or relatives to use that term.

In medical parlance the word "miscarriage" is rarely employed.

THREATENED ABORTION. An abortion is regarded as threatened if a patient in early pregnancy has vaginal bleeding or spotting; this may or may not be associated with mild cramps. The cervix is closed. The process has presumably started but may abate under suitable treatment (Fig. 19-3).

INEVITABLE ABORTION. Inevitable abortion is so called because the process has gone so far that termination of the pregnancy cannot be prevented. Bleeding is copious, and the pains are more severe. The membranes may or may not have ruptured, and the cervical canal is dilating.

INCOMPLETE ABORTION. An incomplete abortion is one in which part of the product of conception has been passed, but part (usually the placenta) is retained in the uterus. Bleeding persists until the retained secundines of the uterus have been passed.

COMPLETE ABORTION. Complete abortion is the expulsion of the entire product of conception.

MISSED ABORTION. In a missed abortion the fetus dies in the uterus, but, instead of being expelled, it is retained indefinitely. The term is generally restricted to cases in which 2 months or more elapse between fetal death and expulsion. During this period the fetus undergoes marked degenerative changes. Of these, maceration, or general softening, is the most common. Occasionally it dries up into a leatherlike structure (mummification) and very rarely it becomes converted into stony material (lithopedion formation). Symptoms, except for amenorrhea, are usually lacking, but occasionally such patients complain of malaise, headache and anorexia. Hypofibrinogenemia, a hemorrhagic complication, may result (see p. 467).

HABITUAL ABORTION. By this term is meant a condition in which spontaneous abortion occurs in successive pregnancies (3 or more). This is a most distressing condition, some women having 6 or 8 spontaneous abortions.

Therapeutic Abortion. Therapeutic or medical abortion refers to the termination of pregnancy by a physician because of a threat to the health of the mother or, in some instances, because of a high risk of fetal malformation. Attitudes of physicians and the public toward pregnancy termination have undergone remarkable changes in recent years, and many states have liberalized their abortion laws. The number of in-hospital abortions in the United States is increasing rapidly as a result of these changes. Policies regarding therapeutic abortion vary from area to area, and in fact from hospital to hospital, and include as indications: threats to the physical or mental health of the patient, rape, incest, and the threat of a malformed child, as in the case of German measles.

Techniques of therapeutic abortion have also undergone change. For a pregnancy of 12 weeks or less, in which dilatation and curettage has been the standard approach, many physicians now employ the suction curet. This instrument is also used by some in completing spontaneous abortion. For the more advanced pregnancy which formerly had to be terminated by abdominal hysterotomy, the use of intraamniotic instillations of hypertonic glucose or saline has provided an alternative. This approach obviates the need for cesarean section in future pregnancies, which would be brought about by hysterotomy. In addition, many investigators are now exploring new techniques, especially medications which might be effective in aborting early pregnancies.

The nurse must recognize that attitudes toward abortion are extremely varied and personal, and that there are strong religious and moral influences in these attitudes. She is entitled to her own conclusions in the matter and should respect those of others.

Criminal Abortion. Criminal, or perhaps better stated, extra-hospital (or extra-clinic) abortion is the termination of pregnancy outside of appropriate medical facilities, generally by non-physician abortionists, regardless of the validity of the indication. The frequency of such abortions is not precisely known but estimates range from 200,000 to 1,200,000 per year in the United States. In most urban areas, abortions are responsible for the majority of maternal deaths, with estimates of 800 to 5,000 abortion deaths per year in this country. Attempts at producing abortion are generally made by the ingestion of drugs such as quinine or castor oil, which usually do nothing, or if taken in sufficient quantities to produce an abortion place the woman in serious jeopardy. Another common approach involves the placement of a foreign body, such as a urethral catheter, into the uterus with or without the instillation of toxic substances. Severe infection, often with shock and kidney failure, is a common consequence of such crude efforts at pregnancy termination. Patients so affected surely are some of the most critically ill the nurse may ever have to care for and, unfortunately, they sometimes succumb in spite of the best efforts of all concerned.

Clinical Picture. About 75 per cent of all spontaneous abortions occur during the 2nd and the 3rd months of pregnancy, that is, before the 12th week. The condition is very common; it is estimated that about 1 pregnancy in every 10 terminates in spontaneous abortion. Almost invariably the first symptom is bleeding due to the separation of the fertilized ovum from its uterine attachment. The bleeding is often slight at the beginning and may persist for days before uterine cramps occur; or, the bleeding may be followed at once by cramps. Occasionally the bleeding is torrential in nature, leaving the patient in shock. The uterine contractions bring about softening and dilatation of the cervix and expel the products of conception either completely or incompletely.

Causes. What causes all these spontaneous abortions—so tragic and shattering to so many women? If the evidence is reviewed with some perspective and with full fairness to all concerned, it is the inevitable conclusion that most of these abortions, far from being tragedies, are blessings in disguise, for they are Nature's beneficent way of extinguishing embryos which are imperfect. Indeed, careful microscopic study of the material passed in these cases shows that the commonest cause of spontaneous abortion is an inherent defect in the product of conception. This defect may express itself in an abnormal embryo, in an abnormal *trophoblast* (p. 77) or in both abnormalities. In early abortions, 80 per cent are associated with some defect of the embryo or trophoblast which is either incompatible with life or would result in a grossly deformed child. The incidence of abnormalities passed after the 2nd month is somewhat lower but not less than 50 per cent. Whether the germ plasm of the spermatozoon or the ovum is at fault in these cases, it is usually difficult, if not impossible, to say. Abortions of this sort are obviously unpreventable and, although often bitterly disappointing to the parents, serve a useful purpose.

Spontaneous abortions may be due to causes other than defects in the product of conception. Severe acute infections, such as pneumonia, pyelitis and typhoid fever, often lead to abortion. Heart failure is another etiologic factor. Occasionally, abnormalities of the generative tract, such as a congenitally short cervix, produce the accident. Retroposition of the uterus rarely causes abortion, as was formerly believed. Many women tend to explain miscarriage on the grounds of injury of one type or another, or excessive activity. Different women exhibit the greatest variation in this respect. In some the pregnancy may go blithely on despite falls from second-story windows and automobile accidents so severe as to fracture the pelvis. In others a trivial fall or merely overfatigue seems to contribute at least to abortion. Since there is no way of telling who is susceptible and who is not it would seem prudent for every expectant mother to follow the dictates of common sense and avoid long automobile trips, lifting heavy weights and any form of activity which involves jolting.

Treatment. The severity of the symptoms manifested in threatened abortion will determine the treatment prescribed. If the patient is having only a slight vaginal bleeding or even spotting, without pain, she should be advised to stay in bed, eat a light well-balanced diet, avoid straining

FIG. 19-4. Sims's speculum for inserting into the vaginal canal so as to expose the cervix to view.

FIG. 19-7. Modified Goodell-Ellinger dilator used for enlarging the canal of the cervix.

FIG. 19-5. Schroeder vaginal retractor for drawing back the vulvar or vaginal walls during an operation.

FIG. 19-8. Uterine sound.

FIG. 19-9. Placental forceps with heart-shaped jaws.

FIG. 19-6. Bullet forceps used in grasping the lips of the cervix.

FIG. 19-10. Sims's sharp curette, a scraper or spoonlike instrument for removing matter from the walls of the uterus.

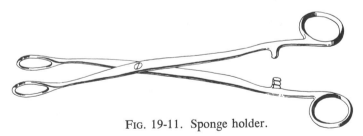

FIG. 19-11. Sponge holder.

at bowel evacuation and the use of cathartics. If she appears to be apprehensive, a mild sedative may be given. She should be further advised to save all perineal pads, as well as all tissue and clots passed, for the physician's inspection. If the bleeding disappears within 48 hours, she may get out of bed but should limit her activities for the next several days. Stair climbing should be avoided for the first 24 hours and then resumed gradually. Coitus should be avoided for 2 weeks following the last evidence of bleeding. In cases in which pain accompanies the vaginal bleeding, the prognosis for saving the pregnancy is poor. Usually bleeding is observed first, and then in a

Fig. 19-12. Hegar dilators, of graduated diameters from 5 to 12 mm. Larger sizes also are used.

few hours, sometimes days later, uterine contractions ensue. This is treated by absolute bed rest, narcotic drugs (paregoric, morphine, etc.) and some preparations of progesterone (see Chap. 3). When the pain and the bleeding increase, the patient should be hospitalized, if this has not already been done. If the abortion is incomplete, ordinarily efforts are made to aid the uterus in emptying its contents. Oxytocin may be administered, but if this is ineffectual, surgical removal of the retained products of conception should be done promptly. Active bleeding may make this urgently necessary. Many times the tissue lies loose in the cervical canal and can be simply lifted out with ovum forceps; otherwise, curettage of the uterine cavity must be done. The instruments commonly used in completing an incomplete abortion are shown in Figures 19-4 to 19-12. The suction curet may also be used. If evidence of infection is present (fever, foul discharge, or suspicious history of criminal abortion), evacuation of the uterus should be delayed only long enough to obtain appropriate studies (especially smears and cultures) and to initiate antibiotic therapy. Such prompt and aggressive management of the patient with an infected abortion will effectively reduce the incidence of more serious complications such as septic shock, thrombophlebitis, and renal failure, and will reduce morbidity and hospital stay as well.

Nurse's Responsibilities in Abortion Cases. Bleeding in the first half of pregnancy, no matter how slight, always must be considered as threatened abortion. The patient must be put to bed and the physician notified. An episode of this nature is indeed distressing to the expectant mother, many times alarming. The nurse should bear in mind that although the emotional support she gives her patient is important, she must never try to reassure her that "everything will be all right," because in fact the patient may lose this pregnancy. Perineal pads and all tissue and blood clots passed by the patient should be saved. The physician will wish to examine these to determine the amount of bleeding and, when tissue has been passed, to examine the products of conception to ascertain, among other facts, whether or not the abortion is complete. If bleeding is so copious as to be alarming, elevate the foot of the bed (shock position) while awaiting the physician's arrival. If surgical completion of the abortion is to be carried out, the same aseptic regimen is carried out as for delivery.

All cases of extra-hospital abortion must be regarded as potentially infected, and strict antiseptic precautions must be carried out to prevent spread of infection to others. In caring for a woman who has had such an abortion recently, or one whose history is suspicious, the nurse may find it difficult to handle her own feelings so that she does not reflect a judgmental attitude. It is helpful to remember that it is not within the province of the nurse to pass moral judgments as she gives nursing care. In such situations the nurse should direct her concern to the gravity of the patient's illness. Occasionally circumstances make it possible for the nurse to be of definite educational help both to her patients and to the public.

Incompetent Cervical Os

Recently, a mechanical defect in the cervix, incompetent cervical os, has gained recognition as a cause of late habitual abortion or premature labor. When repeated termination of pregnancy in the second trimester is due to an anatomic factor such as this, surgical treatment may make fetal salvage possible. One of the various treatments used to prevent relaxation and dilatation of the cervix when it is incompetent to carry on a "good" pregnancy is the modified Shirodkar technique.[2] In this, the vaginal mucous membrane is elevated and a narrow strip of some material such as Mersilene is carried around the internal os of the cervix and tied. Then the vaginal mucosa is restored to its original position and sutured. This is the most popular of several so-called "cerclage" procedures used in the management of the incompetent cervix. The procedure may be done between pregnancies, if the diagnosis is clearly established, or during pregnancy. When done during pregnancy, it is usually elected to wait until the early part of the second trimester (14 to 16 weeks) to avoid the possibility of having to remove the suture if a spontaneous first trimester abortion occurs.

Postoperatively, the main concerns are rupture of the membranes and uterine contractions. If the membranes rupture, the suture must be removed and the uterus emptied because of the risk of infection. If contractions ensue, an effort to control the contractions is in order, and the most effective means for such control is intravenous alcohol. Attempts to control contractions should not be persistent if they are not effective promptly, since there is a risk of uterine rupture. Decisions regarding the type of delivery a patient is to have are generally based upon the position of the suture when the patient reaches term or labor begins. If the suture is in good position, with the cervical closure maintained, cesarean section may be elected to preserve the suture for future pregnancies. If the suture has loosened or rolled down on the cervix, it is not adequate for subsequent pregnancies. In that case, it is removed when labor begins and vaginal delivery is permitted.

Ectopic Pregnancy

An ectopic pregnancy is any gestation located outside the uterine cavity. The majority of ectopic pregnancies are tubal gestations. Other types, which make up about 5 per cent of all ectopic pregnancies, are: interstitial (in the interstitial portion of the tube), cornual (in a rudimentary

---

[2] Durfee, R. B.: Surgical treatment of the incompetent cervix during pregnancy. Obstet. Gynec. 12:91, 1958.

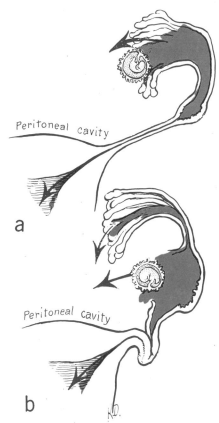

FIG. 19-13. (a) Tubal abortion, showing passage of the products of conception, together with much blood, out the fimbriated end of the tube. (b) Rupture of tubal pregnancy into peritoneal cavity. There is an outpouring of blood into the abdomen from vessels at the site of the rupture.

horn of a uterus), cervical, abdominal and ovarian gestations.

About once in every 300 pregnancies the fertilized ovum, instead of traversing the length of the fallopian tube to reach the uterine cavity, becomes implanted within the wall of the fallopian tube. This condition is known as "ectopic pregnancy" (literally, a pregnancy which is out of place) or as "tubal pregnancy" or "extra-uterine pregnancy." Since the wall of the tube is not sufficiently elastic to allow the fertilized ovum to grow and develop there, rupture of the tubal wall is the inevitable result. Rupture most frequently occurs into the tubal lumen with the passage of the products of conception, together with much blood, out the fimbriated end of the tube and into the peritoneal cavity—so-called "tubal abortion."

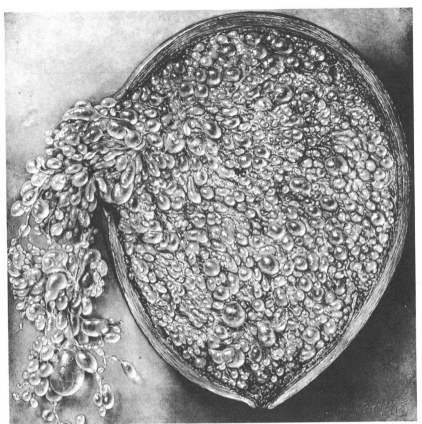

Fig. 19-14. Hydatidiform mole × ½. (Eastman, N. J.: Williams' Obstetrics, New York, Appleton)

Or, rupture may occur through the peritoneal surface of the tube directly into the peritoneal cavity; and, again, there is an outpouring of blood into the abdomen from vessels at the site of rupture (Fig. 19-13). In either case, rupture usually occurs within the first 12 weeks.

Occasionally an ectopic pregnancy may develop in that portion of the tube which passes through the uterine wall, a type known as "interstitial pregnancy." In very, very rare instances, the product of conception, after rupturing through the tubal wall, may implant itself on the peritoneum and develop to full term in the peritoneal cavity. This extraordinary occurrence is known as "abdominal pregnancy." Surprisingly enough, quite a few living infants have been delivered in such cases by means of abdominal incision.

Ectopic pregnancy may be due to any condition which narrows the tube or brings about some constriction within it. Under such circumstances the tubal lumen is large enough to allow spermatozoa to ascend the tube but not big enough to permit the downward passage of the fertilized ovum. Among the conditions which may produce such a narrowing of the fallopian tube are: previous inflammatory processes involving the tubal mucosa and producing partial agglutination of opposing surfaces, such as gonorrheal salpingitis; previous inflammatory processes of the external peritoneal surfaces of the tube, causing kinking, such as puerperal and postabortal infections; and developmental defects resulting in a general narrowing of the tubes.

In cases of ectopic gestation the woman exhibits the usual early symptoms of pregnancy and, as a rule, regards herself as being normally pregnant. After missing one or two periods, however, she suddenly experiences pain which is knifelike in nature and often of extreme severity in one of the lower quadrants. This is usually associated with very slight vaginal bleeding, commonly referred to as "spotting." Depending on the amount of blood which has escaped into the peritoneal cavity, she may or may not undergo a fainting attack and show symptoms of shock.

Ectopic pregnancy is a grave complication of pregnancy and is an important cause of maternal death. Moreover, if a woman has had one ectopic

FIG. 19-15. The 3 types of placenta previa, showing position of the placenta in relation to the internal os (B, C and D) contrasted with normal placental insertion (A). (*Below*, b, c and d) On vaginal examination the placenta can be felt during effacement and dilatation of the cervix in low implantation, partial and complete placenta previa.

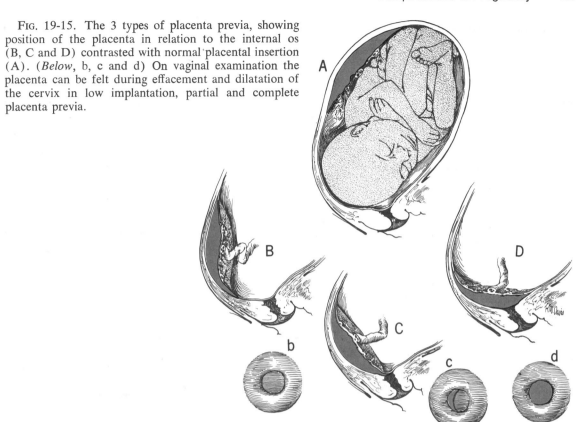

pregnancy and subsequently becomes pregnant, she is more likely than in the case of the average woman to have another such accident.

In the vast majority of cases the tube has already ruptured, and the fetus is dead when the patient is first seen by the physician. It is indeed the rupture which produces the acute clinical picture. The treatment is removal of the tube, supplemented by blood transfusion. Occasionally the ovary must be removed with the tube. Under certain circumstances in which subsequent fertility must be maintained, the tube may be preserved by merely removing the pregnancy. This latter approach, called salpingotomy, is applicable if the contralateral tube is badly diseased or has been previously removed.

During the transportation of such a patient to the hospital or in the interval when the patient is awaiting operation, the nurse can be of immeasurable assistance in combating the shock that is frequently present. Elevation of the foot of the bed and maintenance of body heat by means of hot-water bottles and blankets may help to save the patient's life.

Hydatidiform Mole

Hydatidiform mole is a benign neoplasm of the chorion in which the chorionic villi degenerate and become transparent vesicles containing clear, viscid fluid. The vesicles have a grapelike appearance and are arranged in clusters involving all or part of the decidual lining of the uterus (Fig. 19-14). Although there is usually no embryo present, occasionally there may be a fetus and only part of the placenta involved. Hydatidiform mole is rather an uncommon condition, occurring about once in every 2,000 pregnancies. The pregnancy appears to be normal at first. Then bleeding, a usual symptom varying from spotting to that of a profuse degree, occurs, so that one might suspect threatened abortion. If the patient does not abort, the uterus enlarges rapidly, and profuse hemorrhage may occur, at which time these vesicles may be evident in the vaginal discharge. Vomiting in rather severe form may appear early. Severe preeclampsia, a complication which does not usually occur until the later months of pregnancy, may appear early in the second trimester. The treatment consists in emptying the uterus by dilating the cervix and carefully extracting the uterine contents. There is always great danger of injury to the uterine wall, which is weakened and of spongy consistency due to the growth of the mole. Some physicians advise hysterectomy. The follow-up care is very important because, although this is a benign process, extremely malignant chorioncarcinoma (formerly called chorionepithelioma) sometimes further complicates the picture.

Placenta Previa

Although abortion is the most frequent cause of bleeding early in pregnancy, the most common cause during the later months is placenta previa. In this condition the placenta is attached to the lower uterine segment (instead of high up in the uterus as usual) and either wholly or in part covers the region of the cervix. There are three types, differentiated according to the degree to which the condition is present (Fig. 19-15):

1. *Total placenta previa,* in which the placenta completely covers the internal os

2. *Partial placenta previa,* in which the placenta partially covers the internal os

3. *Low implantation of placenta,* in which the placenta encroaches upon the region of internal os, so that it can be palpated by the physician on digital exploration about the cervix, but does not extend beyond the margin of the internal os.

Painless vaginal bleeding during the second half of pregnancy is the main symptom of placenta previa. The bleeding usually occurs after the 7th month. It may begin as mere "spotting" and increase, or it may start with profuse hemorrhages. The patient may awaken in the middle of the night to find herself in a pool of blood. The bleeding is caused by separation of the placenta as the result of changes which take place in the lower uterine segment during the later months. This separation opens up the underlying blood sinuses of the uterus from which the bleeding occurs.

Fortunately, placenta previa is not a very common condition, occurring about once in every 200 deliveries. It occurs much more frequently in multiparae than in primigravidae. Placenta previa always must be regarded as a grave complication of pregnancy. Until recent years it showed a maternal mortality of approximately 10 per cent. Modern methods of management, plus the more liberal use of blood transfusion, have reduced this figure considerably. The outlook for the baby is always dubious, not only because the placental separation interferes with the infant's oxygen supply, but also because many of these babies are very premature when delivery must necessarily take place.

Treatment. The presence of a placenta previa causes two main problems for the mother: bleeding and obstruction of the birth canal. For the baby, the most significant concern is prematurity. These problems provide the guides to treatment.

1. Conservative management is in order when the fetus is premature (by weight or dates) and the bleeding is not excessive. The natural history of placenta previa is such that uncontrolled bleeding is not likely to occur with the first episode. There may be, in fact, several episodes of bleeding, starting early in the third trimester, before there is sufficient bleeding to force the obstetrician to intervene and terminate the pregnancy. Thus, under such circumstances, bed rest and observation will often result in cessation of the bleeding and provide valuable days for the maturation of the fetus. Often, a technique for placental localization may be employed. Such techniques include isotope scans, amniography, abdominal x-rays and ultrasound. It is also important that the obstetrician rule out other causes of bleeding under these circumstances. He will generally do a speculum examination of the vagina, looking for other sources of bleeding such as cervicitis, cervical polyps, vaginal lacerations, etc. He will *not,* however, insert his finger through the cervix under these circumstances, since such a maneuver might well precipitate bleeding and therefore the delivery of a premature infant.

2. *An active* approach to the patient is indicated if the fetus is at term by size and dates, if labor has begun, or if bleeding is sufficient to threaten the mother. Then, the patient is taken to the operating room where a "double setup" examination is performed. This means that everything is prepared for an immediate cesarean section, should the examination confirm the diagnosis. This precaution is necessary, since digital examination of the cervix might precipitate increased bleeding. In all instances of total and partial placenta previa, and in most instances of low implantation of the placenta, cesarean section is the approach of choice for delivery. In an occasional case of low implantation, especially if the baby is small, the obstetrician may elect to rupture the membranes in the hope that the presenting part may enter the pelvis and control the bleeding by compressing the area of placenta

which has separated. If this does occur, then vaginal delivery may be accomplished.

Bleeding, shock and infection are the main dangers. Before the arrival of the physician, the nurse should keep a solicitous eye on the amount of bleeding and the pulse rate and watch for signs of oncoming shock (pallor, increased pulse rate, cold extremities, etc.). Should the bleeding be profuse, elevation of the foot of the bed and application of external heat may forestall shock. In determining the amount of bleeding, the patient should be instructed to report feeling the escape of fluid from the vulva. The nurse, in turn, should inspect the pad or bed frequently for hemorrhage.

Abruptio Placentae

Abruptio placentae (meaning that the placenta is torn from its bed) is a complication of the last half of pregnancy, in which a normally located placenta undergoes separation from its uterine attachment. The condition is frequently referred to as "premature separation of the normally implanted placenta"; other synonymous terms such as "accidental hemorrhage" (meaning that it takes place unexpectedly) and "ablatio placentae" (ablatio means a carrying away) are sometimes used. Bleeding may be apparent, in which case it is called *external hemorrhage*; or bleeding may be concealed, in which case it is called *concealed hemorrhage*. In other words, if a separation occurs at the margin, the blood is apt to lift the membranes and trickle down to the cervical os and thus escape externally. If the placenta begins to separate centrally, a huge amount of blood may be stored behind the placenta before any of it becomes evident (Fig. 19-16). Although the precise cause of the condition is not known, it is frequently encountered in association with cases of toxemia of pregnancy.

Premature separation of the normally implanted placenta is characterized not only by bleeding beneath the placenta but also by pain. The pain is produced by the accumulation of blood behind the placenta, with subsequent distention of the uterus. The uterus also enlarges in size as the result of the accumulated blood and becomes distinctly tender and exceedingly firm. Because of the almost woody hardness of the uterine wall, fetal parts may be difficult to determine. Shock is often out of proportion to blood loss, as manifested by a rapid pulse, dyspnea, yawning, restlessness, pallor, syncope and cold, clammy perspiration.

Treatment is dependent upon the condition of the fetus and the mother at the time the diagnosis is made. If the fetus is alive, prompt delivery is in order and should be by cesarean section, unless vaginal delivery can be accomplished promptly. If the fetus has already succumbed, this is usually an indication of an extensive placental separation. The complications of abruptio placenta to be described subsequently are all time-related and occur with greater frequency with more extensive separation. Therefore, although a vaginal delivery is desirable with a dead baby, one should not persist for too long.

Further Complications. Hemorrhagic shock is a common complication and demands vigorous treatment with blood replacement and control of the bleeding by emptying the uterus in the most expeditious manner. Occasionally, with a severe abruption, a coagulation defect, *hypofibrinogenemia,* develops. This complication is also seen with other entities such as amniotic fluid embolus, prolonged retention of a dead fetus, and septic abortion. It is brought about by the entry into the circulation of thromboplastin from the uterus and placenta, which causes small fibrin clots in the capillaries and consumes fibrinogen, leaving the patient with nonclotting blood. Treatment involves the use of heparin (to prevent fibrin

FIG. 19-16. Abruptio placentae with large blood clot between placenta and uterine wall.

clots), blood and fibrinogen replacement, and termination of the pregnancy. Also, in severe abruptions, when coagulation is impaired, there is extensive bleeding into the uterine muscle, producing the so-called "Convelaire uterus." Such a uterus occasionally does not contract well after delivery, causing further bleeding and even necessitating hysterectomy. Finally, *renal failure* may result, either on the basis of acute tubular necrosis or bilateral cortical necrosis. In the latter case, the outlook is grave.

Mistaken Diagnosis of Hemorrhage

A false alarm concerning hemorrhage is sometimes due to a normal "show" at the beginning of labor. It simply means that dilatation of the cervix has begun, causing slight bleeding. No treatment is required. However, the nurse should reassure the patient and watch to determine whether or not the bleeding which is present is more than the normal show.

"Supine Hypotensive Syndrome"

Many pregnant women, if placed in the supine position in the last trimester, suffer a fall in blood pressure. In some of these women the drop is so great as to simulate shock due to blood loss. The chief cause of supine hypotensive syndrome is failure of venous return of blood from the legs and the pelvis as a result of the compression exerted by the enlarged uterus on the inferior vena cava. The condition can be corrected promptly by having the patient lie on her side rather than on her back.

HYPEREMESIS GRAVIDARUM

A mild degree of nausea and vomiting, "morning sickness," is the most common complaint of women in the first trimester of pregnancy. This manifestation is considered in the realm of a minor discomfort rather than a complication, and it usually responds to measures discussed in Chapter 8. It is uncommon today for this mild form of nausea and vomiting to progress to such serious extent that it produces systemic effects (i.e., marked loss of weight and acetonuria), but when it becomes thus exaggerated, the condition is known as hyperemesis gravidarum, sometimes called "pernicious vomiting." Because even the gravest case of hyperemesis starts originally as a simple form of nausea, all cases of nausea and vomiting should be treated with proper understanding and judgment, and none should be regarded casually. When simple remedies do not prove to be effective, and symptoms of hyperemesis appear to be imminent, the patient should be hospitalized for more intensive treatment. At the present time less than 1 pregnant woman in 300 has to be admitted to the hospital because of this complication of pregnancy, and, indeed, the grave cases of hyperemesis gravidarum are becoming rare. The recovery of those who are admitted to the hospital is usually rapid.

Cause

It is currently recognized that during pregnancy there are certain organic processes which are basic to all cases of vomiting, regardless of whether the symptoms are mild or severe. The endocrine and metabolic changes of normal gestation, fragments of chorionic villi entering the maternal circulation and the diminished motility of the stomach might well give rise to clinical symptoms.

It has long been thought that hyperemesis gravidarum is in large measure a *neurosis.* The term "neurosis," it will be recalled, is employed very loosely to designate a large array of conditions in which symptoms occur without demonstrable pathologic explanation, the symptoms being due, it is thought, to a functional disturbance of the patient's psyche. Some psychiatrists estimate that 40 per cent of patients who visit physicians belong in this neurotic class. As many examples show (quite apart from pregnancy), nausea is often psychic in origin. For instance, a repellent sight, an obnoxious odor or the mere recollection of such a sight or odor may give rise to nausea and even vomiting. Our general use of the adjective "nauseating" to depict a repulsive object is further acknowledgement that an upset mind may produce an upset stomach.

In all life's encounters there are probably few experiences which are at first more upsetting, mentally and emotionally, than the realization by a young woman that she is pregnant. At the onset are several weeks of anxious uncertainty before she can be sure of the diagnosis. Then, numerous adjustments must be made and plans changed. Emotionally, the implications of pregnancy extend far back into the past when she first met her husband, while its future ramifications are endless. The responsibilities entailed are plain enough, also, and seem, on first thought, perhaps more than can be assumed. These and a thousand other thoughts crowd themselves into the mind; and in women who cannot adjust themselves to all these new circumstances, it is understandable that the groundwork for a neurosis is laid. Beyond question, there is a large neurotic element in most cases of hyperemesis, a factor which looms large in the treatment of the condition.

The neurotic factor, on the other hand, is not the whole cause of hyperemesis, nor in all probability even the basic cause. As has been stated previously, in every case an important underlying organic process is also at work—either the dissemination of toxins into the maternal blood stream or some maladjustment of the metabolism to the changes wrought by the growing fetus. It is this toxic or organic element which is doubtless the fundamental cause of the disease. To what extent the patient reacts to this underlying process by vomiting seems to be determined in large measure by neurotic factors, that is, by her psychic and emotional stability and by the mental stress and strain which pregnancy has imposed.

Clinical Picture

The clinical picture of the patient suffering from pernicious vomiting varies in relation to the severity and the duration of the condition. In any event, the condition begins with a typical picture of "morning sickness." The patient experiences a feeling of nausea on arising in the morning, she may even be unable to retain her breakfast, but she recovers in a few hours and has no further episodes until the next morning. With the majority of these patients this pattern persists for a few weeks and then suddenly ceases.

A small number of patients who have "morning sickness" develop persistent vomiting which lasts for 4 to 8 weeks or longer. These patients vomit several times a day and may be unable to retain any liquid or solid foods, with the result that marked symptoms of dehydration and starvation occur. *Dehydration* is pronounced, as evidenced by a diminished output of urine and a dryness of the skin. In some instances slight jaundice may develop. Further results of dehydration may be observed in the patient's vital signs. The pulse is usually accelerated, often to 130 or over, and a low-grade fever may be present. The temperature seldom rises above 101° F. (38.4° C.), but it may persist despite therapy to combat dehydration.

Starvation, which is regularly present, manifests itself in a number of ways. Weight loss may vary from 5 pounds to as much as 20 or 30 pounds. This is tantamount to saying that the

digestion and the absorption of carbohydrates and other nutrients have been so inadequate that the body has been forced to burn its reserve stores of fat in order to maintain body heat and energy. When fat is burned without carbohydrates being present, the process of combustion does not go on to completion. Consequently, certain incompletely burned products of fat metabolism make their appearance in the blood and in the urine. The presence of acetone and diacetic acid in the urine in hyperemesis is common. In severe cases considerable changes associated with starvation and dehydration become evident in the blood chemistry. There is a definite increase in the nonprotein nitrogen, uric acid and urea, a moderate decrease in the chlorides and little alteration in the carbon dioxide combining power. Then, too, vitamin starvation is regularly present, and in extreme cases, when marked vitamin B deficiency exists, polyneuritis occasionally develops, and disturbances of the peripheral nerves result.

The severe type of vomiting may occur in either acute or chronic form. With prompt, persistent and intelligent therapy, the prognosis of hyperemesis is excellent.

Treatment and Nursing Care

The principles underlying the treatment of hyperemesis gravidarum are as follows: (1) combat the dehydration by liberal administration of parenteral fluids; (2) combat the starvation by administration of glucose intravenously and thiamine chloride subcutaneously and, if necessary, by feeding a high-caloric, high-vitamin fluid diet through a nasal tube; (3) combat the neurosis by psychotherapy, sedatives and "isolation."

Although it may be necessary on occasion to treat cases of hyperemesis in the home, hospitalization is urgently desirable, because isolation from relatives, change of atmosphere and better facilities for intravenous medication confer unusual benefits in this condition. During the first 24 hours in the hospital it is customary to withhold all food and fluids by mouth in order to give the gastrointestinal tract as complete a rest as possible. Glucose solution, usually in 10 per cent concentration, is administered intravenously and, in addition, normal saline solution intravenously. The total fluid intake should approximate or exceed 3,000 cc. in the 24 hours. The nurse must keep a careful record of the exact quantity of fluids given, the amount of urine excreted and the quantity of the vomitus. Sedation is accomplished either by Luminal Sodium hypodermically in dosage of 1 or 2 grains (0.06 to 0.12 Gm.) every 4 hours, or by the rectal instillation of some barbiturate drug such as Amytal Sodium, 3 grains (0.2 Gm.) every 6 hours. Thiamine hydrochloride, 50 mg. daily hypodermically, supplies the most urgent vitamin needs during the first 24 hours. All visitors are excluded during this period, including husband and relatives.

After such a regimen for 24 hours, dry toast, crackers or cereal are given by mouth in small quantities every 2 or 3 hours. Fluids are given on alternate hours in small amounts (not over 100 cc. at a time); hot tea and ginger ale usually are tolerated better than plain water. If no vomiting occurs, the amounts and the variety of the food are increased gradually until the patient is on a regular soft, high-vitamin diet. The intravenous administration of fluids may have to be continued for several days, depending on the oral intake.

The success of the treatment will depend in large measure on the tact, the understanding and the attitude of the nurse. Although optimism must be the keynote of the nurse's approach to the patient, this must be coupled with a plainly avowed determination to conquer the complication. The patient must be led gradually to understand that, in the treatment of vomiting, the nurse knows no such word as "failure." Not a few of these patients are in psychological conflict because of family, financial or social difficulties, and many are averse to the whole idea of pregnancy. If one can only get to the root of these difficulties in a tactful, empathic way, and help the patient to become reconciled to becoming a mother, a great deal will have been accomplished.

The nurse must exercise great care in preparing and serving trays for patients suffering from hyperemesis. The portions should be extremely small and attractively arranged. Cold liquids such as ginger ale or lemonade must be ice-cold; and hot foods, such as soups, cocoa and tea, must be steaming hot, since lukewarm liquids may be nauseating. It is best not to discuss food with the patient, even when serving the tray, but simply to assume that she will enjoy it and talk about other matters. At all times keep the emesis basin out of view, since the sight of it may start vomiting. Likewise, the smell of food may be nauseating; accordingly, the patient's room should be kept well-aired and should be as far from the kitchen as possible.

If vomiting continues despite these measures,

as it rarely does, the physician may institute nasal feeding. A small rubber tube (Levin tube) is inserted by the physician through a nostril and on down into the stomach. The tube is strapped to the patient's cheek, connected with an overhanging bottle and left in place. By this means, large amounts of vitamin-rich liquid foods may be administered. The secret of success with nasal feeding lies in very slow but constant introduction of food into the stomach. The apparatus should be so arranged that the number of drops per minute passing through the tube can be counted. This should not exceed 50 per minute. Even this slow rate, it may be noted, yields about 200 cc. per hour.

Even the most severe cases of hyperemesis usually will respond favorably to the treatment described if patience and persistence are exercised; but, in extremely rare instances, the patient may continue to vomit despite all efforts, and such grave signs may develop that the physician is forced to the conclusion that further continuation of pregnancy will be at the cost of the woman's life. The following signs are grave omens and, especially when several are present, may call for therapeutic abortion if it has been decided that the mother is to be removed from danger: (1) jaundice; (2) delirium; (3) steadily rising pulse rate to levels of 130 or above; (4) fever of 101° F. (38.4° C.) or above which persists despite liberal fluid intake; and (5) hemorrhages in the retina, as observed by the physician during ophthalmoscopic examination.

COINCIDENTAL DISEASES AND PREGNANCY

It has been said wisely that the pregnant woman can have any disease which her nonpregnant counterpart can have except infertility. One must be aware that the abnormal physiology of many disease states is modified by the physiologic changes of pregnancy. This may alter the classical clinical picture of a disease state and require different approaches in treatment. The possible effect on the fetus must of course always be taken into consideration when one is treating a pregnant woman. For most entities, the effects of pregnancy on the disease and the disease on pregnancy are negligible and do not influence the management of either. On the other hand, there are a few complications which have significant effects on the fetus. Those entities are discussed in Chapter 22. Those which have a predominant maternal effect are discussed in this chapter. This is admittedly an artificial separation, since most of these diseases have both fetal and maternal consequences. Such separation does, however, lead to more efficient organization of the material.

General Physiologic Disturbances

Anemia. During pregnancy the blood volume is increased (p. 115). Because of this hydremia, hemoglobin estimations in gestation are likely to be lower than ordinarily considered as normal. This is not a true anemia, since the total amount of hemoglobin in the body remains the same, and sometimes the condition is referred to as the "pseudoanemia of pregnancy." Hemoglobin standards which have been established for non-pregnant women, i.e., 12 to 15 Gm. per 100 cc. of blood, are applicable for normal pregnant women also. The diagnosis of true anemia is made when the hemoglobin falls below 12 Gm., or the hematocrit below 35 per cent.

The hemoglobin levels of pregnant women fall as the result of a number of factors. Most of these cases represent a true anemia due to iron deficiency. The need of the fetus and the growing uterus for iron, inadequate iron intake in the diet and a low hemoglobin level at the start of pregnancy combine to bring about this anemic state. Iron deficiency is more common in the socio-economically deprived, whose general nutrition is poor.

The symptoms are few, but some of these patients complain of becoming tired easily; many are pale; and in a few the pulse rate is fast. Because of the rather frequent occurrence of anemia in pregnancy, hemoglobin determinations are a routine part of antepartal care. The treatment consists of an iron-rich diet (emphasis on liver, meat, eggs, spinach, etc.) supplemented by the administration of some iron compound such as ferrous sulfate. In patients with anemia who do not tolerate orally ingested iron well, as shown by gastrointestinal disturbances, or in whom rapid effects are desired, injections of intramuscular iron in the form of Imferon are most helpful.

Another common cause of anemia in pregnancy is folic acid deficiency. This should always be suspected if an anemic patient does not respond to iron therapy. Patients with abnormal hemoglobins (Sickle cell disease, Sickle cell-C disease and Sickle cell trait) also present with anemia, and in the case of S-S and S-C disease may also have hemolytic crises.

Cardiac Complications. Rheumatic heart disease is a serious complication of pregnancy. Heart lesions, especially those of the mitral valve, may be greatly aggravated by pregnancy. Constant medical supervision of the pregnant woman with any degree of cardiac involvement, however mild, is imperative, for, fortunately, much can now be done to aid cardiac patients. If the patient has placed herself under medical care at the beginning of gestation, and if the physician has made a proper and thorough examination of all her organs at that time, he will be in a position to administer promptly such treatment as may be necessary. In this day of heart specialists, the specialist and the obstetrician must work hand in hand; and each in his own province is of the greatest help to the other. It is also absolutely essential to have close cooperation between the patient and the physician. In this situation the nurse may play an important part—by helping the patient to understand and to observe with care the primary principles of antepartal care.

The treatment of heart disease in pregnancy is governed to a large measure by the functional capacity of the heart. Rest probably will accomplish more than any other single measure, and the amount of rest needed will naturally vary with each individual, some patients having to be kept at rest a great part of the time. Strenuous activity and undue excitement must be avoided during pregnancy. The great majority, however, may safely indulge in moderate activity, and all should be in the fresh air as much as possible. Upper respiratory infections play great havoc in patients with heart disease and may even precipitate heart failure; accordingly, the nurse should advise all such patients to take special precautions against catching cold—that is, they should avoid large gatherings, and people known to have sore throats, colds, etc. All of these safeguards will be advised by the physician, but the nurse may aid greatly in helping the patient to carry out his instructions.

Although heart failure usually occurs suddenly, the onset may be gradual. The nurse should be alert to particular signs and symptoms which may be warning signals and report her observations to the physician promptly. Such symptoms include sudden limitation in the patient's ability to carry on her usual household activities, increased dyspnea on exertion, tachycardia, coughing or attacks of smothering with the cough. It is well to remember that serious cardiac lesions complicating pregnancy may predispose to premature labor or may be responsible for premature death. In the past many cardiac patients have had their pregnancies terminated by therapeutic abortion, but today many such pregnancies are carried to a happy completion by providing thorough medical supervision and nursing care during pregnancy and labor. However, these successes should not lead us to forget that, if not adequately cared for, even mild cardiac disorders as well as the severe types result in definite invalidism or even death.

Urinary Tract Infection. Inflammation of the ureter and the pelvis of the kidney is not uncommon during pregnancy. It seldom occurs earlier than the 4th month, and occasionally an acute attack of great severity occurs in the puerperium, in which case care will be required to distinguish it from peurperal infection. It is due to several causes, each of which may aggravate the condition. Among the possible causes are mechanical pressure on the ureters, hormonal effects acting on the tonus and peristalsis of the ureters, improper intestinal elimination, an increase of colon bacilli, and certain displacements of the bladder due to pregnancy itself. The symptoms may be gradual and slight, or quite acute in their onset, with chills and high temperature, 103° or 104° F. (39.4° or 40° C.). The patient often complains of frequency of urination, pain in the kidney region and malaise. In the acute form the patient is seized suddenly with acute abdominal pain, sometimes attended with chills or shivering; after a few hours the abdomen may become distended, and vomiting may occur. The pain, diffused at first, usually localizes in the right side. It is necessary for the nurse to secure definite instructions from the physician concerning the treatment; but rest, forced fluids and a bland, nonirritating diet (chiefly milk) may be advised in the interim. Heat over the kidneys will relieve pain.

DRUGS. The main aim of treatment in urinary tract infection is to rid the urine and the urinary tract of bacteria. During recent years the treatment of infections of the urinary tract has been revolutionized by the introduction of a variety of antimicrobial drugs. The fluid intake is maintained between 2,500 and 3,000 cc. daily. The physician will follow the results of treatment not only by means of the temperature chart but also by thorough and repeated examinations of the urine. These examinations will entail both a microscopic study of the number of pus cells present and a survey of the bacteria yielded on culture. Accordingly, the nurse will be asked to secure frequent urine specimens. Follow-up of these cases is highly important and must be carried out not only during the remainder of pregnancy but also for several months after delivery, until it is certain that the urine is sterile, and x-ray studies of the kidney reveal a normal state.

Ptyalism. Although this is one of the rarer complications of pregnancy, it is one which is most annoying to the patient and very stubborn in resisting treatment. It is due entirely to altered innervation or changes in nerve control and is characterized by an enormously increased secretion of the salivary glands. Women at times have been known to discharge as much as 2 quarts of saliva daily from this cause. This complication, if it occurs at all, usually appears in the early months of pregnancy and lasts a considerable time, but, fortunately, it is inclined to cease spontaneously. It is seen in highly nervous women of low vitality and is likely to cause great mental depression and interfere with nutrition.

The treatment consists in building up the general health and the administration of such medication as may be prescribed by the physician. The use of astringent mouthwashes often contributes to the patient's comfort. Any treatment may seem to be inadequate, and the condition is most disagreeable.

Infectious Diseases

Certain infectious diseases have no proved specific ill effect on the mother or the baby, but, if possible, any communicable disease should be avoided during pregnancy, for even mild diseases add strain at this particular time.

With infectious diseases two types of effects may occur: (1) on the mother and (2) on the fetus. The diseases which often have serious effects on the infant are discussed in Chapter 23. Among those directly affecting the mother are the following.

The Common Cold. The susceptibility to acute upper respiratory infections is apparently greater during pregnancy. Therefore, the pregnant woman should make every effort to avoid contacts with these infections. When she does acquire a cold, prompt medical attention is usually desirable, because the common cold often precedes more serious conditions affecting the upper respiratory tract. Prescribed medication should be used in preference to the various antihistamine drugs obtainable without a prescription. Rest in bed helps the individual and aids in checking the spread of the disease.

Pneumonia. Pneumonia, which may follow the common cold, can frequently lead to complications of pregnancy. The pneumonia organisms, especially streptococci, also may infect the uterus, causing puerperal infections. Prompt use of antibiotics is most helpful. Since antibiotics have been employed, the occurrence of abortion and premature labor is less common.

Influenza. Serious complications may follow influenza, especially in the pneumonic type in which pregnancy is sometimes interrupted. Sulfa drugs and such antibiotics as penicillin usually are given to help forestall pneumonia, but they do not control the influenza virus.

Measles. Ill effects are not commonly noted in pregnancy, but pregnant mothers who contract measles are said to be more likely to have premature labors. No other definite effects are reported, although eruptions have been noted on infants at birth.

Typhoid fever, which is now relatively rare in this country, may cause serious complications in pregnancy, resulting in abortion, prematurity and infant mortality. Immunization is not contraindicated during pregnancy, and antityphoid vaccine should be administered when necessary.

Brucellosis (Undulant Fever, Malta Fever). These debilitating diseases in humans are contracted mainly from unpasteurized milk. In this country today, conditions for the production and the processing of milk are set by U. S. Public Health Service standards. When these diseases are seen, the bacteria have been found in the human placenta, but abortion in humans is very infrequently traced to this organism, although brucella bacteria do cause abortion in cattle. Good results have been attained with Aureomycin and also with combined streptomycin-sulfadiazine.

Scarlet Fever. There seems to be greater susceptibility to scarlet fever during the puerperium. The cause is a streptococcus, and so the risk of developing puerperal fever is clear. Antibiotics are effective in treating the disease, but sometimes abortion is caused by scarlet fever contracted during early pregnancy, due to the mother's high fever.

Smallpox. Cases of abortion and prematurity increase with the severity of the attack, especially with the hemorrhagic type. As in measles, small pox may be transmitted through the placenta, for eruptions may be present in live births.

Malaria. In more severe cases of malaria the incidence of abortion and premature labor is increased. Prompt therapy is of utmost importance. Malaria organisms have been found in the blood of the cord and the fetus; they are frequently found in the placenta, although no ill effects have been noted on the infants. Quinine or the newer related drugs, such as Atabrine, should be administered to women with malaria history to prevent recrudescence during pregnancy and the puerperium. The decrease in malaria reported (1951) by the Communicable Disease Center of the U. S. Public Health Service makes malaria much less important as a complication of pregnancy.

Tuberculosis. The average case of tuberculosis in itself has only a slight effect on the course of pregnancy, since it rarely predisposes to abortion, premature labor or even stillbirth. (Fortunately, the disease is seldom acquired congenitally, although a small number of authentic cases have been reported in which, in addition to a tuberculous condition of the placenta, tubercle bacilli were found in the cord blood, together with tuberculous lesions in the baby.) Medical opinions differ, but the consensus is that pregnancy does not exert an adverse effect on tuberculosis. Some authorities think that this disease becomes aggravated by pregnancy, and that only a patient in an arrested case should consider becoming pregnant. Pregnancy is undertaken with some risk, for although a tuberculous lesion may remain latent for an indefinite time, provided that the natural resistance is not overtaxed, it must be noted that pregnancy is one of the factors often responsible for overtaxing the resistance sufficiently to convert a latent, inactive lesion into an active one. Maintenance of the proper hygiene, nutrition and excellent surroundings so that health is conserved in every possible way will do much to prevent activity in a latent focus. Other authorities deny that the tuberculosis is necessarily aggravated by pregnancy, basing this belief on statistics of a large series of tuberculous patients who have progressed satisfactorily in pregnancy.

The symptoms of tuberculosis in pregnancy do not differ materially from those that accompany the disease in other conditions. During the early months of gestation the characteristic anemia and general malnutrition of tuberculosis are usually pronounced, but in the latter months there is often considerable improvement. Too often, however, this is followed by a rapid decline after delivery.

Treatment with the modern antituberculosis drugs, streptomycin, INH and PAS, has completely altered management in general, as well as during pregnancy. New advanced cases are rare and a majority of patients are managed as outpatients. Treatment of active cases generally consists of streptomycin, 1.0 Gm. daily for 3 to 4 weeks, then 1.0 Gm. twice weekly. Isoniazide, 300 mg., and PAS (paraamino salicylic acid), 12.0 Gm. daily, are given in divided doses. No deleterious effects on the mother or the infant have been reported. Labor and delivery are conducted in a normal fashion, avoiding inhalation anesthesia, and mother and baby are separated if disease is active. Breast-feeding is unwise even in inactive disease. Some authorities recommend INH therapy in the third trimester and puerperium for the inactive patient who has had active disease within 2 years of pregnancy.

Tuberculosis detection should be the concern of all physicians, and since the obstetrician sees a number of young women who might otherwise have no medical supervision he has a responsible role. If the patient has had a recent chest x-ray (within 6 months), a repeat is not necessary unless there are symptoms which suggest a pulmonic process. Many obstetricians prefer screening patients with a tuberculin skin test. This eliminates the need for an x-ray in non-reactions. Appropriate procedures for shielding the fetus should be used whenever a pregnant woman is x-rayed.

Poliomyelitis generally does not complicate pregnancy or delivery, except in the very unusual cases in which respiratory paralysis develops; in these rare cases cesarean section has given satisfactory results. Fortunately, the fetus rarely contracts the disease. Of about 80 cases reported during pregnancy, less than one fifth occurred in the first trimester. A milder form of infection of poliomyelitis is attributed to a different virus, the Coxsackie virus, which produces less paralysis but is often unrecognized.

Syphilis. The major hazard of syphilis in pregnancy was, in the past, the occurrence of intrauterine infection and late abortion or stillbirth. Congenital syphilis has now been reduced nearly to the point of elimination. The antenatal blood test for syphilis is required by law and, except for the instance in which prenatal care is nonexistent, maternal syphilis should be detected and adequately treated, thereby protecting the fetus.

Syphilis can occur in any stage during pregnancy. The primary and secondary stages are usually apparent because of their lesions. In latent syphilis, the diagnosis is based upon a positive serology; the most difficult problem occurs when the serology is repeatedly positive and the patient denies a history. Biologic false positives do occur in a number of circumstances, but, fortunately, new, more specific tests are now available which can be used in the questionable case.

Treatment is indicated in the following circumstances:

a. When a diagnosis of early syphilis is made, regardless of stage.

b. When late symptomatic syphilis is discovered.

c. When latent syphilis is diagnosed by repeated positive serologic tests and the patient's history corroborates the diagnosis, and when there has been either inadequate or no treatment.

d. When the diagnosis is made by repeated positive tests, even though the history does not confirm, and when either the more specific tests are not available or there is not time for adequate therapy. Retreatment in subsequent pregnancies is necessary if there is any doubt about the adequacy of previous therapy.

The treatment consists of a course of penicillin in the total dose of 6 million units (12 million for neurosyphilis), or a suitable substitute if penicillin allergy exists. Both mother and baby should be carefully followed by serologic tests postpartum. It is important to know that even the unaffected baby will have a positive test because the mother's test is positive; however, the titer in the baby will be lower than that of the mother and will become negative within 3 months.

Gonorrhea. This disease should be studied by the nurse with the other infectious diseases; but, because of the consequences of gonorrheal infection to the mother at the time of labor and during the puerperium, as well as the risk of permanent injury to the baby's eyes at the time of birth, this disease is of special concern to the maternity nurse.

The disease is due to a microorganism, known commonly as the gonococcus organism (*Micrococcus gonorrhoeae* or *Neisseria gonorrhoeae*). It may affect any mucous membrane (e.g., that of the eye), but usually attacks the mucosa of the genital tract, particularly the opening of the bladder and the crypts around the cervix, causing a catarrhal discharge of pus. The usual mode of transfer of this infection is by sexual intercourse. The infection often extends into the uterus and the tubes, causing a very serious localized peritonitis, and may cause sterility by a mechanical blocking of the tubes. Gonorrhea is not commonly considered to be a fatal disease, in the sense that a high proportion of the cases terminate in death, but in the list of diseases causing chronic ill health, especially in the female sex, gonorrhea is most important.

Gonorrhea does not greatly modify the course of pregnancy, and its existence is often unsuspected by the patient. The vaginal discharge may increase, as it normally does during pregnancy, and, with the local congestion of the venous system, the patient may have some irritation in the vulvar region. Pregnancy may act as a barrier to the ascent of the gonococcus, and thus the fetus may be protected during development. The patient may abort, but more commonly she carries the baby to full term and delivers normally. However, after delivery, conditions are quite different. Even when a patient has had a normal labor, the cervix is dilated, and the minute tears and abrasions offer many avenues for the spread of the infection, and the lochial discharge makes an ideal culture medium for the bacteria. This condition may lead to the development of a form of puerperal fever.

It is now routine practice to obtain a specimen of vaginal secretions for culture on the first antepartal visit. In the female, the diagnosis of gonorrhea is confirmed by culturing the organisms from fresh vaginal secretions. If the culture is positive, penicillin is given promptly, for it yields dramatic results in treatment of this disease. Cure may be effected by a single intramuscular injection of suitable dosage of penicillin in at least 90 per cent of the cases. In chronic cases 1 or 2 repeated doses may be necessary.

Gonorrhea is not hereditary, but, if a woman is infected at the time of her confinement, the organism may get into the baby's eyes and cause blindness. This infection of the eyes is called ophthalmia neonatorum. The prophylactic treatment of the baby's eyes at this time never should be neglected (see Chap. 13).

SUGGESTED READING

Barter, R. H., Dusbabek, J. A., Tundac, C. M., and Erkenbeck, R. V.: Further experiences with the Shirodkar operation. Amer. J. Obstet. Gynec. 85: 792, 1963.

Beler, F. K.: Treatment of coagulation disorders in pregnancy. Clin. Obstet. Gynec. 7:372, 1964.

Burwell, C. S., and Metcalfe, J.: Heart Disease and Pregnancy. Boston, Little, Brown, 1955.

Douglas, R. G.: Symposium on bleeding and hemorrhage in late pregnancy. Clin. Obstet. Gynec. 3, September 1960.

Eastman, N. J., and Hellman, L. M.: Williams Obstetrics. ed. 13, New York, Appleton, 1966.

Goldstein, D. P., and Gore, H.: Symposium on trophoblastic disease. Clin. Obstet. Gynec. 10:267-341, June 1967.

Haynes, D. M.: Medical Complications During Pregnancy. New York, McGraw-Hill, 1969.

Marcus, S. L., and Marcus, C. C.: Advances in Obstetrics and Gynecology. Baltimore, Williams & Wilkins, 1967.

Mendelson, C. L.: Cardiac Disease in Pregnancy. Philadelphia, F. A. Davis, 1960.

Rovinsky, J. J., and Guttmacher, A. F.: Medical, Surgical, and Gynecological Complications of Pregnancy. ed. 2, Baltimore, Williams & Wilkins, 1965.

Schwarz, R. H.: Septic Abortion. Philadelphia, J. B. Lippincott, 1968.

Stoddard, F. J.: Case Studies in Obstetrics and Gynecology. Philadelphia, W. B. Saunders, 1964.

Willson, J. R., Jr.: Management of Obstetric Difficulties. ed. 6, St. Louis, C. V. Mosby Co., 1961.

Zuspan, F. P.: Symposium on toxemia of pregnancy. Clin. Obstet. Gynec. 9:859-990, December 1966.

Complications of Labor 20

Mechanical Dystocia • Hemorrhagic Complications • Amniotic Fluid Embolism
Accidental Complications • Multiple Pregnancy

INTRODUCTION

Labor offers a great opportunity to provide "nursing care" in the broadest sense (see Chap. 13). The opportunity is present in an even greater degree in cases of complicated labor. The importance of supportive care of the highest caliber cannot be emphasized enough. Fortunately, the principles of care in these instances usually do not differ significantly from those in normal labor. Some modification, of course, will be necessary at times. Yet because of the stress of the situation, more is demanded of the nurse. Here more than ever, the nurse's ability to make use of the process of clinical judgment is crucial. Her nursing diagnoses and the care that derives from them may have life-saving significance for both mother and infant. Her observations, reporting, technical skills, physical and emotional supportive measures must all be brought into play and carried out with a fine degree of competence, for the labor experience is often prolonged and painful—for all those concerned: mother, father, nurse and physician.

Since modifications of care will be dealt with primarily in this chapter, the student is urged to review in Chapter 13 the basic concepts and components of nursing care during labor.

MECHANICAL DYSTOCIA

Occasionally the nurse will see instances in which hours and hours of labor pass without progress. In such instances there is obviously something wrong with the mechanics or "machinery" of labor. In other words, these are cases of dystocia (difficult labor) in which the mechanics of the process are at fault—cases of mechanical dystocia. But what precisely *is* wrong?

Reduced to its simplest constituents, the process of labor resolves itself into the propulsion by certain *forces* of an irregular object (the infant or *passenger*) through the birth canal (the *passage*). Only three factors are involved in labor therefore—the forces, the passenger and the passage. When, despite many hours of labor, the infant fails to come, one of these three factors or some combination of them must be at fault.

Let us make this clear by a homely example. If a person were trying to force his foot into a boot and was unable to do so, what could be the causes of his failure? First, he might not be pushing hard enough. (The forces are at fault.) Second, he might not be holding his foot in the correct position; the foot cannot be jammed in any way but must be flexed sharply so that the smallest diameters present themselves. (The position is faulty.) Third, the boot may be too small, or (what amounts to the same thing) the foot may be too big. (There is disproportion between the size of the foot and the boot.)

Likewise, when Nature tries to propel an infant through the birth canal and fails to do so, there can be only three causes of the failure —the same three. The forces are inadequate (uterine inertia); or the position of the infant is at fault; or there is disproportion between the size of the infant and that of the birth canal.

Uterine Dysfunction

Definition. The nurse will recall that in normal labor a latent phase of several hours' duration occurs first, in which effacement and a small amount of dilatation take place. An active phase follows this, in which progressive, accelerated dilatation occurs. This is followed by a phase of deceleration or slowing just before full dilatation (see Chap. 11). A significant prolongation of any of these phases is termed uterine dysfunction.

Heretofore, the term "uterine inertia" was used to describe a dysfunctional labor. Inertia was classified as either primary or secondary. Primary inertia occurred at the onset of labor (i.e., the contractions were of poor quality and ineffectual) and was due to unknown causes. Secondary inertia occurred later in labor and was felt to be related to maternal exhaustion. However, increasing knowledge regarding uterine action and the phases of labor indicates that it would be more appropriate to discuss the topic in terms of dysfunction as it relates to the phases of dilatation. The two terms "inertia" and "dysfunction" are used interchangeably to some extent. If the word "inertia" is used, then primary inertia should refer to prolongation of the latent phase and secondary inertia should indicate a prolongation or abnormality of the active phase.[1]

Causes. The chief causes of uterine dysfunction are injudicious use of analgesia (i.e., excessive or too early administration of the drugs), minor degrees of pelvic contraction and fetal malposition of even a small degree such as a slight extension of the head as seen in some occiput posterior positions. Similarly, postmaturity and large size of the infant have been found to be significantly related to dysfunctional labor. These conditions may occur singly or in combination in cases of dysfunction. Other factors that are associated with this condition include overdistention of the uterus, grande multiparity, excessive cervical rigidity and maternal age. The latter group of factors has been shown to play an etiological role although not such an important one as was once believed. Jeffcoate also notes that the fact that one delivery tends to cure a uterus permanently of its dysfunction is so incontrovertible that it makes untenable any theory which invokes an emotional or psychological cause for dysfunctional uterine action. Unfortunately the cause is often unknown. More research at the cellular level will have to be done to obtain increased definitive knowledge concerning the etiologic factors in this condition.

Complications. The complications of uterine dysfunction are unfortunate for both mother and infant. Fetal injury and death are the most serious outcomes of this disorder. For the mother, exhaustion and dehydration may occur if labor is allowed to become too prolonged. The nurse should watch for any elevation of the maternal temperature and pulse, for these are the clinical signs that herald the onset of secondary complications. Acetonuria is another sign of exhaustion and dehydration. These symptoms are to be reported immediately. Generally, in patients having dysfunctional labor, supportive intravenous therapy and electrolyte replacement will have been begun before this syndrome occurs. Intra-uterine infection is another common maternal complication in these types of labor; broad-spectrum antibiotics are the usual choice of treatment. It is particularly important not to allow intra-uterine infection to occur, since it contributes heavily to the increased perinatal mortality. In addition, dysfunctional labor appears to have some long-term consequences. Research[2] has indicated that difficult labors and deliveries have a deleterious effect on future childbearing. Apparently, the more difficult the labor and delivery, the less inclination there is to have future children. In addition, the fear and anxiety that are engendered by a complicated childbirth become a special concern of the health team if these patients do have subsequent children.

Types of Uterine Dysfunction. HYPERTONIC UTERINE DYSFUNCTION. There are two varieties of uterine dysfunction. The first of these is the hypertonic type. Its name is derived from the fact that the muscle of the uterus is in a state of greater than normal muscle tension (i.e., incomplete relaxation). In these instances the contractions are of poor quality in the latent phase of labor, and the force of the contraction also is distorted, that is, one segment of the uterus may contract with more force than another. Although these contractions are inefficient from the standpoint of accomplishing dilatation, they are extremely painful. It is particularly important to help these mothers to distinguish between the anticipation of pain and the actual pain (see Chap. 13), for as labor wears on, and no progress is made, the mother's strength and ability to cope with the contractions diminish, and hence the pain seems to be intensified. The anxiety and fear which are generated can easily lead to panic,

---

[1] Eastman, N. J., and Hellman, L. M.: Williams Obstetrics. ed. 13, p. 826, New York, New York, Appleton, 1966.

[2] Jeffcoate, T. N., et al.: Inefficient uterine action. Surg. Gynec. Obstet. 95:257, September 4, 1952.

which is detrimental to resumption of a successful labor course.

This matter of the intensity of labor contractions is something with which the nurse must familiarize herself so that she may report intelligently. At the height of an excellent uterine contraction it is impossible to indent the uterine wall with one's fingertips, and during a fairly good contraction it may be possible to cause some slight indentation; but if the uterine wall can be indented easily at the height of a contraction, it is a poor one. In evaluating the intensity of a labor contraction, reliance should be placed on this tactile examination and not on the amount of "complaining" done by the patient about her pain.

The nurse should be alert also to signs of fetal distress, since in hypertonic dysfunction fetal distress tends to appear quite early in labor.

Treatment for this type of dysfunctional labor generally consists of rest and fluids. When medication is indicated to produce the needed rest and relaxation, an injection of 16 mg. of morphine may be prescribed, because it usually stops the abnormal contractions. In addition, a 0.1- to 0.2-Gm. dose of a short-acting barbiturate may be administered. Intravenous fluids are utilized to maintain hydration and electrolyte balance, and in most instances normal labor resumes when the patient awakens.

Intrapartal Infection. Occasionally, however, some patients do not respond to this regimen, and labor becomes prolonged. In such patients who have been in labor for 24 hours or more or who have ruptured membranes (whether from uterine dysfunction or other causes), bacteria are likely to ascend into the uterus and give rise to infection. This is known as *intrapartal infection* and is a serious complication. It is signalized by a rise in temperature, often in association with a chill. Because of this danger, it is customary to take temperatures every 2 hours in patients whose labors have lasted more than 24 hours. Even an elevation of half a degree should be reported at once to the physician. Intrapartal infection is much more likely to occur if the membranes have been ruptured for a long time. As previously stated, treatment is usually in the form of antibiotics. Oxytocin also may be used in these cases in spite of its adverse effects (it tends to increase the hypertonicity of the muscle). However, only dilutions of two or three times the usual strength should be employed. Cesarean section is resorted to if fetal distress occurs.

HYPOTONIC UTERINE DYSFUNCTION. The second variety of uterine dysfunction has been designated as hypotonic. Here the tone or tension of the muscle of the uterus is defective or inadequate. In these cases the uterus contracts synchronously, but the force is inadequate to accomplish dilatation. This condition occurs in the accelerated or active phase, or even during the second stage of labor; the contractions become infrequent and of poor quality, and the uterus is easily indentable at the acme of a contraction. Signs of fetal distress usually do not appear until intrapartal infection has developed. Thus, it is important that the nurse be cognizant of the signs and the symptoms of both these secondary complications and report these accordingly.

Treatment. When hypotonic dysfunction is suspected, diagnosis is confirmed by x-ray pelvimetry and sterile vaginal examination in order to ascertain accurate pelvic measurements, abnormalities of presentation and position, state of the cervix and level of the presenting part. It should be stressed that early diagnosis is a chief factor in reducing fetal death and injury. If a marked degree of disproportion exists (see p. 484), or if there is an uncorrectable malposition, then cesarean section will be employed to effect delivery. If these conditions are not present, then supportive therapy together with stimulation of the uterus will be the treatment of choice.

Explanations to Parents. It goes without saying that labors of this type are extremely discouraging for the mother and the father. The diagnostic procedures as well as the therapy will take a certain amount of time, and carrying out these measures will require patience and waiting on the part of everyone concerned. It is essential that the couple know and understand this fact. This will mean that the doctor or the nurse will spend sufficient time with the parents to explain what is happening in depth and in terms that are appropriate for them. It is very possible that repeated reinforcement of the explanations, progress, etc., will be needed. Feedback from the parents should be encouraged, so that their level of understanding and acceptance can be ascertained. The normal tension and anxiety found in any labor certainly will be intensified, and it is important that it not be compounded by fantasy or misunderstanding. Since dysfunctional labor is so variable, it is often impossible (and unwise) to give the parents any ironclad definite reassurances as to when effective labor will commence. Yet some kind of boundaries must be placed on when this ineffective phase will end, and progress will begin, so that the mother will have some goal to look forward to and to work for. Therefore, it is important to reassure the patient, reminding her that her case is not absolutely unique (patients think after many hours that theirs is the longest labor in obstetric history), that certain specific measures are known and can be taken to help effective labor to begin, and that she will be receiving competent medical and nursing care throughout her labor. If possible, the course of action should be explained by the doctor (or by the nurse with the doctor's permission), so that the parents can anticipate more realistically what is in store and therefore can be more reassured that certain definite measures are available to them and are being employed.

Further Treatment and Care. In addition, all the comfort measures which promote relaxation should be utilized. Sponge baths, various positioning, soothing backrubs, clean, dry linen, quiet conversation, reading or other diversionary activities as well as a quiet restful environment are all appropriate. However, the patient should not be isolated in a dark room on the premise that she should "sleep" or "rest"; any patient who is having a difficult or complicated labor should never be left alone unless she is actually sleeping, and then frequent observations should be made to see when she awakens. Human contact is one of the most important items of "treatment" in cases of complicated labor and should never be neglected. The presence of the same person, nurse and/or doctor, is very helpful for the reasons already mentioned in Chapter 13. Coaching the mother in breathing patterns and relaxation techniques also will conserve her strength.

The doctor may want the patient to have fluids by mouth, or he may order intravenous infusions to maintain hydration and electrolyte balance. A total of 2,000 cc. or more of intravenous fluid may be given in 24 hours. Hot soapsuds enemas probably will be ordered from time to time in the hope of stimulating more effectual uterine contractions. In certain cases (in some it may be dangerous) the physician may ask that the patient be allowed to walk about, in the belief that this may favor descent of the head, which in turn will exert greater pressure on the lower uterine segment and thereby stimulate stronger contractions.

Rupturing the membranes often stimulates satisfactory labor. In the case of hypotonic dysfunctional labor, if there is no critical disproportion or uncorrectable malposition, and amniotomy fails to bring about desired results, then an intra-venous infusion of oxytocin usually will be utilized to stimulate the uterus. It should be used with the utmost caution and in very small doses, for the employment of oxytocin in labor can be fraught with dangerous possibilities such as tetanic contraction of the uterus with asphyxiation of the fetus and even rupture of the uterus. (Contractions are termed "tetanic" when the uterus stays contracted continuously with no regular periods of relaxation.)

Because it affords better control of dosage, the intravenous administration of oxytocin by the continuous drip technique, as described on page 271, is being used extensively in the treatment of dysfunctional labor. Sparteine sulfate (Tocosamine) sometimes is used as an alternative to oxytocin to stimulate labor. It is given in repeated doses until satisfactory uterine action is achieved; however, there are limits to the total dosage that can be used (see p. 271). The intramuscular administration of Tocosamine does not assure the precise and controlled blood level of the drug that the intravenous administration of oxytocin does. In addition, the dosage cannot be discontinued or decreased readily, as can the oxytocin infusion.

As stated in Chapter 13, oxytocin is a dangerous drug; hence, the patient must have someone in attendance at all times during the infusion. Every uterine contraction is to be timed and fetal heart tones are to be taken after each contraction or every 5 minutes. Maternal blood pressure and pulse are checked every half hour. As the physician specifies the dosage, the nurse (or other attendant) will make certain that the infusion is running at the prescribed drops per minute and will report any maternal or fetal aberrations immediately. Many institutions have an "Oxytocin Record" or a "Pitocin Sheet" on which there is space for recording times, amount and frequency of the oxytocin given, fetal heart tones, maternal blood pressure and pulse, frequency, intensity and length of contractions, and other relevant comments. This type of sheet gives an easily accessible record of the patient's progress during the infusion.

Recording and reporting the physiological signs and symptoms cannot be stressed enough during these infusions. However, supportive care is also to be maintained. Adequate explanation and reassurance can be given, and since the nurse will be with the mother continuously she can utilize the time to good advantage to establish a relationship of rapport. While the infusion will stimulate contractions (and therefore, discomfort), the mother and her husband often look upon this treatment optimistically for it marks the end of a desultory, ineffective period in labor and brings with it promise of termination of a difficult time. This positive attitude can be especially reinforced if the nurse provides explanation and assurance.

Abnormal Fetal Positions

Persistent Occiput Posterior Positions. As stated on page 26 and illustrated in Figures 2-5 and 2-7, the fetal head usually enters the pelvic inlet transversely and therefore must traverse an arc of 90° in the process of internal rotation to the direct occiput anterior position. In about a quarter of all labors, however, the head enters the pelvis with the occiput directed diagonally posterior, that is, in either the R.O.P. or the L.O.P. position. Under these circumstances the head must rotate through an arc of 135° in the process of internal rotation.

With good contractions, adequate flexion and a baby of average size, the great majority of these cases of occiput posterior position undergo spontaneous rotation through the 135° arc just as soon as the head reaches the pelvic floor. This is a normal mechanism of labor. It must be remembered, however, that labor is usually prolonged, and the mother has a great deal of discomfort in her back as the baby's head impinges against the sacrum in the course of rotating. Nursing intervention is aimed at relieving the back pain as much as possible. Sacral

pressure, backrubs and frequent change of position from side to side can be helpful, and they should be employed to the degree that seems to be well-tolerated by the patient. In a minority of cases, however, perhaps 5 or 10 per cent, these favorable circumstances do not exist, and rotation may be incomplete or may not take place at all. If rotation is incomplete, the head becomes arrested in the transverse position, a condition known as *transverse arrest*. If anterior rotation does not take place at all, the occiput usually rotates to the direct occiput posterior position, a condition known as *persistent occiput posterior*. Both transverse arrest and persistent occiput posterior position represent deviations from the normal mechanisms of labor and may require operative delivery. Sometimes the mechanical problem associated with abnormal uterine action is an abnormal position of the presenting head. Hence, these conditions of posterior or transverse arrest of the occiput appear to have, in some cases, an adverse effect on uterine behavior. Here the malposition is the cause rather than the effect of uterine inefficiency. This conclusion can be verified by the following findings. (1) When the fetal head is rotated or rotates spontaneously, uterine action improves. (2) Oxytocin therapy for dysfunction associated with an occipito-posterior position does not cause the infant's head to rotate.

It should be remembered that the uterus of the multigravid patient usually reacts to mechanical obstruction by becoming more active and ultimately rupturing itself. On the other hand, when

Fig. 20-1. Footling breech.

Fig. 20-2. Frank breech.

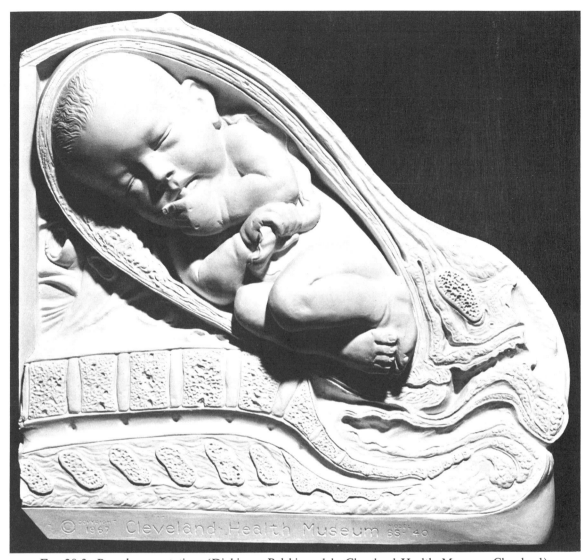

FIG. 20-3. Breech presentation. (Dickinson-Belski model. Cleveland Health Museum, Cleveland)

the primigravid uterus encounters resistance it nearly always responds by inertia or incoordinate behavior. It is imperative then, that the obstetrician rule out mechanical obstruction before deciding that labor is prolonged due to idiopathic faulty uterine action. Since disproportion may be slight and therefore easily overlooked, only the most careful observation and study can disclose the important association between faulty uterine action and smallness of the pelvis or large size of the baby. The nurse can make an important contribution in this diagnosis by her continuous and critical observations of the character and frequency of the contractions, the amount of the mother's discomfort, her vital signs, general condition and the fetal heart rate.

Breech Presentations. These are presentations in which the breech instead of the vertex presents at the pelvic brim. They occur in about 3 per cent of all term deliveries (see Chap. 5). In breech presentation the infant often passes meconium from his rectum during the course of labor, and after the membranes are ruptured, and the liquor amnii has escaped, the nurse may find the black, tar-colored material coming from the patient's vagina. She should make certain that the presentation is, in fact, a breech, for if such a phenomenon occurred in a vertex presentation,

Fig. 20-4. (*Top*) Extraction of posterior shoulder in breech delivery. (*Bottom*) Extraction of head in breech delivery (Mauriceau maneuver).

then it would be an indication of probable fetal distress.

Explanation and appropriate reassurance are important for mothers who have breech presentations, as they are for any patients having an abnormal presentation or complicated labor of any type. Many patients are steeped in old wives' folklore of the fearfulness of a "breech birth" and become exceedingly anxious and terrified as soon as they find out (or overhear) that theirs

is this type of presentation; the same is often true of the husbands, and the anxiety and fear that are communicated from one partner to the other can impede the patient's working effectively with her labor. With modern obstetric techniques and knowledge, labor need not be prolonged or exceptionally painful.

CLASSIFICATION. Breech presentations are classified as follows:

1. *Complete,* when the feet and the legs are

flexed on the thighs, and the thighs are flexed on the abdomen, so that the buttocks and the feet present (see Fig. 5-6).

2. *Footling,* when one or both feet present through the cervix (Fig. 20-1).

3. *Frank,* when the legs are extended and lie against the abdomen and the chest, with the feet meeting the shoulders, and the buttocks present (Fig. 20-2).

DELIVERY. With strong contractions, particularly in multiparae, breech cases may be delivered spontaneously, or at least with very little aid by the attendant. The breech is pushed through the vulva as the result of the mother's bearing-down efforts and rises upward in front of the symphysis pubis. With the emergence of the trunk, the legs descend, the attendant simply receiving them and steadying the breech. With further bearing-down efforts, the shoulders are expelled; then, as the attendant holds up the body, the head is extruded with the face directed back at the perineum (Fig. 20-4).

However, in the majority of breech cases, especially in primigravidae, it is necessary for the physician to give more aid than is indicated above, and, as a rule, this amounts to extraction of the shoulders and the head after the umbilicus has appeared (Fig. 20-4). It is to be remembered that there is a fundamental difference in a vertex and breech presentation. In the former, the head, which is the largest portion of the infant is born first, and is followed by successively smaller portions. In a breech presentation, however, the process is reversed, with successively *larger* portions of the infant being born; thus, the buttocks, shoulders and the head represent, in effect, three "births" each preceded by its own internal rotation.

The frank breech usually is a better dilating wedge than a complete breech because the buttocks impinge more closely on the margins of the dilating cervix. However, the complete breech is more satisfactory for immediate delivery if medical assistance becomes necessary, since a foot can be brought down readily for traction. Converting the other types of breech presentations to a complete breech is not done routinely, however, unless there is some abnormality of the mother or infant that makes immediate delivery likely. Because of the serious perinatal mortality (12 per cent in the United States) the obstetrician will want to be available for immediate medical assistance. Extraction may be employed and the application of Piper forceps to the aftercoming

head is considered a conservative and reliable approach to breech delivery. Similarly, cesarean section is a safer approach and yields better results for the baby than a difficult extraction. It is recommended that cesarean section be employed in cases of breech presentation with concomitant uterine dysfunction, pelvic contractions, large infant and in primigravidae over 35 years of age.

Occasionally, cases of precipitate breech delivery may fall to the care of the nurse. These cases are uncommon and, when they do occur, seldom give rise to difficulty, because the very fact that they are precipitate presupposes a small infant, excellent expulsive forces and a capacious birth canal. As the breech emerges, it is received and is steadied with a sterile towel and sterile hands, and the mother is urged to bear down strongly. This usually will effect delivery of the shoulders in cases of this sort, but if it does not, the arm which is the more posterior is drawn out of the vagina by passing the first and the middle fingers over the infant's shoulder, down the arm to the elbow, and then drawing the forearm and the hand across the face and the chest and out. The other arm is delivered in the same way; and then, to favor the birth of the head, the body of the baby is raised upward in a vertical position. If there is any great delay, the nurse may place two fingers into the baby's mouth, with the trunk resting on the palm of the same hand and the legs straddling her forearm. Then, with the other hand, upward and outward traction is made on the shoulders, while firm down-

FIG. 20-5. Shoulder presentation with prolapse of arm.

ward pressure is made by an assistant on the lower abdominal wall. As with any other emergency delivery by the nurse, the nurse's composure and teamwork with the patient are important cornerstones to a successful outcome (see Chap. 13).

The great danger in breech delivery is to the baby as the result of the trauma which he may sustain in delivery. Tentorial tears and subsequent intracranial hemorrhage are twice as common in these presentations as they are in cephalic presentations. The symptoms and nursing care associated with these conditions are discussed in Chapter 23. Lesions of the spinal cord and extrusion of the medulla into the foramen magnum also account for a goodly portion of deaths. In footling presentations, prolapse of the umbilical cord (see p. 490) is common. Even in the most skilled hands, and considering only full-term infants, about 1 breech infant in 15 succumbs as the result of delivery. The danger to the mother is not appreciably greater than in vertex deliveries, but lacerations of the birth canal are more frequent.

Shoulder, Face and Brow Presentations. In shoulder presentations the infant lies crosswise in the uterus instead of longitudinally (see Fig. 5-8). This complication occurs about once in every 200 cases and is seen most often in multiparae. Not infrequently an arm prolapses into the vagina, making the problem of delivery even more difficult (Fig. 20-5). The physician usually will turn the infant in these cases, bringing a foot or both feet into the vagina, an operation known as "version" (p. 434). Shoulder presentation is a serious complication, occasionally causes rupture of the uterus (p. 489) and carries a much greater risk to the infant than either vertex or breech presentations.

Face presentations are also seen about once in every 200 cases. They usually terminate spontaneously, the face coming through the vulva with the chin anterior. As edema of the scalp is common in vertex presentations (caput succedaneum), so in face presentations the presenting part, the face, becomes greatly swollen and purplish. This disappears within a few days. Brow presentations are even more rare and are much more difficult to deliver because the largest diameter of the fetal head, the occipitomental, presents. They frequently convert themselves into face or occipital presentations. Because the majority of brow presentations occur with premature infants and because of the transient nature of the remainder, spontaneous or forceps deliveries are more usual. In the case of persistent brow presentation at term, Cesarean section becomes the delivery of choice.

Disproportion

Contracted Pelvis. Disproportion between the size of the infant and that of the birth canal (commonly spoken of as cephalopelvic disproportion) is caused most frequently by contracted pelvis. The pelvis may be contracted at the inlet, the midpelvis or the outlet. In the case of inlet contraction the anteroposterior diameter of the inlet is shortened to 10 cm. or less, or the greatest transverse diameter is 12 cm. or less. The sacrum is broader and less concave from side to side, thinner from behind foreward and shorter from above downward. Inlet contraction is most often due to rickets, a fact indicating how much good may be accomplished by the prevention of rickets in infants and children through an adequate intake of vitamin D. Contracted pelvis due to rickets is much more common in the Negro race than in the white. In midpelvic contraction, the distance between the ischial spines is diminished; it is often found in conjunction with outlet contraction. In outlet contraction, the angle formed by the pubic rami is narrow, and the ischial tuberosities are close together; it thus resembles a male pelvis insofar as the outlet is concerned. This type of pelvic contraction occurs with equal frequency in the white and the Negro races, but its cause is not known. It is not only likely to hinder the egress of the infant at the outlet but also may be responsible for deep lacerations, since the narrow pubic rami tend to push the infant's head posteriorly in the direction of the rectum.

One of the main functions of antepartal care is to detect pelvic contraction during pregnancy, so that—long before labor begins—some intelligent decision can be reached about how best to deliver the infant. Of course, in a case of extreme pelvic contraction, cesarean section is obligatory. But all gradations of contracted pelvis are encountered, and, depending on the size of the infant and other factors, many patients with moderate degrees of the condition can be delivered vaginally without difficulty.

In doubtful cases the physician may give the patient a "trial labor," that is, 6 or 12 hours of labor to ascertain whether or not with adequate contractions the head will pass through the pelvis. For these patients labor may be even more anxiety-provoking than usual (depending in part on the extent and the depth of supportive ante-partal counseling), and if cesarean section is the ultimate outcome, there may be a great deal of disappointment and perhaps even a feeling of failure. The warm empathic attitude of the nurse is particularly needed with these patients. Frequent reports on the progress of labor should not be overlooked when the progress is favorable; if it is not, then compensatory reassurance and anticipatory guidance regarding cesarean section may be given if the physician so desires. The health team does the patient a disservice in avoiding the subject if progress is not made in labor.

Oversize Baby. Excessive size of the infant is not commonly a cause of serious dystocia unless the fetus weighs over 4,500 Gm. (10 pounds). About 1 infant in 100 will fall in this class. The trauma associated with the passage of such huge infants through the birth canal causes a decided increase in fetal mortality; this has been estimated as 15 per cent (almost 1 in 6), in contrast with the usual death rate of 4 per cent for normal-size infants. Uterine dysfunction is frequent in labors with excessive-size infants, and at the time of delivery the shoulders may give great difficulty. Even though these infants are born alive, they often do poorly in the first few days because of cerebral hemorrhage and must be watched closely for signs of that condition (see Chap. 23).

One of the common causes of excessive-size infants is diabetes. Large infants are also more commonly seen in older multiparae and after prolonged pregnancies; the majority of such infants are boys.

Despite tales to the contrary, tremendously large infants—weighing over 13 pounds—are extremely rare and almost all are born dead. In 50,000 deliveries at the Johns Hopkins Hospital, there have been only two such cases. Both these infants were boys; the smaller, who weighed 13 pounds, 7 ounces, was the ninth child of a 34-year-old Negro woman; and the larger, 14 pounds, 4 ounces, was the seventh child of a white woman aged 44. The largest infant born at the New York Lying-In Hospital in 100,000 cases weighed 15 pounds. Although there may be rare exceptions, most stories that one hears of infants weighing over 15 pounds at birth are the result of either gross exaggeration or incorrect scales.

Hydrocephalus. Hydrocephalus, or an excessive accumulation of cerebrospinal fluid in the ventricles of the brain with consequent enlargement of the cranium, is encountered in 1 fetus in 2,000, approximately, and accounts for some 12 per cent of all malformations at birth. Associated defects are common, spina bifida being present in about one third of the cases. Varying degrees of cranial enlargement are produced, and not infrequently the circumference of the head exceeds 50 cm., sometimes reaching 80 cm. The amount of fluid present is usually between 500 and 1,500 cc., but as much as 5 liters has been reported. Since the distended cranium is too large to fit into the pelvic inlet, breech presentations are exceedingly common, being observed in about one third of such cases. Whatever the presentation, gross disproportion between the size of the head and that of the pelvis is the rule, and serious dystocia is the usual consequence. This is a tragic and serious complication of labor, and the obstetrician will find it necessary, as a rule, to puncture the cranial vault and aspirate as much of the cerebrospinal fluid as may be necessary to permit delivery. This procedure in itself does not injure the child. Nevertheless, fetal mortality is very high, 70 per cent (this percentage includes very mild forms of the disease).

Births of this type are a terrible tragedy for all concerned; the mother must undergo a difficult labor at great risk to herself, the husband will suffer with her, the fetus may expire, and the physician and the nurse must cope with a grave crisis with a poor prognosis. It is often difficult to describe the emotional climate at this time; perhaps it is impossible if one has not experienced a similar loss or disappointment. A state of emotional shock prevails, in which disbelief, noncomprehension and, sometimes, denial prevail. It seems to the husband and wife that the hopes and the dreams of 9 months and perhaps a lifetime lie shattered around them. This is a situation in which the nurse will be called on to exercise her nursing skill to the utmost, not only during labor but after the delivery, and particularly if there is an obvious abnormality, or if a fetal demise occurs. The components of care that are useful in helping the parents in such a crisis are discussed fully in Chapter 23, Disorders of the Newborn.

HEMORRHAGIC COMPLICATIONS
Postpartal Hemorrhage

It has been said of the three stages of labor that the first stage is the most difficult for the physician and the nurse (because of the patience required during the long hours of waiting), that the second is the most difficult for the infant (because of the trauma and asphyxia it may undergo in passing through the birth canal); and that for the mother the third stage is the most dangerous because of the likelihood of postpartal hemorrhage and shock.

Definition and Incidence. The average blood lost postpartum is about 300 cc. The term "postpartal hemorrhage," as ordinarily used, does not refer to bleeding of this magnitude but only to excessive blood loss; and, by rather general consensus, when postpartal bleeding reaches 500 cc. or more, it is designated as "postpartal hemorrhage." Bleeding of this degree occurs in every 20 or 30 cases despite the most skilled care. Hemorrhages of 1,000 cc. and over are encountered once in about every 75 cases, whereas blood losses of even 1,500 and 2,000 cc. are encountered now and then. In other words, postpartal hemorrhage is a fairly common complication of labor. Moreover, it is one with which the nurse must be intimately familiar, because she will be expected to assume an important role in the prevention and treatment of the condition.

The Three Causes. In order of frequency, the three immediate causes of postpartal hemorrhage are:

1. Uterine atony
2. Lacerations of the perineum, the vagina and the cervix
3. Retained placental fragments

Clotting defects as well as obstetrical accidents such as inversion of the uterus also can be classified as causes but they are much less common and are of a more indirect nature.

Uterine atony is by far the most common cause. Again let us recall that the uterus contains huge blood vessels within the interstices of its muscle fibers, and that those at the placental site are open and gaping. It is essential that the muscle fibers contract down tightly on these arteries and veins, if bleeding is to be controlled. They must *stay* contracted down, for only a few seconds' relaxation will give rise to sudden, profuse hemorrhage. They must stay *tightly* contracted down, because continuous, slight relaxation gives rise to continuous oozing of blood, one of the most treacherous forms of postpartal hemorrhage.

Lacerations of the perineum, the vagina and the cervix are naturally more common after operative delivery. Tears of the cervix are particularly likely to cause serious hemorrhage. Bright red arterial bleeding in the presence of a hard, firmly contracted uterus (no uterine atony) suggests hemorrhage from a cervical laceration. The physician will establish the diagnosis by actual inspection of the cervix (retractors are necessary) and, after locating the source of bleeding, will repair the laceration.

Retained Placental Fragments. Small, partially separated fragments of placenta may cause postpartal hemorrhage by interfering with proper uterine contraction. Careful inspection of the placenta to determine whether a piece is missing will rule out or confirm the diagnosis; the treatment, obviously, it to remove the placental fragment. This is an uncommon cause of postpartal hemorrhage, but occasionally the nurse will encounter cases in which profuse bleeding occurs suddenly a week or more after delivery. These late hemorrhages are usually designated by the term "puerperal hemorrhage." They are often caused by a retained placental fragment.

Predisposing Factors. There are certain factors which predispose to postpartal hemorrhage, so that to a certain extent it may be anticipated in advance. Among these, one of the most important is the size of the infant. With a 9-pound infant, the chances of postpartal hemorrhage are 5 times as great as they are with a 5-pound infant. Excessive bleeding is twice as common in twin pregnancy. Hydramnios (excessive amount of amniotic fluid) is another predisposing factor. It has been shown, however, that with the careful use of oxytocin in the placental stage and special care to achieve effective contraction, in this stage, that the incidence of hemorrhage due to overdistention can be reduced considerably. Operative delivery, with deep general anesthesia, prolonged labor with maternal exhaustion, and mismanagement of the third stage of labor greatly increase the likelihood of this complication. Other conditions in which postpartal hemorrhage is extremely frequent are premature separation of the placenta and placenta previa. Finally, internal podalic version is followed by a very high incidence of hemorrhage. Thus, it is recommended that blood transfusions be ready for *immediate* use if this procedure must be attempted.

Clinical Picture. Excessive bleeding may occur prior to the birth of the placenta, but it is seen more commonly thereafter. Although it is occasionally torrential in character, the most common type is a continuous trickle—minute by minute. These small constant trickles are not alarming in appearance, consequently, no one may become alarmed, and no one may do anything. This is what makes this type of hemorrhage so treacherous. This fact has been emphasized particularly by Doctor Beecham, of Philadelphia, in his survey of 52 deaths from postpartal hemorrhage which occurred in that city. The average interval between delivery and death in this series was 5 hours and 20 minutes. Only 6 patients, 11.5 per cent, died within 2 hours of delivery, and none in less than 1½ hours. In other words, there would have been ample time for intensive treatment in any of these cases, had the attendant been alert to how much blood was being lost.

Treatment. The first and most important thing to do is to grasp the uterus and massage it. This must be continued until the uterus assumes a woody hardness; if the slightest relaxation occurs, the massage must be reinstituted. In many cases the uterus stays contracted most of the time but occasionally relaxes; it is therefore obligatory to keep a hand on the fundus constantly for a full hour after bleeding has subsided. When the uterus is well contracted, care should be taken *to avoid overmassage*, because such practice contributes to muscle fatigue, which in turn further encourages uterine relaxation and excessive bleeding. Even then the danger is not over, since relaxation sometimes occurs 2 or more hours after delivery; in these cases the uterus may balloon with blood, with very little escaping externally. Accordingly, the consistency, size and the height of the uterus should be checked frequently until several hours have elapsed. Ordinarily, the height of the fundus after delivery will be about at the level of the umbilicus. If the uterus becomes distended with blood, or if the bladder becomes full and presses upward against the uterus, causing it to rise in the abdomen, then the fundus can be palpated several centimeters above the umbilicus. The nurse must make absolutely certain that she is actually massaging the uterus and not a roll of abdominal fat or a distended bladder (see pp. 273, 307). When properly contracted, the uterus should feel like a small-to-medium-sized hard grapefruit. Frequently, a big, boggy, relaxed uterus is difficult to outline through the abdominal wall, and it may be necessary to push the hand well posteriorly toward the region of the sacral promontory to reach it. The very fact that the uterus is hard to identify usually means that it is relaxed. If the nurse is not sure that she is feeling the uterus, she should inform the physician at once.

ALLAYING ANXIETY. The frequent massage and deep palpation are often painful to the mother; at best they are disturbing, since they come at a time when the mother wants nothing more than to rest and sleep after her great effort. If she is awake and alert, then the continued attention and scrutiny may increase her anxiety. It must be remembered that apprehension is a natural concomitant of hemorrhage and shock. Therefore the nurse should take pains to make her observations as quickly and efficiently as possible and to allay the mother's (and father's) concern by appropriate explanation and reassurance.

This aspect of nursing care may be difficult to implement. If the mother or the father expresses concern and questions the activity by asking "What's wrong?" then the nurse can say simply, "The uterus has a tendency to relax, and must be massaged so that it will contract down as it should." Usually, such a statement will suffice. This will indicate to the mother and father the reason for the continued activity without associating hemorrhage and its fearsome consequences with the actions of the attendants. If the mother drifts off to sleep between the nurse's observations, then the nurse can gently rouse her by speaking her name before she commences massage, so that the mother is not awakened abruptly to the painful sensation of someone squeezing her abdomen.

OTHER ASPECTS OF CARE. Vital signs will be required every 5 to 15 minutes, and any variation, however slight, is to be reported immediately. One of the most perfidious things about postpartal hemorrhage is the fact that the blood pressure and the pulse may show only moderate alterations until a large amount of blood has been lost. Then, when the vascular system can no longer compensate for the diminished blood volume, the pulse increases rapidly, the blood pressure drops precipitously, and shock ensues.

One way that the nurse can keep a more accurate account of the blood loss is to keep a perineal pad count. In doing this she counts the number of pads saturated, how fully they are saturated, and the time it took for the saturation to occur. Thus, her nurse's notes might read: "Two pads ¾ saturated in 20 minutes." This type of report is more helpful to the physician than a more general, vague statement like, "Saturating perineal pads quickly."

If the bleeding occurs prior to delivery of the placenta, the physician may find it necessary to extract the placenta manually. (A change of gloves as well as gown may be called for to ensure strict asepsis, since the uterine cavity is to be invaded.) Oxytocics will invariably be requested, ergonovine or oxytocin or both intramuscularly. One or the other of these may be given intravenously by the physician. Blood transfusion will undoubtedly be instituted. The blood group of *all* maternity patients should be known before labor and cross-matched blood should be available for those in whom hemorrhage is anticipated or appears imminent. Seeing that the bloodtyping is carried out, ordering and calling for the cross match and the blood to be sent to the unit are all responsibilities of the nurse, and she must fit these additional responsibilities into her full schedule as she attends these patients. Moreover time is of the essence for these patients, therefore the nurse must pre-plan and establish priorities with rapidity.

If oxytocin therapy fails to stop the bleeding, the physician probably will carry out bimanual compression of the organ. This provides the most efficient means of massaging and compressing the uterus. Packing the uterus with gauze, a procedure once considered valuable to promote hemostasis in such cases, is seldom utilized today. It is considered by many authorities (e.g., Eastman, Hellman, Cosgrove, Leff and Berkeley) to be inadequate and conducive to infection. If shock threatens, the Trendelenburg position should be employed, external heat applied, and preparations for blood transfusion made.

In the handling of a case of postpartal hemorrhage, the nurse may be taxed to her utmost. The physician in charge may have to search for and suture a cervical laceration or start a blood transfusion or even resuscitate the infant; another physician may be needed to give the anesthesia. To the nurse, or nurses, will usually fall the important tasks of massaging the uterus, giving oxytocics, helping with the transfusion and caring for the infant. The nurse must be prepared to act quickly and efficiently if the lives of these bleeding mothers are to be saved.

If postpartal hemorrhage should occur after the physician has left, the nurse should grasp the uterus at once, press out as much blood as possible and begin gentle, but vigorous massage, sending word, of course, to the physician. If massage fails to stop the bleeding, the physician usually will not object if the nurse gives the patient an intramuscular injection of ergonovine or oxytocin. If possible, this arrangement should be understood beforehand.

Late Postpartal Hemorrhage. Occasionally, postpartal hemorrhage may occur later than the first day following delivery. These late postpartal hemorrhages may take place any time between the 2nd and the 28th day, are usually sudden in onset and may be so massive as to produce shock. Late postpartal hemorrhage is fortunately uncommon, occurring perhaps once in 1,000 cases. While this condition is relatively uncommon, it is to be remembered that the mother will usually be home, often alone, and without professional attendance. Thus, if the hemorrhage is massive, she may be in immediate danger; even if the bleeding is not great, there is still considerable difficulty getting medical assistance and all of this can produce a great deal of anxiety and fatigue. Arrangements must be made for the care of the infant even if the mother is to be seen only for a short while in the emergency room. Husbands must be contacted, transportation arranged, and often myriads of other details worked through before the mother can receive medical attention. This is why it is so important that the mother know where she can readily contact her doctor should she need him in an emergency situation. Moreover, it becomes clearer why the mother should have help in the person of someone who is readily available and responsible for the first weeks of the puerperium.

Factors which most often cause these late hemorrhages are retention of placental fragments, recurrent bleeding from lacerations or episiotomy and subinvolution of the placental site. The latter condition is especially interesting because as yet, the pathogenesis is unknown. The regeneration of the placental site takes longer than the rest of the uterus. It is accomplished in about 6 weeks as compared with about 21 days for the rest of the endometrium. The regeneration of the placental site begins from the remains of the epithelial glands; if these are not viable, then regeneration must occur from the spread of the surrounding epithelial tissue in the rest of the uterus. Until the site is firmly epithelialized, sloughing of clots may cause bleeding. Certain factors have been found to be associated with clot sloughing and hemorrhage, among them low grade fever, a history of abortion or uterine bleeding during pregnancy, hormonal influences, and the absence of breast-feeding. Often, however, none of these factors are found to be present, and the reason for the subinvolution remains a mystery. The physician will probably want to examine the patient. He may then carry out instrumental dilation of the cervix at which time he will remove any placental fragments that are present with a curet or ovum forceps or repair any lacerations or incisions.

If the mother must return to the hospital, this will no doubt upset to some degree the beginning relationship with the newborn. If the mother is nursing her infant and it is within a two week period after delivery, the physician often can arrange to have the mother room-in with her infant for the short 1 or 2 day hospital stay. If the mother is bottle feeding, then relatives, husband or "mothers' helpers" can help in the interim until the mother's return. The nurse will want to remember that much of the mother's apparent anxiety and/or desire to return home as quickly as possible arises from these often abrupt and temporary arrangements that she has had to make. Understanding and counseling the mother to help her get adequate rest upon her return home is one of the helpful measures that the nurse can offer.

Rupture of Uterus

Rupture of the uterus is fortunately a rare complication, but when it does occur, it constitutes one of the gravest accidents in obstetrics, since almost all of the infants and about a third of the mothers are lost. In this condition the uterus simply bursts, because the strain placed upon its musculature is more than it can withstand. It may occur in pregnancy but is far more frequent in labor. In modern obstetrics the most common cause is rupture of the scar of a previous cesarean section. Accordingly, when observing labor in a patient who has had a previous cesarean section, the possibility of this accident always should be borne in mind. Other contributing factors include prolonged and/or obstructed labor, certain faulty presentations, multiparity, traumatic delivery, such as version and extraction, and the injudicious use of oxytocin in labor. When rupture occurs, the patient complains of a severe, sudden, lancinating pain during a strong labor contraction. The rupture may be complete or incomplete; pain and abdominal tenderness are always present in both cases. If there is complete rupture, regular contractions cease, since the torn muscle can no longer contract. There is an outpouring of blood into the abdominal cavity and sometimes into the vagina. The uterus may be palpated abdominally as a hard mass lying alongside the fetus. The patient soon exhibits signs of shock: her pulse is rapid and weak, her skin cool and clammy, her face may be pale and her nostrils

dilated, a sign of air hunger. If the rupture is incomplete, the contractions may continue, and the signs of shock may be delayed, since the blood loss is slower. As soon as the diagnosis of rupture of the uterus is made, rapid preparations for an abdominal operation should ensue, since hysterectomy is the usual treatment. In addition, antibiotics are administered to combat infection, and blood transfusions are given to replace blood loss and to alleviate shock. Since this accident gravely compromises the lives of both the infant and the mother, prevention, early diagnosis, prompt treatment, blood transfusions and antibiotics are essential components in improving the prognosis. The nursing care will be essentially that for any complicated delivery and postpartum hemorrhage. Whenever possible it is advisable to have the nurse who has been attending the mother during labor remain with her until the anesthetic for the cesarean section is given. This will provide some measure of continuity of care and help in reassurance and comfort of the parents.

AMNIOTIC FLUID EMBOLISM

At any time after the membranes have ruptured there is a possibility that amniotic fluid may enter the gaping venous sinuses of the placental site as well as the veins in the cervix, be drawn into the general circulation and in this way reach the pulmonary capillaries. Since the amniotic fluid invariably contains small particles of matter, such as vernix caseosa, lanugo and sometimes meconium, multiple tiny emboli may reach the lungs in this manner and cause occlusion of the pulmonary capillaries. This complication, amniotic fluid embolism, is almost invariably fatal and, as a rule, causes the death of the mother within 1 or 2 hours. Fortunately, this tragic condition is rare, occurring only once in many thousand labors.

The clinical characteristics of the condition are sudden dyspnea, cyanosis, pulmonary edema, profound shock and uterine relaxation with postpartal hemorrhage. A highly important feature of amniotic fluid embolism is a diminution in the fibrinogen content of the blood, or hypofibrinogenemia. The mechanism is similar to, if not identical with, that which occurs in abruptio placentae and missed abortion, as described on pages 459 and 467.

The treatment consists of oxygen therapy, blood transfusion and the intravenous administration of fibrinogen, but, as indicated, this is usually futile.

ACCIDENTAL COMPLICATIONS

Lacerations of Perineum

Lacerations have already been referred to as a cause of postpartal hemorrhage. In addition, perineal tears may do great damage in destroying the integrity of the perineum and in weakening the supports of the uterus, the bladder and the rectum. Unless these lacerations are repaired properly, the resultant weakness, as the years go by, may cause prolapse of the uterus (called by the laity "falling of the womb"), cystocele (a pouching downward of the bladder) or rectocele (a pouching forward of the rectum). These conditions, which originate from perineal lacerations at childbirth, give rise to many discomforts and often necessitate operative treatment.

Because lacerations of the birth canal sometimes occur during the process of normal delivery, and are sometimes unavoidable even in the most skilled hands, this subject has already been discussed in Chapter 13.

Prolapse of Umbilical Cord

In the course of labor, the cord prolapses in front of the presenting part about once in every 400 cases. It is a grave complication for the fetus, since the cord is then compressed between the head and the bony pelvis, and the fetal circulation is shut off (Fig. 20-6). The accident is usually due to premature rupture of the mem-

FIG. 20-6. Prolapse of the umbilical cord (Bumm). As the head comes down, the compression of the cord between the fetal skull and the pelvic brim will shut off its circulation completely.

branes when the head, the breech or the shoulder is not sufficiently down in the pelvis to prevent the cord from being washed past it in the sudden gush of amniotic fluid. After the membranes rupture, the cord comes down, and it may be either a concealed or an apparent prolapse. In the latter instance, the diagnosis is made when the cord is seen; but when the cord is not visible, the correct diagnosis will not be made unless the patient is examined and the cord is felt, or examination of the fetal heart reveals distress due to pressure on the cord. This is why it *must* be a routine practice to listen to the fetal heart sounds immediately after the membranes rupture and again in about 10 minutes.

If the nurse is alone with the patient, she should send immediately for the physician and then attempt to relieve the pressure on the cord by elevating the patient's hips, thus allowing the head to gravitate away from the pelvis. This takes place in either the "knee-chest position" (see Fig. 15-23) or the Trendelenburg position. In the home the latter is arranged by slipping the back of a straight-backed chair, covered with a flat pillow, under the buttocks and the shoulders, with the knees down over the rungs of the chair. In putting the patient in such a position, her hips must be kept raised above the level of her shoulders. If the patient is unable to remain in either of these positions very long, she may be put in the elevated Sims's position, that is, on her side with the hips elevated by pillows in order to raise the hips higher than the thorax. Any change in position must be carried out slowly!

If the physician is expected to arrive on the scene within the next 15 minutes, this is all that the nurse should do. If he can be reached by telephone in this period, instructions about further therapy should be sought. If no medical advice can be obtained at the end of 15 minutes, and the umbilical cord is protruding from the vagina, the nurse should protect the exposed cord with sterile wet saline dressings, if they are available. In handling the cord, great care must be exercised not to compress it. The nurse should *never* attempt to replace a prolapsed cord into the vagina.

This particular complication is not painful for the mother; however, it can be very frightening, for many patients realize it can result in their infant's death. Also whether they realize the grave implications or not, the various antic positions and quickened responses of the attendants give them an indication that all is not well. Therefore, again, the calmness, warmth and efficiency of the

Fig. 20-7. One-egg and two-egg twins. (Dickinson-Belskie models, Cleveland Health Museum, Cleveland)

nurse can do much to reassure the patient that all possible measures are being taken to bring the situation under control. It goes without saying that these patients never should be left unattended, and the husbands, if they are present, should be treated with consideration. It is difficult, when any crises occur, to deal with the husband or relatives of the patient with appropriate thoughtfulness, since most of the energy is directed toward meeting the pressing (and often lifesaving) demands of the situation. However, it must be remembered that the patient and her husband are considered as a unit, and a few moments usually can be found to apprise the husband of what is being done for his wife.

Inversion of Uterus

Inversion of the uterus is a rare and highly fatal accident of labor in which, after the birth of the infant, the uterus turns inside out. Shock is profound, in many cases causing the death of the mother. This rare complication is mentioned here only to stress the two common causes: (1) pulling on the umbilical cord and (2) trying to express the placenta when the uterus is relaxed. In the former case, the traction on the attached placenta simply pulls the uterus inside out, while in the latter the hand pushes the relaxed muscular sac inside out. The umbilical cord *never* should be pulled on, and the uterus *never* should be pushed upon unless it is firmly contracted.

MULTIPLE PREGNANCY

When two or more embryos develop in the uterus at the same time, the condition is known as multiple pregnancy. Twins occur approximately once in every 54 births in the white race and once in every 39 births in nonwhite races. Triplets occur approximately once in 9,400 births;

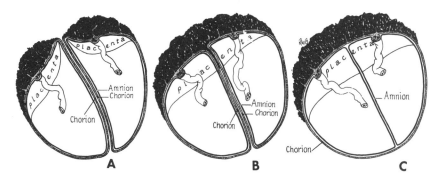

FIG. 20-8. Single- and double-ovum twin differences. A and B, double-ovum twins; there are two chorions; in B the two placentas have fused. C, single-ovum twins; there is only one chorion and one placenta.

and quadruplets, once in 620,000. These statistics have been altered somewhat due to the recent advancements in hormone therapy for infertility. Over 40 cases of quintuplets have been recorded, but with a few notable exceptions, none of these infants has survived more than a few weeks. The Dionne quintuplets, the most familiar case, were exceptional in that they were the first to live to adulthood.

Heredity plays an important causative role in twin pregnancy, and if there are twins in the family of either the expectant mother or her husband, the likelihood of twins is greater.

Twins may be of two kinds: identical and non-identical (fraternal). Identical twins *are* identical because they come from a single egg; hence they are called "single-ovum twins." Fertilization takes place in the usual way, by a single spermatozoon, but then, very early in the ovum's development, it divides into two identical parts instead of continuing as a single individual. Such twins are always of the same sex and, as we have implied, show close physical and mental resemblances. Nonidentical twins come from the fertilization of two ova by two spermatozoa and are therefore known as "double-ovum twins" (Fig. 20-7). Such twins, according to chance, may be of the same sex or of opposite sexes; and the likelihood of their resembling each other is no greater than that of any brother and sister.

Single-ovum twins have 1 placenta and 1 chorion, but there are normally 2 amnions and 2 umbilical cords (Fig. 20-8). In double-ovum twins each fetus has its own chorion, amnion, cord and placenta, but the placentas may be partially fused. These double-ovum twins are much the more common of the two types, making up about 85 per cent of all twins.

In the majority of instances (but not all) it is possible for the physician to make a diagnosis of twins by abdominal examination during the last few months; in doubtful cases, a roentgenogram may be necessary to settle the question. Twins are suspected whenever uterine size is greater than that which is ordinarily expected for any point in pregnancy. In addition, the palpation of three (or four) large parts in the uterus, the appearance of two fetal heart tones, of differing frequency, and the history of twins "running in the family" all serve to alert the obstetrician to the possibility of a multiple pregnancy.

Twins are likely to be born about 2 weeks before the calculated date of delivery. Even though pregnancy goes to full term, twins are usually smaller than single infants by nearly 1 pound; however, the outlook for such infants, provided that the pregnancy continues into the last month, is almost as good as that for single infants.

The patient with a multiple pregnancy faces greater discomforts and greater hazards than does a woman with a single pregnancy. The latter weeks of a twin pregnancy are likely to be associated with heaviness of the lower abdomen, back pains and swelling of the feet and the ankles. Abdominal distention makes sleeping difficult, and therefore the doctor may prescribe a hypnotic. A well-fitting maternity girdle will make daytime more comfortable for her. Because of the excessive abdominal size, the patient may find that frequent small feedings are more suitable than the usual three larger meals a day. The nurse can be very helpful in giving the mother anticipatory guidance regarding these matters during the antepartal period.

Moreover, there are serious complications which these patients are particularly prone to develop: premature labors, toxemia and postpartal hemorrhage. Coitus probably will be restricted during the last 3 months of pregnancy to mitigate against the possibility of early labor. Also travel will be curtailed, since labor may begin at any time without warning, and delivery in strange surroundings may be hazardous. The mother will be encouraged to take frequent afternoon rests and to avoid activities involving physical strain.

The antepartal course of these patients should be followed with special care for signs of toxemia. Thus, the mother's antepartal visits usually will be more frequent to ensure meticulous supervision. A low-salt diet and diuretics will be ordered when indicated. In addition, iron may be prescribed, since anemia is usual in multiple pregnancy.

Postpartal hemorrhage is twice as common in twin pregnancy, although mechanical difficulties in labor are less frequent than might be expected. Uterine dysfunction, however, is encountered rather often. A spontaneous delivery is particularly desired in instances of twins, since this type of delivery results in less blood loss and maternal morbidity and a greater likelihood of healthy, undamaged infants.

At delivery, when the first baby is born, the physician usually has to rupture the membranes of the second twin. Then with combined vaginal and abdominal manipulation, he turns the infant to either a breech or a vertex presentation. *Judicious* abdominal pressure is used to propel the presenting part through the birth canal and effect either a spontaneous delivery or forceps or breech extraction. Occasionally, a version and extraction (see p. 434) may be necessitated if the vaginal and abdominal maneuvers are unsuccessful.

As soon as the second twin is delivered, the doctor will order an oxytocic to be given, and the nurse should assist the obstetrician in observing the fundus carefully for distention due to an accumulation of blood. An intravenous infusion of glucose usually will be administered prophylactically. To guard against uterine atony and blood loss, after the placentae are expressed, oxytocin will be added to the infusion to ensure a firmly contracted uterus.

NURSING CARE. As with any delivery, the nurse will have the responsibility of supportive care for the patient as well as assisting the doctor in whatever activities are indicated. Since these infants are apt to be small, oxygen and/or resuscitative measures may be necessary. The care will be similar to that for the premature baby (see Chap. 17). Any supplies and/or equipment that may be needed (resuscitator, oxygen apparatus, etc.) should be procured early in the delivery and kept in readiness (but out of the patient's

sight, if possible). Maternal vital signs as well as the fetal heart tones should be checked frequently.

Two other points should be considered. Especially in the case of undiagnosed twins (i.e., the presence of twins is not discovered or suspected until labor and delivery), there is a decided psychological and economic (albeit somewhat delayed) shock to the parents. Emotionally, one additional child may be desired and acceptable; two may impose a burden, particularly if this pregnancy was to be "the last." The parents may wonder if they can manage the care of two newborn infants simultaneously. Problems may be compounded in feeding, especially if the mother is desirous of nursing her infant. In addition, two of everything must be provided, instead of one, and this additional cost may put a strain on the budget. In terms of long-range planning, the present housing may be inadequate, especially if the children are of different sexes and eventually will require separate rooms. The cost entailed in additional construction and/or new housing is considerable. None of these problems is insurmountable and can be worked through satisfactorily in time. Some parents need an understanding and empathic person to help them over the initial adjustment period. In some cases they may need the help of a social worker or a public health nurse to help them plan for the unexpected new baby. Many parents seem to adjust nicely with being able merely to ventilate their surprise (and, in some cases, chagrin). Certainly the professional nurse is able and qualified to give this type of support.

SUGGESTED READING

Barter, R. H.: Induction of labor: helpful or harmful. Postgraduate Med. 43:141-144, June, 1968.

Bruce, S.: Reactions of nurses and mothers to stillbirths. Nurs. Outlook 10:88-91, February, 1962.

Cope, E.: Induction of labour. Practitioner 198:207-216, February 1967.

Daly, J. W., and Gibbs, C. E.: Cord prolapse. Am. J. Obstet. Gynec. 100:264-266, January 15, 1968.

Eastman, N. J., and Hellman, L. M.: Williams' Obstetrics. ed. 13, New York, Appleton, 1966.

Farrell, P. J.: Rupture of the uterus. Am. J. Obstet. Gynec. 97:332-337, February, 1967.

Filler, W. W., Filler, N. W., and Zinberg, S.: Spareine sulfate in labor. Am. J. Gynec. 88:737-746, March 15, 1964.

Friedman, E. A.: Labor: Clinical Evaluation and Management. New York: Appleton, 1967.

Goodrich, F. W., Jr.: Obstetrical hemorrhage. Am. J. Nurs. 62:96-98, November, 1962.

Hutchinson, H. T., et al.: Effects of magnesium sulfate on uterine contractility, interauterine fetus, and infant. Am. J. Obstet. Gynec. 88:747-758, March 15, 1964.

Jeffcoate, T. N. A.: The causes of abnormal uterine action in labour. Aust. N.Z.J. Obstet. Gynaec. 5: 222-227, November, 1965.

Keettel, W. C.: Inducing labor by rupturing membranes. Postgrad. Med. 44:199-204, November, 1968.

Kempers, R. D.: The passenger in difficult labor. Postgrad. Med. 42:109-114, August, 1967.

Levine, M. E.: Adaption and assessment—a rationale for nursing intervention. Am. J. Nurs. 66:2450-2453, November, 1966.

Meltzer, R. M., et al.: Brow presentation. Am. J. Obstet. Gynec. 100:255-263, January 15, 1968.

Melber, R.: The nurse's role in obstetrical emergencies in the hospital setting. Nurs. Clin. N. Am. 2:261-269, June, 1967.

Morgan, H. S., and Kane, S. H.: An analysis of 16,327 breech births. J.A.M.A. 187:262-264, January 25, 1964.

Morrison, J. E.: Pathological anatomy of anoxia. Cereb. Palsy Bull. 3:559-565, December, 1961.

Müller, K., and Osler, M.: Induction of labor. A comparison of intravenous, intranasal and transbuccal oxytocin, Acta. Obstet. Gynec. Scand. 46, supp. 9:59-68, 1967.

Pinto, R. M., et al.: Action of estradiol 17 on activity of the pregnant human uterus. Am. J. Obstet. Gynec. 88:59-69, March 15, 1964.

Roberts, C. J.: Incidence of and relation between the common complications of pregnancy and delivery. Brit. J. Prev. Soc. Med. 23:128-131, May, 1969.

Schulman, H.: Prolonged and abnormal labor. Am. J. Obstet. Gynec. 95:732-742, July 1, 1955.

Skipper, J. K., et al.: Barriers to communication between patients and hospital functionaries. Nurs. Forum 11, No. 1:14-23, 1963.

Tucker, J. M.: Nursing care in obstetric hemorrhage. Am. J. Nurs. 62:98-99, November, 1962.

Windle, W. F.: Brain damage at birth. J.A.M.A. 206: 1967-1972, November 25, 1968.

21

Complications of the Puerperium

*Puerperal Infection • Pulmonary Embolism • Subinvolution of the Uterus
Hemorrhage (See Chap. 20) • Vulvar Hematomas • Disorders of the Breasts
Bladder Complications*

PUERPERAL INFECTION

When inflammatory processes develop in the birth canal postpartally, as the result of bacterial invasion of these highly vulnerable areas, the condition is known as puerperal infection. It is really a postpartal wound infection of the birth canal, usually of the endometrium. As is true of other wound infections, the condition often remains localized but may extend along various pathways to produce diverse clinical pictures. Febrile reactions of more or less severity are the rule, and the outcome varies according to the portal of entry, the type, the number and the virulence of the invading organisms, the reaction of the tissues and the general resistance of the patient.

Puerperal infection is one of the most common causes of death in childbearing. Frequently used (but less satisfactory) synonyms are puerperal fever, puerperal sepsis, puerperal septicemia and childbed fever.

Causative Factors

The vast majority of puerperal infections are caused by the streptococcus, but most of the well-known pathogenic bacteria—such as the staphylococcus, the colon bacillus and the Welch bacillus—may be responsible for the disease. The anaerobic streptococcus, of all the various strains of streptococci, has been found to be the most common causative agent of puerperal infection. This organism is often found in the vaginas of normal pregnant women and offers no symptomatology. Since these microbes are nonpathogenic, normal inhabitants of the birth canal, the determining factor in their becoming pathogenic appears to be trauma and devitalization of the maternal tissues. This finding bodes for greater gentleness and restraint during the labor and delivery process. It is to be remembered that hemorrhage at the time of labor or thereafter also takes its toll of maternal strength and tissue resource. Therefore, *hemorrhage and trauma during labor and delivery are to be considered the two main predisposing causes of puerperal infection.*

The late Dr. John Osborne Polak, of Brooklyn, N. Y., used to teach that there are "eleven direct causes" of puerperal infection—the 10 fingers and the nasopharynx. He meant by this that the attendants themselves are most likely to carry infection to the parturient uterus. The physician may inadvertently do so in two ways. In the first place, gloved and sterile though his hands may be during the vaginal examinations or the operative manipulations, he may carry bacteria already in the vagina upward into the uterus. In the second place, his hands and the instruments he uses may become contaminated by virulent streptococci as the result of droplet infection, dispersed by himself or some of the attendants, and in this manner he may be responsible for introducing bacteria into the birth canal. Even in modern obstetrics, the latter is a very common mode of infection, and unless the utmost vigilance is used in masking all attendants in the delivery room (both nose and mouth) and in excluding therefrom all persons suffering or recovering from an upper respiratory infection, it is a constant source of danger.

Although a less common means of transfer today than a few decades ago, careless physicians and nurses have been known to carry bacteria to the parturient from countless extraneous contacts—from other cases of puerperal infection, from suppurative postoperative wounds, from cases of sloughing carcinoma, from patients with scarlet fever, from infants with impetigo neonatorum, and from umbilical infections of the newborn. The physician himself may have the infection on his own person, such as an infected hangnail or felon.

Coitus late in pregnancy is more common than ordinarily believed and may introduce extraneous organisms to the birth canal or carry upward bacteria already present on the vulva or in the lower vagina.

During the second stage of labor, the chances of fecal matter being transferred to the vagina are great, another constant source of danger.

Following completion of the third stage of labor, the site of previous placental attachment is a raw, elevated area, deep red in color and about 4 cm. in diameter. Its surface is nodular, due to the presence of numerous gaping veins, many of which are occluded by clots. These form excellent culture media for bacteria. Furthermore, at this time, the condition of the entire endometrium is peculiarly favorable to bacterial invasion, since it is less than 2 mm. thick, is infiltrated with blood and presents numerous small wounds. Since the cervix rarely escapes some degree of laceration in labor, it is another ready site for bacterial invasion. Vulvar, vaginal and perineal wounds offer still other possible portals of entry.

Puerperal infection is much more likely to occur if the mother has had a traumatic labor or a postpartal hemorrhage. Therefore, hemorrhage and trauma must be regarded as important predisposing causes of this infection. Other causes in this respect are prolonged labor, prolonged rupture of the membranes, retention of placental tissue and pre-existing conditions, such as anemia, which lower the mother's general resistance to disease.

Prevention of Infection

The prevention of infection throughout the maternity cycle has been emphasized in foregoing sections as an important factor in the maintenance of health and the prevention of disease. During pregnancy, blood studies are done routinely and iron prescribed as necessary, not only for the immediate value but also because anemia predisposes to puerperal infection. A great deal of emphasis is placed on health teaching at this time, particularly in regard to general hygiene. The patient is advised to avoid all possible sources of infection. Some physicians advise against tub baths in the last weeks of pregnancy, because the bath water may introduce surface bacteria from the body into the vagina, particularly in multiparas. It is well for the nurse to recognize that this idea is still prevalent in many circles, although it is now believed to have little validity. The greatest hazard of tub baths in these last weeks of pregnancy arises because climbing in and out of the tub is awkward and sudden changes in balance might result in a fall and, thus, the likelihood of physical trauma. Coitus is usually avoided during the last two months of pregnancy, and vaginal douches after the fifth month. Contacts with upper respiratory infections should always be avoided.

During labor, care should be exercised to limit bacteria from extraneous sources. In the hospital, cleanliness and good housekeeping are imperative, but, nevertheless, individual care technique reduces the chance of contamination from other patients. Each patient should have all of "her own" equipment, which includes her own bedpan. This bedpan should be cleansed after each use and sterilized once a day. Scrupulous hand washing on the part of all personnel after contacts with each patient will do much to prevent the transfer of infection from one patient to another. The strictest rules should be enforced for surgical cleanliness during labor and delivery. No one with an infection of the skin or the respiratory tract should work in the maternity department. The nasopharynx of attendants is the most common source of contamination of the birth canal. Masks usually should be worn any time that the external genitalia are exposed for examination or treatments, in the labor room as well as in the delivery room. To be effective, masks must cover the nose and the mouth and be clean and dry; thus they must be changed frequently and should not hang around the neck when not in use.

During the puerperium the same careful precautions should be carried out. For many days following the delivery, the surface of the birth canal is a vulnerable area for pathogenic bacteria. The birth canal is well protected against the invasion of extraneous bacteria by the closed vulva, unless this barrier is invaded. Patients, therefore, are to be taught the principles of perineal hygiene and how to give themselves self-care. The nurse should remember never to use her fingers to separate the labia in giving perineal care, because this permits the cleansing solution to enter the vagina.

Types of Puerperal Infection

Generally speaking, puerperal infection can be divided into two main types: (1) *local lesion processes* and (2) *extensions of the original lesion process*. When a lesion of the vulva, the perineum, the vagina, the cervix or the endometrium becomes infected, the infection may remain localized in these wounds. However, the original inflammatory process may extend along the veins (the most common way) and cause thrombophlebitis and pyemia, or through the lymph vessels to cause peritonitis and pelvic cellulitis.

Lesions of the Perineum, the Vulva and the Vagina. These lesions are highly vulnerable areas for bacterial invasion in the early puerperium and so may become infected. The most common of these is a localized infection of a repaired perineal laceration or episiotomy wound. The usual symptoms are elevation of temperature, pain and sensation of heat in the affected area and burning on urination. The area involved becomes red and edematous, and there is profuse seropurulent discharge. If a wound of the vulva becomes infected, the entire vulva may become edematous and ulcerated. Infections involving the perineum, the vulva and the vagina cause the patient considerable discomfort and alarm. These local inflammatory processes seldom cause severe physical reactions, provided that good drainage is established, and the patient's temperature remains below 38.4° C. (101° F.). To promote good drainage, all stitches may be removed so that the surface is laid open. Because the drainage itself is a source of irritation and contamination, the wound must be kept clean and the perineal pads changed frequently. Care must be exercised in cleansing the wound to see that none of the solution runs into the vagina. It is understood, of course, that vaginal douches would never be given at this time. Treatments by such means as sitz baths or the perineal heat lamp are generally used for the relief of pain. Antibiotics or one of the sulfonamides is prescribed to combat the infection. If drainage is impaired, the patient not only will have more pain but also may have a chill, followed by a sudden elevation of temperature.

Endometritis. This is a localized infection of the lining membrane of the uterus. Bacteria invade the lesion, usually the placental site, and may spread to involve the entire endometrium. When endometritis develops, it usually manifests itself about 48 to 72 hours after delivery. In the milder forms the patient may have no complaints or symptoms other than a rise in temperature to about 38.4° C. (101° F.) which persists for several days and then subsides. On the other hand, the more virulent infections are often ushered in by chills and high fever, with a comparable rise in pulse rate. In the majority of severe cases the patient experiences a chilly sensation, or actual chills, at the onset and often complains of malaise, loss of appetite, headache, backache and general discomfort. It is not unusual for the patient to have severe and prolonged after-pains. The uterus is usually large and is extremely tender when palpated abdominally. The lochial discharge may be decreased in amount and distinguished from normal lochia by its dark brown appearance and foul odor. In some cases, particularly those caused by the hemolytic streptococcus, the lochia may be odorless. If the infection remains localized in the endometrium, it is usually over in about a week or 10 days. But when extension of the infection occurs to cause peritonitis, pelvic thrombophlebitis or cellulitis, the disease may persist for many weeks, often with dramatic temperature curves and repeated chills.

TREATMENT depends on the severity of the condition. Mild cases with temperature under 100° F. and no chills are best handled by simple measures. Fowler's position facilitates lochial drainage. Ergonovine 4 times daily for 2 days promotes uterine tone, and forced fluids provide additional support. However, isolation is desirable to protect other patients and to afford the mother greater rest. In this group it is unnecessary to discontinue breast-feeding.

In severe cases breast-feeding is discontinued not only because it exhausts the mother but also because it is usually futile in the presence of high fever. In addition to the routine measures, antimicrobial drugs may be indicated.

Pelvic Cellulitis, or Parametritis. This is an infection which extends along the lymphatics to reach the loose connective tissue surrounding the uterus. It may follow an infected cervical laceration, endometritis or pelvic thrombophlebitis. The patient will have a persistent fever and marked pain and tenderness over the affected area. The problem is usually unilateral but may involve both sides of the abdomen. As the process develops, the swelling becomes very hard and finally either undergoes resolution or results in the formation of a pelvic abscess. If the latter occurs, as the abscess comes to a point, the skin above becomes red, edematous and tender. Recovery is usually prompt after the abscess is opened.

Thrombophlebitis. This is an infection of the vascular endothelium with clot formation atttached to the vessel wall. It may be of two types: pelvic thrombophlebitis, an inflammatory process involving the ovarian and the uterine veins, or femoral thrombophlebitis, in which the femoral, the popliteal or the saphenous vein is involved. The latter type of thrombophlebitis has been spoken of as phlegmasia alba dolens (painful white inflammation) and also very frequently as "milk leg"—a term once given to the condition by physicians in the belief that it was due to the collection of milk in the affected leg. Early ambulation may be a factor in preventing this complication.

FEMORAL THROMBOPHLEBITIS. This condition presents a special group of signs and symptoms. It is a disease of the puerperium characterized by pain, fever and swelling in the affected leg. These symptoms are due to the formation of a clot in the veins of the leg itself, which interferes with the return circulation of the blood. When this condition develops, it usually appears about 10 days after labor, although it may manifest itself as late as the 20th day. As in all acute febrile diseases occurring after labor, the secretion of milk may cease when phlegmasia alba dolens develops.

The disease is ushered in with malaise, chilliness and fever, which are soon followed by stiffness and pain in the affected part. If it is in the leg, the pain may begin in the groin or the hip and extend downward, or it may commence in the calf of the leg and extend upward. In about 24 hours the leg begins to swell, and although the pain then lessens slightly, it is always present and may be severe enough to prevent sleep. The skin over the swollen area is shiny white in color.

The acute symptoms last from a few days to a week, after which the pain gradually subsides, and the patient slowly improves.

The course of the disease covers a period of 4 to 6 weeks. The affected leg is slow to return to its normal size and may remain permanently enlarged and troublesome.

The prognosis is usually favorable. However, in some of the very severe cases, abscesses may form and the disease may become critical and produce fatality. Since the clot tends to be attached to the vessel wall somewhat loosely, there is a tendency for the clot to dislodge and produce a pulmonary embolism which also is fatal in the majority of cases.

The treatment of femoral thrombophlebitis consists in rest, elevation of the affected leg, and analgesias as indicated for pain. Anticoagulants, such as Heparin and Dicumarol, may be prescribed to prevent further formation of thrombi. Antimicrobial drugs may be used in the cases where more generalized infection is known or suspected. A "cradle" is used to keep the pressure of the bedclothes off the affected part. Some physicians prefer to use a light in the cradle believing that the heat promotes comfort. Others use icebags along the course of the affected vessels. Surgical treatment may be indicated in some severe and/or nonresponding cases and consists of incision of the affected vessel, removal of the clot, and repair of the vessel. Ligation of the major vessels is sometimes resorted to as a preventive measure for pulmonary embolism. Under no circumstances should anyone rub or massage the affected part. The leg should be handled with the utmost care when changing dressings, applying a bandage, making the bed or giving a bath. As the acute stage subsides, nourishing food and the most carefully regulated hygienic conditions are needed to build up the patient's strength. As recovery is usually tedious, skillful nursing care is required to preserve the tissues of the body.

PELVIC THROMBOPHLEBITIS. This is a severe complication in the puerperium. The onset usually occurs about the 2nd week following delivery with severe repeated chills and dramatic swings in temperature. The infection is usually caused by anaerobic streptococci, and although it is difficult to obtain a positive blood culture, bacteria are present in the blood stream during chills. Antimicrobial therapy is used, and is effective in treating most strains of this organism; as long as the chills and the fever persist, blood transfusions may be given. Heparin and Dicumarol may be prescribed to prevent the formation of more thrombi. A further problem is likely to arise with metastatic pulmonary complications, such as lung abscesses or pneumonia.

These patients are often depressed, discouraged and feel physically unwell. Their nursing may have been interrupted and all of the great emotional and physiological changes discussed in Chapter 15 are compounded by the illness. Astute nursing care at this time is particularly essential.

Accurate observing, recording and reporting, and paying particular attention to details of the physical care aspects are extremely important in helping to resolve the disorder and to prevent further complications. Supportive care to help the mother (and family) work through the depression and discouragement is another crucial aspect of care. The principles outlined in the discussion of grief are appropriate here.

Peritonitis. Peritonitis is an infection, either generalized or local, of the peritoneum. Here, as a rule, the infection reaches the peritoneum from the endometrium by traveling via the lymphatic vessels; but peritonitis may result also from the extension of thrombophlebitis or parametritis. The clinical course of pelvic peritonitis resembles that of surgical peritonitis. The patient has a high fever, rapid pulse and, in general, has the appearance of being profoundly ill. She is usually restless and sleepless and has constant and severe abdominal pain. Hiccups, nausea and vomiting, which is sometimes fecal and projectile, may be present. Antimicrobial therapy is given to combat the infection, analgesic drugs for discomfort and mild sedative drugs to relieve the restlessness and apprehension. If there is intestinal involvement, oral feedings are withheld until normal intestinal function is restored; meanwhile, fluids are administered intravenously. Blood transfusions and oxygen therapy may be indicated for supportive treatment. The record of intake and output must be kept, and, in order to be of value to the physician, the elimination of fluids from the skin by sweating should be estimated.

Signs and Symptoms

It is highly important that the nurse recognize and report early signs and symptoms of puerperal infection so that proper treatment may be instituted without delay. When puerperal infection develops, one of the first symptoms usually seen is a rise in temperature. Although temperature elevations in the puerperium may be caused by upper respiratory infections, urinary tract infections and the like, the majority are due to puerperal infection. Puerperal morbidity is the term used to include all puerperal fevers. The Joint Committee on Maternal Welfare in this country has defined puerperal morbidity as a "temperature of 100.4° F. (38° C.), the temperature to occur on any two of the first ten days postpartum, exclusive of the first 24 hours, and to be taken orally by a standard technique at least four times daily." The symptoms may vary, depending on the loca-

tion and the extent of the infectious process, the type and the virulence of the invading organisms and the general resistance of the patient. The affected area is usually painful, reddened and edematous and the source of profuse discharge. The patient may complain of malaise, headache and general discomfort. As mentioned above, the temperature is elevated, and in the more severe infections, chills and fever may occur. In its typical form each of the clinical types of puerperal infection presents a very characteristic set of signs and symptoms, although occasionally one form of the disease is combined with another. The distinctions between these different types of infections are of importance, because the clinical course, the treatment and the prognosis depend on the particular form of infection. For this reason these aspects of the various puerperal infections have been discussed in the preceding pages.

Treatment

The use of the sulfonamides and antibiotic therapy has brought about radical changes in the treatment and the prognosis of puerperal infection. These drugs are effective in combating most of these infections, but, nevertheless, the management and the care of patients with puerperal infections are highly important and demand the utmost in skill. Penicillin is effective against the hemolytic streptococcus, the Welch bacillus and the staphylococcus. Since penicillin is not effective against the colon bacillus and certain strains of staphylococci, sulfadiazine or Gantrisin (sulfisoxazole) and/or a broad spectrum antibiotic may be prescribed for infections caused by these organisms. Resistant staphylococcal infections are often vulnerable to erythromycin used in conjunction with Gantrisin. Many types of antimicrobials exist these days, some specifically for the gram positive or negative organisms, and the penicillin resistant organisms; therefore, the physician has a wide range of products in his armamentarium upon which to draw. The selection and dosage of these drugs will depend upon the severity of the disease and the type of offending organism. Sensitivity series often will be done to help determine the above. Wound cultures are frequently taken to gain information about the organism; and in severe cases blood cultures may be taken, but if they are to be of real diagnostic value they must be taken at the time of the chill. The infected lesions are treated the same as those of any surgical wound. Drainage must be established, and since this discharge is of a highly infectious nature, care must be taken to see that it is not spread, and that all contaminated pads and dressings are wrapped and burned.

The curative treatment, of course, will be directed by the physician, but good nursing care is essential. The patient should be kept as comfortable and quiet as possible, for sleep and rest are important. Conserving the patient's strength in every way, giving her nourishing food, increased amounts of fluids, fresh air and sunshine will help to increase her powers of resistance. To promote drainage the head of the bed should be kept elevated, a measure which also contributes to the patient's comfort.

Care must be exercised to prevent the spread of the infection from one patient to another. Isolation of infected patients from others is desirable in order to protect the healthy maternity patients. Ideally, the patient with puerperal infection should be away from the maternity divisions. If it is impossible to arrange for such complete segregation, the nurse must consider every patient with puerperal infection as "in isolation" and follow scrupulous technique accordingly. Regardless of the situation, the nurse who is caring for a patient with puerperal infection (or any infection, for that matter) should not attend other maternity patients. The hands of all attendants need special attention and should be scrubbed thoroughly after caring for a mother who has an infection. In certain cases strict isolation technique, with special gowns, masks and rubber gloves, is essential. Clean isolation gowns, masks and gloves should be available for all persons who attend the isolated patient and after being used should be left in the room and disposed of in special hampers or containers. Under no circumstances should this apparel be worn outside the patient's room. Since it is assumed that the nurses who care for these patients are fully acquainted with principles of good isolation technique, this aspect of care will not be pursued further here.

PULMONARY EMBOLISM

Pulmonary embolism is usually due to the detachment of a small part of a thrombus which is washed along in the blood current until it becomes lodged in the right side of the heart. In many cases the thrombus originates in a uterine or a pelvic vein, although its origin may be in some other vessel. When the embolus occludes the pulmonary artery, it obstructs the passage of blood into the lungs, either wholly or in part, and the patient may die of asphyxia within a few minutes. If the clot is small, the initial episode may not be fatal, although repeated attacks may prove so. The condition may follow infection, thrombosis, severe hemorrhage or shock, and it may occur any time during the puerperium, especially after sudden exertion.

Symptoms. The symptoms of pulmonary embolism are sudden intense pain over the heart; severe dyspnea; unusual apprehension; syncope; feeble, irregular or imperceptible pulse; pallor in some cases, cyanosis in others; and eventually air hunger. Death may occur at any time from within a few minutes to a few hours, according to the amount or degree of obstruction to the pulmonary circulation. If the patient survives for a few hours, it is likely that she may recover.

Treatment. The treatment consists, first of all, in preventing the accident by careful attention to all details of surgical asepsis and to the proper management of labor and delivery. Following delivery, early ambulation may be an additional prophylactic measure, since circulatory stasis is undoubtedly a causative factor. In some instances it is almost impossible to prevent a fatal attack, because the patient may be recovering without elevation of temperature and without complications and yet, on the 7th or 10th day, suddenly cries out, passes into a coma and succumbs.

When embolism occurs, rapid emergency measures to combat anoxia and shock must be carried out promptly. Oxygen is administered without delay, and anticoagulants are given. Morphine may be helpful to relieve the patient's apprehension and usually is given. It is essential that the patient be kept absolutely quiet and on her back, for the slightest movement may cause fatal results. If the patient survives the attack, absolute rest is mandatory, in the hope that meanwhile the clot may be absorbed. Dicumarol and Heparin therapy will be continued to prevent recurrent emboli. During this time the patient must be kept warm, quiet, comfortable and as free from worry as possible. She may be given a light, nourishing diet during early convalescence.

SUBINVOLUTION OF THE UTERUS

Subinvolution is the term used to describe the condition which exists when normal involution of the puerperal uterus is retarded. The causes contributing to this condition may be (1) lack of tone in the uterine musculature, (2) imperfect exfoliation of the dicidua, (3) retained placental tissue and membranes, (4) endometritis and (5) presence of uterine fibroids. Subinvolution is characterized by a large and flabby uterus; lochial discharge prolonged beyond the usual period, sometimes with profuse bleeding; backache and dragging sensation in the pelvis; and disturbance of general health until corrected. Since this abnormality is the result of local conditions, an important phase of the treatment rests in correcting the causative factor. Oxytocic medication, such as methergine or ergonavine, may be administered to maintain uterine tone and prevent the accumulation of clots in the uterine cavity. Curettage is employed to remove any retained placental tissue or secudines. Endometritis will require antimicrobial therapy. If the uterus is displaced, it may delay normal involution and is usually corrected by a suitably fitting pessary.

Early ambulation is believed to have decreased the incidence of subinvolution. And, since it is recognized that breast-feeding stimulates uterine contractions, the fact that the mother is *not* breast-feeding plus the fact that she is usually taking a lactogenic supressing drug, may be influencing factors when subinvolution occurs.

HEMORRHAGE

These complications are discussed in Chapter 20.

VULVAR HEMATOMAS

Blood may escape into the connective tissue beneath the skin covering the external genitalia or beneath the vaginal mucosa to form vulvar and vaginal hematomas, respectively. The condition occurs about once in every 500 to 1,000 deliveries. These hematomas may develop shortly after labor, but more frequently they occur in the first few days of the puerperium. Vulvar hematomas manifest themselves by severe perineal pain and the sudden appearance of a tense, fluctuant and sensitive tumor of varying size covered by discolored skin. When the mass develops in the vagina, it may temporarily escape detection but pain and the patient's inability to void should alert the nurse to this complication. Since these symptoms also may be indicative of other types of complications, the nurse will want to make a careful examination of the perineum so that she may make an accurate report to the physician. As we have already seen the new parturient has

great difficulty in localizing any pain that she may have. Therefore the nurse usually will have to explore with the mother as to the nature and location of her discomfort, gradually moving from more general statements to those which are specific and more accurate. When the doctor has been informed of the situation, he will undoubtedly perform a vaginal examination which confirms the diagnosis. Small hematomas are usually treated supportively and allowed to resolve of their own accord. However, if the pain is severe or the tumor enlarges, incision and evacuation of the blood, with ligation of bleeding points, will be required.

DISORDERS OF THE BREAST

Certain aspects of many of the following subjects have been presented in Chapters 14 and 15. Here the discussion is centered on complications.

Engorgement of the Breasts

Any time after the 3rd postpartal day, after lacteal secretion has been established, engorgement of the breasts may occur. The onset is usually rapid, and, as the breasts become distended, dilated veins may be visible under the skin, and on palpation the breasts feel hard and nodular. This condition, commonly called "caked breasts" by the laity, is likely to occur in mothers who are breast-feeding as well as in those who are not. At one time it was believed that this was brought about because the lobules of the breast gland became overdistended with milk, but engorgement is really an exaggeration of the normal venous and lymph stasis of the breasts which occurs in relation to lactation (see The Breasts in Chap. 14). The breasts become tense and swollen for a day or so, with the result that the mother experiences throbbing breast pains which may extend into the axilla. The breasts are sometimes so immensely distended and painful that some analgesic medication, such as codeine, may be required. The condition may be relieved by supporting the breasts properly with a firm uplift breast binder or brassière, worn day and night, and by applying icecaps at intervals over the affected areas. When the breasts are well supported, they are not only more comfortable but also, if pendulous, the support aids in preventing congestion caused by the interference with the circulation (see Fig. 15-6). Immediate treatment of engorged breasts is important, because if the condition is allowed to persist, it may threaten the nursing mother's future milk supply. With prompt attention the engorgement usually subsides after 24 to 48 hours. If the mother is breast-feeding, the regular emptying of the breasts by suckling and adequate breast care then will be all that is necessary.

The mother who is desirous of breast-feeding may have additional problems when she is trying to nurse her infant. Because of the fullness of the breasts and the simultaneous flattening of the nipple, the infant may be unable to get a proper grasp on the areola and nipple. Sometimes the use of the breast pump [at very low pressure,] for only a few minutes prior to the feeding will bring the nipple out sufficiently to permit the infant to grasp it. It must be remembered that too vigorous use of the breast pump or frequent and prolonged nursing periods are irritating to the breast, as well as highly discomforting to the mother. When the engorgement is pronounced, it may be helpful to apply hot compresses to the breasts for about 15 minutes before the nursing period.

Drying Up the Breasts

When the mother is not breast-feeding, for one reason or another, measures are usually taken to inhibit lacteal secretion. This is discussed in Chapter 15.

Abnormalities in Mammary Secretion

It is obvious to the nurse who has had experience taking care of new mothers and their infants that there are marked individual variations in the amount of milk secreted by the breast in almost every case. In most instances it depends on the degree of development of the glandular portions of the breast rather than on the individual's general health or the physical appearance of these organs. A mother with large, well-formed breasts may be eager to breast-feed her infant but produces such a meager quantity of breast milk that she is unable to do so. On the other hand, another mother with small, flat breasts may have a remarkably good milk supply and be able to suckle her infant successfully. Obese women with exceedingly large breasts, the bulk of which is fatty tissue, usually do not have a good supply of breast milk for their infants.

When there is an absolute lack of mammary secretion, the condition is called *agalactia*. This condition rarely occurs and is seldom seen. As a rule, there is at least a small amount of mammary secretion, but it is so scant that, despite all efforts to stimulate lactation, the quantity would be inadequate to supply the nourishment required for the infant. Since in the latter instance it is a case of hyposecretion rather than an absolute lack of it, perhaps in time it will be more properly called hypogalactia. One point should be made clear here. When one speaks of abnormalities in mammary secretions, this does not refer to temporary episodes which may momentarily affect lactation but in no way affect the mother's ability to continue with breast-feeding. For example, many new mothers, especially primiparas, who have been breast-feeding their infants quite successfully in the hospital find that when they are discharged home there is a sudden diminution in their milk supply. More than likely this is due to the anxiety and fatigue involved with the experience, because once they are settled and rested at home, the milk supply usually resumes normally. This happens so frequently, in fact, that the nurse will want to apprise the mother of this possibility and include planning for adequate household organization and rest for the mother as part of her regular postpartum counseling.

Occasionally the other extreme in lactation is observed (i.e., the mammary secretion is excessive, so-called *polygalactia*). When this secretion is so copious that it constantly leaks from the nipples, it is called *galactorrhea*. The latter condition is not common, but when it does occur, it may be hazardous to the mother's health if it continues over a prolonged period. The condition is best treated by measures which are similar to those used to "dry up the breasts." In addition, the failure to empty the breasts completely at each feeding may help to check the excessive secretion.

Abnormalities of the Nipples

Variations in what is considered to be normal in the nipple, which is cylindrical in shape and projects well beyond the center of the areolar surface, are not unusual and present no difficulty until the mother wants to breast-feed her infant. The *flat nipple* (i.e., a slightly rounded projection above the breast surface) or the *depressed nipple* (i.e., one which is slightly depressed below the breast surface) are difficult for the infant to grasp with its mouth. The *inverted nipple* is the most pronounced variation, because this nipple is actually inverted, and in this state it is impossible for the infant to grasp it. When these abnormalities exist, the mother should begin corrective measures during pregnancy, such as described by Hoffman (p. 155). Afterward, the use of an electric breast pump or a rubber nipple shield at the beginning of each nursing period may be of value to help draw the nipple out. This may require considerable patience and persistence on the part of the mother, but with encouragement and help from the nurse, she may be successful. However, a real danger may arise if persistent efforts at breast-feeding are attempted and are unsuccessful, because the breasts become engorged and/or the nipples become sore, with resultant fissures or erosions on the surface. These raw, cracked surface areas make breast-feeding a very painful experience for the mother and, moreover, provide a portal of entry for pathogenic bacteria which may give rise to mastitis.

Mastitis

Mastitis, or inflammation of the breast, may vary from a "simple" inflammation of the tissues around the nipple to a suppurative process which results in abscess formation in the glandular tissue. Mastitis is always the result of an infection, usually caused by *Staphylococcus aureus* or hemolytic streptococcus organisms. The disease in most instances is preceded by fissures or erosions of the nipple or the areola, which provide a portal of entry to the subcutaneous lymphatics, although under conducive conditions organisms present in the lactiferous ducts can invade the tissues and cause mastitis.

Symptoms. Puerperal mastitis may occur any time during lactation but usually occurs about the 3rd or 4th week of the puerperium. There is usually marked engorgement of the breast preceding mastitis, although engorgement per se does not cause the infection. When the infection occurs, the patient complains of acute pain and tenderness in the breast and often experiences general malaise, a chilly sensation or, in fact, may have a chill followed by a marked rise of temperature (to 105°) and an increased pulse rate. On inspection the breast appears hard and reddened. The obstetrician should be notified at once and treatment instituted promptly in the hope that resolution may take place before the infection becomes localized as an abscess.

Treatment. Puerperal mastitis is preventable, for the most part, by prophylactic measures. An important measure is initiated when the expectant mother learns about breast hygiene and begins to take special care of her breasts during the latter months of pregnancy (see Chap. 8). After delivery, appropriate breast care will further help to prevent the development of lesions, but if they do occur, proper treatment must be given promptly. Any time the mother complains of sore, tender nipples, they should be inspected immediately. At this time there may be no break in the surface, but if the condition is neglected, the nipple may become raw and cracked. The alert nurse often can detect even a very small crack in the surface of the nipple if she inspects it carefully. Once a break in the skin occurs, the chances of infection mount, because pathogenic organisms are frequently brought to the breast by the hands or may reach the breast from the patient's nightgown or bedclothes.

With early treatment by antibiotics or chemotherapeutic agents, the inflammatory process may be brought under control before suppuration occurs. Penicillin or a broad spectrum antibiotic is effective in treating acute puerperal mastitis if the therapy is started promptly, and often symptoms subside within 24 to 48 hours. The breasts should be well supported with a firm breast binder or well fitted brassière. While the breasts are so painful, small side pillows used for support may give the mother some measure of comfort. Icecaps may be applied over the affected part, but if in time it becomes apparent that suppuration is inevitable, heat applications may be ordered to hasten the localization of the abscess. Most obstetricians advise that breast-feeding be discontinued immediately in cases of mastitis.

If the treatment outlined above is unsuccessful, measures will have to be taken to remove the pus when abscess formation occurs. The obstetrician may prefer in some cases to aspirate the pus rather than resort to incision and drainage. When incision and drainage are done, the abscess should be well walled off. The operation is performed under general anesthesia, so the nurse must prepare the patient for surgery accordingly. In operating the incision is made radially, extending from near the areolar margin toward the periphery of the gland, in order to avoid injury to the lactiferous ducts. After the pus is evacuated, a gauze drain is inserted. Following the operation the care of the patient is essentially the same as that for a surgical patient. Complete recovery is usually prompt.

Epidemic Puerperal Breast Abscess

During the last decade a type of puerperal breast abscess has been seen, both in this country and abroad, which is unlike the type described above. In this new manifestation the offending organism is also *Staphylococcus aureus,* but an antibiotic-resistant strain which has been identified by bacteriophage typing as 52/42B/80/81 and called the "epidemic" strain. Another difference is related to the portal of entry of these microorganisms. In these cases there is no history of nipple lesions, and the infection is introduced through apparently normal lactiferous ducts in the breast, not through the connective tissue. An infant who has been exposed to the epidemic strain of the staphylococcus, and has the organisms present in his nose and throat, can introduce the infection to the mother's breast in the process of nursing. Once these organisms are introduced into the mother's breast, milk provides a superb culture medium for them. Efforts to prevent puerperal mastitis cannot be limited to the care of the mother's breasts but must extend to the hospital nursery, where the infant may acquire the virulent organism. In the nursery such equipment as soap-solution containers, cribs, mattresses, blankets, linens and floors can harbor the organisms. Some methods to help control the spread of infection at its source include rigid nursery aseptic technique on the part of all personnel, measures to prevent the spread of organisms from infant to infant, such as proper spacing of cribs, and the exclusion of carriers from the maternity divisions as soon as they are identified. It should be remembered that in maternity hospitals the nasopharynx of newborn infants tends to become readily infected with *Staphylococcus aureus,* and, moreover, the infection may persist for some weeks after the infant leaves the hospital. Where intensive studies have been carried out and puerperal mastitis or breast abscess appeared after discharge from the hospital, the cultures of the mothers' nares on admission to the hospital did not show evidence of the epidemic strain of the organism. In these cases the infants were the source of infection, because the offending organism was cultured from the nose, the throat and the skin of the infants. The routine pHisoHex infant bath now recommended by the American Academy of Pediatrics has helped greatly in cutting down the amount of colonization in the newborn.

Symptoms. The symptoms of epidemic puerperal breast abscess develop slowly and subtly and usually appear about the 3rd or the 4th week after delivery. The condition is characterized by high fever; the breast becomes very tender, swollen and indurated and suppurates rapidly. The surface of the breast may not be consistently reddened because the abscess is often deep. In some cases the infection may involve more than one portion of the breast, or both breasts.

Treatment and Care. The underlying principles for the care of this form of breast abscess are essentially the same as those described in puerperal mastitis. Breast-feeding should be discontinued immediately, for obvious reasons. Since the offending organism here is antibiotic-resistant, the effects of antibiotic therapy are of questionable value. Nearly all of these infections are susceptible to chloramphenicol, erythromycin and bacitracin but have identical antibiotic sensitivity with resistance to tetracycline, streptomycin and penicillin. The staphylococcus develops antibiotic resistance easily. In the beginning, the treatment of these infections with erythromycin usually resulted in prompt improvement in the condition, but now erythromycin-resistant strains of coagulase-positive staphylococci have been isolated from infections of mothers and their infants. When suppuration occurs in the breast, incision and drainage are usually done as soon as localization of the abscess becomes evident, in order to limit the extent of tissue destruction. When this has been done, special measures must be employed for the control of infection. To protect the surrounding area of the breast, it should be washed with a soap containing hexachlorophene, because such cleansing reduces the occurrence of staphylococci to some degree. This soap is also advocated for hand washing and baths. When warm moist applications to the wound are prescribed, vigilance and care must be exercised so that the underlying skin does not become macerated. Aside from the unnecessary discomfort that this would cause the mother, such maceration would provide another portal of entry for microorganisms. When such infections occur, either in the mother or her infant, the nurse should emphasize health teaching in her care of the mother, not only concerning hygienic measures for the prevention of skin infections but also the urgency for prompt treatment of any member of the family if carbuncles, boils, burns or other skin lesions develop.

The *epidemiologic aspects* of antibiotic-resistant infections of infants and their mothers are far-reaching and a major problem, because when these infections occur, nearly all the hospitals in the community may be affected for varying periods of time. A few years ago this was considered a "hospital" infection, but now it may be found throughout a general community. Once the organism is introduced into a family, this organism can be the cause of disease in the family over a long period of time. For example, the infant may acquire the infection in the maternity nursery, 4 weeks later the mother may develop a breast abscess, and 5 months later the father may develop a boil—all caused by this epidemic strain of staphylococcus. Flaws in nursery "clean technique" in hospital nurseries have long been cited as the cause of spreading skin infections in the newborn, but when these epidemic infections have occurred in hospital nurseries, and the staff has scrutinized their technique and improved it whenever possible, the results have not been as gratifying as one would hope for, because the epidemics have disappeared and appeared again after a period of time. In fact, large numbers of infections have occurred despite meticulous nursery technique. It must be remembered that these infections are not confined to the maternity service but may be spread by carriers to or from other clinical services in the hospital as well as to other members of the family and the community. The infection is thought to be airborne and is easily spread by droplet contamination from the nasopharynx of carriers of these microorganisms. Scrupulous technique in giving patient care in the hospital is undoubtedly an important factor in prevention and control, both in the nurseries or on postpartal divisions, but this alone will not solve the problem. Washing with hexachlorophene has already been mentioned as a means to reduce the occurrence of staphylococcal infections, but this has not reduced the colonization of the organisms in the nasopharynx of individuals. The housekeeping functions which are routine in every institution are of vast importance, both from the standpoint of procedure and personnel, and should be investigated and improved as much as possible. The nurse will find it advantageous to pursue the current literature regarding antibiotic-resistant staphylococcal infections, because there is a wealth of information in the professional journals, and space here does not permit an adequate discussion of the subject. Some references have been listed in the Suggested Reading at the end of this chapter.

BLADDER COMPLICATIONS

The two most common bladder complications in the puerperium are retention of urine and residual urine. In the former, the patient is unable to void at all; in the latter, she is able to void certain amounts of urine but is unable to empty the bladder. If these conditions are allowed to persist, then infection of the bladder (cystitis) and/or the kidneys (pyelitis) may develop.

The nurse will remember that the overhydration of the mother that was necessary for the growth and development of the fetus during pregnancy diminishes rapidly after delivery. The two main avenues for the diminution of the circulating blood volume are the skin and the kidneys. Consequently, the newly delivered mother perspires copiously and excretes large quantities of urine within 24 to 48 hours of delivery. As much as *500 cc. to 1000 cc.* may be voided at *each* urination; that is, as we know, 2 to 3 times what is usual in the nonparturient. The nurse will want to be particularly careful of bladder hygiene at this time because of the above increase in urinary production and the danger of overdistention. Thus, she will not wait for any designated time to elapse to indicate when the bladder should be emptied; rather she will observe for evidence indicating the degree of bladder distention, because the bladder may fill in a shorter span of time than has been specified. This fact should be reported to the physician if the patient is unable to void since a catheterization order will be needed.

Retention of urine, or the inability to void, is more frequently seen after operative delivery. It often lasts 5 or 6 days but may persist for 2 weeks or longer. The main cause is probably due to edema of the trigone muscle, which may be so pronounced that it obstructs the urethra. Very temporary urinary retention may be due to the effects of analgesia and anesthesia received in labor. As already stressed, the nurse should make every effort to have the patient void within 6 hours after delivery (see Chap. 15). If the patient has not done so within 8 hours, the physician usually will order catheterization. In some hospitals this is routine if voiding has not occurred within 8 hours postpartum.

Because of the trauma of labor and/or operative delivery the bladder usually is not as sensitive to distention as it was prior to pregnancy and delivery. Overdistention and incomplete emptying may occur; thus, the problem of residual urine frequently results. Repeated catheterization may be necessary for several days although in these persistent cases, the physician may request that an indwelling catheter be inserted which will provide constant drainage.

When the mother continues to void small amounts of urine at frequent intervals, the nurse may suspect that these voidings are merely an overflow of a distended bladder, and that there is residual urine there. The physician will order catheterization for residual urine, and, to be completely accurate, this must be done within 5 minutes after the patient voids. If 60 cc. or more of urine still remains in the bladder after the patient has voided, it is usually considered that the voiding has been incomplete. It is not uncommon for the catheterization to yield 800 cc. or more of residual urine. Large amounts of urine (from 60 to 1,500 cc., as shown by catheterization) may remain in the bladder, even though the patient may think she has completely emptied her bladder when she voided. The condition is due primarily to lack of tone in the bladder wall and is more likely to occur when the mother's bladder has been allowed to become overdistended during labor. A distended bladder requires prompt attention because of the resultant trauma; moreover, it may be a predisposing cause of postpartal hemorrhage.

In many cases of residual urine the patient is without symptoms other than scanty urination, but in others there may also be suprapubic or perineal discomfort. The treatment of this condition is usually confined to catheterization after each voiding until the residual urine becomes less than 30 cc. as previously stated; in severe cases constant drainage by means of an indwelling catheter may be employed.

The normal bladder is very resistant to infection, but when stagnant urine remains in a traumatized bladder, and infectious organisms are present, there is danger of cystitis. When cystitis occurs, the patient often has a low-grade fever, frequent and painful urination and marked tenderness and discomfort over the area of the bladder. The physician will order a catheterized specimen of urine for microscopic examination, and if pus cells are present in association with residual urine, the diagnosis of cystitis is confirmed. Since it is important in the presence of bladder infection to avoid accumulations of stagnant urine in the bladder, an indwelling bladder catheter may be inserted. In addition, chemotherapeutic agents are prescribed, and fluids should be forced.

If the infection spreads and involves the ureters and kidneys, the patient has a high fever and chills and a good deal of pain over the affected kidney(s). Diagnosis and treatment are essentially the same as for cystitis.

It will be the nurse's responsibility to obtain the urine specimens which are used for the microscopic examinations and occasionally cultures. The technique of catheterization already has been discussed in Chapter 15.

However, some physicians do not wish their patients catheterized, especially if the mother is having no particular difficulties in voiding. They feel that this procedure only enhances the possibility of promoting more infection. Therefore a "clean catch" specimen may be requested. Different terminology exists for this procedure in various parts of the country; but the procedure is essentially the same. It consists of the collection of a "clean" urine specimen that is uncontaminated by lochia. One method for this type of collection is as follows: The patient is requested not to void for at least 2 hours and to drink as much fluid as she can in the meantime. Then she is taken to the bathroom (or placed in a sitting position on a bedpan if she cannot ambulate) and the vulva and introitus are cleansed carefully with a solution of pHisoHex and water. A large sterile cotton ball is placed over the introitus. The mother is then requested to void a little urine forcefully into the toilet or bedpan; but *not to empty her bladder*. Next, a sterile urine specimen or sterile basin is placed under the stream and a specimen of urine is caught. It is sent to the laboratory for examination. Surprisingly, this method yields very good results with respect to uncontaminated specimens, if done carefully with the continued supervision of the nurse.

SUGGESTED READING

Baird, Sir D.: Combined Textbook of Obstetrics and Gynaecology. Edinburgh, Livingstone, 1969.

Bhose, L.: Postpartum eclampsia. Am. J. Obstet. Gynec. 89:898-902, August 1, 1964.

Boesky, D., *et al.*: Postpartum psychoses, Report of a clinical conference at the University of Michigan. Am. J. Obstet. Gynec. 80:1209-1217, December, 1960.

Bussche, G. V.: Treatment of postpartum bacteriuria with a combination of Kanamycin and Penicillin. Curr. Ther. Res. 10:432-440, September, 1968.

Carrington, E. R., and Sivak, A. M.: Epidemic puerperal breast abscess: I. Preventive and therapeutic aspects; II. Nursing care. Am. J. Nurs. 58:1683, 1958.

Daniels, R. S., *et al.*: Severe postpartum reactions; an interpersonal view. Psychosomatics 5:21-26, January-February, 1964.

Eastman, N. J., and Hellman, L. M.: Williams Obstetrics. ed. 13, New York, Appleton, 1966.

Eckerling, B., *et al.*: The use of hypothermia in puerperal sepsis. Int. Surg. 50:34-38, July, 1968.

Gibbs, C. E., and Misenhimer, H. R.: The use of blood transfusions in obstetrics. Am. J. Obstet. Gynec. 93:25-31, September 1, 1965.

Goodrich, F. W., Jr.: Obstetric hemorrhage. Am. J. Nurs. 62:96-98, November, 1962.

Greenhill, J. P.: Obstetrics. ed. 13, Philadelphia, W. B. Saunders, 1965.

Jewett, J. F., *et al.*: Childbed fever—a continuing entity. J.A.M.A. 206:344-350, October 7, 1968.

Leifer, G.: Rooming in despite post-partal complications. Am. J. Nurs. 67:214-219, October, 1967.

Paffenbarger, R. S.: Epidemiological aspects of parapartum mental illness. Brit. J. Preventive Med. 18:189-195, 1964.

Plueckhahn, V. D., and Banks, J.: Breast abscess and staphylococcal disease in a maternity hospital. Brit. Med. J. 2:414-418, August 15, 1964.

Qureshi, M. A., and Hafner, C. D.: Postpartum intestinal volvulus. Am. J. Obstet. Gynec. 89:1080-1081, August 15, 1964.

Ringrose, C. A. D.: A five-year study of massive obstetrical hemorrhage at the Royal Alexandra Hospital, Edmonton, 1958 through 1962. Am. J. Obstet. Gynec. 90:232-235, September 15, 1964.

Robson, J. S., *et. al.*: Irreversible post-partum renal failure. Quarterly J. Med. 37:423-435, July, 1968.

Southwick, H. W., *et al.*: Surgery of the Breast. Chicago, Year Book Medical Publishers, 1968.

Steiner, G. J., and Plasha, M. K.: Late postpartum eclampsia: report of a case. Obstet. Gynec. 24:594-596, October, 1964.

Thomas, W. O.: Postpartum hemorrhage and postpartum hematomas. Clin. Obstet. Gynec. 5:655-669, September, 1962.

Thompson, W. B., and Budd, J. W.: Erroneous diagnoses of amniotic fluid embolism. Am. J. Obstet. Gynec. 91:606-620, March 1, 1965.

Tucker, J. M.: Nursing care in obstetric hemorrhage. Am. J. Nurs. 62:98-99, November, 1962.

Tully, J. G., and Smith, L. G.: Postpartum septicemia with Mycoplasma hominis. J.A.M.A. 204:827-828, May 27, 1968.

Williams, B.: Sleep needs during the maternity cycle. Nurs. Outlook 15:53-55, February 1967.

Wysham, D. N., *et al.*: Staphylococcal infections in an obstetric unit: I. Epidemiologic studies of pyoderma neonatorum: II. Epidemiologic studies of puerperal mastitis. New Eng. J. Med. 257:304, 1957.

CONFERENCE MATERIAL

1. What provisions are made in regard to the care of the infant when the mother develops a puerperal infection in the hospital? At home? What are the implications for the nurse making a home visit?

2. As you consider the situation in which you are working, what measures could be instituted by the hospital or public health agency to further the prevention and the control of infection? What is the role of the nurse in this endeavor?

3. If the mother develops a rash 3 days after delivery and a diagnosis of scarlet fever has been made, what would you consider to be the method of managing this problem?

4. An infant has been exposed to infection caused by staphylococci of the epidemic strain while in the hospital nursery. What instructions should be given the mother concerning the prevention and the control of infection following their discharge from the hospital?

5. How do you account for the maternal mortality rate due to postpartal complications? What contribution can the nurse make toward improving these conditions?

6. If you have a patient whose pregnancy was complicated by cardiac disease (or tuberculosis, or syphilis or diabetes), and who is discharged from the hospital in satisfactory condition following delivery, what would be the responsibility of the hospital and the public health agency in the community for this patient's health supervision? Who has the responsibility for initiating referrals to related health agencies?

7. What routine procedures are employed in maternity care for the detection and the control of venereal disease? How would you go about finding out which states in the United States have legislation governing premarital and antepartal health examinations? What is the existing legislation in your state?

Study Questions

Unit Seven: Maternal Disorders Associated with the Childbearing Cycle

Read through the entire question and place your answer on the line to the right.

1. Which of the following signs and symptoms should the nurse anticipate when a pregnant patient has a history of heart disease?

    A. Dyspnea
    B. Slow pulse rate
    C. Decrease in blood pressure
    D. Hemorrhage

    Select the number corresponding to the correct letter or letters.
    1. A only
    2. B only
    3. A, C and D
    4. All of them

    _____

2. Which of the following factors influence the answer which you have given in Question No. 1?

    A. Increased need for oxygen intake
    B. Increased blood volume
    C. Toxic damage to the heart
    D. Failure of kidneys to excrete

    Select the number corresponding to the correct letters.
    1. A and B
    2. A and C
    3. B, C and D
    4. All of them

    _____

3. Which of the following signs and symptoms would the patient with a ruptured fallopian tube manifest?

    A. Hegar's sign
    B. Intense pain
    C. Profound shock
    D. Irregular fetal heart tones
    E. Vaginal bleeding

    Select the number corresponding to the correct letters.
    1. A and B
    2. A, C and D
    3. B, C and E
    4. B, D and E

    _____

4. Which of the following factors must exist before an erythroblastotic infant can be produced?

    A. Rh-negative mother
    B. Rh-positive father
    C. Rh-positive fetus

D. Rh-positive substance from the fetus must find its way into the mother's blood stream to build up antibodies.

E. Mother must have had a previous Rh-positive pregnancy or transfusion.

Select the number corresponding to the correct letters.

1. A and D
2. A, C and D
3. B, C and E
4. All of them   _____

5. Which of the following statements concerning diabetes complicated by pregnancy are correct?

A. The size of the placenta tends to be in direct relationship to the size of the infant.
B. Toxemia occurs more frequently than in nondiabetic pregnancies.
C. Deliveries are always performed by cesarean section, usually 2 weeks prior to term.
D. The fetus tends to be large.
E. Hypoglycemia occurs in the infant following delivery.

Select the number corresponding to the correct letters.

1. A and B
2. B, D and E
3. B, C, D and E
4. All of them   _____

6. Which of the following are causes of bleeding in the first and second trimesters of pregnancy?

A. Menstruation
B. Abortion
C. Abruptio placentae
D. Placenta previa
E. Ectopic pregnancy

Select the number corresponding to the correct letters.

1. A and B
2. A, B and D
3. A, B and E
4. B, C, D and E   _____

7. How is inevitable abortion distinguished from threatened abortion?

A. Dilatation of the cervical canal
B. Rupture of the membranes
C. Pain
D. Bleeding

Select the number corresponding to the correct letter or letters.

1. A only
2. B only
3. A, B and D
4. All of them   _____

8. What is the effect of tetanic contractions on the pregnant uterus?

A. Descent and rotation are hastened.
B. Ruptured uterus is imminent.
C. Fetal distress may occur.
D. Uterine inertia may follow.
E. Perineal lacerations may occur.

Select the number corresponding to the correct letter or letters.

1. A only
2. B only
3. A, C and D
4. B, C and E   _____

9. Insofar as the toxemias are concerned, which of the following symptoms during labor should be reported to the physician promptly?

A. Hard, painful uterine contractions
B. Epigastric pain
C. Dimness of vision
D. Headache
E. Decrease in urinary excretion

Select the number corresponding to the correct letters.
1. A, C and D
2. A, C and E
3. B, C and D
4. B, C, D and E   _____

10. Which of the following conditions contribute to postpartal hemorrhage?

A. Toxemias of pregnancy
B. Overdistention of the uterus due to twins or hydramnios
C. Unwise management of the third stage of labor
D. Involution
E. Retained placental fragments

Select the number corresponding to the correct letters.
1. A and C
2. A, B and D
3. B, C and E
4. All of them   _____

11. A patient in the first stage of labor develops secondary uterine inertia. Which of the following are important in the treatment of this condition?

A. Pitocin
B. Sedation
C. Fluids
D. Bed rest
E. Ambulation

Select the number corresponding to the correct letters.
1. A, B and D
2. A, C and E
3. B, C and D
4. B, C and E   _____

12. To which of the following causes may urinary tract infections during the puerperium be attributed?

A. Poor hygiene
B. Urinary retention
C. Uterine inertia
D. Subinvolution
E. Trauma sustained during delivery

Select the number corresponding to the correct letters.
1. A and B
2. A, B and E
3. B, D and E
4. All of them   _____

13. Which of the following are the chief dangers from sore, cracked nipples?

A. Infection of the infant from nursing
B. Invasion of bacteria resulting in abscess of the nipple
C. Invasion of bacteria through the nipple into the breast tissue

D. Formation of scar tissue which will prevent normal nursing thereafter

E. Formation of a permanent fissure in the nipple

Select the number corresponding to the correct letters.

1. A and C
2. B and C
3. B, D and E
4. B, C, D and E   _____

14. Which of the following veins is likely to be involved in puerperal thrombophlebitis?

A. Splenic vein

B. Popliteal vein

C. Renal vein

D. Ovarian vein

E. Saphenous vein

Select the number corresponding to the correct letters.

1. A, B and D
2. B, C and E
3. B, D and E
4. All of them   _____

15. In the spaces provided in Column 2, write the term or the phrase which best fits each statement in Column 1.

Column 1	Column 2
A. A suppurative process in the glandular structure of the breast	A._____
B. A localized infection of the lining membrane of the uterus	B._____
C. An infection of the loose connective tissue which surrounds the uterus	C._____
D. Failure of the puerperal uterus to be restored to its normal proportions as rapidly as expected	D._____
E. Exaggeration of the normal venous and lymphatic stasis of the breasts following the development of lacteal secretion	E._____

Note: The key to the correct answers to these questions is given on page 613.

UNIT EIGHT
Abnormalities of the Fetus and the Newborn

Fetal Diagnosis and Treatment

Disorders of the Newborn

Richard H. Schwarz, M.D., F.A.C.O.G.
*Associate Professor and Director of the
Jerrold L. Golding Division of Fetal Medicine,
Department of Obstetrics and Gynecology,
University of Pennsylvania School of Medicine*

Fetal Diagnosis and Treatment

22

Fetal Diagnosis and Treatment   Richard H. Schwarz, M.D.

Fetal Diagnosis   •   Specific Fetal Problems   •   Fetal Treatment

As recently as 20 years ago, evaluation of the fetus and its environment was virtually limited to the animal laboratory or the vivid imaginations of a few obstetricians. There were some exceptions such as the transabdominal aspiration of amniotic fluid, which was practiced before the turn of the century; but at that time, the procedure was used therapeutically, in cases of severe polyhydramnios. Amniography, an x-ray technique with radiopaque dye placed in the amniotic fluid, was introduced in 1930, but fell into disrepute because the dye used was irritating and caused premature labor. Thus, until recently, obstetricians relied almost entirely upon physical observations such as palpation and measurement of the uterus to assess fetal growth, and auscultation of the fetal heart tones to evaluate fetal distress. X-rays were used to determine fetal position and the presence of major bony abnormalities. However, little can be determined about fetal well-being from such a technique.

In the past decade, the amniotic cavity has been invaded with increasing frequency, and a battery of fetal diagnostics has been developed. But the practice of intrauterine medicine has advanced beyond diagnostics, now covering treatment and genetic assessment, as well. Although research is rapidly expanding and changing our knowledge about the subject, the following discussion will serve to indicate the present status of fetal medicine.

FETAL DIAGNOSIS

Physical Measurements

All obstetricians record the patterns of uterine growth in their prenatal records. Measurements of fundal height and estimates of fetal weight, although far from precise, serve to alert the obstetrician to failure of fetal growth or to causes of excessive size, such as twins or hydramnios. The validity of such observations is obviously related to the consistency of the observer and his accuracy.

Blood Studies

Several studies have been suggested as being useful in assessing pregnancy progress. Of all those tried, only the alkaline phosphatase of placental origin and diamine oxidase determinations have demonstrated some worth. Both display patterns of rising values during normal pregnancy; in the abnormal pregnancy, values rise at less than the expected rate, or not at all.

Physiologic Studies

If there is one area which one would most like to assess, it is the physiologic functions of the placenta in relation to the fetus. Unfortunately, at the present stage of technology, it is not possible clinically to measure oxygen and carbon dioxide or amino acid and carbohydrate transfer in the human. At least these things cannot be assessed until the fetal scalp or buttocks are available for blood sampling during labor. Gross attempts to evaluate this area have been made by using the radioisotope Sodium 24. It is injected intravenously, and the uptake over the uterus is measured. Correlations have been less than excellent; and because of concern about the use of radioactive substances, the technique is not clinically acceptable.

Fetal Electrocardiography

The first fetal ECG was accidentally recorded over half a century ago, but the practical use of the method has had to await technologic advances. The source of the technical difficulty

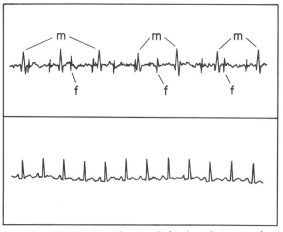

FIG. 22-1. Superimposed fetal and maternal ECG (smaller fetal components marked "f").

lies in the fact that the strength of the electrical activity of the fetal heart is so much less than that of the maternal heart that any approach except direct application of an electrode to the fetus is difficult to interpret. With electrodes applied to the maternal abdomen, one gets a superimposed maternal-fetal tracing (Fig. 22-1). Attempts to "subtract" the maternal tracing electronically with a computer are not practical at present. In order to apply an electrode directly to the fetus, the cervix must be dilated

and the membranes ruptured. With a direct electrode, a pure fetal ECG can be obtained, or the signal can be transformed by an electronic device called a cardiotachometer to give a numerical heart rate recording instead. This approach is the basis for the best available fetal monitoring systems. Very often the heart rate tracing is combined with an intrauterine pressure recording so that heart rate changes can be evaluated in relation to labor contractions. Although some attention has been paid to the pattern of the fetal ECG tracing, clinical usefulness of the ECG is limited to determining the rate and evaluating the patterns of rate change. The fetal heart rate recording may be used in conjunction with the administration of atropine or the breathing of reduced oxygen concentrations (12 per cent), in order to evaluate the adequacy of placental support. If the placenta is functioning well, atropine will quickly cross the placenta and speed the fetal heart rate; if the placenta is not functioning at its best, the rate will not change. Having the mother breathe reduced oxygen will cause a slowing of the fetal heart, if placental function is subnormal. If placental insufficiency is suspected because of past history, maternal complications, or because the fetus is not growing at a normal rate, it would be well to establish the adequacy of placental function and tolerance of the fetus for the stress of labor. This may be done

FIG. 22-2. Doppler probe being used to monitor fetal heart rate in a patient in labor.

FIG. 22-3. Abdominal x-ray showing a fetus with calcification of both the distal femoral and proximal tibial epiphyses (arrows).

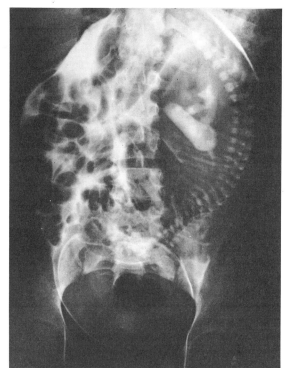

FIG. 22-4. Amniogram showing dye in the fetal G. I. tract.

through the initiation of uterine contractions by oxytocin infusion, while carefully monitoring the fetal heart rate. Each time a uterine contraction occurs, the pressure of the contraction is transmitted to the vessels supplying the placenta. If placental function is less than normal, fetal distress, as evidenced by a slowing heart rate, may occur.

Fetal Phonocardiography

The amplification of the fetal heart sounds by applying a microphone to the maternal abdomen has also been suggested as a means for monitoring the fetal heart rate. This system has the advantage of not requiring direct fetal contact, but it also has the disadvantage of amplifying other sounds (muscular, maternal heart, etc.) and of requiring accurate aiming of the microphone.

Doppler Probe

A low energy ultrasound flow probe is now commercially available (Fig. 22-2). This instrument has the capability of detecting fetal cardiac activity in very early pregnancy and also can be applied externally for fetal heart monitoring in late pregnancy and in labor. As is a phonocardiograph, this instrument is directionally sensitive, requires constant positioning, and picks up maternal as well as fetal pulses. It is, nonetheless, useful in detecting hard-to-hear fetal heart tones and also in localizing the placenta.

Fetal Electroencephalography

The fetal EEG can be recorded once the cervix is dilated and the membranes are ruptured; however, interpretation and clinical value are not established at this time.

Ultrasound

The use of ultrasonic measurements has been applied to the fetal head; since the biparietal diameter of the fetal head is related to fetal size and maturity, this technique has been applied not only when suspicion of cephalo-pelvic disproportion exists, but also when the maturity of the fetus is in doubt.

X-ray Studies

X-ray studies of the fetus are among the oldest approaches. Some of the x-ray changes in the

FIG. 22-5. Technique of amniocentesis indicating the direction of the needle in relation to the fetal position, to avoid fetal injury.

fetus occur only after fetal death and are not of prognostic value, except by their absence. On the other hand, the demonstration of calcification of distal femoral and/or proximal tibial epiphyses (Fig. 22-3) is a rather reliable positive indication of fetal maturity. However, the absence of calcification does not rule out maturity.

Measurements of the fetal head by x-ray (cephalometry) are notoriously unreliable, while measurements of the pelvis (pelvimetry) are more likely to be precise. Gross abnormalities of the fetus such as hydrocephalus and anencephalus are obvious, while many other malformations are not detectable.

In recent years, the technique of amniography has become popular. This involves the instillation of a water soluble radiopaque material into the amniotic fluid, which then outlines noncalcified structures such as the placenta, cord, soft tissue fetal anomalies, and uterine anomalies. In addition, the dye is swallowed by the healthy fetus and concentrated in its G. I. tract, thus performing a fetal G. I. series (Fig. 22-4). The presence of this dye provides evidence of fetal well-being. Amniography is also helpful in establishing a diagnosis of fetal hydrops, by outlining the fetal soft tissues.

Amniotic Fluid Studies

The transabdominal aspiration of amniotic fluid (amniocentesis) (Fig. 22-5) is a safe and accepted procedure which can be done on an outpatient basis. Although it should obviously be done only upon specific indication, the risks of infection, fetal injury, and fetal hemorrhage are extremely small. They are in the range of one complication in 1,000 procedures. Careful attention to aseptic technique, accurate palpation of the fetal position and, when possible, localization of the placenta are the precautions in this procedure. Once the fluid has been aspirated, there are several evaluations to be made.

Color. The presence of meconium staining indicates fetal defecation, which is a way in which the fetus responds to stress such as a reduced oxygen supply. This is especially ominous in a pregnancy which has gone more than two weeks beyond the due date. Regardless of the suspected etiology of fetal distress, the demonstration of clear amniotic fluid is reassuring.

Cytology. Desquamation of the fetal skin occurs in the amniotic fluid, and as the fetus approaches maturity there are an increasing number of fat-containing cells from the sebaceous glands of the more mature skin. These are readily demonstrated by the use of a special fat stain (Nile Blue Sulfate). In addition, some workers are now studying the maturation index (ratio of more mature squamous cells to the basal cells) as a means of determining maturity.

Creatinine. Early in fetal development, the amount of creatinine in the amniotic fluid is merely a reflection of the amount in maternal serum. As the fetus matures, its kidneys develop, and fetal urination causes the concentration of creatinine in the amniotic fluid to be higher than that in maternal serum. An absolute value of > 1.8 mg. per cent, or a ratio of

FIG. 22-6. Tracing from spectrophotometer demonstrating the bilirubin peak at 450 millimicrons.

amniotic fluid to maternal serum creatinine of > 2:1 is indicative of fetal maturity.

Bilirubin. Estimations of the amount of bile pigment in the amniotic fluid are important, especially in the case of Rh sensitization. Before the use of this technique, judgments were based upon the increasing amounts of antibody present in maternal serum. This approach occasionally correlated poorly, or not at all, with the status of the fetus and its degree of anemia due to red cell destruction. Since the mother clears the bilirubin from the fetus and the amniotic fluid with increasing efficiency during the course of pregnancy, the amount present is small in the fluid of an unaffected fetus and gets smaller as term is approached. This decrease can in fact be used as an index of maturity. Technically, because of the small amounts present, chemical determinations are difficult. Hence, optical density analysis is used as an alternative approach. When amniotic fluid is examined in a recording spectrophotometer, bilirubin produces an optical density peak at a specific wave length (450 millimicrons). The height of this peak or $\triangle$ OD_{450} (Fig. 22-6) correlates directly with the degree of fetal involvement in hemolytic disease and is currently the most reliable guide to management.

Genetic Studies. Desquamated fetal epithelial cells in the amniotic fluid can be examined for the presence or absence of sex chromatin (Barr Bodies); therefore, the sex of the fetus can be determined with increasing certainty as term approaches. This study is of course not indicated merely to satisfy idle curiosity, but may be important in advising patients with certain sex-linked genetic defects. In addition, these desquamated cells can be grown in tissue culture and then subjected to chromosome analysis (Karyotyping). This is of obvious value in the antepartum diagnosis of certain genetically determined defects.

Other Studies. There have been a great many other determinations made on amniotic fluid, including pH, oxygen, and carbon dioxide tensions, which are at present of undetermined value. The possibilities for additional studies are literally limitless in this rapidly developing area.

Amnioscopy

In order to evaluate the color of the amniotic fluid without rupturing the membranes, a technique of transcervical amnioscopy has been utilized. This involves the introduction of an endoscope (similar to the cystoscope) into the cervical canal,

Blood

To operator's mouth

FIG. 22-7. Technique of obtaining blood samples from the fetal scalp during labor.

through which the color of the amniotic fluid can be evaluated. The major risk of this technique is inadvertent rupture of the membranes. An additional disadvantage is that although one can evaluate color of the fluid, none is available for chemical or cytologic analysis.

Fetal Blood Studies

It becomes obvious in any discussion of fetal diagnosis that it would be ideal if the obstetrician had ready access to the fetal circulation for sampling. Unfortunately, such access does not exist except under very limited circumstances. It is possible to obtain small samples of blood from the fetal scalp (Fig. 22-7) or, less desirably, the buttocks, if the patient is in active labor, with a cervical dilatation of 3 to 4 cm. or more, the membranes ruptured and the presenting part (preferably the vertex) well down in the pelvis. Although several analyses can be done with these samples, the most useful studies are pH, pCO_2 (carbon dioxide tension), and pO_2 (oxygen tension). These studies are especially helpful in

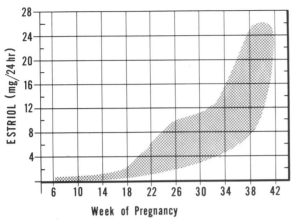

FIG. 22-8. Pattern of urinary estriol excretion in normal pregnancy.

evaluating a fetus during labor when fetal distress is a concern. In the case of a compromised fetus, the pH and the pO_2 fall and the pCO_2 rises. If these values (especially the pH) are normal, the obstetrician can pursue a conservative course with confidence and perhaps avoid a cesarean section.

Endocrine Studies

Estrogens. Levels of all three of the basic estrogens, estradiol, estrone and estriol, rise progressively in the mother's blood and urine, during the course of normal pregnancy. Prior to accurate chemical assays, biological tests for these compounds led to considerable confusion because of their relative potency, estradiol being extremely potent, estrone intermediate, and estriol biologically weak. However, with chemical assay, the level of estriol shows the greatest rise during pregnancy.

In recent years, the origin of estriol in pregnancy has been well worked out. The precursors are formed in the fetal adrenals, modified to some extent by the fetal liver, and then converted to estriol by the placenta. Also, in order to have normal amounts of estriol in the urine, maternal renal function must be normal. Thus, urinary estriol determinations in late pregnancy are not just an index of placental function, but really of the feto-placental unit, and also may be modified to some extent by maternal kidney function. The pattern of normal estriol excretion is illustrated in Figure 22-8. It should be borne in mind that the values will vary from laboratory to laboratory. Urinary estriol studies are of value in assessing fetal well-being in a number of conditions, including diabetes, hypertension, and post-date pregnancy. They are not of value in problems of Rh immunization. Blood estriol determinations are now becoming more readily available and have two distinct advantages. First, the nuisance of the 24-hour urine collection is eliminated, and second, the levels are not influenced by maternal renal function. However, one must be aware of the diurnal variation (high in the morning, lower in the afternoon) in blood estriol levels, and specimens should be obtained at the same time each day. The pattern for blood estriol levels during pregnancy is essentially the same as that of urinary values; however, the quantities are in micrograms rather than milligrams.

Progesterone. This steroid hormone is also produced in progressively increasing amounts during a normal pregnancy, at first by the corpus luteum, but later, predominantly by the syncytial trophoblasts of the placenta. Although blood assays are available, the most practical assay is for urinary pregnanediol, the major metabolite of progesterone. Levels of pregnanediol rise progressively throughout pregnancy and fall off with delivery. However, pregnanediol assays are not as useful in the management of problem pregnancies, since progesterone does not require fetal precursors. Therefore, production can continue and be normal even after an intrauterine fetal death has occurred.

Human Chorionic Gonadotropin (HCG). This hormone, produced by the trophoblast, normally peaks in early pregnancy and falls off to relatively low levels in the second and third trimesters. It is the basis for most pregnancy tests, as well as for the follow-up of hydatid moles and choriocarcinoma, but is of limited value in problem pregnancies. An exception occurs in the case of severely affected erythroblastotic infants. Because of placental hypertrophy, HCG values may be quite high; however, by the time these values are reached, the fetus is usually beyond salvage.

Human Placental Lactogen (HPL). The most recent addition to the endocrine assessment is HPL, a hormone produced specifically by the placenta, which has many characteristics of human growth hormone. Serum assays are available, and levels rise progressively during pregnancy. Levels are especially high in diabetics and are low in patients with placental insufficiency. Although a helpful study in a problem pregnancy, HPL assay does not seem to be replacement for urinary estriol determinations, which remain the most useful endocrine study in pregnancy.

SPECIFIC FETAL PROBLEMS

There are a number of complications of pregnancy which have particularly serious effects on the fetus. In this group are conditions which may have a chronic effect, and several others which may be grouped together under the heading of acute fetal distress. The latter may cause sudden problems, most often in the course of labor and delivery.

Acute Fetal Distress

The fetus signals its distress to observers in two ways: By an altered heart rate and, in certain instances, by the presence of meconium in the amniotic fluid. The most important signal is an altered heart rate, either tachycardia (above 160/min.) or, more ominously, bradycardia (below 120/min.). The presence of meconium in the amniotic fluid indicates distress when the fetus is in a cephalic presentation. This is a result of increased peristaltic activity in the G. I. tract of the fetus. The presence of meconium-stained fluid is not significant with a breech presentation, especially during labor, since the compressive forces often squeeze meconium out. The forces of uterine contractions are transmitted to the arteries and veins supplying the placenta, and these forces, if excessive, may interfere with the normal perfusion of the placenta. Therefore, the relationship between alterations in fetal heart and uterine contractions is quite important. Two types of fetal bradycardia may be seen (Fig. 22-9). Type I, in which the slowing is simultaneous with the contraction, and recovery is prompt, is thought to be due to compression of the fetal head and stimulation of the vagus nerve of the fetus. This pattern of change in the fetal heart rate is much less ominous for the fetus than is bradycardia (Type II) in which the slowing

Fig. 22-9. Patterns of fetal bradycardia (Type I and Type II dips).

begins at the peak of the contraction and persists for some time following the cessation of the contraction. This pattern indicates failure of adequate fetal oxygenation and is associated with an increase in infant death rate.

Fetal distress may be related to one of the following:

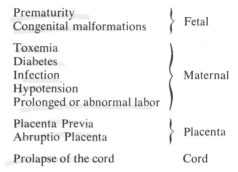

Prematurity Congenital malformations	} Fetal
Toxemia Diabetes Infection Hypotension Prolonged or abnormal labor	} Maternal
Placenta Previa Abruptio Placenta	} Placenta
Prolapse of the cord	Cord

Management is based upon the cause and in most instances involves prompt delivery of the infant, either by cesarean section or vaginally, whichever can be accomplished most quickly. This is true unless the cause is readily and completely reversible, as would be the case in hypotension due to caudal or spinal anesthesia. The cause must be searched for quickly and thoroughly, if it is not readily apparent. Supportive measures such as supplemental oxygen and intravenous glucose should be started simultaneously with more specific treatment. Continuous monitoring of the fetal heart rate is desirable, once evidence of distress has been detected, or in any patient with an obstetrical problem which may lead to distress. This monitoring should be accomplished by the most efficient means available, whether it be simple auscultation with the fetal stethoscope, a doppler probe, or a fetal ECG. If equipment for continuous monitoring is not available, attendants should listen to the fetal heart during and following each contraction. In addition, if the distress is questionable and the circumstances favorable, a fetal scalp blood sample for pH, pCO_2, and pO_2 may aid in the decision as to management.

Chronic Fetal Problems

Although some of the causes of chronic fetal problems were listed also as causes of acute fetal distress, it is more appropriate that they be discussed in relation to their long-standing influence on pregnancy and the fetus. There are other maternal and/or fetal conditions whose effects are exclusively chronic. A number of these pregnancy complications also have significant maternal effects, which are discussed in other parts of the book.

Hemolytic Disease. This is one of the complications of pregnancy in which there may be devastating fetal effects with virtually no maternal risk. Although the fetal pathology of severe hemolytic disease had been described before the turn of the century, the exact nature of the problem was not known until after the discovery of the Rh factor in 1940. The disease is most unusual in that within 30 years the cause, treatment and methods for prevention have been worked out. Most of the attention has been focused on the Rh factor as a cause, but the ABO blood groups may also cause a form of hemolytic disease, as do other lesser-blood groups.

The incidence of hemolytic disease is related to the occurrence of blood groups. In the Caucasian population, 15 per cent are Rh negative, while in Negroes this figure is only 5 per cent; therefore, the frequency of Rh hemolytic disease is much less in Negroes. Approximately 13 per cent of American marriages have the "setup" for Rh problems (Rh negative wife, Rh positive husband), and 22 per cent have the combinations for ABO disease. Ninety-eight per cent of all fetal hemolytic disease is related to either Rh or ABO incompatibilities. Fetal involvement with hemolytic disease occurs from 1 in 100 to 1 in 150 deliveries. These figures will be reduced in the future with the preventive measures now available.

The pathogenesis of Rh hemolytic disease is based upon the fact that, even though the maternal and fetal circulations are normally completely separated, breaks in this barrier permit the entry of fetal red cells into the maternal circulation during the second and third trimesters and at delivery in up to 50 per cent of pregnancies. Such breaks also occur with abortions beyond 6 to 8 weeks of pregnancy. If these cells are Rh positive (containing the Rh+ or D antigen), the mother may react to this mismatched "mini-transfusion" by forming protective antibodies. Since the formation of antibodies takes time, and since the unsensitized woman probably does not react until after she delivers, there is rarely a problem in the first pregnancy, unless the patient has received a mismatched transfusion in the past. Antibodies formed as the result of the first exposure persist for life. When the woman becomes pregnant again, and the fetus is Rh positive, she will respond with rapid antibody formation as soon as she is exposed to Rh positive cells. Thus, once antibodies have been formed, all subsequent pregnancies with Rh positive infants will be a problem.

There are two types of Rh antibodies. The larger (gamma M, or 19S) type does not cross the placenta as readily as the smaller (gamma g, or 7S). In the case of ABO disease where the mother who lacks the antigen has the antibody (e.g., type O has neither A nor B antigen, but has both Anti-A and Anti-B antibodies; type A has A antigen and Anti-B antibody, etc.), these naturally occurring antibodies are the large 19S variety. Also, since these antibodies require a break in the placental barrier to get into the fetal circulation, and since this is most likely to occur at the time of delivery of the placenta, ABO disease is almost always more mild than Rh, and rarely is the child stillborn or severely affected at birth. In addition, because the AB antigens are present in all body cells, this tends to absorb excess antibody and reduce the effect on the red cells. However, in Rh disease, there are both 19S and 7S antibodies (the result of sensitization). The smaller 7S antibodies cross readily into the fetal circulation and are responsible for the destruction of the fetal red blood cells. This produces anemia, and if it is severe enough, heart failure results in an edematous, hydropic infant, and possibly a stillbirth. While the fetus is in utero, the mother is able to remove the breakdown products of the red cells (bilirubin) and handle them in her own liver; therefore, the baby is not born jaundiced. However, once separated from the mother, the baby must handle the continuing breakdown of red cells, and its liver, especially in prematures, lacks the necessary enzymes to do this efficiently. The affected newborn rapidly develops jaundice and, if untreated, brain damage may result from the deposition of the bile pigments in vital areas of the brain (Kernicterus). This is the severest form of pathology, but it must be kept in mind that it is not only possible but likely that an Rh negative woman may have one, two or even more pregnancies without significant difficulty.

The inheritance of Rh blood type follows the simple dominant recessive rules, with Rh+ being a dominant. Each individual receives two genes (one from each parent) to determine Rh blood type. It is necessary to receive two Rh negative genes to be negative, whereas one can be Rh positive with one Rh positive and one Rh negative gene (heterozygous), or two Rh positive genes (homozygous). Thus, if the husband

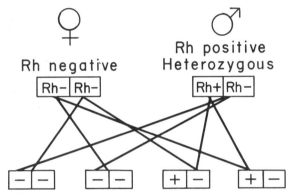

FIG. 22-10. Inheritance patterns for the Rh factor.

FIG. 22-11. Technique of intra-uterine transfusion.

is heterozygous, there is a 50-50 chance of having an Rh negative child (Fig. 22-10) and, therefore, an unaffected one. If the father is homozygous, all offspring will be Rh positive and subject to hemolytic disease.

In the ABO system, an individual may have genes for A, B, AB, or no antigens. Thus, the contribution to the offspring may be either A or B, or none. For example: Type O individuals receive neither A nor B genes from the parents; a type A individual may receive an A gene from each (AA), or an A from one and none from the other (AO). The same is true for the type B individual (BB or BO). The AB individual receives an A from one parent and a B from the other.

All pregnant patients should have a blood group determination, at least with the first pregnancy. If adequate records are available, this need not be repeated with subsequent pregnancies.

Should the patient be Rh negative or type O (the most common maternal type for ABO disease), the husband's blood should also be typed. If he is Rh positive, a genotype may be done to determine whether he is homozygous or heterozygous. Also, the Rh negative woman's blood should be examined for the presence of antibodies to the Rh factor (D). This is accomplished by the indirect Coombs test and is reported in dilutions (e.g., positive 1:2, 1:4, 1:8, etc.). If the initial screening or titer is negative (i.e., shows no antibodies), this should be repeated at approximately 30 and 36 weeks of pregnancy. If both of those titers are negative, it is safe to assume there will be no significant problem and to permit the pregnancy to run its normal course. If the titer is positive, it then becomes necessary to decide how seriously the fetus is affected (i.e., how anemic it is). Since we are unable to approach the fetus directly and do a hemoglobin or hematocrit, we must use less direct means. In the past, we merely repeated the antibody titer, watching for a rise and, combining this with the patient's past history, arrived at a plan of management. Now, with the use of amniocentesis and spectrophotometric analysis of this fluid for bile pigments (see section on fetal diagnosis), it is possible to assess the fetal status much more accurately and decide the appropriate course of action.

If the fetus is seriously affected before 32 weeks of gestation, as evidenced by amniotic fluid analysis, then it is too immature to survive if delivered, and intrauterine transfusion is indicated. This dramatic procedure was first described in 1963 by Liley and involves the instillation (Fig. 22-11) under fluoroscopic control of Rh negative red cells into the peritoneal cavity of the fetus in utero. The fetus is able to absorb these intact cells. If the procedure is repeated successfully every 10 to 14 days until the point of maturity (approximately 34 to 35 weeks), a stillbirth may be avoided. Only 40 to 50 per cent of treated fetuses can be salvaged, because the procedure is rather gross, especially in the smaller fetus, and often the fetus is very sick when the procedure is initiated. Of course, these results are far better than no survivors—which could be anticipated without the procedure.

If the analysis of amniotic fluid indicates severe fetal anemia at a gestational period beyond 32 weeks, then delivery by either induction of labor or cesarean section is indicated, and the pediatrician assumes the care, using exchange transfusion, or other means, as described below. If the amniotic fluid analysis indicates that the fetus is only mildly affected, or not at all, then the pregnancy may be permitted to go to term.

The pediatric management of the newborn involves the use of exchange transfusion to correct the anemia and to reduce the concentration of bilirubin, which averts the brain damage caused by Kernicterus. Recently, there has been a surge of interest in the use of so-called phototherapy (i.e., the jaundiced baby is placed under a special blue light to reduce the concentration of bilirubin).

One of the most promising developments in the field of hemolytic disease is the prospect of prevention and virtual elimination of the problem, at least that due to the Rh system. It has been possible to isolate a human Anti-D (Anti Rh+) gamma globulin (known commercially as Rhogam) from women with high Anti-D titers, or from deliberately sensitized male volunteers. If this is administered to the unsensitized Rh negative woman who has delivered an Rh positive infant in the previous 3 days, the antibody combines with the Rh antigen, neutralizing it. Thus, it can clear Rh positive cells from the maternal circulation and eliminate the possibility of sensitization. Unfortunately, it is of no use in the woman who already has been sensitized. Rhogam should also be given to unsensitized Rh negative women with abortion or ectopic pregnancies, even though the blood group of the conceptus is unknown.

Diabetes Mellitus. In contrast to hemolytic disease, the effects of diabetes are both fetal and maternal. A few years ago it was rather common for diabetics to be relatively infertile. Now, with better control of the diabetes, more patients are able to conceive. In addition, we are recognizing a sizable group of women whose diabetes becomes obvious only during pregnancy, the so-called gestational diabetics. In both groups, there is an increase in perinatal wastage. Pregnancy increases the severity of diabetes throughout gestation. This is the result of insulin antagonism (perhaps by the placenta) which increases the requirements for insulin, often as much as four-fold during the course of pregnancy. Because of the increasing hyperglycemia and the inherent tendency of the pregnant woman toward acidosis, the probability of development of a diabetic keto-acidosis is increased, and if it occurs, the condition of the fetus may be severely compromised. Also, the complications due to toxemia and hydramnios are much more frequent.

In regard to the fetus, the incidence of congenital malformations is increased in the offspring of diabetics. There will be a certain number of fetuses carried by both pre-pregnancy diabetics and gestational diabetics which will die in utero as the result of placental insufficiency. It is not surprising that diabetes, which seems to have a predilection for the blood vessels, might well cause the placenta to age prematurely. To avoid this, it has been customary to deliver all pre-pregnancy diabetics three to four weeks prior to the due date and to do the same with those gestational diabetics who have had previous stillborns or neonatal deaths. This would seem, in the case of the pre-pregnant diabetic, to subject a number of infants to premature delivery in order to salvage the one affected by placental insufficiency. In the case of the gestational diabetic, this approach would appear to require the patient to suffer a perinatal loss before the timing of delivery would be altered. To avoid this dilemma, a reliable means for determining the well-being of the fetus was needed. This has been provided by the use of 24-hour urinary estriol determination and, in some clinics, by the use of serum estriol measurements. If these values are normal for the period of gestation, then it is permissible to allow the pre-pregnancy diabetic to carry her pregnancy closer to term, avoiding the hazard of prematurity. This often also eliminates the need for delivery by cesarean section. In the case of the gestational diabetic, this method can identify the occasional fetus at risk, permit early delivery and avoid a potential perinatal death.

Babies born to diabetic mothers have a tendency to high birth weights, and there is an increased risk of mechanical difficulties in labor and delivery, with an increased chance of birth injury, and an increased need for cesarean section. The reasons for the high birth weights of these babies are not definitely known. Some have suggested that it is due to the fact that the fetus lives in a hyperglycemic environment during pregnancy. Others have pointed to the increased levels of a substance similar to growth hormone which is produced in large quantities by the placenta in diabetic patients. This is called human placental lactogen (HPL). Interestingly, however, excessively large babies are not usually born to diabetics who are well-controlled throughout pregnancy, but more commonly to gestational diabetics who often go undetected until late in pregnancy. These fetuses have lived in a hyperglycemic environment throughout the pregnancy.

When toxemia of pregnancy occurs in a diabetic, there is an increased risk of fetal death. In general, if the toxemia is severe, the pregnancy must be terminated for fetal as well as maternal reasons. Hydramnios (excessive accumulation of amniotic fluid) is exceedingly common in pregnant diabetics and does not seem to have a deleterious effect on the fetus, unless the degree of hydramnios is sufficient to produce premature labor. Both toxemia and hydramnios can be minimized by careful control of sodium intake and the use of diuretics. Meticulous diabetic control reduces the frequency of these complications.

The newborn of the diabetic faces a number of problems, including a high incidence of respiratory distress syndrome (hyaline membrane disease). In addition, because the insulin-forming islets of the fetal pancreas hypertrophy during pregnancy, the newborn of the diabetic produces an excess of insulin and is therefore prone to low blood sugar (hypoglycemia) during the first few days of life. Along with the problems of the neonatal period, the child with one diabetic parent has a 10 to 15 per cent chance of developing diabetes in his lifetime, and if both parents are diabetic the risks are even higher.

Although the perinatal wastage (stillbirths and neonatal deaths due to the causes just described) is often as high as 10 to 12 per cent in good

clinics, it is at least theoretically possible to reduce this by good diabetic and obstetric care. The patient must be seen frequently (at least every 2 weeks) throughout pregnancy, with careful attention paid to diet, the progressively increasing insulin requirement and the prevention of fluid retention. The more closely the patient is maintained in a euglycemic (normal blood sugar) state, the more like a non-diabetic her obstetric performance will be.

Prolonged Pregnancy. The average duration of pregnancy is 280 days from the first day of the last menstrual period, or 267 days from the time of conception, if the menstrual cycle is of average length. Only 5 per cent of women deliver on the actual due date, although most will deliver within 10 to 14 days in either direction from the date. Since the placenta has a normal life span equal to the duration of pregnancy, one may justifiably be concerned that if the due date is exceeded by more than 2 weeks, the aging placenta may no longer be able to support the fetus adequately. Fortunately, in most instances, the placenta is capable of such support. In fact, in a great number of patients who are theoretically late, the date represents a miscalculation or faulty memory. In addition to those post-mature pregnancies in which there is placental insufficiency, there is another group of late pregnancies in which the placenta functions well and the fetus becomes oversized, creating potential mechanical problems in labor and delivery.

If the circumstances, including the status of the cervix, the size and position of the baby, and the size of the maternal pelvis are all favorable, induction of labor should be carried out when a pregnancy exceeds the due date by two weeks. If there is any question about the dates, some of the methods for determining fetal maturity suggested in the section of fetal diagnosis should be applied. If, on the other hand, conditions are not favorable for the induction of labor, then one must have some means for ascertaining the well-being of the fetus. Twenty-four-hour urinary estriol determinations are helpful in this regard. If the values are in the normal range, interference is not necessary, and one may await more favorable conditions for induction. If the value is low and this is confirmed by a repeat determination, delivery by cesarean section is indicated. Evaluation of amniotic fluid is also helpful in these cases. The fluid around the fetus affected by post-maturity is scant in volume and heavily stained with meconium. Thus, amniocentesis can provide additional confirmatory information.

The affected post-mature (sometimes called dysmature) newborn has a typical appearance. It is long for its weight, appearing to have lost weight. The finger- and toenails are long and stained with meconium, as are the cord and membranes. These infants are especially prone to distress during labor and to respiratory problems in the neonatal period.

On the surface, it would seem simple to determine the due date and when a pregnancy has gone beyond that point, but there are a number of pitfalls. Many patients do not record or cannot recall when they had their last period. Others have long cycles, with ovulation and conception occurring later than the 14th day. This is especially true in patients discontinuing oral contraceptive therapy, in whom the first ovulation may not occur until 4 to 6 weeks after the last withdrawal flow. One must assess these factors carefully before overtreating a patient for supposed post-maturity.

Preeclampsia—Eclampsia. (See Chapter 19 for maternal aspects.) Although the signs of preeclampsia (hypertension, edema, and proteinuria) and eclampsia (convulsions in addition to the above) are primarily maternal, fetal interests cannot be ignored. In fact, once a full-blown preeclampsia is manifest, a progressive placental insufficiency develops rather rapidly. If the pregnancy is not terminated, the fetus may fail to grow and even die in utero. On occasion, a patient with severe preeclampsia may seem to be so well-controlled that one is tempted to allow the fetus to remain in utero and mature. This decision is fraught with the risk of failure of the fetus to prosper, and possibly a stillbirth; and in most cases it is unwise. Should such a course be elected, one must use some index of fetal well-being such as urinary estriol to follow the pregnancy. The perinatal wastage in preeclampsia is largely dependent upon the stage of pregnancy at which the process develops and, therefore, on the degree of prematurity of the infant delivered. If toxemia does not develop until after the 36th week of gestation, the perinatal loss should be quite low. Perinatal loss is high when convulsions (eclampsia) occur. The older studies give the rate as 50 per cent, while more recent reviews place it at 20 per cent.

Chronic Hypertension. Approximately 75 per cent of women with benign essential hypertension go through pregnancy with no problems, either maternal or fetal. Unfortunately, some 15 per cent develop preeclampsia. When this happens, the fetal prognosis is very poor, especially if it occurs at a time when the fetus is significantly premature (at the end of the second trimester, for example). The perinatal mortality rate in this group is approximately 20 per cent. In the case of the hypertensive mother without superimposed preeclampsia, the fetal risk is not great, but it is greater than that for women with normal blood pressure. Because of this, it is recommended that all hypertensive patients be followed with estriol determinations in the third trimester, in order to identify that occasional benign hypertensive patient whose fetus is in jeopardy, and for whom pre-term delivery is indicated. There is, in addition, an increased frequency of abruptio placenta in these hypertensive patients, with the added perinatal wastage of that problem.

Infections Affecting the Fetus. There are a number of infectious diseases which are significant if they occur during pregnancy. Some are important because of their direct effects upon the fetus; others have an indirect effect. The indirect effect is usually abortion or premature labor in the presence of, or as a result of, a high fever in the mother. The most well-documented infection with a fetal effect is German Measles (rubella).

The overall risk of congenital malformation in the newborn of the woman who gets rubella in the first trimester is 20 per cent. This risk is greatest in the first 4 weeks (60%), gradually falling off up to 12 weeks, and then decreasing even more dramatically. The common defects involve the heart, the eyes and hearing, although there are a number of others. The question of therapeutic abortion is one which is somewhat controversial, but many feel it is justified if a documented case of rubella occurs in the first 8 weeks, and probably up to 12 weeks, of pregnancy. When a woman is exposed to rubella in the first trimester, it is important to determine whether the woman has had the disease and is, therefore, immune. This can be done by an examination of the patient's blood for the presence of antibodies to the virus. If the antibody level or titer is high enough, this means the patient is immune and need not worry. If the titer is below the critical level, the patient is not immune and must be carefully watched for the development of the infection. Most authorities do not recommend the use of gamma globulin for the patient exposed to rubella, because the gamma globulin may only modify or mask the infection without preventing the effects on the fetus. Fetal infection with the rubella virus may also occur beyond the first trimester. Such infections do not result in congenital malformations but, often, in viremia with hemorrhagic manifestations. The future is now much brighter with the recent development of the rubella vaccine. Large-scale immunization has been started in children and should in time eliminate the problem. For the time, the use of the vaccine in adults should be limited to those women who are not immune (as evidenced by antibody studies) and are at particular risk because of occupation, such as school teachers or pediatric nurses. Since the teratogenic properties of the attenuated virus in the vaccine are unknown, pregnancy must be avoided for three months after its administration.

Other infections which have at least a potential for producing congenital malformations include mumps and toxoplasmosis. Intrauterine infection may occur with the Coxsackie virus, cytomegalovirus, herpes simplex, poliomyelitis and syphilis. Premature labor and abortion are increased in measles, cholera, typhoid, pneumonia, pyelonephritis, and influenza.

Intrauterine infection as the result of premature rupture of the membranes is one of the most common threats to the fetus. It is now well recognized that the frequency of such infection parallels the length of the latent period (time from rupture of the membranes to the onset of labor). Infection of the fetus occurs by way of the amniotic fluid to the tracheo-bronchial tree, as well as from the membranes and placenta through the cord vessels, producing fetal sepsis. The organisms most commonly involved are anaerobic streptococci, and gram-negative bacilli. Since it is difficult to obtain therapeutic levels of antibiotics in the amniotic fluid, once the patient becomes febrile, the treatment is delivery by either induction or cesarean section. More important is prevention of infection. This involves delivery (most often by induction, but by section if necessary) of any patient with premature rupture of the membranes whose fetus is larger than 1500 to 1800 Gm. This weight range is selected because in most clinics the survival data for babies of that size are such that the risk of delivery and prematurity is much less than the risk of intrauterine infection.

Fetal Growth Retardation. This is one term applied to a clinical syndrome in which the fetus fails to prosper in utero. The terms dysmaturity, placental insufficiency, small-for-date babies, utero-placental insufficiency, and stunted fetus have all been applied. Although this syndrome may occur with certain maternal diseases, such as diabetes with severe vascular involvement, chronic renal disease, and chronic hypertension with renal involvement, many cases have no demonstrable etiology and are classified as idiopathic. Idiopathic fetal retardation may recur in the same patient with subsequent pregnancies. These babies, at birth, appear to have lost subcutaneous fat, their skin is often wrinkled, and the finger- and toenails are long. The amniotic fluid, cord, and nails are heavily stained with meconium. The stillbirth rate is high if the situation is not recognized, and the frequency of respiratory problems in the newborn is also increased. The most significant management problem from the obstetrical viewpoint is the antepartum differentiation of such a fetus from a premature. After delivery, this differentiation is simpler and can be based on weight (particularly weight patterns), certain developmental criteria such as ear cartilage development and plantar skin creases, and behavior patterns. The question of erroneous menstrual dates often arises, and this necessitates the use of many of the methods described under fetal diagnosis. Treatment is based upon, first, suspicion of the diagnosis, and then timing of delivery, which is determined by some index of fetal well-being, such as serial urinary or plasma estriol levels. The affected fetuses generally do not tolerate labor well, and fetal distress is very common. If the estriol value is low, a cesarean section may be necessary.

Disproportionate Twin Development. Twins with disparity in size may be accounted for by the fact that there can be a connection between the two circulations. This is especially true in single-ovum twins, but occurs occasionally in two-egg twins. When this happens in early pregnancy and one heart pumps more strongly than the other, there may be monopolization of a larger area of the placenta by one twin and thus a disparity in size. Such twins are not only greatly different in size at birth, but the smaller one is often anemic and may require transfusion. The larger twin may be hypervolemic and require a phlebotomy to prevent heart failure and jaundice. This type of placental anastomosis, when it occurs in double-ovum twins, accounts for those rare situations known as "chimerism," in which an individual may have two populations of cells, as evidenced by blood groups or sex chromatin. The other important clinical significance of disparity in twin sizes is that difficulties may be encountered in delivery if the smaller of the twins is delivered first through a cervix that is not completely dilated.

FETAL TREATMENT

Although, at this time, the practice of fetal medicine is largely diagnostic, an important development is the use of intrauterine fetal transfusion in pre-viable fetuses severely affected by hemolytic disease. However, the most common form of fetal treatment for preventing stillbirths is delivery. In the case of the fetus at jeopardy, this may be accomplished by either induction of labor, or cesarean section, and in many cases involves a compromise between prematurity on the one hand, and the source of fetal jeopardy on the other. Occasionally, this approach only results in a neonatal death.

We certainly make other efforts at fetal treatment, such as the administration of oxygen to the mother in cases of fetal distress. This may be of transient value, as is the use of concentrated glucose solutions intravenously. The problem is whether, in the face of some compromise in placental function, the concentrations of oxygen and glucose can be significantly increased in the fetus.

Similar comments can be made about most drugs, since anything administered to the mother, with the intent that it serve as fetal treatment, requires adequate placental function in order to permit transfer. In general, any substance with a molecular weight of 500 or less can traverse the placenta by simple diffusion. Although some larger molecules do cross, in general, they do not. More often, when one considers giving a drug to the fetus through the mother, the fetal problem for which the treatment is being considered is so serious that delivery is a better solution.

Surgical treatment of the fetus is used now only in the experimental animal. Extraordinary technical feats have been accomplished in the fetal monkey and lamb, such as adrenalectomy, gastrectomy, and craniotomy, but in the human fetus there has been little experimentation. The only efforts at fetal surgery in humans have been attempts to expose a limb for the purpose of venous cannulation and transfusion. These attempts have been almost uniformly unsuccessful, since we have been unable to prevent labor, once the uterus has been opened.

The future undoubtedly holds many advances in this area—from the prenatal correction of congenital defects to the even more unbelievable unscrambling of genetic mishaps. There may well be treatments of maladies which are presently unknown in this rapidly developing area of fetal medicine.

SUGGESTED READING

Adamsons, K.: Diagnosis and Treatment of Fetal Disorders. New York, Springer-Verlag, 1968.

Barnes, A. C.: Intra-uterine Development. Philadelphia, Lea & Febiger, 1968.

Birch, P. K.: Hormonal cytology of pregnancy. Clin. Obstet. Gynec. 4:1062, 1961.

Charles, A. G., and Friedman, E. A.: Rh Isoimmunization and Erythroblastosis Fetalis. New York, Appleton, 1969.

Curtis, C. G., and Philpott, O. S., Jr.: Prenatal syphilis. Med. Clin. N. Am. 48:707, 1964.

Eastman, N. J., and Hellman, L. M.: Williams Obstetrics. ed. 13, New York, Appleton, 1966.

Fuchs, F.: Genetic information from amniotic fluid constituents. Clin. Obstet. Gynec. 9:565-573, June 1966.

Greene, J. W., Jr., Smith, K., Kyle, G. C., Touchstone, J. C., and Duhring, J. L.: The use of urinary estriol excretion in the management of pregnancies complicated by diabetes mellitus. Am. J. Obstet. Gynec. 91:684-688, March 1, 1965.

Greene, J. W., Jr., and Tweeddale, D. N.: Endocrine indices of fetal environment. Clin. Obstet. Gynec. 11:1106, 1968.

Hellman, L. M., and Fillisti, L. P.: Analysis of the atropine test for placental transfer in gravidas with toxemia and diabetes. Am. J. Obstet. Gynec. 91:797, 1965.

Hibbard, L. T., and Anderson, G. V.: Clinical applications of ultrasonic fetal cephalometry. Obstet. Gynec. 29:842-847, June 1967.

Kyle, G. C.: Diabetes and pregnancy. Ann. Intern. Med. 59 (Suppl. 3):1, 1963.

———: Diabetes and Pregnancy in Textbook of Gynecologic Endocrinology, Gold, J. J. (ed.), Hoeber Medical Division, pp. 621-640, New York, Harper and Row Publishers, Inc., 1968.

Queenan, J. T.: Amniocentesis and transamniotic fetal transfusion for Rh disease. Clin. Obstet. Gynec. 9:491-507, June 1966.

———: Modern Management of the Rh Problem. New York, Hoeber, 1967.

Saling, E.: Foetal and Neonatal Hypoxia. Baltimore, Williams and Wilkins, 1968.

Schwarz, R. H., Fields, G. A., and Kyle, G. C.: Timing of delivery in the pregnant diabetic patient. Obstet. Gynec. 36:787-791, December 1969.

Sever, J. L., Nelson, K. B., and Gilkeson, M. R.: Rubella epidemic 1964: Effect on good pregnancies. Am. J. Dis. Child. 110:395, 1965.

Smith, K., Greene, J. W., Jr., and Touchstone, J. C.: Urinary estriol determination in the management of prolonged pregnancy. Am. J. Obstet. Gynec. 96:901-906, December 1, 1966.

Vasicka, A., and Hutchinson, H. T.: Oxygen tension in amniotic fluid and fetal distress. Am. J. Obstet. Gynec. 88:530, 1964.

Disorders of the Newborn

23

Parental and Staff Reactions to Defects and Disorders • Neonatal Respiratory Distress • Injuries Infections • Malformations (Genetic Abnormalities) • Inborn Errors of Metabolism Hemolytic Disease of the Newborn • Miscellaneous Disorders

INTRODUCTION

The care of the newborn infant and the developing relationship between the mother and her infant have been discussed previously. In this section the focus will be on certain disorders of the neonate that are encountered at times in the maternity unit. Fortunately for all concerned, these usually are not seen frequently; yet their appearance, however infrequent, is traumatic for both parents and staff. The principles of supportive care which were delineated in Chapters 16, 17 and 20 are appropriate here; at times modification will be needed, especially when separation of mother and infant is necessary, or when parental response makes the acceptance of the infant difficult. As the various disorders are discussed, the particular aspects, modifications, etc., which are peculiar to the condition will be described. It is important to remember that the parents of babies with disorders have all the usual tasks of adjusting to the coming of a new infant; in addition they must cope with all the restrictions, limitations and complications that the disorder imposes.

PARENTAL AND STAFF REACTIONS TO DEFECTS AND DISORDERS

There are certain characteristics inherent in the maternity unit that tend to give rise to and intensify certain interactional elements of the doctor-patient-nurse relationship. First, the maternity patient usually comes to the hospital, to be assured of a safe delivery for herself and her infant. This means, among other things, freedom from infection and hence the primary orientation of the unit is toward the control and prevention of infection. To this end the ward is "restricted," that is, it may be actually physically set apart from the other units of the hospital, only obstetric patients are admitted to the unit, personnel (and often patients) are especially gowned, scrubbed and cleansed in a particular manner, visitors and traffic are restricted. All of this protocol tends to make patients and staff feel isolated. Secondly, the maternity unit is set apart from other units by the rather unique service it offers. In our culture, the childbirth process is considered part of the normal reproductive function of a woman. This normality as a life process together with the predictability of events leads to a set of expectations with consequent standardization and routinization of the technical and organizational aspects of the units. Thirdly, the overall expectation is that a healthy patient arrives in anticipation of a happy outcome. Usually *two* healthy persons are returned to the community instead of only the one who entered, and the maternity staff often derives from this tangible production a sense of acheivement and satisfaction so highly valued in our society.

It could be hypothesized, then, that the social interaction will be influenced by the interrelatedness of the above characteristics. When a traumatic event occurs, such as the birth of a defective child, both the parents and the staff will be affected in different ways and degrees.

Working Through a Crisis

Many parents, as we have said, think of labor and delivery as "the end" of something rather than the beginning of a whole new phase in the family cycle. Probably the enormous responsibilities involved in being parents are responsible in part for this psychological adaptation. One can say with certainty, however, that becoming a parent is a turning point in life, and it is particularly so for the parents of a child who has a disorder. They can emerge from this crisis less mentally and emotionally healthy than they were, or they can move on to increased maturity. If they utilize maladaptive coping mechanisms to deal with the crisis, then the former no doubt will occur; if they can be helped to work through positively, then this experience will stand them in good stead for future stressful situations.

It is the responsibility of the members of the health team to help them cope with this situation adequately. However, staff members, too, are only human, and at times they are hampered by their own anxieties, feelings and fantasies. Thus, it is especially important for the staff to understand the psychodynamics that are occurring in both the parents and themselves so that they may choose a therapeutic course of action to help the parents.

Avoiding Negative Communication. In the delivery room, the doctor, patient and nurse are intensely involved with one another as we have seen in Chapter 13. The patient needs guidance, coaching, and explanation at this time. Since the time span in the delivery room is short, and the events that occur very important, tensions rise with the imminence of birth. The interactions, therefore, are characterized by intense alertness to behavioral cues. Moreover the mother is encouraged verbally by the staff that she is "doing well" and that everything is going along "well." Whenever a disorder is apparent at birth, especially if it is of any magnitude or of a long-term nature (an anomaly, acute respiratory distress, etc.), the tension in the delivery room may be prolonged and intensified instead of being released in the more customary ways. The doctor and the nurse will know about the disorder immediately or shortly thereafter. Both their verbal and nonverbal behavior are apt to convey their shock and disappointment to the mother. Their posture may become rigid or they may use their bodies to shield the baby from the mother; their conversation may dwindle or cease or if an emergency ensues their actions quicken and conversation is directed to each other and away from the mother and is of a technical nature. If the mother is conscious, she may sense this heightened tension and become increasingly aware and terrified that all is not well. As was stated, it is not always possible for the staff to stop their activities and to respond to the mother's questions; not only are their efforts often going into lifesaving measures for the infant, but they are having to cope with their own emotional reactions. For instance, it is not unnatural for the staff (and the parents later) to have, and perhaps to express, death wishes for a severely defective child. They feel frustrated and resentful toward a situation that they can neither control nor in many cases change. It may be an extremely difficult time for the physician, for it may seem to him that he has "failed" somehow, since he cannot heal the patient. The mother, in turn, may sense the attendants' frustration and misinterpret it as hostility or resentment toward her—that she also has "failed." This negative communication only intensifies the trauma that is experienced by all concerned. In addition, the new mother feels sadness, a completely different emotion than the joy she had anticipated; furthermore, it comes at a time when she may be physically and emotionally exhausted (see Chap. 13).

Forming a Relationship of Trust. The total response of the mother will depend on the type and the severity of the disorder and on her past experiences with stress and life in general. During this immediate period when the disorder or defect may become apparent, the nurse can be a key person in easing the concern. She should utilize the relationship with the patient that hopefully she has established in the labor room, for it is vitally important that a trust relationship be formed with the patient if she and her husband are to weather this hardship. She can try to communicate her concern and empathy in any way that seems acceptable to the patient. This may be by just staying with the patient and/or holding her hand. Certainly allowing and encouraging the mother to express her feelings, either verbally or by crying, or by letting her be silent, are constructive measures on the part of the nurse. The nurse should never underestimate the importance of her mere presence; she is someone to share the mother's burden. However, she sometimes has to cope with her own inclinations to flee or to avoid the topic.

Telling the Parents. Many physicians agree that the mother and father should be informed as soon as possible (preferably immediately) of the disorder. However, research has indicated that many physicians tend to seek or develop strategies for delaying the announcement of "bad" news (see Suggested Readings). If this occurs, it can mean significant and far reaching consequences for the mother and father. Since the mother has the expectation that she will see or at the very least be told about her infant, if this does not happen, she will become suspicious and alarmed and eventually mistrustful. The important immediate establishment of a "trust" relationship will be impeded. Moreover, there will be implications for the attainment of the future goals of the professional services and for the parents' image of professional workers in general.

Sometimes, however, the abnormality makes the condition of the infant so critical that he must be transferred immediately to more suitable facilities. Thus, for entirely different reasons, the mother may not receive a glimpse of her baby. Therefore, *what* the couple is told about the condition and *how* they are told become critical issues. All too often one hears parents complain bitterly about the "bluntness," "coldness" and "unconcern" that the staff demonstrated. Worse still is the "conspiracy of silence" that tortures the already overwrought pair, in which each professional avoids saying anything, pretending or assuming that the other will handle the matter, or that it is better left alone. It is important to recognize that the so-called "coldness," avoidance, etc., are not really manifestations of the staff's true feelings, but rather are unsuccessful coping mechanisms on their part to allay their feelings of helplessness, anxiety and inadequacy. However, it is part of the nurse's professional responsibility to explore her feelings in these matters and to develop more effective ways of handling them.

Most physicians want to tell the parents of the disorder themselves; on rare occasions the telling may be delegated to the nurse. In any case it is imperative for her to confer with the doctor, so that each can be aware of what is being told to the parents, and thus effective communication is fostered. Moreover, the nurse should maintain communication with the rest of the health team, so that a coordinated effort can be made for comprehensive care.

REALISTIC APPRAISAL AND REASSURANCE. In order to give the parents a realistic appraisal of the situation, many authorities feel that the parents should be informed immediately of the disorder and the prognosis, especially if repair or long-term care is involved. This information, of course, must be explained in terms that the couple can understand, and reinforcement over the days probably will be necessary.

Whatever specifics are told, it is important that two aspects of realistic reassurance be given the mother and father: first, that they and their child are acceptable, and second, that the hospital and personnel are there to render any assistance possible. Particularly in the cases of some defects and deformities (e.g., phocomelia or myelomeningocele) the parents must understand that although their child may not be made whole, he usually may be helped to some degree. This kind of reassurance demonstrates an attitude of understanding and sharing of the parents' feelings of hurt and loss, and at the same time it does not minimize the gravity of the situation.

Acceptance of the Infant by the Staff. It is generally the doctor who determines when the parents, and especially the mother, will see and care for her infant. The parents' first encounter with their infant is another crucial time. Particularly in cases in which there is an obvious anomaly, it is vitally important that the physician or the nurse who is showing the baby demonstrate an attitude of warmth and acceptance of the infant; if revulsion or rejection is manifested, then the parents' own feelings of despair and ostracism will be intensified.

One of the ways that the staff can demonstrate to the parents that their child is valuable and important is to hold him close, cuddle him and call him by name. At this time, if it seems to be indicated, the positive points in the prognosis can be reiterated or reinforced. This may be a difficult time for all concerned, since the staff, too, is trying to cope with their own possible feelings of rejection. Therefore, an attempt should be made to avoid a common type of destructive behavior that tends to be demonstrated unconsciously, that of isolating the patient under the guise of "protecting" the mother. In this kind of destructive behavior the mother may not be allowed to see her infant at all (or very infrequently) until she is "stronger"; no one talks to her of her child's handicap or death, because it will "upset" her, visitors are often restricted, and so on. The baby, in turn, is isolated and often overtreated (i.e., time- and energy-consuming procedures are employed which lead to very little change in the infant's condition). All this only emphasizes the enormity of the problem for the parents and hinders them in attaining a successful resolution of the problem.

Grieving. Grief can be considered a response to loss. It is most often known to us as a response to a loss through death or separation of a loved person, but it can occur following the loss of anything, tangible or intangible, which is highly valued. This may be such things as a material possession, a highly valued expectation (such as a well, whole infant), a position of status, a prized faculty, or even a place one is forced to leave. The ability to experience grief is gradually formed in the course of normal development and the capacity for grieving is closely related to the person's capacity to develop meaningful object relationships. Therefore, those who are able to form relationships at all become attached even to situations and places which are less than optimal and grieve for them (however briefly), even when moving to better conditions. Grief, then, is a universal, normal, developmentally evolved adaptive process. It progresses through three predictable phases which we will discuss and this progress enables the individual to deal adaptively with the disturbance of his psychological equilibrium which is inevitably caused by object loss. Fortunately it is self-limiting if not allowed to deteriorate into deep-seated depression, and gradually diminishes over a period of a year. Only the very early, acute phase is actually incapacitating, and even this phase, with appropriate professional help, may not grossly interfere with the person's normal functioning in many areas of his life. The staff can expect the parents to show signs of grieving when a substantial defect (or death) occurs. The couple must come to terms with a difficult and perhaps unexpected situation, one in which the prognosis may be poor. Both parents will demonstrate grief, and the father's needs should not be forgotten. He is particularly vulnerable, since it is on him that the early decisions, making arrangements, etc., usually fall, and he often does not have the time or the privacy to express his own sorrow.

SEVERAL PHASES are encountered in the grief reaction,[1] and how intensely the parents experience these will vary according to the nature and the gravity of the disorder and their capacity for grieving.

In the first phase are shock and disbelief; this phase may be manifested by a refusal to accept or to comprehend the fact of the disorder or the loss. The person may appear stunned, immobilized, or may try to carry on ordinary activities; intermittent flashes of anguish and despair occur as reality penetrates. Occasionally, there is an overtly intellectual response to the reality of the situation: the mother or father may try to comfort the other, make any necessary arrangements,

etc. This type of response takes place only if the full emotional impact is not allowed to reach the consciousness. The loss, etc., is recognized, but its painful character is muted. This phase may last minutes to days; the longings for a "perfect child" may be recalled, felt intensely and discharged gradually. This process serves to free the parents' feelings so that they may proceed to the next phase. The nurse's presence is beneficial at this time, for it helps the parents to feel that they are not entirely alone.

The second phase, that of developing awareness, involves a *feeling* of loss and disappointment, accompanied at times by affective and physical symptoms (i.e., emptiness in the epigastric or chest regions, sadness, etc.). Now the painful feelings are allowed to become conscious. The parents (particularly the mother) may cry, express anger toward a variety of persons and things, talk about the situation, or they may be unable to express any verbal emotions, although they want to. A relationship between the nurse and the parents that is based on helping is most effective at this time; the nurse's approach should be dictated by the parents' reactions. When she is accepting and encourages the expression of feelings (and provides privacy for their expression), she is helping to prepare the way for the next phase. Developing awareness may take a long time—days or months, in fact. The nurse in the hospital usually will see its beginning, but very infrequently will she see its termination.

The third and final phase of grieving involves restitution and resolving the experience. During restitution mourning occurs, in which mutual grief and loss are expressed by the parents and sympathetic friends and relatives. At this stage religious beliefs and rituals are helpful, for they help to clarify the ambiguity about suffering, eternity and death. In this, the final phase of grief, resolution of the problem gradually occurs; this phase may take 6 months to a year. Here memories and expectations are intensely experienced by repeated questioning, ruminating and recalling the experience to mind. The wise nurse will listen empathically in this phase, reflect what is being said, and gently probe to help the parents arrive at reality.* As already implied, the nurse

---

[1] Engel, G. L.: Grief and grieving. Am. J. Nurs. 64: 93-98, September, 1964.

* The articles in Suggested Reading that deal with grief, stillbirth, deformities, etc., will help the student gain more explicit insight into the process of grief and the species of effective communication and intervention that are necessary in these cases.

in the community health agency will be in the best position to do this, and enlisting her help will entail appropriate referral on the part of the hospital staff.

The Interdisciplinary Team

Many institutions are now employing an interdisciplinary team when the disorder is grave and/or of a long-term nature. In the case of a child who is born with a cleft palate, a pediatrician, plastic surgeon, otologist, orthodontist, psychologist, maternity nurses and public health nurses may all be involved in the care. Since the parents easily can become lost in a maze of appointments, it is wise to have one central person (e.g., the private physician or a social worker) to be the mother's liaison with the other members of the team. The nurse can be instrumental in helping to arrange this.

Stillbirth or Neonatal Death

Occasionally, parents and staff will be faced with the unfortunate circumstance of a stillbirth or a neonatal death. All of the responses of both personnel and parents that have just been described may be apparent in these cases. Grief and mourning will be noted particularly, and it will become the nurse's responsibility to provide an environment in which the mother and father can express their feelings. Nursing care is essentially the same as that just described.

DECISIONS will be difficult for the parents, and whenever possible, especially in everyday mundane matters concerning hospital routine, the nurse should try to structure the situation so that the mother is not overburdened with choices. It is often easier for the mother to respond to "I thought you would like your bed made now," than to "Would you like to shower now, or should I make your bed?" One other point needs special consideration. The nurse must be careful not to offer the mother unhelpful platitudes, such as, "Please don't feel so bad. You have such lovely children at home." Or "You can always have another baby." Statements of this kind are not only unhelpful but are detrimental to the situation, since they convey to the patient the nurse's great lack of understanding and/or her disinterest in the situation. The parents will trust the nurse to the degree that they perceive her understanding and empathic perception of their problem, and to this same degree will they trust her and permit her to help them arrive at a positive solution of their problem.

Getting Help From Instructors and Supervisors

All of the responses that have been described (both for parents and staff) are related to emotionally charged areas (e.g., disappointment, loss and death). As previously implied, these topics often are not discussed easily, and the nurse may encounter resistance on the patient's part in the form of hostility when she attempts to speak of these subjects. It is one thing to *talk* about letting patients express their feelings; it is quite another to permit them to *do* this. At times the inexperienced nurse may become very uncomfortable if a response of resistance is not anticipated. Since the student must have consistent and supportive help to plan effective care (and to manage her feelings and responses adequately) in these cases, she should turn to her instructors and other supervisory personnel for help in this regard. Faculty and supervisors who make themselves readily available as "supportive listeners" to students and anticipate the need for this role can be key persons in helping all concerned to resolve the trauma associated with a disorder or a loss.[2]

In the foregoing section some general aspects related to parental and staff reactions as well as nursing care have been described. In the following pages the specific disorders and principles of care related to them will be discussed. The student may benefit from review of this section as she proceeds with the specific disorders.

NEONATAL RESPIRATORY DISTRESS

Asphyxia Neonatorum

Normally, the infant cries immediately after delivery—often when the shoulders are being born. If respiration has not begun within 30 seconds or so after birth, the condition usually is referred to as *asphyxia neonatorum*. This complication may show various gradations from brief, transitory apnea (absence of respiration) to fatal respiratory failure. In the milder cases the infant's face and often the entire body are of a livid hue, and the vessels of the umbilical cord are distended with blood; the tone of the muscles is good, so that any attempt to move the extremities or open the mouth will meet with some resistance. This stage of the process is known as *asphyxia livida*. In severe

[2] Quint, J. C., and Strauss, A. L.: Nursing students, assignments and dying. Nurs. Outlook 12:24-27, January, 1964.

Quint, J. C., *et al.*: Improving nursing care of the dying. Nurs. Forum 6:369-378, 1967.

ENDOTRACHEAL TUBE

AIRWAY

STILET

SUCTION TUBE

LARYNGOSCOPE AND PREMATURE BLADE

Fig. 23-1. Tray-resuscitation apparatus. (Special Committee on Infant Mortality of the Medical Society of the County of New York: Resuscitation of the Newborn, rev. ed., p. 5, Fig. 4, Philadelphia, Smith Kline & French Laboratories, 1963)

cases the infant's face and body are of a deathlike pallor, the vessels of the cord empty and the muscles relaxed so that the infant is entirely limp. This stage is known as *asphyxia pallida*.

Failure of the infant to breathe at birth usually is due to one of three main causes, or to a combination of them:

1. Anoxia (deprivation of oxygen)
2. Cerebral injury
3. Narcosis

Anoxia. Since the infant in utero is entirely dependent on the placenta for its oxygen supply, any interference with the function of that organ or with that of the umbilical cord will put the infant in grave danger because of anoxia. If the oxygen supply is entirely cut off for more than a very few minutes, fetal death in utero results; if only partially curtailed, the infant is born in an asphyxiated state and (like all asphyxiated persons) does not breathe.

Intra-uterine asphyxia may be produced in a number of ways. The umbilical cord may prolapse and become pinched between the pelvic brim and the fetal head, with the result that the umbilical vein becomes compressed and unable to carry oxygen to the infant. Premature separation of the placenta often disrupts placental function entirely, so that the baby suffers complete deprivation of oxygen. Extremely severe uterine contractions may so squeeze the placental site as to jeopardize the infant's oxygen supply.

Cerebral Injury. This is a very common cause of apnea at birth, particularly after difficult deliveries. Not only may the associated brain hemorrhage damage the respiratory center itself, but other vital centers may be injured. Cerebral injury at birth may be caused by difficult operative delivery, such as midforceps operations, version and extraction, and breech extraction. Likewise, disproportion between the size of the head and that of the pelvis may bring about such compression of the fetal skull as to damage the brain. Cerebral injury may result also from long, difficult labor when no instruments are used.

Narcosis. The narcosis produced in the fetus by analgesic and anesthetic drugs given to the mother is a frequent cause of sluggish respiration at birth. As a rule, however, this is quite transitory, and statistics indicate that these infants do as well subsequently as infants whose mothers received no such drugs. This explains why nurses with adequate experience should supervise these patients closely.

Prevention of Asphyxia Neonatorum

Preventive treatment is very important but is largely the responsibility of the obstetrician. It begins with the first antepartal visit when he measures the pelvis and makes sure that it is large enough to allow passage of the infant's head without compression. Good diet and hygiene contribute greatly to the health of the infant at birth. During labor, the physician can do much to prevent asphyxia of the infant by care in the use of analgesic and anesthetic drugs and by avoiding as much as possible the more difficult types of operative delivery. Moreover, by listening regularly to the fetal heart tones, the attendant may detect early signs of impending fetal distress (slow and/or irregular rate), and, with this warning, it may be possible for the physician to deliver the infant before serious trouble develops. The passage of meconium-stained amniotic fluid is another sign of fetal distress but is of no value in breech presentations, since the passage of meconium—ordinarily pure meconium—is the rule in breech cases.

In the past many phsyicians believed that the administration of vitamin K to the mother late in pregnancy and during labor tended to prevent cerebral hemorrhage in the newborn by improving the clotting power of the fetus' blood. This antihemorrhagic vitamin passes readily through the placenta and raises the prothrombin concentration of the fetal plasma, which ordinarily is low. Recent studies indicate, however, that hyperbilirubinemia is associated with the parenteral administration of a vitamin K analogue antepartally; this is particularly true in the case of premature infants. Therefore, the prophylactic administration of this drug to the mother during labor should be viewed with caution. Current practice is to administer a small dose (1.0 mg.) of water-soluble vitamin K to the infant immediately after birth as a prophylaxis against the coagulation defect related to vitamin K deficiency.

Treatment of Asphyxia Neonatorum

It has been recommended[3] that all members of the delivery room team be trained in methods of resuscitation for mother and baby since both may have difficulty at the same time. Indecisive or ineffective therapy may lose precious moments in which the infant's life can be saved. All equipment necessary for resuscitation (Fig. 23-1) should be checked before each delivery and should include a suction apparatus, a plastic oropharyngeal

airway, a laryngoscope equipped with a premature blade (and working batteries) and a Cole plastic endotracheal tube with a stilet. In addition, oxygen should be available.

Generally, the anesthesiologist will assume responsibility for the maintenance of the resuscitation equipment per se. Since he is usually responsible for the immediate measures of resuscitation, it will fall to the nurse to assist him in any way that she can. Moreover, it is the nurse's function to keep the delivery room prepared for adequate and prompt treatment of asphyxia neonatorum (as well as other emergencies), whether it is expected or not. Therefore, she should have supplies and equipment in readiness. These may include the resuscitator, warm blankets, oxygen and the aforementioned equipment. She is to be prepared to position the infant during the procedures, if necessary, and to make and to report accurate observations. Her skill and competence in assisting the physician in caring for the infant and the mother will go far in giving the mother the reassurance and the support that she needs at this time.

Any infant who has an Apgar score (see Chapter 13) of 0, 1, or 2 is severely depressed and deserving of immediate treatment. In treating an infant who does not breathe at birth, there are five main principles to keep in mind.

1. Gentleness. These infants are often in a state of shock, and rough attempts to resuscitate them—as by vigorous spanking or other overvigorous methods of external stimulation—may do more harm than good. Methods of physical stimulation should be limited to gentle rubbing of the back and, at the most, to light patting of the buttocks. When anoxia is present, oxygen is necessary to overcome it, and the use of measures which act as external irritants will not oxygenate the tissues.

2. Warmth. Heated cribs and other means of maintaining body warmth, such as hot-water bottles and warm blankets, must be in readiness. This is particularly important to remember, because the measures employed to resuscitate infants, unless care be taken, tend to expose their completely naked bodies (accustomed to the temperature in utero) to room temperature; and this may aggravate the state of shock. The body of the infant should be kept covered as much as possible.

3. Posture. Some obstetricians hold the infant up by the feet momentarily after birth in order to expedite drainage of mucus from the trachea, the larynx and the posterior pharynx. Others cradle

[3] Manual of Standards in Obstetric-Gynecologic Practice. p. 25, Chicago, The American College of Obstetricians and Gynecologists, 1963; and Special Committee on Infant Mortality of the Medical Society of the County of New York: Resuscitation of the Newborn. rev. ed., p. 5, Philadelphia, Smith Kline & French Laboratories, 1963.

FIG. 23-2. Catheter and glass bulb with a trap, for aspirating mucus in the treatment of asphyxia. (Chicago Lying-in Hospital)

the baby in the arm with the hand supporting the head, which is held down. The baby is then placed on his back in a slight Trendelenburg position (head turned aside, lower than buttocks), also to favor gravity drainage of mucus.

4. Removal of Mucus. Cleansing the air passages of mucus and fluid is essential, since effective respiration cannot be accomplished through obstructed air passages. The head-down position will promote drainage of mucus and fluid from the respiratory passages, but postural drainage alone is often not adequate for this purpose, and suction of one type or another is frequently necessary. An ordinary catheter is used, size 12 to 14 French; in premature infants a smaller size (8 to 10) is advisable. A glass trap (Fry) is inserted into the catheter to arrest mucus which otherwise might be drawn into the operator's mouth (Fig. 23-2). Milking the trachea upward will help bring mucus and fluid into the posterior pharynx, where it may be aspirated by the catheter. Gentleness is essential, since the mucous membrane of the infant's mouth is delicate. Although the physician occasionally does so, the nurse should not introduce the catheter farther than the posterior pharynx. Mechanical suction devices are provided with most of the modern machines for infant resuscitation and are very convenient.

5. Artificial Respiraton. If a newborn infant fails to respond to other resuscitative measures within 1½ minutes after delivery, oxygen must be administered promptly, since diminished muscle tone and lowered heart rate usually result from the progressing asphyxia. The infant should be positioned with his head lower than his torso to facilitate drainage, and with his neck extended as if in a "sniffing posture." Consequently, the infant's natural air passage is straightened (see Fig. 23-3). As oxygen is administered by mask, the infant's chin should be supported by pressing upward with the 4th and the 5th fingers under the angles of the baby's jaw. Because the adult fingers are large in comparison with the smallness of the infant's jaw, *extreme care* must be taken not to allow the fingers to slip toward the midline under the chin. If this happens, it only contributes to further obstruction of air passages by the infant's tongue. The most effective way to prevent obstruction by the tongue is by insertion of a small oropharyngeal airway into the mouth. Mechanical devices for the controlled administration of oxygen are the most efficient, but resuscitation may be carried out in a number of ways when such equipment is not available.

Probably the oldest method of resuscitation is mouth-to-mouth insufflation, but this is disapproved by some physicians because the method

FIG. 23-3. Closed-chest cardiac massage in the newborn infant. *Note:* The infant is placed on a flat surface which is tilted so that his head is on a lower level than his body, facilitating drainage of his airway. In addition, the infant's neck is extended; thus, his natural air passage is straightened.

may be dangerous, both from the possibility of rupturing pulmonary alveoli and the risk of infection. Although this procedure is ordinarily performed by the doctor, the nurse may be asked to carry it out if the available physicians are busy attending the mother. The operator stands or sits back of the infant's head. After placing 3 or 4 layers of gauze on the infant's nose and mouth, the operator bends over the infant and puts his opened mouth over the infant's mouth and nose, the gauze intervening. He now exhales gently into the infant's respiratory tract. It is advantageous to follow this with light compression of the chest, insufflation and compression being alternated. One does not "blow" into the baby's mouth but simply exhales more or less naturally. As mentioned above, blowing into the baby's mouth with any degree of force is highly dangerous and may rupture pulmonary alveoli.

A modification of mouth-to-mouth breathing for resuscitation, using instead a mouth-to-airway technique, has been described.[4] This method is accomplished with the use of an S-shaped instrument assembled from two standard rubber oropharyngeal airways in such a way as to provide both an oropharyngeal airway for the infant and a mouthpiece for the operator. In the resuscitation of the newborn infant, the operator must "puff" gently into the mouthpiece, a No. 0 airway, using only the air from his oral cavity and not the air from his lungs. It is done in this manner to avoid damage to the infant's lungs. As soon as the chest rises, the operator takes his mouth off the mouthpiece and allows the infant to exhale passively before proceeding with the next "puff" of breath into the airway.

Many hospitals are now using mechanical devices for the resuscitation of the newborn. Such apparatus permits the administration of pure oxygen to the baby's lungs at pressures which are controlled mechanically within safe limits.

Gentle compression of the chest with the *fingers* (external cardiac massage) is usually initiated if the infant's heart has not begun to beat after the administration of oxygen (Fig. 23-3). External manual compression of the heart between the chest wall and the vertebral column forces blood into the aorta. When the pressure is relaxed, the heart is allowed to fill with venous blood. When compression is combined with proper ventilation, the blood pressure and adequate oxygenation can

often be maintained until spontaneous cardiac activity is resumed.

Only a person who fully understands this technique of resuscitation should attempt it, since the procedure *differs* from that used for the adult patient—both in the *manner of applying pressure* and in the *degree of pressure exerted* on the heart (see Suggested Reading at end of chapter).

A RELATIVELY SIMPLE TECHNIQUE FOR CLOSED-CHEST MASSAGE OF THE NEWBORN has been described as follows:

1. Immediately on delivery the baby is placed in a bassinet with its head on a lower level than its torso in order to facilitate drainage of the airway.

2. The presence or absence of a heartbeat is determined by auscultation.

3. The oropharynx is cleared of meconium so that the vocal chords are visible.

4. Intubation of the trachea is performed under direct vision to ensure access to the pulmonary tree.

5. The trachea and bronchi are rapidly aspirated and cleared of meconium and secretions in order to obtain adequate ventilation.

6. The tracheal tube is held firmly in one hand, and the lungs are expanded by blowing gently down the tube. This is continued intermittently at a rate of 20 per minute.

7. Immediately after filling the lungs, the fingers of the free hand are applied flatly on the midthorax at the level of the sternum, and the latter is compressed firmly in the direction of the vertebral column, and immediately released. This is continued at a rate of approximately 80 to 100 per minute. The degree of pressure exerted on the heart should be enough to obtain a femoral pulse. It is expected that this will suffice to obtain adequate circulation, and yet not inflict trauma on the heart, large vessels, liver, and surrounding tissues. If necessary 0.1 to 0.2 mg. of epinephrine can be injected into the heart.

8. Immediately on the appearance of spontaneous heartbeats, cardiac massage is interrupted, but positive pressure aeration is continued until the baby gasps spontaneously, or under direct external stimulation.

9. Prior to extubation, the trachea, oropharynx, and nasal passages are again aspirated in order to clear any remaining meconium or secretions that may have appeared in the course of treatment.[5]

[4] Safar, P., and McMahon, M.: Mouth-to-airway artificial respiration, J.A.M.A. 166:1459, 1958.

[5] Mathews, D. H., *et al.*: Closed-chest massage in the newborn infant. J.A.M.A. 183:964-966, March 16, 1963.
Barnett, H. L.: Pediatrics. p. 65, New York, Appleton, 1968.

No drugs have been found to be effective as respiratory stimulants for the infant. However, if the infant's respiratory depression is related to maternal narcosis from opiates, then the physician may administer levallorphan (Lorfan, 0.25 mg.) or nalorphine (N-allylnormorphine: Nalline, 0.1 mg. per kilogram of body weight) into the umbilical vein. Respiration may be improved. These drugs should be used only when a specific opiate has been used for the mother, as they otherwise will act as respiratory depressants for the baby (see Suggested Reading).

Investigators have found that, in experimental animals, the rapid correction of the pH during asphyxia by the rapid intravenous infusion of an alkali together with glucose prolongs gasping and delays cardiovascular collapse. Resuscitation also appears facilitated if the alkali and glucose are infused at the same time that artificial ventilation is started. *Tris*-(hydroxymethyl) aminomethane (THAM), has been effectively used in experimental animals. It appears safe when administered in a 0.5 molar solution adjusted to a pH of 8.85 (12 ml./kg.) over a 2-to-4 minute period. The beneficial effects of this alkali administration both to asphyxiated newborn monkeys and human adults suffering from cardiac arrest, suggest that this treatment would be of value if used in newborn infants. Some physicians do attempt this treatment on depressed infants; by and large, however, indications and exact dosage schedules have not yet been determined.

Continued Observation. It is important that close observation be continued after resuscitation methods have ceased. Generally, the baby's condition will improve; occasionally, however, it will worsen, especially if the difficulty is due to mucous obstruction or to drugs administered to the mother. The Apgar method of infant evaluation, as well as the other observations described in Chapter 13, can be utilized in these cases. The continuing observations that should be made when the infant is transferred to the nursery are described in Chapter 16.

Atelectasis

Prior to birth the lungs contain no air and are in a state of collapse. With the first breath, expansion of the lung tissue begins and continues progressively for several days until all parts of the lung are expanded. Feeble respiratory action after birth, incomplete development of the lung, or blockage by mucus or amniotic debris in the small ducts leading to the air sacs may expand the lungs only partially, leaving large areas in a collapsed state. This condition is known as atelectasis. It is particularly common in premature infants. Cyanosis is usually present, because the small areas of expanded lung are inadequate to oxygenate the blood properly. When extensive areas of the lung are involved, there will be irregular, rapid respiration with respiratory grunt, flaring nostrils, intercostal and suprasternal retractions and weakness, in addition to cyanosis.

Atelectasis is treated best by maintaining a clear airway, continuous administration of oxygen, high humidity (to liquefy the secretions so that the infant may cough them up), frequent changes of position, and occasional attempts to stimulate deeper respiration, e.g., short whiffs of carbon dioxide gas. Antibiotics may be utilized, since the inactive portions of the lung are susceptible to infection.

Pneumonia

This condition is the largest pulmonary cause of death in infants dying after 48 hours and is noted in as many as 22 per cent of all newborn autopsies. The incidence is usually bimodal, that is, two peaks occur. One is in the first 12 hours of life and is usually secondary to maternal infection. The second peak comes after 48 hours of life, and is probably acquired in the nursery. In the newborn the condition may be due to bacteria or viruses and is usually of the bronchopneumonic variety rather than the lobar. The birth process itself as well as infection after birth can be etiologic factors. For instance, infection may come from aspiration of infected amniotic fluid or aspiration of secretions from the mother's vagina during delivery, or it may be acquired through the blood stream. Colds are the most common source of infection after birth.

One of the first signs that alerts the nurse is that of rapid respiration (80 per minute or more), accompanied by flaring of the nostrils. The baby is listless, pale or cyanotic and may refuse his feedings; in addition, his temperature may be higher or lower than is usual for him. Oxygen and antibiotics are the treatment of choice. If the pneumonia is due to aspiration of feedings, the first symptom is usually an episode of choking or coughing. The other symptoms soon follow. Careful feeding is a key in prevention. If the infant does choke, he should be placed in a head-down position and the trachea milked to encourage the aspirated fluid to drain from the lungs. After feedings it is wise to place infants on their abdomens or sides to avoid aspiration if regurgitation occurs.

Since many newborn nursery units transfer a baby to a pediatric unit if the infant is born with or develops a serious disorder or infection, separation from her infant may be a problem for the mother. The principles regarding this aspect of nursing care will be essentially the same as those described in Chapter 17.

Idiopathic Respiratory Distress Syndrome (Hyaline Membrane Disease)

Hyaline membrane disease is a syndrome of neonatal respiratory distress in which the alveoli and the alveolar ducts are filled with a sticky exudate, a hyaline material, which prevents aeration. Although it is known that the hyaline material is a protein, the cause of hyaline membrane formation is not definitely known. Three main theories are now under study. The first proposes an alteration in the fibrinolytic enzyme system in the lung or blood which leads to the proliferation of the protein (fibrin) exudate. The second suggests an absence or alterations of the pulmonary surfactant which reduces alveolar ventilation and promotes atelectasis. The third indicates pulmonary hypofusion rather than surfactant deficiency. This hypofusion begins with intrauterine asphyxia and also results in reduced alveolar ventilation and atelectasis.

The greatest incidence occurs in premature infants weighing between 1,000 and 1,500 Gm., and it is observed in about 10 per cent of all premature infants. It also occurs in about 50 per cent of all infants of diabetic mothers and also in infants whose mothers experienced antepartal vaginal bleeding. The condition has also been noted in infants born by cesarean section; however, cesarean section in otherwise *uncomplicated* full-term deliveries is probably not associated with any increased incidence of the disease. This disease is not found in stillborn infants.

It was formerly believed that a free interval existed after birth before the onset of symptoms. However, when infants are observed closely and examined carefully, symptoms can be noted immediately after birth. A chest x-ray usually confirms the diagnosis and rules out congenital cardiovascular disease. Expiratory grunting or whining (observable when the infant is not crying), sternal and subcostal retractions, nasal flaring, rapid respirations (more than 70 per minute) and low body temperatures are seen early and are diagnostic clues. Grunting, which is the most important and useful clinical sign, may be the only and earliest indication of the disease. Conversely, cessation of grunting is often the first sign of improvement. The infant may be cyanotic in room air. Infants who are badly affected may be cyanotic even with oxygen therapy yet paradoxically exhibit a normal respiratory rate. Auscultation of the chest reveals poor air entry, decreased breath sounds, and at times, fine rales. Bowel sounds are often absent in the early hours of the illness and the urine output is low during the first 2 or 3 days of life. If the disease progresses, respiratory rate increases, chest retractions become more marked, and see-saw respirations (see Fig. 17-1) ensue. Peripheral edema increases, and muscle tone decreases. With the increase in cyanosis, the body temperature tends to drop and short periods of apnea are noted. The heart rate is often fixed except for periods of bradycardia accompanied by severe cyanosis and grunting. Many symptoms are related to asphyxia which depresses the respiratory center and causes apneic episodes as well as changes in the blood distribution throughout the body. This latter fact accounts for the pale gray skin color of the severely affected infant. In addition the rate of heat production is also decreased. If treatment is instituted promptly, modern care has resulted in about a 50 to 70 per cent salvage rate for these infants. If treatment is not prompt and/or the infant is small or does not respond to treatment, death may occur within 48 hours.

It is important that the nurse make meticulous observations and recordings about the respiratory signs and symptoms, especially of infants who are born prematurely or who are delivered by cesarean section. The outcome for the premature is usually poorer and depends a great deal on his birth weight: the smaller he is, the graver is the prognosis. For example, infants who weigh 1,000 Gm. or less generally succumb, since their lungs are not developed enough to make the adjustment to extrauterine life.

Treatment. Mortality from this condition has been reduced not so much because of any new advances in technique but rather because of an increased interest in the care of these infants, and a standardized approach and properly equipped facilities. Treatment primarily consists of prompt placement of the infant in an incubator to facilitate the administration of oxygen and the maintenance of high humidity as soon as the first symptoms appear. These infants must be watched carefully and the nurse is a key person in this sphere. Accurate recording and reporting includes rate and quality of respiration, cardiac rate, temperature, and intake and output of fluids. The most severely affected receive respirator therapy. If sepsis or infection is suspected antibiotics are utilized. The acid-base status is corrected as necessary with the use of intravenous fluids. By 72 hours, infants with this condition will usually show either marked improvement or definite deterioration. When the infant remains stable for 12 to 24 hours in terms of acid-base and clinical status, small feedings of clear fluids may be instituted and the intravenous feedings discontinued if the oral feedings are retained.

Since infants delivered by cesarean section who have had a stormy labor are prone to develop this complication, many physicians prescribe that they be placed in an incubator with oxygen and high humidity immediately on delivery as a prophylactic measure. The stomach contents may be aspirated, and the oropharyngeal suctioning is done to remove mucus and fluid from the nose and the mouth.

Recent work indicates that exchange transfusion may also help infants with severe respiratory distress syndrome. This is based on evidence that the addition of adult hemoglobin raises levels of an enzyme, 2,3-diphosphoglycerate, which facilitates the unloading of oxygen from hemoglobin at the tissue level.

INJURIES

Caput Succedaneum

Prolonged pressure on the head during a protracted first stage of labor, where the membranes rupture before the cervix is fully dilated, causes an edematous swelling of the soft tissues of the scalp over the area where it is encircled by the cervix (Fig. 23-4). This is called "caput succedaneum," and in its milder forms is very common —so common that it may be regarded as normal.

It is due to an extravasation of serum into the tissues of the scalp at the portion surrounded by the cervix. The term is not confined to vertex cases; the corresponding swelling which forms on any presenting part is also, for the sake of uniformity, known as caput succedaneum. The condition always disappears within a few days without treatment. A prompt and simple explanation should be given to the parents, since this condition, although benign, can be somewhat disfiguring. Once the parents know that the caput will disappear of its own accord, they usually are reassured and will not press for "treatment."

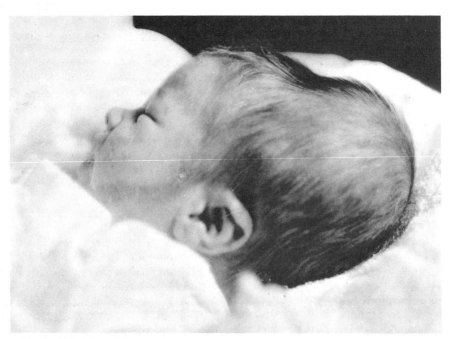

FIG. 23-4. Caput succedaneum. (MacDonald House, University Hospitals of Cleveland)

Fig. 23-5. Cephalhematoma. (Mac-Donald House, University Hospitals of Cleveland)

Cephalhematoma

Another swelling of the scalp which resembles caput succedaneum in certain respects is caused by an effusion of blood between the bone and the periosteum (Fig. 23-5). This explains why the swelling appears directly over the bone. It is most common over the parietal bones. It is seldom visible when the infant is born and may not be noticed for several hours or more after delivery, since subperiosteal bleeding occurs slowly. The cephalhematoma increases gradually in size until about the 7th day after labor, when it remains stationary for a time and then begins to disappear. The infant usually recovers without treatment. It may be due to pressure in normal labor, or by forceps; but also it is seen occasionally in breech cases in which no instruments were used or prolonged pressure exerted on the aftercoming head. Such cases, however, are not common. Again, the parents should receive assurance regarding the temporary nature of this condition and its spontaneous disappearance.

Intracranial Hemorrhage
(Cerebral Hemorrhage, Brain Hemorrhage)

In contradistinction to the two conditions just described, intracranial hemorrhage is one of the gravest complications encountered in the newborn. It may occur any place in the cranial vault but is particularly likely to take place as the result of tears in the tentorium cerebelli with bleeding into the cerebellum, the pons and the medulla oblongata. Since these structures contain many important centers (respiratory center, etc.), hemorrhage in these areas is very often fatal.

Intracranial hemorrhage occurs most often after prolonged labor, especially in primiparae, and is particularly likely to take place in difficult forceps deliveries and in version and extractions. It is also seen more commonly in precipitate deliveries as the result of the rapid propulsion of the infant's head through the birth canal. It is due primarily to excessive or unduly prolonged pressure on the fetal skull. This causes excessive molding of the head and such overriding of the cranial bones that the delicate supporting structures of the brain (tentorium cerebelli, falx cerebri, etc.) are torn, with consequent rupture of blood vessels.

The development of symptoms in cerebral hemorrhage may be sudden or gradual. If the hemorrhage is severe, the infant is usually stillborn; if less marked, apnea neonatorum may result, often with fatal outcome. Many infants who are resuscitated with difficulty at birth succumb later from brain hemorrhage. On the other hand, the infant may appear normal after delivery and develop the first signs of intracranial hemorrhage several hours or several days later.

The nurse should be familiar with the common signs of cerebral hemorrhage, which are described as follows. Any such signs should be reported immediately.

1. Convulsions. These may vary from mild, localized twitchings to severe spasms of the whole body. Twitching of the lower jaw is characteristic, particularly when associated with salivation.

2. Cyanosis. This may be persistent but is more likely to occur in repeated attacks.

3. Abnormal Respiration. Grunting respiration is characteristic; or it may be irregular, of Cheyne-Stokes type, or very rapid and shallow, or very slow. Very slow breathing, usually associated with cyanosis, suggests respiratory paralysis due to pressure on the medulla oblongata and is a grave sign.

4. A Sharp, Shrill, Weak Cry. This is similar to that seen in meningitis.

5. Flaccidity or Spasticity. If the preceding condition is present, it usually portends a fatal outcome. Somnolence also may be present. In other cases there may be generalized spasticity with backward arching of the head and neck and extension of the legs (opisthotonos).

Treatment. Prevention is most important and is largely the responsibility of the physician. It consists in protecting the infant from trauma, particularly in difficult operative delivery. As stated previously, many obstetricians believe that the administration of vitamin K to the mother before delivery decreases the likelihood of cerebral bleeding. This is done less frequently now due to the possibility of hyperbilirubinemia. A small dose of water-soluble vitamin K_1 (1.0 mg.) may be given the infant after birth, however (see p. 276).

Curative treatment can be effective if damage is not too extensive.

Complete rest, with the very minimum amount of handling, is imperative. Infants suspected of having a cerebral hemorrhage should not nurse the breast and should not be weighed or bathed. Since shock often is present, external heat frequently is indicated. Feeding should be carried out in such a manner as to impose on the infant the least possible effort; some of these infants have to be gavaged. Usually the physician will order some form of sedative for convulsions and will prescribe the administration of oxygen for cyanosis. Vitamin C and water-soluble vitamin K may be used to control the hemorrhage, and antibiotics may be given prophylactically. The head of the infant is kept a few inches above the level of the hips, because this position is believed to lower intracranial pressure. Moreover, the infant should *not* be placed in Trendelenburg position after delivery.

The parents, of course, will need and deserve adequate explanation and reassurance. Since it is difficult to prognosticate in this condition (as well as in several of the other disorders) until the extent and the severity of the injury can be determined, personnel will not want to give the parents false hopes nor yet seem to be unduly pessimistic. The physician and nurse, however, as they report to the parents, can always add an expression like "today" or "at this time" to their explanations, even if the news seems to be unfortunate (e.g., "The baby is responding satisfactorily to the medicines today." "He is progressing at this time."). This will give the parents a more realistic reassurance and yet subtly alert them to the fluidity of the situation.

Facial Paralysis

Pressure by forceps on the facial nerve may cause temporary paralysis of the muscles of one side of the face so that the mouth is drawn to the other side. This will be particularly noticeable when the infant cries. The condition is usually transitory and disappears in a few days, often in a few hours. Since the infant can look grotesque, the parents will need an explanation concerning the temporary nature of this affliction. If the mother is allowed to feed the baby, the nurse will want to be with her more consistently during the first feedings to help her as necessary. Sucking may be difficult for the infant, and the mother will need to develop patience and skill in the feeding of her baby. If one eye remains open because of the affected muscles, the doctor will prescribe such treatment as is appropriate. Any necessary instruction regarding this continuing care after discharge should be given the mother before she leaves the hospital. Very often parents are afraid to handle their infants when disorders occur for fear of hurting the child; this may happen even if the condition is short-term and fairly innocuous. Thus, parents should be encouraged to hold and cuddle their infants whenever the condition permits.

Arm Paralysis
(Erb-Duchenne's Paralysis, Brachial Palsy)

This condition results from excessive stretching of the nerve fibers that run from the neck through the shoulder and down toward the arm (brachial plexus). It is a result of forcible pulling of the shoulder away from the head during delivery, usually during a breech extraction. Generally, only the muscles of the upper arm are involved, and the infant holds his arm at the side with the elbow extended and the hand rotated inward. The hand and fingers may not be involved. If the nerves are merely stretched, recovery occurs in several weeks; if they are broken within their sheaths, then healing will not be complete for several months. If healing fails to occur within that time, then surgery is indicated; the outcome for recovery in these cases is guarded. In order to reduce tension on the brachial plexus, the physician usually will place the arm in a splint or cast in an elevated, neutral position. While the arm is healing, the doctor will order gentle manipulation and massage of the muscles to prevent contractures. The mother is to be instructed in these procedures so that she may continue the care.

Fractures and Dislocations

Fracture of a long bone or dislocation of an extremity may be the result of a version; or it may occur following a breech delivery in which the arms were extended above the head and are brought down into the vagina. Fractures of the clavicle or of the jaw, or dislocation of either of these bones, may follow forcible efforts to extract the aftercoming head in cases of breech presentation. Fracture or dislocation of the cervical spine, usually accompanied by damage to the spinal cord may also be the consequence of a difficult breech extraction. The vertebra most usually affected are C5 and C6. If the cord is not completely severed, surgical repair is often effected. These babies will have a flaccid paralysis of the trunk and extremities and breathe abdominally since the diaphragm is innervated by the nerves which have been injured in the dislocation or fracture.

Fractures in the newborn baby, particularly in the long bones usually heal rapidly, but it is often difficult to keep the parts in good alignment during repair. Immobilization of the part often can be achieved by swaddling and positioning the infant on his side. Splints, slings and other apparatus are useful. However, these often make handling the infant difficult and cumbersome; hence parents tend to avoid touching the infant for fear of "hurting" him. Care should be taken by the staff to encourage the parents to give their infant adequate love and attention if these are used. This will mean that the parents will have to be shown how to manipulate the apparatus effectively so that they will not traumatize the injury. Dislocation should be reduced at once, or there will be great danger of permanent deformity in the joint. Follow-up supervision is necessary in order to prevent permanent deformity. Physiotherapy under orthopedic direction is important.

INFECTIONS

Most institutions have an area designated as an isolation nursery where any infant who has or is suspected of having an infection is placed immediately. Once the infant has been transferred to the isolation nursery, he should not be returned to the newborn nursery even though the infection has been treated and/or cured. Strict aseptic technique is used in the care of these babies, and therefore the principles of communicable disease nursing must be understood and carried out by all personnel coming in contact with the infants. Separation of the mother and the infant may be necessary, depending on the type and the severity of the infection. This may require consequent nursing action that has been discussed in Chapter 13.

Ophthalmia Neonatorum (Gonorrheal Conjunctivitis)

This is a serious condition which may result in total blindness, but if suitable treatment is adopted at the very outset of the disease and intelligently carried out; usually the sight can be saved. The entire treatment is, of course, under the direct supervision of the physician.

Fortunately, state laws making the use of an antibacterial prophylaxis compulsory for all infants at birth have reduced the incidence of this infection immeasurably. Before eye prophylaxis became mandatory, however, 25 to 30 per cent of all children in schools for the blind suffered impaired sight as the result of the infection. This condition is of gonorrheal origin and is characterized by a profuse, purulent discharge in the eyes due to infection, generally from the genital canal at the time of birth. However, the causative organism, *Neisseria gonorrhoeae,* can be transmitted also on the hands of personnel working with infected mothers and by articles (e.g., towels, tissues, etc.) that come in contact with the infection. Thus, the importance of proper hygiene for those working with infected persons cannot be stressed enough. Prompt diagnosis and treatment of those suspected of having the disease is also vital, since the mother may reinfect her infant as she handles him.

If the infection occurs at the time of birth, the disease appears within 2 or 3 days; but as the septic discharge may be introduced into the eye at a later period by neglect of the proper care of the infant, the onset may be later. Both eyes are usually affected; and at first they are suffused with a watery discharge and considerable inflammation of the eyelids. Within 24 hours the lids become very much swollen, and a thick, creamy, greenish pus is discharged. Later, unless treatment has been instituted early, the swelling becomes so marked that the eyes cannot be opened, opacities of the cornea occur, the conjunctiva is ulcerated and then perforated, and the eye collapses and finally atrophies.

The preventive treatment consists in the use of an antibacterial agent, usually 1 per cent silver nitrate, or penicillin ophthalmic ointment, which is instilled immediately after birth. However, if infection does occur, penicillin intramuscular injections may be given. If the infection persists, intensive penicillin administration should be carried out. Thanks to this drug, gonorrheal ophthalmia, which used to be one of the most stubborn and grave afflictions and demanded the utmost in elaborate and prolonged nursing and medical care, is now cured within 12 to 24 hours. The swelling and the pus usually disappear in even less time than this.

Ophthalmia neonatorum is a distinctly infectious disease, and there is extreme danger of conveying it to others. This applies not only to other infants' eyes but to the genital tract of other mothers. Even the eyes of the nurse herself may become infected, unless she is most conscientious in her methods. The infant should be isolated, and all articles used should be sterilized.

Staphylococcus of resistant types occasionally cause purulent discharge; all such cases require the care of a physician until recovery.

Impetigo

Impetigo is a skin disease of infectious origin and not infrequently occurs in epidemic form in the nursery. For this reason it is often called "impetigo contagiosa." The condition manifests itself by the eruption of small, semiglobular vesicles or pustules. Although these may appear on any part of the body, they are most frequently encountered on moist opposing surfaces, such as the folds of the neck, the axilla and the groin. Thence they may spread rapidly by auto-inoculation to any part of the body. The lesion is small and varies from the size of a pinhead to a diameter of half an inch. It contains yellow pus. The bacterium involved is usually the staphylococcus or the streptococcus.

The treatment is essentially preventive, and cases rarely occur if the nursery technique has been meticulous. The nurse and the physician must wash their hands carefully before handling any infant, and every possible source of skin infection must be eliminated. Constant vigilance is necessary if these cases are to be prevented. Treatment consists of prompt isolation of the infant and local treatment of the lesions. Since these lesions tend to appear on moist or opposing skin surfaces, the infant is kept clean and dry. Daily baths using hexachlorophene (pHisoHex) may be given. Usually the blebs are broken, and the denuded areas are exposed to dry heat. Gentian violet, alcohol, bacitracin, or neomycin oint-

ment may be applied locally. Systemic antibiotic therapy may be required.

As soon as a lesion develops which resembles impetigo even slightly, strict isolation of the infant is imperative. The physician should be notified at once. If properly treated, the superficial lesions heal quickly and with little scarring. Parenteral antibiotic therapy may be given prophylactically. A high nutritional level must be maintained, and scratching should be controlled. It is important for the nurse to remember that it is the fluid within the bleb which spreads the infection. When impetigo develops in a nursery, it may be stubborn to eradicate, and occasionally it may even become necessary to close the nursery for a few weeks.

Thrush

Thrush is an infection of the mouth caused by the organism *Candida albicans,* the organism which causes monilial vaginitis in the mother (see Chap. 8). The infant may acquire the infection as it passes through the birth canal of a mother so infected. However, the infection may be transferred from infant to infant on the hands of attendants and is favored by lack of cleanliness in feeding, in the care of the mother's nipples, or in the care of the bottles and the nipples. It is most likely to occur in weak, undernourished babies. The condition appears as small white patches (due to the fungus growth) on the tongue and in the mouth. These white plaques may be mistaken at first for small curds of milk. The infant's mouth must be kept clean, but great gentleness is required to avoid further injury to the delicate epithelium, and any attempt to wipe away the plaques will usually cause bleeding.

Some physicians advise painting the spots with an aqueous solution of 1 per cent gentian violet, in which case the spots are touched gently with a sterile, soft cotton swab saturated with the medication. Another method of treatment is with nystatin, an antibiotic specific for infections caused by the monilial organism, *Candida albicans.* Mycostatin, an oral suspension of nystatin (200,000 units per cc.) is dropped into the infant's mouth and thus comes in contact with the affected areas. The usual dosage of Mycostatin is 1 to 4 cc. 3 or 4 times daily, as prescribed by the physician. The nurse will recall that nystatin is poorly absorbed from the gastrointestinal tract and is excreted almost entirely in the feces after oral administration.

Special care must be taken with the bottles and nipples used for infants who have thrush. These bottles and nipples must be kept separated from the others in the nursery until they are soaked in antiseptic solution, washed thoroughly and boiled before they are cared for in the routine way with bottles and nipples of other infants.

Epidemic Diarrhea of the Newborn

During recent years a number of highly fatal epidemics of diarrhea have occurred in nurseries for the newborn throughout the country. Among infants so affected, almost half have died. The mortality rate in premature infants is twice the rate in full-term infants. The onset is sudden, with profuse, watery yellow stools which increase in frequency. Associated with the diarrhea, a precipitous weight loss occurs—often a pound within 24 hours. The appearance of the infant changes rapidly from that of a healthy baby to one of a markedly dehydrated and emaciated infant. In a severe case, death may occur in a day, but more often the baby lingers on in a semi-comatose condition for 4 or 5 days. The spread of the disease is very rapid, and half the infants in a nursery may succumb within a fortnight. Many of the epidemics accordingly are described as "explosive" in character.

The most common offending organisms are strains of a common inhabitant of the intestinal tract, *Escherichia coli*. These pathogenic strains are carried by healthy adults who handle the newborn infant; unfortunately, it is very difficult to diagnose these carriers by the usual means and thus prevent their coming in contact with the newborn.

The symptoms and the mortality rate differ from bacterial types of dysentery or diarrhea. One of the most important predisposing factors is overcrowding in the nurseries. Faulty nursery technique is another—that is, failure to wash the hands before touching a baby, failure to sterilize rubber nipples properly, etc. The guiding principle involved is that everything coming in contact with the baby's mouth and nose should be in a surgically aseptic condition. All obstetric and nursing techniques must be planned accordingly. Various health departments have set up rigid regulations along these lines in the hope of preventing epidemics.

Treatment and Prevention. When a case is discovered, immediate and absolute isolation is necessary; therefore, the infant is transferred from the newborn nursery. A culture of the stools is done to find out the causative organism. This is done so that specific therapy can be instituted as soon as possible.

Neomycin and Colimycin given orally have been found to be most effective against the *E. coli* organisms. These drugs may be given prophylactically to exposed but uninfected infants until their discharge. Penicillin and streptomycin are sometimes administered to prevent or control the secondary infection that might occur in the debilitated infants. Supportive fluid therapy by the intravenous or the subcutaneous route also may be utilized. Oral fluids—water, 5 per cent glucose in water, or Lytren (a commercially prepared electrolyte fluid replacement for oral use)—are given in small amounts. Whole blood is given by transfusion if indicated.

If necessary, the nursery is closed to new admissions until the epidemic clears up. These nurseries are washed and sometimes even painted before being opened again for new admissions. In the prevention of this disease there seems to be nothing more effective than strict aseptic nursery technique. Hand washing with soap or pHisoHex and water after changing diapers, before feeding the infant and after handling the infant or any of its equipment is a rigid rule that should be stressed.

If an outbreak occurs, there should be a followup of all infants discharged in the preceding 2 weeks, and any infants needing treatment are readmitted to the pediatric service of the hospital. All infants exposed at the time of an outbreak are given prophylactic therapy. Complete control of this disease, which formerly led to closing of the nursery, can be gained by prompt reporting, rigid techniques and immediate treatment.

Because of the "explosive" and virulent character of this disease and the startling debilitation of the infant, the parents usually become very anxious about their baby and with good reason. The baby is usually not allowed to go out to the mother, as a measure to prevent the spread of the infection and to guard against secondary infection of the infant. Thus, breast-feeding is interrupted for a time at least. The nurse can be helpful in keeping the mother and father informed about the status of the infant and helping the mother to work through her anxiety and grief positively. If it appears that breast-feeding can be resumed shortly, then the nurse can also show the mother how to empty her breast by manual expression to keep the milk supply available until nursing is resumed.

Syphilis

Even with the rise in the rate of this disease in the general population in recent years, syphilis in the newborn can be prevented when antepartal care is adequate. It has decreased greatly in the 42 states where serologic tests on the blood of all pregnant women are required. This condition shows lesions only if the infant has early prenatal syphilis. They may be present at birth or may appear from a few days up to 4 months of age, predominantly on the face, the buttocks, the palms and the soles. Mucous patches occur in the mouth, and condylomata about the anus. These lesions are highly infectious. The eruption is usually maculopapular and not quite so generalized as in acquired syphilis. Bullae may appear on the palms and the soles, a type of lesion never found in acquired syphilis. The palms and the soles may desquamate as a result of the lesions. Less frequently seen are papular lesions or purely macular or, very rarely, vesicular or somewhat pustular ones. The nails may be deformed, and alopecia may be persent. In such cases the blood test for syphilis is usually strongly positive. In addition to the cutaneous manifestations of syphilis, other signs and symptoms may arouse suspicion of the presence of the disease. The infant becomes restless, develops rhinitis (snuffles) and a hoarse voice. The baby does not gain weight as it should. The lymph nodes are enlarged, especially the epitrochlear nodes. The liver and the spleen are enlarged, as are also the ends of the long bones.

In the treatment of syphilis of the newborn, the physicians will rely chiefly on penicillin. The broad-spectrum antibiotics may be used if sensitivity makes the use of penicillin inadvisable. Usually additional therapy is unnecessary; however, most of these infants are kept under surveillance for 1 or 2 years after treatment.

Babies born to mothers who have been treated early in the antepartal period for syphilis are seldom born with the disease.

Staphylococcal Infection

There continues to be growing concern about the spread of staphylococcal infection in hospitals and its increasing resistance to antibiotic therapy. The newborn nursery is one of the most vulnerable areas because of the infants' low tolerance to infections.

In recent studies of staphylococcal infection of the newborn, the epidemic strain of the organism has been found not only in skin lesions of the infected infants but also in the nasopharynx of a high percentage of apparently well infants. Nurseries at this time must be considered potential epidemic centers. Many factors contribute to the large numbers of infants found to harbor these organisms. *Crowding* of infants in a nursery has always been a serious problem and a contributing factor in any epidemic disease outbreak. The usually recommended minimum of 24 to 30 square feet of space per infant may actually not be adequate to prevent spread of infection. *Hospital personnel* have been found to be carriers of staphylococcus coagulase-positive organisms. These organisms are highly resistant to most antibiotics in current use, and when they are transmitted to infants, they may result in such manifestations as skin lesions (impetigo; p. 544), pneumonia, septicemia, conjunctivitis, omphalitis, osteomyelitis and other forms of infection from mild infections to those of extremely serious nature. In many studies there appears to be a direct transmission of the offending organisms from hospital personnel to infant, from infant to infant, from infant to mother and to the family at home, and even into the community (see Chap. 21). Hospital sanitation must be critically appraised, since these organisms may be air-borne and can exist in many contaminated or unclean surfaces of the nurseries, wards and other hospital areas. The type of walls, floors and equipment used must be of materials which can be easily and satisfactorily cleaned. Housekeeping personnel, their equipment and methods are to be constantly evaluated and supervised. There is no substitute for cleanliness, aseptic technique and isolation of infected patients and staff in controlling the spread of infection.

Manifestations of staphylococcal infection of the newborn frequently appear as pyoderma, stuffy noses, pneumonia and conjunctivitis. Few infants develop serious staphylococcal disease without preceding or accompanying pyoderma. Treatment usually consists of antimicrobial drugs given parenterally.

MALFORMATIONS (GENETIC ABNORMALITIES)

In approximately 1 out of 200 cases, infants are born with anomalies incompatible with life. The incidence of these disorders has not changed greatly over the decades; however, the techniques of repair and correction have improved immensely, thus offering a great deal of hope and consolation to the parents and the children who are afflicted with these conditions. Congenital deformities may range from minor abnormalities such as supernumerary digits to grave malformations incompatible with life, such as anencephalia (absence of brain), hydrocephalus (excessive amount of fluid in the cerebral ventricles with tremendous enlargement of head) and various heart abnormalities. In 1963, 20,817 infant deaths (excluding fetal deaths) were attributed to congenital malformations (rate, 11.0%). In the case of hydrocephalus, grave dystocia may occur because of the inability of the huge head to pass the pelvic inlet. Congenital malformations of the heart are a common cause of cyanosis in the newborn. Clubfoot, imperforate anus and meatus, cleft lip and cleft palate are other fairly frequent congenital deformities.

Since these conditions are so numerous and varied, this section will present selected disorders —those more commonly seen that are apparent at birth or soon thereafter and/or those with which the maternity nurse will have to deal. As we indicated on pages 529 to 533, the care of these infants and their parents presents a great challenge to the nurse. She must give competent and, at times, complex nursing care to the babies, and she must help the parents to convert their feelings of disappointment and, often, despair to constructive efforts of habilitation of the infant. In addition, the negative feelings that are aroused in the nurse must be handled. The young student will find that discussing these feelings with her instructor or supervisors will help her to cope with them.

Congenital Heart Disease

At the time of birth and for weeks thereafter, there are great changes in the circulation of the newborn. When the cord is clamped and expansion of the lungs occurs, the pulmonary circulation increases in volume. The foreamen ovale, the ductus arteriosus and the ductus venosus are no longer needed and therefore close gradually over a period of several months. Usually the foramen ovale is closed by the third month of life and the ductus by the second; during the period of closure, signs or symptoms of patency rarely occur. When they do, they may be an indication of defects in these structures or other parts of the heart. Congenital heart disease has an incidence of about 3 per cent per 1000 at birth and 1 per cent per 1000 at the age 10. Cardiovascular malformations account for approximately 50 per cent of the deaths from congenital defects in the first year of life. The role of heredity as an etiologic agent is not as yet well understood. Congenital lesions may be recorded in as many as three generations and siblings seem to manifest the disease more often than in the preceding or succeeding generations. *Maternal disease* during pregnancy influences the bodily structures of the developing fetus, yet the etiology and dynamics of cardiovascular lesion are not known definitively. However, there is a higher incidence of other congenital defects among infants with congenital heart disease. Thus, the infant may suffer from multiple disorders.

Distress from congenital heart disease is often hard to distinguish from the distress that is secondary to pulmonary disease such as respiratory distress syndrome. Yet accurate diagnosis is essential so that effective cardiac surgery can be instituted when indicated. Because no murmur per se is apparent in about one third of the cases, the diagnostic problem is further accentuated. Often respiratory distress and/or cyanosis are the presenting symptoms. Closer scrutiny may disclose other signs which are indicative. These include ready tiring, reluctance to feed, constant or sporadic respiratory embarrassment of varying degrees, shallow "panting" respirations, sudden periods of distress accompanied by crying suggestive of pain, changes in color characterized by pallor, grayishness or intense cyanosis. The older infant may exhibit a failure to thrive syndrome. These symptoms can occur in any combination at any time after birth.

Diagnosis is established from the history, physical findings, roentgenographic and electrocardiographic examinations. If doubt still exists, cardiac catheterization, angiocardiography and aortography usually supply the needed confirmatory data. These latter procedures are strenuous and if the child is severely distressed or in danger of circulatory failure, they may very well threaten his life. Therefore, great effort is made to utilize astute observation, history findings, and the roentgen and electrocardiograph findings.

Nursing care of these infants is directed to offset those factors observed to aggravate symptoms. Severely affected infants may be transferred directly to the pediatric facility; however, less distressed infants may remain on the maternity unit especially during the time a diagnosis is being established. Every precaution is taken to keep the infant from exposure to infection. The principles discussed in the care of the premature infant apply here. In addition, unnecessary disturbance is to be kept at a minimum as startling, or physical effort often distresses these babies. When the infant shows signs of severe respiratory embarrassment, relief is sometimes achieved by raising the head and shoulders. When these episodes are accompanied by crying which is suggestive of pain, the baby is sometimes eased if a warm hand is applied over his abdomen and he is very gently inclined over the upper margin of the supporting hand. In the case of severe distress, the baby may lie with his head loosely retracted; this should not be corrected as the infant assumes a position most suitable for aeration. Restlessness is often apparent and hence clothes and positioning should allow for maximum freedom of movement. Profuse diaphoresis is often seen and sponge baths with tepid water can supplement the daily pHisoHex bath. Oxygen is to be ready at all times for these babies and the doctor may want to prescribe digitalis if heart failure appears imminent. Feedings are usually given more frequently and in less amounts than to the healthy term infant. The aim, of course, is to avoid undesirable pressure of a distended stomach on the diaphragm and heart. If the infant can suck without distress, then a bottle is the feeding method of choice. If bottle feeding does result in cyanosis or impaired respiration, then a spoon or gavage tube may have to be utilized. Breast-feeding is almost always discouraged because of the suddenness and capriciousness of the respiratory difficulties.

Supportive care is necessary for the parents of these babies; keeping lines of communication open between the parents and the staff (i.e., obstetrician, pediatrician, heart surgeon, nursery nurses, pediatric nurses) will do much to help alleviate anxiety and help in the adjustment. As with infants with other types of defects or the premature infant, there is no contraindication for the parents to "visit" their infant. He usually is viewed through a window to prevent exposure to infection. When the parents indicate a desire for a visit the nurse can arrange for it.

Cleft Lip and Cleft Palate

These deformities, which may occur separately or in combination, result from the failure of the soft and/or boney tissues of the palate and the upper jaw to unite during the 8th to 12th weeks of gestation. The defect may be unilateral or bilateral (Fig. 23-6). Only the lip may be involved, or the disunion may extend into the upper jaw or into the nasal cavity. About 1 in every 1,000 births is so affected; thus, the anomaly is considered to be one of the most common of human birth defects. In some cases heredity seems clearly to be implicated, but in others there is no definite etiologic cause. It occurs in near relations of persons with the defect more often than in the general population.

The plan of treatment and outcome will depend on the severity of the condition. If only the lip is involved, surgery may be performed as early as 12 hours after birth. If the maxilla is involved as well, then surgical repair usually is done within the first few weeks of life. Repair of defects of the palate usually is deferred until about the 2nd year to take advantage of the developmental changes that occur. When surgery is done later, a prosthetic speech device usually is fitted so that speech development may not be hindered. Cleft palates usually involve other difficulties, frequent respiratory infections, orthodontia and speech problems, etc.; therefore, the care of these children involves the coordinated activities of the pediatrician, plastic surgeon, orthodontist, hos-

FIG. 23-6. Cleft lip and complete cleft palate. In this case surgical closure of the harelip was performed less than 18 hours following birth, with excellent results. (MacDonald House, University Hospitals of Cleveland)

pital and public health nurses, speech therapists and, very often, the social worker. Fortunately, modern treatment is so effective that this defect becomes a relatively minor handicap.

Nevertheless, the parents require a great deal of supportive help initially, as mentioned earlier, especially since this disorder is so disfiguring. In our culture a high value is put on physical attractiveness and beauty; and when this condition occurs, particularly if the baby is a girl, it may come as a tremendous shock and burden to the parents. However, repair is generally successful, and it is very helpful if the parents know and understand this. The nurse should emphasize the essential normality of the infant. Babies with this condition may be transferred to the pediatric ward, especially if surgery is to be performed. This will mean separation and loneliness for the mother. If possible, arrangements should be made for the parents to visit the infant whenever possible. (See Chap. 17.)

Feeding is usually one of the most immediate and difficult problems in the daily care of the infant. It can best be accomplished by placing the infant in an upright position and directing the flow of milk against the side of the mouth. This will decrease the possibility of aspiration as well as the amount of air swallowed during feeding. Since sucking strengthens and develops the muscles needed for speech, a nipple is used for feeding whenever possible. A variety of nipples may be tried, including a regular nipple with enlarged holes, a soft rubber nipple, a cleft palate nipple, or a duck bill nipple. The last two are more expensive and should be used only after the others have been tried. Specific instructions are necessary with their use. If the infant cannot use any of the nipples, then a spoon or a rubber-tipped medicine dropper may be tried. The flow of milk will have to be adjusted to the infant's swallowing and should not be released until the infant attempts to suck. The feedings are given at a pace which will neither cause the infant to become unduly tired nor result in aspiration of the liquid. Since these infants tend to swallow a large amount of air, they should be bubbled at frequent intervals, and the mother will need to be instructed in this technique. The nurse will want to help the mother to attain ease in feeding her baby and should arrange to stay with her during at least several of the sessions. She then can ascertain by demonstration and observation how well the mother is progressing. Gavage feeding usually is unnecessary and should be used only when the other methods fail, since it does not stimulate the sucking and swallowing reflexes and promotes aspiration.

The mother may want to breast-feed her infant, and there is no contraindication as long as the milk can be given the baby in a way that is appropriate. This may mean that the mother will have to pump or express her milk and offer it in a bottle or a medicine dropper. After surgery has been performed, and the infant's sutures have healed, the mother may resume breast-feeding.

Frenum Linguae

The frenum linguae is a vertical fold of mucous membrane under the tongue which is normally short and tight in the newborn infant. If this membrane is *too* short, the activity of the tongue is limited, so-called "tonguetie," and this interferes with sucking and later with the child's speech. This condition is observed at the time of the initial physical examination or during the inspection bath. The physician will "snip" the margin of the membrane with sterile blunt scissors if necessary.

Hypospadias and Epispadias

In hypospadias the urethra opens on the under surface of the penis proximal to the usual site. Minor degrees of this condition are quite common, and no surgical intervention is necessary. If the opening is at the base of the penis or far back on the shaft, then plastic surgical repair will be necessary. In epispadias the urethral opening is on the dorsal surface of the penis. If the defect is pronounced, then it also will require repair. Surgery usually is deferred in these conditions until childhood or puberty to take advantage of the maturation of the structures. Urination with the penis in the usual elevated position is impossible in these cases when they are severe. Very infrequently the condition occurs in females; in these instances the urethra opens into the vagina. Newborn with hypospadias or epispadias should not be circumcized until after correction, since the foreskin may be useful to the urologist in the urethral reconstruction.

Spina Bifida

Spina bifida is a rather common malformation and is due to the congenital absence of one or more vertebral arches, usually at the lower part of the spine. When the membranes covering the spinal cord bulge through the opening, the condition is known as meningocele. It forms a soft, fluctuating tumor filled with cerebrospinal fluid.

The tumor can be diminished by pressure and enlarges when the baby cries. The extrusion of the cord along with the coverings is known as meningomyelocele. When the tumor is very small and shows no signs of increasing in size, it may merely be protected from injury and infection by carefully applied dressings; but the more severe cases must be treated surgically. Unfortunately, the outlook for surgical repair is discouraging, since hydrocephalus usually occurs, if it is not already present, and fatalities are common. The situation and the prognosis for the infant is discouraging, and the parents will need a good deal of support and instruction about the continuing care of their infant. (See Suggested Reading.) The physician will prescribe regarding the care that is to be carried out at home.

Umbilical Hernia

Umbilical hernia, or rupture at the umbilicus, may appear during the first few weeks of life. The associated protrusion of intestinal contents may be made to disappear entirely on pressure, but it reappears when the pressure is removed, or when the baby cries. This is due to a weakness or an imperfect closure of the umbilical ring and is often associated with nonunion of the recti muscles. The condition usually disappears spontaneously by age 1. If the protrusion of omentum persists, the abdomen may be strapped by using broad bands of interlocking adhesive after reducing the hernia by finger pressure and drawing each side of the adjacent abdominal wall together. Some authorities feel that the strapping technique is useless and some feel it may even be deleterious. Surgery is usually avoided unless the hernia persists until the age of 3 to 5 years, causes symptoms, becomes strangulated or enlarges. Some mothers may need to be discouraged from placing a coin or button beneath the adhesive or a home fashioned umbilical dressing; this practice was used for many years as a "home remedy." It has no value and prohibits adequate approximation of the margins of the abdomen.

Obstructions of the Alimentary Tract

Atresia of the Esophagus. This condition, although less common than some which have been mentioned, is quite serious, and immediate steps must be taken to prevent aspiration. The defect, which occurs during embryonic development, results in the esophagus ending in a blind pouch rather than a continuous tube to the stomach. A fistula usually occurs into the trachea near the bifurcation of the esophagus and the trachea. When the baby attempts to swallow liquids or even normal secretions, there is an overflow into the trachea from the blind pouch. This malformation should be suspected whenever the infant demonstrates excessive drooling, coughing, gagging or cyanosis during feeding. The nurse must report these symptoms immediately; unless necessary surgery to correct the defect is prompt, the baby will contract bronchitis or pneumonia from repeated aspiration of milk and secretions. The infant is placed in the supine position, with his head elevated 30 degrees or more to prevent any gastric secretions from rising into the trachea through the fistula. The baby usually is placed in a heated, humidified incubator after surgery. This atmosphere is needed to liquefy the tenacious mucus that collects. Nasopharyngeal suction is necessary, and the nurse should watch carefully for any cyanosis or labored respiration that indicates the need for this. Blood, plasma, parenteral fluids and antibiotics also are given. The extent of the repair and the condition of the baby determine when oral feeding will be begun.

Pyloric Stenosis. This is a congenital anomaly and usually manifests its symptoms from the first few days to the 2nd or 3rd week by the onset of vomiting which becomes projectile in character and occurs within 30 minutes after every feeding. The infant loses weight, the bowel elimination lessens, highly colored urine becomes scanty, and the symptoms of dehydration appear. Upon examination, gastric peristalsis is found to be present, and the pyloric "acornlike" tumor can be palpated. Usually, thick cereal feedings are prescribed. If no improvement is noted, it is necessary to resort to surgery. Since it is not usually an emergency operation, there is sufficient time for supportive treatment to prepare the infant for surgery by vein and hypoclysis. The preoperative preparation includes intravenous blood and plasma. If the hemoglobin is below 70 per cent, transfusion is indicated. Gastric lavage, from 1 to 2 hours before operation, should be done until returns are clear. Maintaining body heat before and after the operation is essential. Transfusion should be given if indicated. The physician usually orders from 5 to 10 cc. of water to be given within a few hours, then alternated with 10 cc. of milk. As soon as the baby is gaining and consuming from 3 to 4 onuces at each feeding, he is ready for discharge.

Obstruction of the Duodenum and the Small Intestine. These conditions are relatively easy to diagnose. Vomiting occurs with the first feeding, and no meconium is eliminated. The vomitus may or may not be bile-stained, depending on whether the obstruction is high or low in the intestinal tract. If the obstruction is low, usually there is marked distention. A roentgenogram is used to confirm the diagnosis, and immediate surgery is indicated. However, the newborn infant should be allowed at least 12 hours for the respiration and kidney function to become stabilized. The operation is usually accompanied by continuous venous drip and plasma, and blood should be available if needed. Postoperative care includes maintaining body temperature, intravenous fluids until peristalsis is established (about a week), followed by feedings as given in pyloric stenosis. If distention occurs, nasoduodenal suction may be necessary. If the distention is severe, the infant is placed in an oxygen tent.

Intussusception. Acute intussusception is the most frequent type of intestinal obstruction and often may be unrecognized. There is usually intermittent abdominal pain, mild or severe, accompanied by blood and mucous intestinal elimination; and the baby may vomit. Upon abdominal examination a mass can be palpated. Immediate surgery is usually indicated. In preparation for surgery a gastric lavage is done, and an indwelling gastric catheter is inserted. Shock, if present, should be treated. Fluids are replaced by the intravenous route. Hypoclysis may be given for 24 hours, followed by water by mouth. Feedings may be started on the 3rd day if retained. Antibiotics may be ordered for the first 3 to 5 days and vitamin C to stimulate healing.

Imperforate Anus. This abnormality consists of atresia of the anus, with the rectum ending in a blind pouch. Careful examination of the infant in the delivery room usually reveals the condition, but it may be discovered by the nurse when attempting to take the first rectal temperature. Surgical treatment is, of course, imperative.

Chromosomal Abnormalities

In the past decade, several striking chromosomal abnormalities have been found. When a particular chromosome is in triplicate rather than the usual duplicate (pair) it is called trisomy. Three such trisomies have been identified in man—trisomy 13-15, trisomy 17-18, and trisomy 21-22 (Down's Syndrome). The clinical pictures of these conditions are so distinct that they can be recognized in the delivery room or the nursery and hence are included here for consideration by the maternity nurse.

As we have seen in Chapter 4, in the normal person, there are 46 chromosomes which are found in 23 pairs: one pair of sex-determining chromosomes and 22 pairs of autosomes. It is not yet possible to distinguish which chromosome is present in triplicate in a specific trisomy, thus, the numerical designations of suspect pairs are included in each particular trisomy aberration. Nor has the mechanism by which the offending chromosome produces its particular abnormality been determined. However, three distinct clinical patterns appear at birth. The extra chromosome found in trisomy results from nondisjunction (see Chap. 4) which can occur at any time in a cell's lifetime. Two different cytologic pictures emerge in trisomic cells. In the first, there is a free extra chromosome giving 47 chromosomes. In the second case, the extra chromosome is translocated, that is, attached to another chromosome. The total number is 46 but one of the chromosomes is the size of two chromosomes put together. There is an increased incidence of all three types of trisomy with advanced maternal age. This phenomenon is thought to be related to the long storage of oocytes in the mother. These germ cells are laid down during the mother's own fetal life; they wait, however, until the time of their individual ovulation to complete their meiotic divisions. Thus, it appears that nondisjunction tends to occur in older oocytes.

Trisomy 13-15 or D. This trisomy is characterized by an extra chromosome in the D group which includes pairs 13 through 15 (see Chap. 4). Infants with this abnormality frequently have difficulty establishing and maintaining respiration. One of the most striking features is the abnormal cranial development. The cranium is usually small with a sloping forehead. The ears may be malformed and low set and the eyes usually have some defect (cataracts, iris defects, unusual smallness) often bilaterally. Cleft palate and lip are commonly present. In addition, the hands and feet are often grossly deformed. Extra digits are common on both hands and feet. The thumbs may be retroflexible (double jointed) and the foot frequently has a posterior prominence of the heel sometimes accompanied by a convex sole known as "rocker bottom" foot. Other defects may include a bulbous nose, umbilical and diaphragmatic hernias, abnormal genitalia, scalp defects and extensive capillary hemangiomata far in excess of what is usually found in the normal newborn. Neurologic examination reveals these infants to have a weak or absent Moro reflex and little or no response to loud noises hence they appear to be deaf. They are prone to develop myoclonic seizures and all suffer from apneic spells of unknown origin. Autopsy often reveals the complete absence of olfactory nerves and tracts. All of these infants are mentally retarded and the majority have severe cardiac defects (dextroposition of the heart, ventricular septal defects) which are the major contributors to death in these infants. The average life span for these youngsters is less than a year, although several have lived to the age of five years.

Trisomy 17-18 or E Trisomy. This trisomy is characterized by an extra chromosome in the E group, which includes pairs 17 and 18 (see Chap. 4). These babies are usually born at term but are small, averaging about 5 pounds. Their placentas are often very small. The head is small with a prominent occiput but in proportion to the body size. The eyes are usually normal but the ears are generally malformed and low-set. The mouth appears small because of the short upper lip and the mandible is small giving a receding chin. The hands of these babies are always malformed but in a different way from the trisomy 13-15, and they give the best diagnostic clue to the condition. These babies keep their fists clenched most of the time, with the index finger overlying the third finger. Profuse lanugo covers the forehead, back and extremities and the skin usually has a mottled appearance. The sternum is very short, hence the abdomen appears long. The pelvis is small with limited abduction of the hips. There also may be abnormal genitalia. Inguinal and umbilical hernias are frequent; diaphragmatic eventration (elevation of a thinned portion of the diaphragm) rather than frank hernia occurs more often in these patients. Neurologic examination reveals abnormal muscle tone; these babies progress from a hypertonic state to frank opisthotonus. Since the sucking reflex is poor, gavage feeding is often instituted. Unlike trisomy 13-15, no gross brain abnormalities can be demonstrated, although cardiac abnormalities are common and either these or aspiration account for the demise of these babies. Their survival rate is less than 6 months on the average. During this time they become progressively undernourished and present a failure to thrive syndrome. As with trisomy 13-15, some infants have survived to childhood, so that death in infancy cannot be predicted.

Trisomy 21-22 or Down's Syndrome. In this condition an extra chromosome belonging to either pair 21 or 22 or a translocation of 15/21 is found (see Chap. 4). Although these babies are apt to have congenital defects and are more susceptible to infection, they can be expected to live much longer and have less severe mental retardation (although it can be very severe) than the other trisomies. The reader may be more familiar with the term "mongolism" used in reference to this syndrome, but recently this has lost favor, because it bears a connotation which is not only unfortunate but incorrect.

For many years the term "mongolism" has been given to the condition of infants who present a definite clinical picture, the configuration of their faces resembling that of a Mongol or an Oriental. Their eyes are set close together, are slanting, and the palpebral fissures are narrow. The nose is flat. The tongue is large, fissured, and usually is very obvious as it protrudes from the open mouth. The head is small, and posteriorly the occiput appears flat above the broad, pudgy neck. The hands are short and thick, especially the fingers (the little finger is curved), with simian creases apparent on the palmar surfaces. In addition to having defective mentality and the deformities mentioned above, these infants have underdeveloped muscles, loose joints, heart and alimentary tract abnormalities. Although these infants sometimes live past the age of puberty, the majority succumb earlier to some infection.

Incidence and Etiology. The incidence of Down's syndrome has been estimated at 1.5 in 1,000 births. Advanced maternal age has been known to play a very important role in the etiology of this condition, over a third of these children being born to mothers who are 40 years of age or older. Several decades ago it was suggested that this condition might be associated with a chromosomal aberration, but it was not demonstrated until recently that the etiologic factor in Down's syndrome is the result of one of the three chromosomal abnormalities.

Types. The most common chromosomal defect of the ovum in Down's syndrome is trisomy of the chromosome 21 or 22, resulting in a total chromosomal count of 47 instead of the normal number of 46. This type, commonly referred to as standard trisomy, usually occurs in infants born to older women and is rarely familial. The incidence of standard trisomy is 1 in 600 births. The second type of abnormality results from a 15/21 translocation; in this type the actual chromosomal count is 46. The translocation type of Down's syndrome usually occurs in infants born to younger parents, is the familial type and is rare. The third type of the disorder, mosaicism, is very rare. A unique factor in mosaicism is that one individual may have cells with different chromosomal counts. Laboratory tests may demonstrate that the affected person's blood cells, for example, have 47 chromosomes, whereas his skin cells may show 46 chromosomes. This is not a familial type of Down's syndrome, and, moreover, the abnormalities may be less.

The usual causes of death in these babies are heart defects and infectious illnesses. The average survival rate with effective antibiotic treatment has been extended to beyond 9 years. Children with Down's syndrome are essentially retarded but have been found to be far more educatable than was previously thought. Thus the decision to institutionalize the child is an exceedingly difficult one and should not be forced on the parents by well-meaning professionals.

The key approach to trisomy conditions lies in prevention since treatment does not alter the long range prognosis. With respect to prevention, education of the public regarding the effect of maternal age is the key issue. As we have seen that the incidence of all three trisomies goes up with increased maternal age. The later *thirties* and *forties* are less safe for childbearing (from many points of view) and elective childbearing is better done when the mother is younger. Genetic counseling is another aspect of public education. Parents who have had a trisomic child (or if trisomy has appeared among their siblings) would do well to talk to their physician concerning the risk of producing more of these children. In some families, trisomies are not the result of nondisjunction and hence have an appreciable chance of recurring, depending on the interaction of the variables of family history, maternal age and chromosomal arrangement. For instance, if a couple produced a trisomy infant in their twenties, the child may have received a translocated chromosome from one of them. If they continue to produce children, then these children would stand a high chance of also inheriting the translocated chromosome. Parents clearly deserve to be told the facts of the matter so that they may be in a better position to make valid decisions regarding future childbearing. A young patient who has had a translocation (hereditary type) child may be a candidate for amniocentesis with cell culture and karyotyping in a subsequent pregnancy. This may be done as early as 14 weeks and thereby provide the option of therapeutic abortion, should the abnormality be present again. This approach of antenatal diagnosis can now be applied to an ever increasing number of chromosomal abnormalities as well as biochemical disorders.

Immediate care will be supportive for the infant. Warmth, prevention of infection, fluid and electrolyte balance, and often oxygen therapy will be under the supervision of the physician. Nursing therapy will be aimed primarily at support of the parents and helping them to work through their grief. This latter aspect is particularly important because of the grave prognosis for these babies. It is often helpful to institute public health and/or visiting nurse referrals since the parents may need technical help upon arriving home with the infant. If a fetal demise occurs, supportive help from a public health nurse is also helpful.

Phocomelia

In 1961-62 many thousands of newborns in Germany were afflicted with an extremely pitiful type of malformation characterized either by total absence of the arms and the legs or by such stunting of the extremities that they were mere nubbins. The deformity is known as *phocomelia*. Investigation revealed that practically all the mothers who gave birth to such infants had taken a certain sedative drug, *thalidomide,* during the first part of pregnancy, and that this drug was undoubtedly the cause of the malformations.

Largely as the result of the thalidomide tragedy, the United States Food and Drug Administration, a Federal agency authorized to approve new drugs, tightened greatly the regulations concerning new drug approval. But from the viewpoint of nurses and physicians, the most important lesson to be drawn from this sad experience is that *no pregnant woman should take any drug whatsoever* unless, in the opinion of her physician, it is urgently necessary for her health (see Chaps. 8 and 19). This rule does not apply to the routine administration of vitamins and iron, nor to the use of laxatives when indicated, but it does apply very strongly to most other drugs, particularly those often employed in the treatment of insomnia and nausea.

The child with deformed or missing limbs has special rehabilitation problems that do not occur in the treatment of adults who undergo a loss of a limb (see Suggested Reading). His physical characteristics and contours are different from those of an adult, and they are constantly changing as he grows. This complicates fitting an adequate prosthesis. Furthermore, his psychosocial adjustment demands continued attention, for he does not have the chance to make his adjustment to society as a whole person, and he therefore is likely to have some feelings of inadequacy and devaluation in a culture geared to the nonhandicapped. Fortunately, there are about 15 child amputee clinics throughout this country. They are located in Alabama, California, Connecticut, Florida, Georgia, Illinois, Maryland, Michigan, New York, North Carolina, Oklahoma, Pennsylvania and Washington. These clinics are invaluable in helping parents to learn that their child can be fitted with a functional prosthesis and achieve satisfaction in its use. Even when the deformity is multiple, the child can achieve at least limited function with proper training. Since much of the success of the plan of treatment depends on the parents, it is particularly important that they be informed and reassured of these positive aspects in the situation. It has been demonstrated that the sooner the parents receive this knowledge, the more chance there is of an effective prosthetics program.

The newborn infant with a congenital amputation will be discussed here since nurses in the maternity unit will have initial contact with these infants and will need to instruct parents on various aspects of daily care. (For a thorough, interesting discussion of amputations in children of all ages, see the Steele article in the Suggested Readings.)

The usual sleeping position for the newborn is prone with the pelvis raised and the knees tucked under the abdomen. When the lower extremities are missing, the infant is unable to assume this position and, in addition, will not be able to indulge in the kicking behavior which appears to give a good deal of gratification. The baby with missing upper extremities presents other problems. Prior to feeding, the infant is usually occupied with a good deal of hand to mouth contact and this of course, will be altered. If both hands are missing the infant will be deprived of one of his major sources of sucking gratification. We know that the need for sucking and the need for feeding often do not coincide and hence the normal infant uses his fingers to complete the gratification of this need. Therefore the nurse will want to offer a pacifier to these infants. Clinging behavior in the human infant is not clearly understood, but it is observed that as the infant matures he tends to grasp things and bring them to his mouth possibly for further identification. In the absence of both upper limbs, this behavior also will be altered.

The nurse will also want to instruct the parents, that when the infant is older, he may not be able to lift his head up (while in the prone position) since he can not raise up on his elbows to look around. A wedge shaped pillow or thick folded blanket placed under the infant's chest will correct this handicap a great deal.

The development of body image begins in infancy and will play an increasingly important role in the development of these youngsters. The normally developed infant first perceives his moving arms (and legs) as part of the outside world; as he grows, he incorporates them into his body image and hence, his self concept. The infant amputee may not be aware that his body is different from others', but as he matures, he begins to compare himself with others and his concept about himself changes as he slowly integrates his defect into his existing body image. Obviously, the more positive attitudes he encounters with respect to his defect, the more positive his concept of himself can become. It is important for the nurse to remember that while the defect may seem rather minor to her (in comparison to some of the life-threatening conditions recently discussed), in the parents' eyes, it may be catastrophic. The principles of care, as given at the beginning of the chapter, especially with regard to how the nurse actually handles the baby are especially germane here. Guilt may be present, especially if the defect is thought to be the result of taking drugs or from contact with viral diseases. Denial also may be apparent, with the parents actually refusing to look at or admit, the defect. The nurse's warm, accepting attitude in this case is very helpful since the parents' denial is often related to their apprehension regarding how others will view their infant. Fortunately, these infants are usually in apparent good health in other respects and will thrive if given the chance. They do not seem to be handicapped by multiple abnormalities as is the case with some of the other disorders. Calling attention to the positive aspects of the baby's growth, development and general features will help the parents place the amputation in its proper perspective after the initial shock and grief have been worked through.

INBORN ERRORS OF METABOLISM

Numerous metabolic disorders, so-called "inborn errors of metabolism," are now known to originate from mutations in the genes which alter the genetic constitution of an individual to the extent that normal function is disrupted. These biochemical disorders arise because of the disturbance (mutation) in a *molecule of the gene* itself. They *do not* stem from some mishap or alteration during the embryonic development of tissue or organs. The mode of transmission of these "inborn errors" usually is recessive; that is, a child must receive a pair of defective genes (one from his mother and one from his father) to be affected. The mother and the father in these cases would be carriers of the defective genes but would not be affected by the resulting disorder per se. Fortunately, defective genes are found rather infrequently in the general population, and the chance of their joining is even rarer; hence, the diseases they produce are commensurately rare. Some of the more familiar hereditary metabolic disorders and resulting conditions include:

1. Defects in metabolism and transport of amino acids
   A. Phenylketonuria
   B. Maple sugar urine disease
2. Defects in protein metabolism
   A. Agammaglobulinemia
3. Defects in metabolism and transport of carbohydrates
   A. Diabetes mellitus
   B. Gargoylism (Hurler's disease)
   C. Galactosemia
   D. Arachnodactyly (Marfan's syndrome)
4. Defects in metabolism and transport of lipids
   A. Cerebroside lipidosis (Gaucher's disease)
   B. Ganglioside lipidosis (Tay-Sach's disease)
   C. Sphingomyelin lipidosis (Niemann-Pick disease)

It is important to remember that these inborn errors of metabolism *do not produce symptoms* that are apparent at birth. Therefore, the maternity nurse rarely will see evidence of these disorders. However, two conditions do concern us here. The one directly because nursery personnel play an important role in the early detection of the condition; this disorder is phenylketonuria. The other is more indirect since it is the babies of mothers with the condition that we must attend; this latter condition is diabetes mellitus.

Phenylketonuria

This disease, commonly known as PKU, is an inborn error of metabolism of the essential amino acid phenylalanine, characterized by a deficiency in the liver enzyme phenylalanine hydroxylase, which is essential in phenylalanine metabolism. High blood levels of phenylalanine occur, and phenylketone bodies are excreted in the urine. Phenylalanine makes up 5 per cent of the protein factor of all foods. Normally, phenylalanine is converted to tyrosine in the liver and then is further metabolized. The phenylketonuric child is able to digest protein and to absorb the resulting amino acids. However, there is a block in the normal metabolic pathway at this point, and the excess dietary phenylalanine, unable to be converted to tyrosine, builds up in the tissues (blood levels of this amino acid reach as high as 60 mg. per 100 ml., as compared with the normal 1 to 3 mg. per 100 cc.) and spills into the urine in the form of phenylpyruvic acid, excess phenylalanine, phenylacetic acid and orthohydroxyphenylacetic acid. These components, excreted in the urine and the perspiration, give the child a characteristic musty odor.

Without treatment, the condition usually results in mental retardation, although the rest of the clinical picture will vary. Typically, the child with PKU is hyperactive and demonstrates unpredictable erratic behavior. Usually he does not relate well in interpersonal contacts, either within the family or with strangers, and he appears very immature and overly dependent. The three R's, routine, relaxation and repetition (as used with other mentally retarded youngsters), are effective in helping him make a more satisfactory social adjustment. The main foci of management, however, is early detection of the condition and dietary management restricting the phenylalanine intake. If treatment is initiated before 6 months of age, the child probably will fall into the borderline-to-normal range of intelligence (70 to 100 I.Q.).

Diagnosis. This disorder may be diagnosed from both blood and urine tests. The former are more advantageous, since they can be done before the infant leaves the hospital, and they give a low rate of false positive reactions. One of the easiest and most efficient to perform is the microbiological assay (MIA), more commonly known as the Guthrie method. In this test 1 or 2 drops of blood are secured from the infant's heel on the day of discharge and are placed immediately on filter paper. The laboratory then uses a bacterial inhibition assay method on the serum phenylalanine to determine the phenylalanine level. A result of 8 mg. per cent or above is considered to be diagnostic of PKU. The nurse may be asked to collect the specimen for this test and/or to prepare the infants for the doctor. Usually several babies will be tested at one time, therefore, she can facilitate matters by placing the infants in the prone position, which makes the heels easily accessible. The babies then can be covered loosely with a blanket so that they will remain accessible but will not be unduly exposed. After the heel has been wiped with a disinfectant solution, pricked (usually with a disposable blood lancet), and the specimen obtained, the infant should be observed for bleeding from the heel. The test must be repeated in 4 weeks. The test equipment usually is given to the mother at the time of discharge. She should be instructed to take the baby to her physician or baby clinic so that testing may be completed. The other blood tests require 1 to 5 cc. of blood; they are as reliable as the Guthrie method, but many laboratories do not have the facilities required to perform the analysis.

The urine tests utilize ferric chloride as the testing agent; this solution is dropped on a freshly saturated diaper. A green reaction indicates probable phenylketonuria. The urine tests are effective only after the infant is 6 weeks old; they are useful in screening large populations of infants and are most often done in well-baby clinics. Since early diagnosis is imperative, the blood tests are becoming the tests of choice.

Treatment. Restriction of phenylalanine intake is the basis of treatment, and yet enough protein must be available for growth and development; hence the child's diet becomes all-important. Commercial products (e.g., Lofenalac, a special food, which is mixed with water) are available that provide adequate protein for growth with minimal phenylalanine content. The plan of dietary treatment should be reviewed carefully with both parents, so that they have an understanding of how to prepare the formula, use the meal guides and food exchange lists (see Suggested Reading) and prepare menus from them.

Requesting the parents to review their understanding of the problem, diet, etc., often will elicit the areas that need clarification. The parents must be supported until they feel comfortable in discussing the problem; until this happens, they cannot be receptive to further teaching. Since this is a long-term condition and requires consistent counseling and follow-up, the need for a referral to the public health nurse becomes evident.

Care should be taken so that the parents of an affected child are not led to believe that all babies treated will have the usual pattern of growth and development (intellectual development may be slow, for instance). This cannot be guaranteed. *Early detection* and *prompt treatment* prevent mental retardation. The control of this condition demands consistent and disciplined supervision and follow-through on the part of the parents.

The Infant of the Diabetic Mother

The successful control of diabetes with insulin has led to the survival and fertility of an increasing number of diabetic women (see Chap. 22). The infants of these women and women who have a prediabetic condition exhibit certain characteristics that are distinctive. In addition to having distinctive characteristics, these infants have a higher incidence of intra-uterine deaths after the 36th week of gestation and a higher neonatal mortality rate than the general population. These babies are large, often 10 pounds or over; their increased body weight is due to a combination of obesity and edema. The former is thought to be related to excessive insulin production, and the latter, to excessive intracellular glycogen deposition. Hypoglycemia, hyperbilirubinemia and hypocalcemia also are common. The infants appear to be bloated and tend to be jumpy or trembly after the first 24 hours of life. They are subject to unexplained cyanotic attacks, and the respiratory distress syndrome (see p. 539) is common. The tremulousness appears to be due to the hypoglycemia and hypocalcemia. The increased perinatal mortality is thought to be secondary to such maternal factors as ketosis, hydramnios, preeclampsia and vascular degeneration, which are common accompaniments of the diabetic and prediabetic state.

The management of these infants is all-important. A pediatrician is usually in attendance at the time of delivery, which may be done vaginally, but is often accomplished by cesarean section (to prevent intra-uterine death, which can occur after 36 weeks of gestation). He will institute resuscitation measures in cases of respiratory distress, treat hyperbilirubinemia or infection, if they are present, and examine the infant for congenital anomalies. The infant is usually given an Apgar rating, which gives a more accurate indication of the prognosis than other classifications (see Chap. 13). Aspiration of the infant's gastric contents is done immediately after the airway has been cleared. This procedure is thought to be helpful in reducing the incidence of respiratory distress syndrome through removal of swallowed amniotic fluid, which may be regurgitated and aspirated and contribute to the formation of the syndrome.

The child may be transferred to the premature nursery and a low concentration of oxygen given to facilitate respiration. Early feeding (4 to 12 hours after birth) of glucose in water or sodium chloride solution may be instituted to reduce the hypoglycemia. If convulsions occur, especially within the first 6 hours of life, blood will be drawn for sugar determination and a glucose solution started intravenously; intravenous feeding will be continued until the infant is feeding well by mouth.

Nursing Care. The importance of accurate observation and reporting by the nurse regarding these infants cannot be stressed enough. Vital signs must be watched carefully and respiratory function closely observed. Nursing care is similar to that for a premature infant and that for a baby who is being observed for respiratory difficulty. The nurse will want to remember that even though these infants have robust birth weights, they are often delivered before term. Moreover the weight is a good deal edema; therefore the strong emphasis on preventing infection and maintaining body temperature is as applicable here as it is in the case of the premature. Appropriate explanation and reassurance of the parents also are necessary. This disorder is a recessive hereditary trait and thus, the parents could benefit by counseling regarding future childbearing. There is no prevention of the problems in these infants as long as diabetes or a prediabetic condition exists. However, careful control of the maternal diabetics does markedly reduce perinatal morbitity and mortality. The baby's prognosis is good if he survives the first 48 hours of life; his subsequent progress will be the same as that of an infant of his gestational age.

HEMOLYTIC DISEASE OF THE NEWBORN
Hemolytic Disease Due to Rh Incompatibility

This condition is a severe hemolytic disease of the newborn due to Rh iso-immunization. It occurs in cases of Rh incompatibility (see Chap. 22). The term "erythroblastosis fetalis" has been applied rather generally to all cases in which there is Rh incompatibility; actually, it is somewhat of a misnomer when used in this way. Erythroblastosis fetalis should be used to designate an illness in the infant which is due to Rh iso-immunization, since this disorder is neither specific nor always present in all instances of Rh incompatibility. The name is derived from *erythros,* red, and *blastos,* a formative cell. It occurs approximately once in every 200 deliveries. The disease may manifest itself in different degrees of severity. About one fifth of the Rh-positive infants born of sensitized Rh-negative mothers may have no clinical manifestations. Others may be mildly or severely affected. If the mother's antibody titer is low, the infant will likely have a mild form of the disease. In mild cases of erythroblastosis fetalis, slight jaundice and anemia may be present at birth or may become evident within a few hours thereafter. These symptoms may be the only clinical manifestations. In more severe cases the jaundice and the anemia are more exaggerated, and the liver and the spleen may be enlarged. Marked anemia with consequent pallor is a characteristic feature due to the destruction of the erythrocytes (see Chap. 22). In making observations the nurse should bear in mind that if the jaundice is pronounced, it may mask the developing pallor. Jaundice and anemia which are present at birth or appear during the first 36 hours are the cardinal clinical symptoms of erythroblastosis. Therefore, the nurse is to notify the doctor immediately if any infant is jaundiced on the 1st or the 2nd day of life.

Severe jaundice is a manifestation of hyperbilirubinemia. This condition becomes critical when the level of indirect bilirubin (unconjugated) in the blood reaches 20 mg. per cent. Normal values range between 0.2 and 1.4 mg./100 cc. of blood. Even at the peak of physiologic jaundice, often seen in normal newborn infants, the bilirubin level does not exceed 5 to 13 mg./100 cc. of blood. This high serum bilirubin level is caused by the inability of the liver to handle the large amount of bilirubin that is liberated with the destruction of the erythrocytes. So that the indirect bilirubin (free bilirubin) may be excreted after birth properly, it must be converted to direct bilirubin by enzymes in the liver. These enzymes are deficient during the infant's first few days of life. Thus, when hemolysis is excessive (as it is in erythroblastosis), and the bilirubin cannot be converted to the excretable direct variety, the bilirubin accumulates in the blood in such concentration as to cause jaundice and in severe cases to stain the brain cells, causing irreparable damage.

This latter condition is known as *kernicterus.* The infant who has symptoms of kernicterus (jaundice of the nuclear masses of the brain) will take its feedings poorly and show increasing signs of lethargy and loss of normal Moro reflex. It may have convulsions and opisthotonos, often accompanied by a shrill high-pitched cry. Kernicterus due to Rh incompatibility is often fatal, and if the infant survives, it almost always suffers from severe forms of mental retardation and spastic paralysis, and its hearing may be impaired.

Even when kernicterus is not present, the infant with erythroblastosis is usually lethargic, due to the anemia and generalized weakness, and he should have his position changed frequently to prevent atelectasis. Furthermore, special precautions must be exercised to protect these infants from intercurrent infection.

There is some disagreement as to whether or not mothers giving birth to erythroblastotic infants should breast-feed their babies. One well known authority feels, however, that erythroblastosis fetalis is not a contraindication to breast-feeding if the infant's general condition allows it. The antibodies in the mother's milk are inactivated in the intestinal tract and therefore do not contribute to further hemolysis of the infant's red blood cells.

1. CHILD receives from FATHER an "Rh-positive" gene, and begins to produce "Rh-positive" blood, shown by symbol ⊕

2. MOTHER'S blood is "Rh-negative," shown by symbol ⊖

3. Some of the CHILD'S "Rh-positive" blood substance travels through placenta into MOTHER

4. MOTHER'S blood begins producing ANTIBODIES to attack hostile substance*

5. ANTIBODIES FROM MOTHER ENTER CHILD AND BEGIN DESTROYING ITS BLOOD CELLS

*If "Rh-negative" mother has had previous "Rh-positive" pregnancies, or transfusions with "Rh-positive" blood, antibodies already are present.

Fig. 23-7. Effect of the Rh factor. (Scheinfeld, Amran: The New You and Heredity, Philadelphia, Lippincott)

The most severe manifestation of erythroblastosis affecting the newborn is *hydrops fetalis*. With this condition the infant is tremendously edematous, has marked anemia, jaundice and enlargement of the liver and the spleen. Such infants may be stillborn; otherwise they invariably succumb shortly after birth.

Erythroblastosis fetalis is very likely to repeat itself in subsequent pregnancies, and some unfortunate mothers give birth to a series of such infants. Its cause is immunologic in character and is based on the fact that the mother in these cases develops in her blood certain antibodies which attack a substance in the baby's red blood corpuscles known as the "Rh factor" (see Fig. 23-7).

Treatment in Erythroblastosis. When hemolytic disease is suspected, the infant is carefully observed at birth for clinical signs of the disorder. His skin color, the color of the vernix, and the size of his liver and spleen are noted. In addition, a specimen of umbilical cord blood is obtained for the following tests: Coombs' test, Rh determination, blood group, serum bilirubin, reticulocyte, erythrocyte and nucleated red blood cell count, and hemoglobin level. The direct Coombs' test (direct antiglobulin test) is important in accurate diagnosis of hemolytic disease. It reveals the presence of maternal antibodies attached to the red blood cells of an Rh-positive baby (see Chap. 22). The red blood cells of a baby with hemolytic disease may be coated with anti-Rh antibodies, and these antibodies will cause hemolysis of the baby's red blood cells. A positive direct Coombs' test indicates the presence of antibodies on the surface of the infant's blood cells. A negative direct Coombs' test indicates that no antibodies are present on the baby's red blood cells. Depending on the results of the laboratory reports and/or the presence and the severity of the clinical signs, treatment will be instituted.

In live births, that is, except in *hydrops fetalis,* the life of the infant may be saved by exchange transfusion with Rh-negative blood. This provides new red cells and removes the harmful maternal antibodies and products of hemolysis which produce jaundice. Transfusions should be given promptly. The exchange transfusion is accomplished through a polyethylene catheter inserted into the umbilical vein, or other large vein, such as the saphenous. Small amounts of the infant's blood are withdrawn (approximately 10 to 15 cc. at a time) and equal amounts of the Rh-negative donor's blood injected. This procedure is continued until most of the circulating blood of the infant is replaced.

When there is any possibility that exchange transfusion may be required for the infant, the obstetrician invariably will leave the umbilical cord stump longer than usual.

Those infants with hemolytic disease who do not require exchange transfusion should be observed carefully for development of anemia for at least 3 weeks following birth, even when they appear to be doing satisfactorily. The physician will continue to have scheduled determinations of hemoglobin levels done during this period.

The prognosis is favorable for the infant with erythroblastosis fetalis if he survives the first week without developing signs of kernicterus, provided that the severe anemia is given watchful attention and treatment. One may anticipate that hemoglobin and erythrocyte levels will be normal by the time the infant reaches the age of 5 months.

Very recently, a new concept in the management of the Rh problem (i.e., *amniotic fluid evaluation* and *intra-uterine fetal transfusion*) has been introduced to improve the perinatal mortality from erythroblastosis fetalis. It has been found that by the examination of the amniotic fluid of Rh-negative sensitized women, it is possible to predict the presence and the severity of the hemolytic process in the fetus.

The amniotic fluid is obtained by abdominal amniocentesis on pregnant women suspected of bearing infants with erythroblastosis. Then, since there is a relationship of the amniotic fluid bilirubin concentration to the presence of erythroblastosis fetalis in utero, the amniotic fluid can be evaluated by spectrophotometric analysis. Once this has been done, the further management of the pregnancy is determined almost entirely by the results of amniotic fluid analysis, irrespective of the height of the mother's antibody titer levels.

Intra-uterine fetal transfusion is indicated when the fetus is likely to die otherwise before becoming mature enough to survive premature delivery. The fetal transfusion is done on the basis of the mother's past history of having a severely affected infant at birth or a fetal death in utero due to erythroblastosis, in addition to the appearance of an amniotic fluid absorption curve in the spectrometric tracings suggesting a severely affected infant.

ABO Incompatibility

A relatively mild type of hemolytic disease of the newborn is associated with ABO incompatibility. In this disease the father's blood group is A, B or AB and the mother's is Type O. At the time of conception the fertilized ovum receives the genes from both parents, and because the A and B genes are dominant over O, the infant will develop Type A or B blood. During the placental exchange of intra-uterine life, the anti-A or anti-B agglutinins of the mother's blood cross the placental barrier and attack the red blood cells of the infant. Hemolysis of these cells occurs, resulting in severe jaundice and anemia.

This disease occurs in first as well as in subsequent pregnancies, but rarely is it as severe as the hemolytic disease caused by Rh incompatibility. The Coombs' test is usually negative.

Exchange transfusions are done, as necessary, to keep the serum bilirubin level below 20 mg. per 100 cc. The blood for transfusion should be of appropriate Rh type and Type O, the mother's blood group and not the infant's.

Hyperbilirubinemia of the Newborn

Hyperbilirubinemia, as previously stated, is present beyond physiologic bounds when the total serum bilirubin levels reach 18 to 20 mg. per 100 cc. of blood. This may occur particularly in premature infants as an exaggeration of physiologic jaundice or as a consequence of excessive hemolysis, such as severe hemolytic disease of the newborn. Occasionally, this condition is found in term infants who have no blood group incompatibilities. Therefore some authorities suggest that this term, "hyperbilirubinemia of the newborn," be applied only to those infants whose primary problem is a deficiency or inactivity of bilirubin transference rather than an excessive load of bilirubin for excretion. Certain conditions of the mother (e.g., diabetes, as well as neonatal conditions arising from the use of certain drugs, bacteremia and prolonged cyanosis) appear to be implicated in causing this condition. Occasionally this disorder appears among breast-fed infants during the 2nd week of life. For some reason the mother manufactures a substance in her milk that inhibits the conjugation of bilirubin. If breast-feeding is discontinued, serum bilirubin levels return to normal within 5 days, and apparently no lasting damage is done to the infant. The significance of hyperbilirubinemia, of course, lies in the high incidence of kernicterus associated with it, which, as previously explained, can be lethal to the baby.

Fortunately, clinicians recently have confirmed that infants with this condition responded to exposure to light (phototherapy). This exposure to sunlight or artificial light results in a reduction of the serum bilirubin level. Either fluorescent or the usual G.E. daylight 20-watt bulbs have been used. Apparently the bilirubin is converted by light into a colorless, polar, water-soluble compound, which is excluded from the nervous system and readily excreted in the urine. It is important to note that jaundice in the premature (other than Rh and ABO) can usually be treated successfully with phototherapy. In all cases the infant's eyes are bandaged to protect him from the direct light. Some physicians suggest phototherapy after exchange transfusion of Rh sensitized babies, since this may prevent the need for further transfusions.

MISCELLANEOUS DISORDERS

Hemorrhage from Cord

Hemorrhage from the cord may be of two types: (1) primary, due to the slipping or loosening of the ligature or umbilical clamp, and (2) secondary, coming from the base of the cord when it separates from the body of the baby. In the first instance, the bleeding is from the end of the cord and not from its base and can be controlled by the proper application of a fresh ligature. The secondary hemorrhage, from the base of the cord, occurs at about the 5th to the 8th day when separation takes place. It is often preceded by a slight jaundice; it is not an actual flow of blood but a persistent oozing which frequently resists treatment. This variety of hemorrhage, which is of rare occurrence, is usually due to one of two causes: (1) the baby may be syphilitic, or (2) the peculiar condition known as hemorrhagic diathesis may be present. In this condition the baby's blood shows no disposition to coagulate, and bleeding from any denuded surface is persistent and often profuse.

The nurse's responsibility in the treatment of secondary hemorrhage from the cord consists in applying a sterile dressing to the bleeding surface. The physician should be notified promptly; and if, by the time he arrives, the use of the dressing has not effectually controlled the oozing, he will doubtless ligate the base of the umbilicus. When this form of bleeding is at all severe and persistent, recovery is doubtful; and even if the umbilical hemorrhage is controlled, bleeding may appear in the nose, the mouth, the stomach, the intestines or the abdominal cavity; or purpuric spots may develop on various parts of the body. The prompt administration of vitamin K has greatly improved the prognosis in these cases.

Retrolental Fibroplasia

Retrolental fibroplasia is an acquired disease, associated with prematurity, in which retinal pathology occurs in those infants receiving continuous oxygen therapy in high concentration. The incidence of the condition depends on (1) the concentration of oxygen given, (2) the degree of immaturity of the eyes at the time when oxygen is given (see Chapter 17). The disease is characterized by spasm, then obliteration, of the developing retinal vessels which is followed by neovascularization, hemorrhage and retinal detachment. The disease has both an acute and a cicatricial phase; both eyes are affected, although different stages may be present in the two eyes; spontaneous arrest may occur at any stage.

The onset of the acute stage is usually between the ages of 3 weeks and 3 months and the smaller the birthweight, the *later* the onset. Dilation and tortuosity of the retinal blood vessels occur, with the fundus becoming pale. Hemorrhages appear adjacent to the vessels and spread into the vitreous; separation of the retina follows. After several weeks, the acute stage passes into the cicatricial stage, characterized by formation of the retrolental membrane. The anterior chamber becomes shallow and impairment of vision may be accompanied by squint, photophobia and nystagmus. In severe cases, microphthalmia and secondary glaucoma may be sequelae. Because most of the damage is mechanical, one cannot determine the extent of detachment that will occur. When the condition is detected early, and proper measures are instituted promptly (i.e., reduction in concentration of oxygen administered) the condition in the infant may regress at any stage of the disease, or, on the other hand, partial or complete blindness may result.

Retrolental fibroplasia is no longer considered to be a major problem, because it rarely occurs today. Extensive research, carried on within the past two decades since retrolental fibroplasia was first described, has established the cause and the means of prevention of the disease. It is now a fact that almost all cases of retrolental fibroplasia in the premature infant are the result of intensive oxygen therapy. Today oxygen is administered to an infant in the lowest concentration compatible with life and is discontinued as soon as feasible. The maximum oxygen concentration of the incubator housing the premature infant is kept at less than 40 per cent, with rare exceptions, and this is done only for as long as it is *absolutely* necessary (see Oxygen Therapy, p. 415).

Drug Addiction in the Newborn

Although this condition is still rare, it is seen more frequently with the rise of drug addiction in the general population. Furthermore, it is the nurse who may be the first to discover this condition. The symptoms of the infant are due to withdrawal rather than narcosis; they may appear almost immediately after birth, or they may be delayed for several hours, depending on the time of the mother's last injection of narcotic, the dose, and the interval between the administration of the narcotic and the delivery. The infant may manifest restlessness, tremors, shrill crying, convulsions, or twitchings of the extremities and/or face. The Moro reflex may be incomplete, and the deep tendon reflexes may be increased. Diarrhea, vomiting, anorexia, yawning, sneezing and excessive mucus also may be present. These symptoms parallel somewhat those found in the adult undergoing withdrawal symptoms from narcotics. If the signs of withdrawal are unrecognized, the baby may die; if the infant is treated (hydration, supportive measures, and diminishing doses of sedatives), then recovery and permanent cure are assured since the infant does not have a psychic dependence on narcotics. However, some physicians believe that the infant should be removed from the mother's environment if it carries a threat of readdiction. This possibility will present a problem that will require a multidisciplinary approach, and the nurse can be helpful in beginning the process through appropriate and accurate reporting and recording. Recent evidence indicates that withdrawal symptoms in the newborn can be avoided if the mother can be treated with methadon substitution antepartum. Another drug problem, perhaps of a more indirect but nevertheless important nature, concerns abuse in the use of the drug lysergic acid (LSD-25). This drug, a consciousness expander, was developed for research use and was never intended for indiscriminate use by the general population. Recent research has documented that LSD-25, when taken by mothers during pregnancy results in a significant increase in chromosomal abnormalities in her babies. This fact is also true, but to a lesser degree of children of mothers *who took the drug before, but not during pregnancy.* How and in what manner any malformations will be manifested as a result of these chromosomal abnormalities is as yet uncertain. However, it is recommended that any agent capable of inflicting chromosomal damage should be treated with extreme caution until all the genetic implications are understood. Antenatal chromosomal analysis might also be of help in this group of patients.

SUGGESTED READING

Apgar, V.: Drugs in pregnancy. Am. J. Nurs. 65: 104-105, March, 1965, reprinted from J.A.M.A. 190:840-841, 1964.

Ascari, W. Q., et al.: Incidence of maternal Rh immunization by ABO compatible and incompatible pregnancies. Brit. Med. J. 1:399-401, February 15, 1969.

Asnes, R. S., and Lamb, J. M.: Neonatal respiratory depression secondary to maternal analgesics, treated by exchange transfusion. Pediatrics 43:94-96, January, 1969.

Banatvala, J. E., et al.: Rubella syndrome and thrombocytopenic purpura in newborn infants. New Eng. J. Med. 273:474-478, August 26, 1965.

Barnett, H. L.: Pediatrics. New York, Appleton, 1968.

Basara, S. C.: The behavioral patterns of the perceptually handicapped child. Nurs. Forum 5, No. 4:24-39.

Bessolo, R. J., and Vincent, W. R.: Diagnosis of congenital heart disease in the first two weeks of life. Calif. Med. 110:200-206, March, 1969.

Bordley, J. E., et al.: Prenatal rubella. Acta Oto-Laryngologica 66:1-9, July-August 1968.

Bowes, W. A., et al.: Amniocentesis and intrauterine fetal transfusion in erythroblastosis. Am. J. Obstet. Gynec. 93, No. 6:822-841.

Braverman, S. J.: Death of a monster. Am. J. Nurs. 69:1682-3, August, 1969.

Brody, J. A., et al.: Prevention of rubella by gamma globulin during an epidemic in Barrow, Alaska, in 1964. New Eng. J. Med. 272:127-129, January 21, 1965.

Brooks, M., et al.: The child with deformed or missing limbs—his problems and prosthesis. Am. J. Nurs. 62:88-92, November, 1962.

Bruce, S.: Reactions of nurses and mothers to stillbirths. Nurs. Outlook 10:88-91, February, 1962.

Caplan, G.: The mental hygiene role of the nurse in maternal and child care. Nurs. Outlook 2:14-19, January, 1954.

Carson, M. J.: Diabetes mellitus in infants and children. Postgrad. Med. 36:67-75, July, 1964.

Caylor, G. G.: A new approach to neonatal cardiac diagnosis. Med. Times 9:953-957, October, 1968.

Coffelt, R. W.: Unexpected finding from a PKU newborn screening program. Pediatrics 24:889-890, December, 1964.

Cohen, M. M., et al.: The effect of LSD-25 on the chromosomes of children exposed in utero. Pediat. Res. 2:486-492, November, 1968.

Committee on Handicapped Child: Statement on treatment of phenylketonuria. Pediatrics 25:501-503, March, 1965.

Connon, A. F.: Improved accuracy of prediction of severity of hemolytic disease of the newborn. Obstet. Gynec. 33:72-78, January, 1969.

Cooper, L. Z.: Rubella: A preventable cause of birth defects, Birth Defects. Original Article Series 4, No. 7:23-25, The National Foundation—March of Dimes, December, 1968.

Craig, W. S.: Care of the Newly Born Infant. Edinburgh, Livingstone, 1966.

Crosse, V. M.: The Premature Baby and Other Babies of Low Birth Weight. London, J. and A. Churchill, 1966.

Cunningham, G. C.: Two years of PKU testing in California. Calif. Med. 110:11-16, January, 1969.

Davens, E.: A view of health services for mothers and children. Children 12:47-54, March-April, 1965.

Davidson-Buchanan, D. J.: Erythroblastosis neonatorum. Am. J. Nurs. 64:110-112, April, 1964.

Davis, L.: PKU testing in older children—follow-up report. Nurs. Outlook 12:55, April, 1964.

da Sa, D. J.: Analysis of certain factors in the etiology of respiratory distress syndrome of the newborn. J. Obstet. Gynec. British Commonwealth 76:148-153, February, 1969.

Diamond, I., et al.: Prevention of hyperbilirubinemia and kernicterus by exposure to light: studies in newborn guinea pigs and premature infants, Trans. Am. Neurological Assoc. 93:70-74, 1968.

Diller, L.: Psychology of disabled children. Am. J. Nurs. 64:131-136, July, 1964.

Eastman, N. J., and Hellman, L. M.: Williams Obstetrics. ed. 13, New York, Appleton, 1966.

Editors: Saving life before birth. Med. World News 6:43-53, January 1, 1965.

Engle, G. L.: Grief and grieving. Am. J. Nurs. 64: 93-98, September, 1964.

Falconer, M. W., et al.: The Drug, the Nurse, the Patient. ed. 3, Philadelphia, W. B. Saunders, 1966.

Firm to make live vaccine for measles. Los Angeles Times 88, No. 189: Part I, p. 5, June 10, 1969.

Fishbein, M. (ed.): Birth Defects. Philadelphia, J. B. Lippincott, 1963.

Fleming, J. W.: Recognizing the newborn addict. Am. J. Nurs. 65:83, January, 1965.

Fox, H. P., and Robertson, W. O.: Closing the information gap. Northwest Med. 68:124-125, February, 1969.

Freda, V. J.: The Rh Problem in obstetrics and a new concept of its management using amniocentesis and spectrophotometric scanning of amniotic fluid. Am. J. Obstet. Gynec. 92:341-371, June 1, 1965.

Freda, V. J., and Robertson, J. G.: Amniotic fluid analysis in Rh iso-immunization. Am. J. Nurs. 65: 64-68, August, 1965.

Gardam, J. W.: Diarrheal diseases. J. Med. Society New Jersey 66:27-30, January, 1969.

Gingras, G., *et al.*: Congenital anomalies of the limbs —medical aspects. Canad. Med. Assoc. J. 91: 67-72, July 11, 1964.

Glaser, B. G., and Strauss, A.: The social loss of dying patients. Am. J. Nurs. 64:119-121, June, 1964.

Glynn, E. M.: Nursing support during intrauterine transfusion. Am. J. Nurs. 65:72-73, August, 1965.

Graw, R. J., Jr., and De'ak, W. R.: Respiratory distress syndrome—protocol for management. Clin. Pediat. 7:510-517, September, 1968.

Guthrie, R., and Stewart, W.: Phenylketonuria. Children's Bureau Publication No. 41, Washington, D.C., U.S. Government Printing Office, 1964.

Hall, J. G., and Heicht, F.: Autosomal trisomies, Am. J. Nurs. 64:87-91, November, 1964.

Ingles, T.: Maria, the hungry baby. Nurs. Forum 5, No. 2:36-47, 1966.

James, L. S. (ed.): The newborn II. Pediatric Clinics of North America 13, No. 4, November, 1966.

Jolly, H.: Diseases of Children. Oxford, Blackwell Scientific Publications, 1968.

Kallaus, K.: The child with cleft lip and palate—the mother in the maternity unit. Am. J. Nurs. 65:120-123, April, 1965.

Krause, S. O., *et al.*: Heroin addiction among pregnant women and their newborn babies. Am. J. Obstet. Gynec. 75:754-758, April, 1958.

LaDu, B. N.: Inborn errors of metabolism. Am. J. Obstet. Gynec. 90:1024-1034, December 1, 1964.

Larsen, G. L.: What every nurse should know about congenital syphilis. Nurs. Outlook 13:52-54, March, 1965.

Latham, H. C., and Heckel, R. V.: Pediatric Nursing. St. Louis, C. V. Mosby, 1967.

Lepow, M. L., *et al.*: Effect of Sabin Type I poliomyelitis vaccine administered by mouth to newborn infants. New Eng. J. Med. 264:1071-1078, May 25, 1961.

Liley, A. W.: Intrauterine transfusion of foetus in haemolytic disease. Brit. Med. H. 2:1107, November 2, 1963.

Lin-Fu, J. S.: Histidinemia. Washington, D.C., U.S. Children's Bureau, 1964.

McDermott, M. M.: The child with cleft lip and palate: the pediatric ward. Am. J. Nurs. 65:122-123, April, 1965.

McDonagh, B. J.: Congenital atrial flutter. Arch. Dis. Child. 43:731-733, December, 1968.

McDonald, J. C.: Gamma-globulin for the prevention of rubella in pregnancy. Brit. Med. J. 5354:416-418, August 17, 1963.

McKendry, J. B. J.: Jaundice in the newborn infant. Clin. Pediat. 3:209-214, April, 1964.

McLenahan, I. G.: No baby to take home. Am. J. Nurs. 62:70-71, April, 1962.

Maple Syrup Urine Disease. Washington, D.C., U.S. Children's Bureau, 1964.

Marlow, D. R.: Textbook of Pediatric Nursing. ed. 2, Philadelphia, W. B. Saunders, 1965.

Mathews, D. H., *et al.*: Closed chest massage in the newborn infant. J.A.M.A. 183:964-966, March 16, 1963.

Nelson, W.: Textbook of Pediatrics. ed. 8, Philadelphia, W. B. Saunders, 1964.

New York State Dept. of Health: PKU in expectant mothers. Health News 45, No. 8:i, 1968.

Nursing Education Service: The Nursing Management of Neonatal Respiratory Distress. Ross Laboratories, 1960.

Odell, G. B.: Hyperbilirubinemia in the neonatal period. Postgrad. Med. 36:280-286, September, 1964.

Owens, C.: Parents' reactions to defective babies. Am. J. Nurs. 64:83-86, November, 1964.

Parmalee, A. H.: The doctor, and the handicapped child. Children 9:189-193, September-October, 1962.

Peeples, E. H., and Francis, G. M.: Social-psychological obstacles to effective health team practice. Nurs. Forum 7, No. 1:28-37, 1968.

Queenan, J. T.: Intra-uterine transfusion for erythroblastosis fetalis. Am. J. Nurs. 65:68-72, August, 1965.

Queenan, J. T., and Douglas, R. G.: Intrauterine transfusion: a preliminary report. Obstet. Gynec. 25:308-321, March, 1965.

Questions and Answers on Rubella. National Communicable Disease Center, Health Services and Mental Health Administration, Public Health Service, U.S. Dept. Health, Education and Welfare, Atlanta, Georgia.

Quint, J. C., *et al.*: Improving nursing care of the dying. Nurs. Forum 6, No. 4:368-378.

Quint, J. C., and Strauss, A. L.: Nursing students, assignments and dying. Nurs. Outlook 12:24-27, January, 1964.

Ravitch, M. M., and Rowe, M. I.: Surgical emergencies in the neonate. Am. J. Obstet. Gynec. 103:1034-1057, April 1, 1969.

Ripley, I. L.: The child with cleft lip and palate: through his years of growth. Am. J. Nurs. 65:124-127, April, 1965.

Rubella vaccine "race" nears finish. J.A.M.A. 207:1615, 1617, March 3, 1969.

Schild, S.: Parents of children with phenylketonuria. Children 11:92-96, May-June, 1964.

Semoff, M.: Neonatal hyperbilirubinemia and phototherapy. Arizona Med. 25:803-806, September, 1968.

Serologic Testing for Rubella—A Warning. reprinted by the U.S. Dept. of Health, Education, and Welfare, Public Health Service, from MMWR, 18, No. 15, April 12, 1969.

Steele, S.: Children with amputations. Nurs. Forum 7, No. 4:411-423, 1968.

Strassman, S. S.: The respiratory distress syndrome. Ohio Med. J. 60:556-558, June, 1964.

Symposium on congenital defects, Am. J. Obstet.

Gynec. 90:part 2:983-1250 (entire issue), December 1, 1964.

Taylor, A.: Autosomal trisomy syndromes: a detailed study of 27 cases of Edwards Syndrome and 27 cases of Patoy's Syndrome. J. of Med. Genetics 5:227-252, September, 1968.

Thaler, O. F.: Grief and depression. Nurs. Forum 5, No. 2:8-22, 1966.

Ujhely, G. B.: Grief and depression—implications for preventive and therapeutic nursing care. Nurs. Forum 5, No. 2:23-35, 1966.

U.S. Children's Bureau: Galactosemia: A Selected Bibliography. compiled by Donough O'Brien, Washington, D.C., U.S. Government Printing Office, 1963.

U.S. Children's Bureau: The Clinical Team Looks at Phenylketonuria. Washington, D.C., U.S. Government Printing Office, 1964.

Van Leeuwen, G., and Jackson, R. L.: Infants of diabetic mothers. Clin. Pediat. 4:315-319, June, 1965.

Warner, R. A., and Cornblath, M.: Infants of gestational diabetic mothers. Am. J. Dis. Child. 117:678-683, June, 1969.

Westberg, J. A., and Margolis, A. J.: Amniotic fluid evaluation and intrauterine transfusions for erythroblastosis fetalis, Am. J. Obstet. Gynec. 92:583-591, July 1, 1965.

Which women can safely receive the rubella vaccines? J.A.M.A. 207:1804-1805, March 10, 1969.

White, P.: The pregnant diabetic. Virginia Med. Monthly 91:102-105, March, 1964.

Wolman, I. J., and Freedman, A. R. (eds.): Clinical pediatrics handbook, drug dosages for the newborn infant. Clin. Pediat. 5:26 B-C, February, 1966.

————: Clinical pediatrics handbook, management of neonatal disease. Part III: The exchange transfusion. Clin. Pediat. 7:16 B-C, June, 1968.

————: Clinical pediatrics handbook, screening infants for phenylketonuria (PKU). Clin. Pediat. 5:36 B-B. September, 1966.

CONFERENCE MATERIAL

1. In your own hospital setting, evaluate the facilities for and the care of the newborn infants in relation to the prevention of infection.

2. A mother's firstborn infant has a cleft lip and cleft palate. The infant is apparently normal otherwise. The distraught mother can see only "my poor deformed baby girl" and blames herself for this "tragedy," because she did not follow her physician's instructions during pregnancy, particularly in relation to good nutrition. How might the nurse handle the nursing problems in this situation?

3. How do you account for the high infant mortality during the neonatal period?

4. What community agencies in your city render services for handicapped children? What is the procedure for making the referral to such agencies? How can the public health nurse function most effectively in such cases?

5. What legislation in your city or state has contributed to reducing the incidence of congenital syphilis?

6. What methods are used by your hospital, well-baby clinics, and/or other community agencies for the detection of phenylketonuria?

Study Questions

Unit Eight: Abnormalities of the Fetus and the Newborn

Read through the entire question and place your answer on the line to the right.

1. When the newborn infant does not breathe at birth, and modern equipment for infant resuscitation is not available, which of the following procedures are sometimes resorted to?
   A. Hold the infant in the palm of one hand, with head, legs and arms hanging forward, thus compressing the chest wall. Then turn the infant over on its back, in the other hand, in which position the head, legs and arms hang backward, thus expanding the chest.
   B. With one hand grasp the infant by the ankles and hold him suspended head downward, while the other hand is used to "milk the trachea" or gently rub the infant's back.
   C. Mouth-to-mouth insufflation, exhaling through clean dry gauze directly into the infant's mouth at intervals corresponding to those of normal respiration.
   D. Alternately, plunge the infant into tubs of hot and cold water.
   E. Immerse the infant's body in a tub of hot water (110° F.) to prevent chilling and simultaneously dash a little cold water upon the infant's face and chest.

   Select the number corresponding to the correct letters.
   1. A and C
   2. B and C
   3. B and D
   4. C and E
   _____

2. The nurse sometimes observes swelling of the newborn infant's scalp which may be due to caput succedaneum or cephalhematoma. Which of the following statements are true concerning cephalhematoma?
   A. It is due to an extravasation of serum into the tissues of the scalp.
   B. It is seldom visible when the infant is born and may not be noticed for several hours or more after delivery.
   C. The infant usually recovers without treatment.
   D. It always disappears within a few days.
   E. It gradually increases in size until about a week after the infant's birth, when it remains stationary for a time and then begins to disappear.

   Select the number corresponding to the correct letters.
   1. A and B
   2. A, C and D
   3. B, C and D
   4. B, C and E
   _____

3. What are some of the signs of cerebral hemorrhage which may be observed by the nurse caring for infants in the newborn nursery?
   A. Convulsions
   B. Slow, deep, rhythmic respiration
   C. Twitching of extremities
   D. Flushed face with circumoral pallor
   E. Weak, whining cry

   Select the number corresponding to the correct letter or letters.
   1. A only
   2. A and C
   3. B, C and E
   4. All of them
   _____

4. A newborn infant develops respiratory distress several hours after birth, and the diagnosis of hyaline membrane disease is made. Which of the following statements have bearing on this condition?
   A. The infant was born prematurely.
   B. The infant is cyanotic and dyspneic.
   C. Progressive respiratory difficulty is evidenced by increased cyanosis and marked sternal retractions.
   D. Treatment primarily consists of the administration of oxygen and maintenance of high humidity.
   E. A protein material is obstructing the flow of air and the exchange of oxygen and carbon dioxide in the lungs.

   Select the number corresponding to the correct letters.
   1. A, B and C
   2. B, D and E
   3. C, D and E
   4. All of them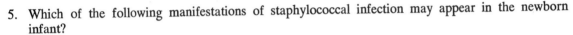

5. Which of the following manifestations of staphylococcal infection may appear in the newborn infant?
   A. Impetigo
   B. Milia
   C. Conjunctivitis
   D. Erythema toxicum
   E. Breast engorgement

   Select the number corresponding to the correct letters.
   1. A and C
   2. A and D
   3. B, C and E
   4. All of them

6. Which of the following conditions are congenital disorders?
   A. Phimosis
   B. Chloasma
   C. Frenum linguae
   D. Retrolental fibroplasia
   E. Seborrhea capitis

   Select the number corresponding to the correct letters.
   1. A and C
   2. B, C and D
   3. B, D and E
   4. All of them

7. The most effective treatment of erythroblastosis is accomplished by blood transfusion. Which one of the following is the best method to use?
   A. Exchange transfusion with Rh-negative blood
   B. Exchange transfusion with Rh-positive blood
   C. Exchange transfusion with blood plasma
   D. Repeated small transfusions with Rh-negative blood
   E. Repeated small transfusions with Rh-positive blood
   F. Repeated small transfusions with blood plasma

8. Hemolytic disease of the newborn may be produced by the union of parents with which of the following blood types?
   A. Rh-positive mother with Rh-negative father
   B. Rh-negative mother with Rh-negative father
   C. Rh-negative mother with Rh-positive father
   D. Type O mother with Type A father
   E. Type A mother with Type B father

Select the number corresponding to the correct letters.
1. A and C
2. B and D
3. C and D
4. All of them

9. Which one of the following infectious diseases, when contracted by the mother during the first trimester of pregnancy, will most often produce congenital anomalies in the infant?
   A. Scarlet fever
   B. Rubella
   C. Diphtheria
   D. Rubeola
   E. Typhoid fever

10. Some disorders which affect the infant in the neonatal period are manifestations of inborn errors of metabolism. Which of the following conditions would this include?
   A. Phenylketonuria
   B. Icterus neonatorum
   C. Galactosemia
   D. Down's syndrome
   E. Erythroblastosis fetalis

Select the number corresponding to the correct letter or letters.
1. A only
2. A and C
3. B, C and D
4. B, D and E

11. What has recently become the best method to prevent erythroblastosis fetalis?
   A. Injection of the mother soon after delivery with Rh immune globulin to prevent maternal sensitization.
   B. Transfusing the mother during pregnancy.
   C. Transfusing all Rh-negative fathers.
   D. Transfusing all Rh-negative babies.
   E. Repeated small transfusions of Rh-positive blood to the mother.

Select the number corresponding to the correct letter or letters.
1. A only
2. A and B
3. B, C and D
4. C, D and E

Note: The key to the correct answers to these questions is given on page 613.

UNIT NINE
Related Information

Nurse-Midwifery
Obstetrics During Emergency
History of Obstetrics

NURSE-MIDWIFERY

The 15th Congress of the International Confederation of Midwives, held in Santiago, Chile the week of November 15, 1969 was attended by 1400 midwives representing 47 countries. The theme of the Congress was "The Role of the Midwife in a National Program of Maternal and Child Care." This theme was developed through a series of papers presented by speakers from various parts of the world. On the first day midwives from Chile, The United Kingdom and World Health Organization discussed "The Planning of Midwifery Services at the National, Regional and Local Level" and "Midwifery Services in Practice." During the week of the Congress, midwives from Germany, Argentina, Sweden, France, Switzerland, Greece, Ghana and Peru discussed subject matter about prenatal care, postnatal care of the infant and family planning. Other programs included papers presented by physicians representing several other countries. These presentations provided excellent media to study socioeconomic problems and cultural backgrounds, as well as differences in midwifery training and education.

The President of the American College of Nurse Midwives, Lucille Woodville, was elected President of the International Confederation of Midwives for the next three years. Since it is customary to hold the ICM Congress in the country of the current president, the October, 1972 ICM Congress will be held in Washington, D.C.

NURSE-MIDWIFERY IN THE UNITED STATES

Organizations

Frontier Nursing Service. The first use of the trained nurse-midwife in this country was made in 1925, when an organization was established in the mountains of eastern Kentucky to handle the maternity problem in the rural and isolated areas of that territory—the now famous Frontier Nursing Service. This organization was founded by the late Mrs. Mary Breckinridge at Wendover, Ky., the headquarters of the public health nurse-midwifery service. Today, FNS is organized with Hayden Hospital, which has a full-time Medical Director (an M.D.), and 5 outpost clinics, each staffed with nurse-midwives. These nurses often travel by horseback from the outposts to serve families in the even more remote areas, but along the highways and roads they travel today by jeep or station wagon. This organization has demonstrated clearly that graduate nurses prepared in midwifery can help to lower mortality rates in a large population in rural and isolated areas.

Frontier Nursing Service gives a wide range of medical care to 10,000 patients annually. In slightly more than the last decade, during which more than 5,000 mothers have been safely delivered by these nurse-midwives, there have been no maternal deaths. In the fall of 1939, the Frontier Nursing Service inaugurated the Frontier Graduate School of Midwifery in Hayden, Ky.

The Maternity Center Association was founded in New York in 1918, and in 1932 the Center established its school of nurse-midwifery for graduate nurses. The Lobenstine Midwifery Clinic was established to provide a field service for this school. It trained about 12 students a year in a 6-month course which provided obstetric theory and supervised practice by an obstetrician and by graduate nurse-midwives. In 1935, the Maternity Center Association and the Lobenstine Midwifery Clinic applied to the State of New York to consolidate under the name of Maternity Center Association. The progress achieved in this endeavor can best be explained by citing an excerpt from the Center's recent annual report:

WHITHER NURSE-MIDWIFERY?[1]

One of the major projects of the Maternity Center Association since 1932 has been the education of nurse-midwives. These are professional nurses with graduate education in the science and art of obstetrics. The Center's school was the first in the United States.

Working within the framework of organized obstetric services, nurse-midwives provide warm, human, scientific care to mothers in clinics, in labor and delivery rooms, in homes, in parents' classes. They direct maternal and child health programs at different levels of government. They are professors of graduate and undergraduate nursing education. These are superior, dedicated women, a majority of whom have a bachelor's degree, and many their master's degree in Nursing or Public Health. They enter nurse-midwifery because they want to serve well where the need is great.

Wherever nurse-midwives have worked, at large universities and medical centers, in the backwoods of Kentucky or the deserts of the Southwest, the bush country of Africa or the bleak hills of Korea, they have helped to bring confidence and comfort to patients and their families.

In an article in the *American Journal of Nursing,* Dr. Mary I. Crawford, who heads the nurse-midwifery program at the Columbia-Presbyterian Medical Center, explained how nurse-midwives can improve maternity care in a large urban hospital. She pointed out that teams consisting of a resident doctor, a nurse-midwife and nurses, working in shifts in prenatal clinics and labor and delivery rooms, could provide greater continuity of care for the mother and more job satisfaction for the professional workers. Nurse-midwives in the United States, she went on to say, are not trying to be poorly prepared doctors but expertly prepared nurses.

Dr. Louis M. Hellman, Professor of Obstetrics and Gynecology at the State University of New York (Downstate Medical Center) and Director of the Department of Obstetrics at Kings County Hospital, recently estimated that by 1975 as many babies will be born in the *hospital ward services* as were born in the whole country in 1950. He foresaw also a rapidly declining number of general practitioners, with only a moderate increase in the number of obstetricians—not nearly enough to provide good care for the oncoming flood of newborn babies.

Who can provide this care? Since the nurse-midwives have been at Kings County Hospital, Dr. Hellman said, the capacity of the hospital has risen from 5,000 to 7,000 deliveries a year, and the perinatal mortality rate is an incredibly low 0.96.

---

[1] Maternity Center Association: Forty-fifth Annual Report (1918-1963). pp. 6-11, New York, Maternity Center Association, 1964.

Since 1958, Maternity Center Association's School of Nurse-Midwifery has conducted a joint program with the Downstate Medical Center of State University of New York and Kings County Hospital. In this time it has certified 89 nurse-midwife graduates. Most are Americans planning to practice in this country; some come from other parts of the world. Since the Center's School of Nurse-Midwifery was founded in 1932, 413 graduates have been certified.

The New York City Department of Health provides for the licensing of nurse-midwives, and qualified nurse-midwives, working as such, are employed in two municipal hospitals. The position of nurse-midwife is spelled out on the city's line budget.

If maternity care is to profit fully from what the nurse-midwife can contribute, the existing personnel-structure within the hospital should be restudied and recast. Is the nurse-midwife primarily a nurse working under the director of nurses? Or should she work under the medical director of obstetrics? Dr. Hellman believes she provides "third-party care," that is, between medicine and nursing, and a new pattern for work relationships among the professions must be developed. Unless this is done, most nurse-midwives will continue to work as consultants, educators and administrators rather than in direct patient care.

The American College of Nurse-Midwifery was established in 1955 as an organization of nurse-midwives to study and evaluate the activities of nurse-midwives, to plan and develop educational programs meeting the requirements of the profession, and to perform other related functions. In 1957, the College became a member of the International Confederation of Midwives, a midwifery organization with members from some 31 countries throughout the world.

At the annual meeting of the College in May, 1962, the definitions of the nurse-midwife and nurse-midwifery were accepted by the membership and stated as follows:

The Nurse-Midwife is a Registered Nurse who by virtue of added knowledge and skill gained through an organized program of study and clinical experience recognized by the American College of Nurse-Midwifery, has extended the limits (legal limits in jurisdictions where they obtain) of her practice into the area of management of care of mothers and babies throughout the maternity cycle so long as progress meets criteria accepted as normal.

Nurse-Midwifery is an extension of nursing practice into the area of management of care of mothers and babies throughout the maternity cycle so long as progress meets criteria accepted as normal.

This was a major step in the formulation of a basic policy for the College as a professional organization.

FIG. 24-1. Postpartal care and teaching in the home provided by the certified nurse-midwife. (Catholic Maternity Institute, Sante Fe, New Mexico)

The American College of Nurse-Midwives had its inception in 1969 when the American College of Nurse-Midwifery amended its Articles of Incorporation.[2]

The objectives of the American College of Nurse-Midwives are as follows:

1. To enable nurse-midwives to concentrate their efforts in the improvement of services to mothers and newborn babies in cooperation with other allied groups.

2. To identify the area of nurse-midwifery practices as they relate to the total service and educational aspects of maternal and newborn care.

3. To study and evaluate the activities of the nurse-midwife in order that qualifications for these activities may be established.

4. To plan and develop with the assistance of allied educational groups educational programs in nurse-midwifery that will meet the qualifications of the profession.

5. To establish channels for communication and interpretation of midwifery to allied profes-

sional and nonprofessional groups on a regional, national, and international basis.

6. To sponsor research and develop literature in the field of nurse-midwifery.

What is a Nurse-Midwife?

A nurse-midwife is a registered professional nurse who has successfully completed a recognized program of study and clinical experience leading to a certificate in nurse-midwifery. She is prepared to provide prenatal, intrapartum and postpartum care geared to the individual needs of each mother and family. She cares for the mother during pregnancy and stays with her in labor, providing continuous physical and emotional support. She evaluates progress and manages the labor and delivery, always watchful for signs requiring medical attention. She evaluates and provides immediate care for the newborn. She helps the mother to care for herself and for her infant, to adjust the home situation to the new child, and to lay a healthful foundation for future pregnancies. The nurse-midwife is prepared to teach, interpret and provide support as an integral part of her service.

The American nurse-midwife always functions

[2] American College of Nurse-Midwives: Articles of Incorporation of American College of Nurse-Midwives, amended April, 1969, New York, N.Y.

FIG. 24-2. Newspaper pad made of 12 thicknesses of newspaper sewed together at the outer edges and covered with unbleached muslin (viewed from underside). The muslin covers are mitered at the corners so that they may be removed, laundered and used again.

within the framework of a medically directed health service: she is never an independent practitioner.

Midwifery Programs

At the present time there are 12 schools of nurse-midwifery in the United States with several programs reported to be in the planning stage. All of the schools provide programs of study leading to a Certificate in Nurse-Midwifery for registered nurses (graduates from accredited schools of nursing). Six of the schools have their programs designed in conjunction with graduate study in nursing, leading to a Master of Science degree in addition to a Certificate in Nurse-Midwifery.

The American College of Nurse-Midwives has published the following list of schools in the U.S.A. having programs in nurse-midwifery:[3]

Programs leading to a certificate in nurse-midwifery:

Nurse-Midwifery Program
Maternity Center Association,
48 East 92nd Street, New York, New York 10028
 affiliated with
Downstate Medical Center
State University of New York and
Kings County Hospital

Catholic Maternity Institute
School of Nurse Midwifery
417 East Palace Avenue
Sante Fe, New Mexico 87501

Frontier Nursing Service
School of Nurse-Midwifery
Wendover, Leslie County
Kentucky 41775

Ponce School of Maternity and Nurse-Midwifery*
Ponce District General Hospital
Ponce, Puerto Rico 00731

Puerto Rico Nurse-Midwifery Program
University District Hospital
Department of Health
Caparra Heights, Puerto Rico 00922

University of Mississippi*
Nurse-Midwifery Program
2500 North State Street
Jackson, Mississippi 39216

Programs leading to a Master's degree and a certificate in nurse-midwifery:

Presbyterian Hospital
Columbia University Graduate Program in Maternity Nursing
Department of Nursing Faculty of Medicine
Columbia Presbyterian Medical Center
630 West 168th Street
New York, New York 10032

---

[3] The American College of Nurse-Midwifery, 50 East 92nd Street, New York, New York 10028.

---

* New program—evaluation pending.

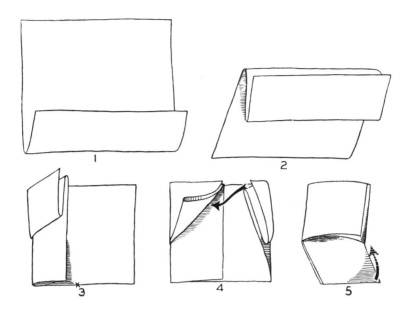

FIG. 24-3. Steps in making a newspaper bag. These are useful receptacles for waste material. They may be made in small and large sizes.

The Johns Hopkins University
Nurse-Midwifery Program
Room 151, Woman's Clinic
601 North Broadway
Baltimore, Maryland 21205

The Catholic University of America
Washington, D.C. 20017
    affiliated with
Catholic Maternity Institute
Sante Fe, New Mexico

Yale University School of Nursing
Nurse-Midwifery Program
Yale University School of Nursing
New Haven, Connecticut 06520

Graduate School of Nursing
New York Medical College
Nurse-Midwifery Program
Fifth Avenue and 106th Street
New York, New York 10029

Nurse-Midwifery Program
University of Utah Medical Center
50 North Medical Drive
Salt Lake City, Utah 84112

The authors believe a brief orientation to nurse-midwifery should be included in this textbook. Since it is impossible to deal more fully with this subject here, references have been categorized in the Suggested Reading at the end of this chapter to assist the students.

HOME DELIVERY

Even though at the present time the vast majority of mothers in this country are delivered in hospitals, there is still a small percentage of deliveries attended by physicians and qualified midwives at home, the majority of which take place in rural areas. Therefore, the nurse should know how a home delivery is conducted. In an emergency, too, the nurse may need this knowledge and experience. For the nurse who is interested in obtaining special preparation for this aspect of maternity care, a small number of schools in this country offer nurse-midwifery programs that include education and training for the conduct of home deliveries.

When a home delivery is preferred, such factors as the normalcy of the patient, accessibility of the obstetrician, facilities at home and available care are important considerations.

Preparations for Home Delivery

Preparations for home delivery should be begun early in pregnancy to enable the family to make adequate preparations. Today in many areas the public health nurse visits the patient in her home routinely during the antepartal period and assists the physician in the management and care of the mother. When there is a home delivery service, these nurses may attend the delivery with the physician. The nurse can be most helpful with preparations for delivery because of her special knowledge.

Many obstetricians give their patients a list of supplies that they will need for delivery at home, but where the matter is left to the parents and the nurse, the following suggestions may be helpful. Even when the mother has been able to avail herself of the opportunity of attending a Mothers' Club or expectant parents' classes and of obtaining suggestions, she may desire to discuss some of them, along with personal problems, with the obstetrician and the nurse.

Supplies for the Mother

The supplies provided by the mother will necessarily vary in the individual situation. The following list contains supplies which will be needed:

Sheets and pillowcases (4)

Bath towels and washcloths (4)

Waterproof material—large enough to protect the mattress (about 1½ yards square). Rubber sheeting, plastic or white table oil-cloth are preferable, although heavy brown paper can be used.

Receiving blanket for the infant

Delivery pads (4 to 6). These bed pads are made from 12 thicknesses of newspaper opened to full size (sewed together at the edges) and covered with freshly laundered old or new muslin. The corners of the cover may be mitered, so that it can be removed and laundered when necessary and fresh newspaper inserted (Fig. 24-2).

Quilted pads or large-size paper diapers may also be purchased for this purpose.

Newspapers. A supply of clean newspapers should be saved for the many uses to which they can be put at this time.

Newspaper bags. The large newspaper bags are especially useful at the time of delivery (Fig. 24-3).

Small enamel wash basins (2 or 3) for solutions and sponges used in cleansing the patient's genitals, to receive the placenta, and a hand basin.

Large pail with cover

Covered kettles or stew pans (2), one for cooled boiled water and one for boiling water

Ladle or dipper

Enema can with tubing and rectal tip

Board for placing under mattress of delivery bed (table leaf or ironing board without legs may be used)

Hot-water bottle and cover

Bedpan

Pair of white stockings (may be inexpensive variety)

Nightgowns or pajama tops (3 or 4)

Brassières (3 or 4) (may be improvised from straight binders, 10 in. wide, or large smooth cotton towels)

Sanitary pads (2 to 3 doz.). If they cannot be purchased, they may be made from freshly laundered, soft, absorbent material, folded and ironed ready for use.

Sanitary belts or T-binders (3 or 4)

Safety pins: 1 doz. small and 1 doz. large

Pitcher or Mason jar with cover

Sterile absorbent cotton (1 lb.) in original package, unopened

Sterile gauze squares 4″ x 4″ (1 doz.)

Mineral oil

Plain white petroleum jelly (tube)

Soap

New nail brush and orangewood stick

Umbilical tape or bobbin tape (narrow cotton) for tying cord (1 yd.)

Scissors

Roll of toilet tissue, unopened

Home Preparations

In preparing for a home delivery, the nurse should explain and demonstrate to the mother how to prepare the articles that are to be used during delivery (viz., sheets to be used for the bed and draping, towels and bed pads of the homemade variety). These articles should be washed with soap and water, dried in the sun if possible, ironed and folded so that the ironed surfaces are folded upon each other. The ironed surface should be used for the field of delivery. These articles should be put away in a pillow-case or wrapped in a piece of ironed paper. The other articles needed at the time of delivery should be laid aside ready for use. Packages of absorbent cotton, gauze squares, sanitary pads and toilet tissue should be put away unopened.

Packages of sterile delivery supplies may be available from a local health agency, or it may be possible to have a package, assembled at home, autoclaved at a local hospital. Although auto-claving is most desirable, it is possible to sterilize dressings, etc., in the oven at home. The simplest method is to place the materials in small muslin bags, or bags of some other heavy white cotton material, and then place these bags in an old pillowcase and pin it shut (double wrapped). This package should be baked on the top shelf in a moderate oven, 325° for 1 hour. If an oven thermometer is not available, place a large white potato (washed and scrubbed) in the oven, and when it is done, the supplies in the pillowcase should be sterilized. The pillowcase should not be opened until the time of delivery, and if it has not been used within a month, it must be resterilized.

The more simple and carefully prepared the preparations are, the more efficient will be the results. The important factor to be achieved in a home delivery is cleanliness. Soap and water, sunshine and a hot iron have proved to be effective. On the whole, only a few articles must be sterile.

Room for Delivery

Deciding on the room in which the patient is to be delivered is one of the "preparations." It should be the room in which the patient will be most comfortable. Many mothers during this period have to assume certain responsibilities for the management of the household, so it means much to be where the household affairs can be directed with the least exertion.

Ideally, it should be a room that is light, airy, quiet, cheerful and comfortable, conveniently near a bathroom. The room furnishings should be simple, so that they are easy to keep clean, as cleanliness is one of the first essentials of good obstetric care. The bed should be so placed that it can be approached from either side, and so that the light is convenient either day or night. Ample light is a necessity.

The nurse may help select the room, but the choice is limited or even fixed by the possibilities of the house. Naturally, the nurse will avoid putting the family to any unnecessary inconveni-ence, but always her first thought must be in the interest of her patient.

The nurse should make sure that the room has not been occupied recently by a patient suffering from any contagious, infectious or sup-purative disease. The instructions set forth in the manual *The Control of Communicable Disease in Man,* American Public Health Association, regulate the isolation, quarantine and disinfection practiced in the care of the patient with com-municable disease. In case of such disease, adaptation of procedures to facilities in the home is made as necessary.

In any event, the room should be cleaned thoroughly, and all unnecessary furniture re-moved, only enough being left to make the room comfortable and cheerful. The obstetrician will need a plain table or a substitute. The nurse will need a table or chair for supplies, unless perhaps the top of the bureau may be used. A card table may be very practical.

Preparation of the Delivery Bed

The mother's bed should be comfortable. The springs should be in good condition, and the mattress firm and level. A single bed is prefer-able to the wider or double bed, because it is easier for the obstetrician and the nurse to care for the mother. If the bed is low, it may be raised to a more convenient height by using blocks. The bed should be so arranged that after the labor the mother may be made clean and comfortable without too much disturbance. The best way to accomplish this is first to prepare the bed as it is to be used after delivery and then to add the necessary preparations on top for the labor and the delivery.

The mattress should be supported by means of boards placed between it and the springs, so that it will be perfectly firm and level and not sag. Table leaves, a flat ironing board or plain board may be used for this purpose. Such supports should lie crosswise under the mattress at a point directly under the mother's buttocks and should be removed at the conclusion of the delivery. A firm, flat mattress helps to prevent the patient's hips from sinking into the bed.

The mattress should be covered with a piece of waterproof material, if available; if not, heavy brown paper, newspaper or water-repellent paper may be used. Over this covering, a white cotton sheet should be placed and tucked in securely

Fig. 24-4. The evolution of a newspaper Kelly pad. When used under a patient, it is lined with a piece of waterproof material and a towel.

along the edges. The top sheet, the blanket and the spread should be fan-folded to the foot of the bed, where they will be convenient to cover the mother immediately after the delivery. Covered newspaper or moistureproof pads afford excellent protection and are so arranged that they protect the bed at the time of delivery, and a fresh one is left under the mother after delivery.

If these preparations are first demonstrated and their uses explained to the patient and her husband, they may be better able to make adequate preparations and have them ready at the time of labor.

Special Equipment

The physician and the nurse probably will have all the supplies needed for the delivery other than those provided by the mother. As stated previously, sometimes these supplies are provided by a local health agency. The Maryland State Department of Health, Division of Public Health Nursing, provides its staff with a nurse's bag and, since it provides a home delivery service, also makes available a nurse-midwife's delivery bag which contains the following:

1. Newspaper pads
   Safety pins
2. Sterno outfit
3. Box of medicines:
   A. Syntocinon (2 amp.)
   B. Methergine (2 amp.)
   C. Ergotrate tablets (50)
   D. Silver nitrate 1 per cent (2 wax amp.)
   E. Vitamin K_1 (2 amp.)
   F. File
   G. Chromic catgut #2 (2 tubes)
4. Sterile gloves:
   Size 7 (2 pairs)
   Size 7½ (2 pairs)
5. Sterile pack containing:
   A. Hand towel (1)

B. Doctor's gown (1)
C. Leggings (2) with towel clips (2)
D. Towels (6)
E. Gauze squares 3″ x 3″ (12)
F. Cord dressings (2) with cord ties (4)
G. Perineal pads (package)
H. Towels for pelvic examination (package of 5)
6. Case of instruments:
   A. 1–2 cc. syringe with No. 25 needles (2)
   B. Mayo scissors (1)
   C. Metal box with needles
   D. Sponge holder (1)
   E. Kelly clamps (2)
7. Muslin case with scales, tape measure, bottle of cord tape, 3″ x 3″ gauze squares (2 pkgs.)
8. Large basins (2)
   Liter cup (1)
   Bag of cotton (to be placed in cup)
9. Enamel covered container
10. Muslin case containing:
    A. Applicators, tongue depressors, razor and box of blades, and finger cots
    B. No. 14 catheters (2):
       1 for bladder catheterization
       1 for suctioning the infant
    C. No. 28 rectal tube with glass connecting tip (1)
    D. Rubber bulb syringe (1)
11. Muslin case containing enema equipment
12. Muslin case containing:
    A. Aprons (2)
    B. Caps (2)
    C. Masks (4)
13. Brown folder containing:
    A. Delivery bag list
    B. Labor and delivery procedure
    C. Standing orders
    D. Procedure for care of premature infants
    E. Birth certificate book

FIG. 24-5. Delivery room in the home, in readiness for the mother in labor.

A. Bureau (newspaper protecting the surface, cloth on top):
    1. Flashlight
    2. Perineal pads
    3. Paper waste bag
    4. Clock
    5. Basin
    6. Enamel tray containing: (a) Thermometer in solution in glass tube, (b) Thumb forceps, (c) Cotton balls in tray

B. Chair at head of bed for enema equipment. *Note.* This chair will be moved down toward the center of the bed later to support the mother's legs for the actual delivery.

B[1]. Second chair to be moved toward the center of the bed to support the mother's legs for the delivery.

C. Bed protected with paper pad, Kelly newspaper pad and cloth cover for the delivery. Sheet fanned-folded to foot of bed, extra blanket and sheet. (Bed is made for delivery with the mother lying crosswise.)

D. Table (protected with newspaper covered by cloth):
    1. Basin of antiseptic solution
    2. Basin with sterile cotton balls in water
    3. Sterile gloves and towels
    4. Sterile pack (for contents see Special Equipment in this chapter)

E. Small table (protected with newspaper) for nurse's bag and delivery bag (see Special Equipment for contents)

F. Crib containing small bundle of infant's clothes and blankets. *Note.* The crib is moved in place of chair B when that space is available.

G. Improvised toilet tray for the infant:
    1. Jars (3) for boiled water, cotton balls and small cotton swabs
    2. Soap dish
    3. Dish for mineral oil

Note. This tray should be readily available for use when needed for the infant's initial care. Before this time there may be no place for it because the bureau and small table surfaces are occupied by the essentials for the delivery.

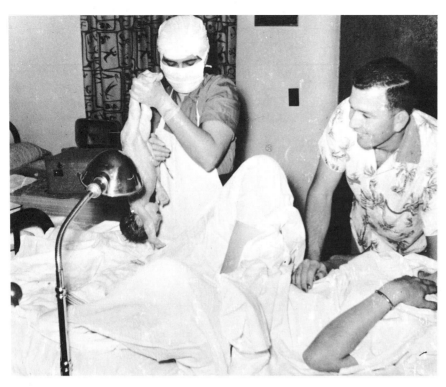

FIG. 24-6. The certified nurse-midwife conducting a home delivery. The father at the bedside encourages his wife and simultaneously derives considerable satisfaction from his participation in the birth of their baby. (Catholic Maternity Institute, Sante Fe, N. Mex.)

F. Labor and delivery records (12)
G. Infant records (6)
H. Baby's care (6)
I. Small envelopes (12)
J. Scratch pad and pencil
K. Laundry lists (12)
14. Side pockets of bag:
No. 1. Thermometers
   A. Mouth thermometer
   B. Rectal thermometer
No. 2. K. Y. jelly
No. 3.
   A. Alcohol 70%
   B. Green soap
   C. Bottle of antiseptic No. 3
   D. Mercury cyanide
   E. Brush and orangewood stick
   F. Paper napkins (12)
   G. Paper towels (12)
   H. Aromatic spirits of ammonia

If an anesthetic other than Trilene is to be given, the nurse may need to cover the wire mask. A cone may be improvised with a wire sieve, but should not be made from newspaper because of the danger involved (see Chap. 12, Analgesia and Anesthesia in Labor).

Delivery in the Home

During the antepartal period the patient and her husband will have prepared the needed sup-plies and made preparations so that labor should be conducted with comparatively little incon-venience and confusion. They have been instructed concerning the symptoms of labor and when to call the physician and the nurse. Many physicians wish to be with the mother from the onset of labor; however, this will have been arranged beforehand, and if the nurse's arrival precedes that of the physician, she will make her observa-tions of the mother's condition and proceed accordingly.

A few preparations cannot be made until labor begins, such as boiling the two kettles of water (for 20 minutes) in covered vessels and setting 1 aside to cool. It is a good idea also to boil a ladle or dipper in the kettle that is set aside to cool. The bed and the crib should be prepared and the delivery supplies arranged (Fig. 24-5). The nurse should also see that the provisions for lighting the room are ample, and that the room is warm and as comfortable as possible.

The underlying principles for the care of the mother being delivered at home are the same as those for hospital delivery (see Chap. 13), although procedures will necessarily have to be modified because of the home situation. The patient will probably have taken a warm sponge bath, but it may be necessary to assist her with it if this is necessary and time permits. The patient should have special preparation for delivery. These preparations may seem strange to the patient, so the nurse should explain procedures and any developments carefully, so the mother will have less cause to become anxious. According to the physician's specific orders, a low soapsuds enema may be given to empty the lower intestine in order to make more room for the descending head and to prevent fecal discharge during the delivery. The vulva should be shaved and the external genitalia cleansed with aseptic technique. The mother may need to have it explained that the former practice of keeping a perineal pad on while in labor has been largely discarded because of the danger of carrying infection, notably the colon bacillus, to the parturient canal from the anal region.

During the first stage of labor the mother is usually allowed to be up and about until labor becomes very active, or the membranes rupture. The physician may suggest liquids to be given freely and that light nourishment be offered, such as tea and toast or crackers, if delivery is not imminent. As labor progresses, careful explanation will provide comfort and reassurance.

The nursing care of the mother in labor at home is essentially the same as in the hospital. Observations of the mother's temperature, pulse, respirations, blood pressure, intake and output and the progress of labor are made consistently. The fetal heart tones should be checked routinely, and the mother should be watched closely for any complication which might develop. If membranes rupture in the first stage of labor, the danger of prolapse of the cord must be kept in mind. In addition, if the physician is not present, he should be notified immediately, as would be the case if anything unusual developed. If the physician needs to be called for this reason, it should be done without alarming the mother, especially if this is her first labor. From the beginning of true labor, the mother should use a commode or bedpan and should be encouraged to empty her bladder at fairly frequent intervals to avoid bladder distention, as well as to keep her more comfortable.

As soon as it is apparent that the mother is nearing the second stage of labor, she should be put to bed, if she has not been already. The nurse should now have everything in readiness for delivery, if possible. On the arrival of the physician, he will, in all probability, want to make a rectal or a vaginal examination at once to determine the amount of dilatation of the cervix and the progress the mother has made.

For the examination the patient should be in lithotomy position, lying on the side of the bed convenient for the physician. The nurse should drape the mother so that she is well protected, but with the perineal region well exposed. Some physicians prefer to make the examination with the patient lying on her back, but across the bed, with the buttocks resting on the edge of the mattress and the patient's feet supported by two chairs. A pillow may be placed under the patient's head for comfort. When a vaginal examination is to be made, the preparation of the perineal area will be according to the wishes of the physician. Although the technique for local preparation of the patient for vaginal examination varies, if the nurse always regards the perineal region as a site for operation and cleanses the immediate area accordingly, she has followed an important principle for safe care.

All instruments required for the delivery are usually provided by the physician and are brought to the home in sterile packages. However, if such equipment as catheters, hypodermic syringes and needles and the various instruments are not sterile, these are boiled in a tightly covered container for 20 minutes. Sterile packages should not be laid open, or sterile equipment laid out, until just before they are to be used for the delivery.

The Delivery. The activities of the nurse in assisting the physician at delivery will vary. Because of the vast differences in home situations, the details in each case are so variable that it would be impossible to describe them here. In general, the conduct of normal labor, as described in Chapter 13, should serve as a guide for the care of the mother and her infant.

Delivery by the Nurse

In certain cases the nurse will find it necessary to manage the entire labor herself, either because of precipitate delivery or through delay in securing the services of a physician.

It is needless to say that labor in such cases progresses rapidly, and that almost before anything else can be done, the contractions are recurring with such frequency and severity that the mother must be put to bed and be given the undivided attention of the nurse. If time permits, much can be done for the comfort of the mother while preparations are made for delivery. Undoubtedly, the calmness of the nurse at the bedside will be transferred to the mother.

It seldom happens that the nurse and her patient are entirely alone; usually the husband, some relative or friend in the home can be called upon to assist and bring the necessary things to the bedside. In an emergency, when there has been no previous preparation, an ordinary pair of scissors and pieces of clean, soft, white cord or tape may be boiled and used for tying and cutting the cord. As there is usually never any special hurry about tying and cutting the umbilical cord, there is time for scissors and tape to be boiled. Time may be saved by using only enough water to cover the instruments, but it must be sufficient to allow for evaporation. Also, anything which will float, such as the tape, should be weighted down with the scissors. The pan may be covered with a second pan, thus sterilizing both.

If the patient is fully dressed, as may be the case in precipitate delivery, the nurse should do what she can to protect the patient's clothing and the bedding and maintain cleanliness to the best of her ability. The procedure is, of course, the same as when the physician is present; but since the nursing care is wholly different, it may help her to have the steps described as they are in the section on Emergency Delivery by the Nurse in Chapter 13, in order to aid her until help arrives.

SUGGESTED READING

Definition of Nurse-Midwife

Statements of functions, standards and qualifications for the practice of nurse-midwifery. Bull. Am. College of Nurse-Midwifery 11:55-61, July, 1966.

Education of the Nurse-Midwife in the United States

Bull. Am. College of Nurse-Midwifery. Education issues. 10, No. 1 and 2, 1965.

Functions, Standards and Qualifications for the Practice of Nurse-Midwifery in the United States

Statement of functions, standards and qualifications for the practice of nurse-midwifery. Bull. Am. College of Nurse-Midwifery, 11:55-61, July, 1966.

Historical Background of the Nurse-Midwife in the U.S.

Fox, C. G.: Toward a sound historical basis for nurse-midwifery. Bull. Am. College of Nurse-Midwives 14:76-82, August, 1969.

Harris, D.: The development of nurse-midwifery in New York City. Bull. Am. College of Nurse-Midwifery 14:4-12, February, 1969.

Midwifery Practice Throughout the World

Barnes, A. C.: The World Health Organization report —midwife in maternity care. Bull. Am. College of Nurse-Midwifery 12:19-27, February, 1967.

Cavero, C.: Nurse-midwife in a developing country. Bull. Am. College of Nurse-Midwifery 13:134-138, November, 1964.

Joint Study Group of the International Federation of Gynecology and Obstetrics and the International Confederation of Midwives. New York: Pergamon Press, 1966.

Nurse-Midwifery Legislation in the U.S.

ANA statement on nurse-midwifery. Bull. Am. College of Nurse-Midwifery 13: 26-27, February, 1968.

Crawford, M.: Nurse-midwifery—Licensure or certification. Bull. Am. College of Nurse-Midwifery 13:18-22, May, 1968.

Hellman, L. M.: Nurse-midwifery in the United States. Obstet. Gynec. 30:883-888, December, 1967.

Nurse-midwifery legislation: pro and con. Bull. Am. College of Nurse-Midwifery 11:62-68, July, 1966.

Swartz, D. P.: Nurse-midwifery from the viewpoint of one obstetrician. Bull. Am. College of Nurse-Midwives 14:111-117, November, 1969.

Objectives of the American College of Nurse-Midwives

American College of Nurse-Midwives: Articles of Incorporation of American College of Nurse-Midwives, New York, The College, April, 1969.

Leppert, P. A.: The merger and the birth of the American College of Nurse-Midwives. Bull. Am. College of Nurse-Midwives 14:68-70, August, 1969.

Role of the Nurse-Midwife in the U.S.

Boone, P.: The nurse-midwifery service at Harlem Hospital Center. Bull. Am. College of Nurse-Midwifery 13:13-18, February, 1968.

Jones, G. W.: Will there be a place for nurse-midwives? Virginia Med. Monthly 93:173-175, March, 1966.

Lang, D. M.: Providing maternity care through a nurse-midwifery service program. Nurs. Clin. N. Am. 4:509-520, September, 1969.

Linder, E. M.: Nurse-midwife—a nurse clinician. Bull. Am. College of Nurse-Midwives 14:53-59, May, 1969.

Nurse-midwifery statistics. Bull. Am. College of Nurse-Midwives 14:70-75, August, 1969.

Okrent, S.: The nurse-midwife in a family planning clinic. Bull. Am. College of Nurse-Midwifery 11: 48-54, July, 1966.

Runnerstrom, L.: The effectiveness of a nurse-midwife in a supervised hospital environment. Bull. Am. College of Nurse-Midwives 14:40-52, May, 1969.

Sundberg, A.: Nurse-midwife in an urban health department. Bull. Am. College of Nurse-Midwifery 11:102, October, 1966.

Swenson, N.: The role of the nurse-midwife on the health team as viewed by the family. Bull. Am. College of Nurse-Midwifery 13:128-133, November, 1968.

Obstetrics During Emergency

Commonalities of Disaster Situations • Thermonuclear Disaster
Disaster Insurance for Mothers and Babies • Psychological Reactions in Emergency Situations

INTRODUCTION

When any large-scale emergency arises, it is usually sudden and calls for immediate action, whether it is caused by hurricane, flood, fire or war. In the event of such catastrophe, babies are likely to be born rapidly, and many women may abort. When organized rescue work is hampered, it may fall to those who are in the immediate area to manage as best they can. The nurses in the area should be able to assist with measures for the safety and the welfare of maternity patients and their newborn infants.

All nurses who have completed the basic course in maternity nursing are familiar with antepartal care, the conduct of labor and the immediate care of the newborn infant, but their preparation has been carried out, for the most part, in an organized environment (such as a hospital) where supplies, equipment and medical direction are available. It requires considerable imagination on the part of the nurse to conceive of an emergency situation in which she might be required to work without the availability of these facilities. Yet in any large scale disaster, whole communities may be isolated and left to their own resources when telephone and radio communications are wrecked; roads may become impassable if they are inundated by water and blocked by debris, and an area may be without safe water, means of power and light and medical supplies.

COMMONALITIES OF DISASTER SITUATIONS

It has been established that all disaster emergencies have certain similarities and differ only in scope, intensity, and effect. It has also been demonstrated that there are usually two kinds of peo-ple remaining, those who *need* help and those who *are able* to help. It is safe to assume that in any extreme, large scale emergency, the medical-health requirements of the surviving population will lead to an unprecedented need for hospital space (improvised if necessary) and for skilled professionals to care for the ill and injured and to keep the well well.

In extreme disaster conditions nursing care is usually administered on an austere basis, but, whenever possible, in accordance with established medical principles designed to save life, prevent the spread of disease, alleviate suffering and promote recovery. If the emergency is dire but confined to an area, the resources and manpower of the unaffected regions can be brought to bear upon the situation, thus allowing all health care to proceed along the above lines. In the case of a thermonuclear holocaust involving a whole nation, then survival will depend upon self- and buddy-help, with only life-sustaining care provided by the necessarily limited resources which must be conserved for a prolonged period.

Every responsible practitioner will want to familiarize herself with basic emergency and disaster nursing techniques (see Suggested Reading). It is well to remember, however, that the required knowledge and skills for nursing under these conditions are essentially the same as those required in daily patient care; *only the priorities change*. Thus, treatment will be based on available personnel, drugs, supplies and equipment.

THERMONUCLEAR DISASTER

This type of catastrophe is given particular attention since of all the disaster situations it is without a doubt the most severe.[1] Moreover, the medical and health problems which arise from it require special physical facilities and particular attention with respect to modification of priorities.

Fallout Shelters

The advent of the nuclear age and the continuing development of thermonuclear weaponry has brought with it not only the possibility of war, but also the risk of nuclear accidents and the hazards of radioactive fallout. To meet these contingencies, the United States Government enacted the Federal Civil Defense Act in 1950; each state followed with similar legislation soon after. Thus, Civil Defense has come to represent government in emergency and its guide principle is that disaster preparedness is a responsibility of each citizen, assisted by the local, state, and Federal government. Original civil defense planning provided for mass casualty care which utilized emergency medical facilities that could be mobilized in a short time. With the threat of fallout, however, concepts have changed and it is now the policy to provide shelter against radiation for as many persons as possible. These "fallout" shelters are marked and stocked with emergency equipment by the Federal Government. Supplies include survival biscuits, water, sanitation kits, and basic medical supplies sufficient to provide for total capacity of the shelter and to last 14 days. Each community is responsible for providing any additional supplies it can to make living more comfortable.

Special Health Problems of the Shelter. A catastrophe of the magnitude to require the population to utilize shelters will automatically subject all of us to very unusual pressures never before experienced in this country. Moreover, immediate care of the sick and the injured will focus on life-sustaining survival techniques, dependent upon self-help and buddy-help, both of which are basic principles in disaster nursing. Hopefully, each shelter will have a shelter manager and staff, but this is not a certainty. During the crisis the nurse may find she is the only medically oriented person in the shelter and therefore its health leader.

Certain health related problems will arise which are basic to the general care of the maternity patient as well as all inhabitants of the shelter. For instance, waste disposal and personal hygiene will

---

[1] The following discussion is adapted from Eicherly, E. E.: Nursing in thermonuclear disaster. Nurs. Clin. N. Am. 2:325, June, 1967.

be of major importance. The sanitation kit includes an improvised toilet which is about the height of a kitchen stool; its construction is such that it requires an even distribution of weight, so that the user must place his feet firmly and squarely on the floor. This will be difficult for many and impossible for some; thus, foot rests may have to be improvised from a spare cardboard carton. Alternate methods will have to be devised for the very small child or the handicapped. Privacy and odor control present additional problems and must be solved. Water will be required for drinking purposes and this purpose *must remain a top priority*. Thus, alternate measures to maintain personal hygiene and to keep the living area clean will need to be devised. Ready made "wipes" and disinfectant sprays are suitable if they are available. Unfortunately not even general statements can be made regarding solutions to these myriad problems since the sites chosen for the shelters vary so with respect to space, number and type of inhabitants, and the possibility of improvising facilities. The key principles to remember are improvisation and flexible priority setting.

The total diet consists of biscuits augmented by a carbohydrate supplement (in the form of candy) and a ration of water. Obviously this is a *subsistence* diet which provides the basic caloric intake necessary to keep functioning. Dietary problems will arise, including those relating to infant feeding, the nursing mother, and individuals requiring special diets. Shelter inhabitants, particularly the weak and the young, will need to be checked to make sure they are consuming their ration, since the monotony and tastelessness of the diet will tend to curtail appetite.

The medical kits usually found in the shelters weigh 26 pounds apiece and provide supplies for 50 people for the two-week period. There are three categories of supplies: medications, dressings, and miscellaneous materials. Instruction booklets are included. Medical supplies are comparable to medical items usually found in the average household. In addition, there are three prescription drugs: sulfadiazine, phenobarbital, and penicillin G tablets. These are to be considered "life saving" drugs and are to be utilized only in extreme cases. General discomfort is not to be considered an extreme case. Operating the medical treatment area may become the responsibility of the nurse. Therefore the location of supplies should be ascertained as quickly as possible and located as far as possible from the general living area.

As soon as possible after entry into the shelter, a check of the inhabitants is to be made to ascertain any contagious diseases, impending deliveries or abortions, and vermin infestation. Acute casualties, of course, are considered top priority. Later, when some routine is established, a daily sick call will do much to survey the routine complaints and the general level of health. It will also provide for the enforcement of health and environmental rules and shelter regulations.

Certain psychological disruptions and manifestations will become apparent. Grieving, depression and anxiety reactions will be seen in abundance particularly in children reflecting their parents' anxieties and in those who are alone because of the disaster. This aspect will be discussed more fully later in the chapter.

Minor injuries and major health emergencies will occur especially among those with chronic health and/or social disability. Other additional and related difficulties will occur as a result of the limited supplies, lack of water, inadequate light and heat, poor ventilation, and from discomfort and boredom. These problems will tax the ingenuity, skill and emotional fortitude of those who accept the responsibility of the care of others. Needless to say, the life and well being of all of the shelter inhabitants will depend largely upon the shelter staff and/or upon its nurse.

The Packaged Disaster Hospital

These hospitals are units stored at various sites throughout the country. They contain sufficient supplies to set up an emergency disaster hospital and keep it in operation for 30 days. There is an admitting and sorting area (triage), operating rooms, wards, an x-ray, a laboratory, a pharmacy and a central supply. In addition, each hospital has its own generators, water pump and storage tank. The hospitals belong to the Federal government and are loaned to various states for use primarily in nuclear emergency. Community medical-health and government leaders are responsible for the storage of the hospital unit, and unless otherwise arranged, are also responsible for preparing for its use.

Packaged Disaster Hospitals are used in major emergencies to augment existing hospital facilities or to establish independent hospital facilities. It is planned that in the case of a nuclear catastrophe, these units will be in the forefront when the stage of post-shelter rehabilitation is begun. There is no way to predict the conditions under which this type of hospital will be used. However, any dis-aster of the magnitude requiring its activation is bound to make severe demands on the staff. Hours will be long, staff and supplies short. The basic objective of an emergency unit of this type is to assist in meeting the health needs of the surviving population. The actual situation may vary from *early activation* with a large number of traumatic injury casualties to *delayed activation* with less injuries but more illness. These units must conserve their resources and so casualties will undergo triage by a physician who will establish priorities for patient care and the possible methods of treatment.

While each packaged unit has its own basic supplies, the continued use as well as the general functioning of the unit, depends on services originating in the community. These would include such things as ambulance and transportation services, communication facilities, decontamination capabilities, refuse and body waste disposal, mortuary services, and food and laundry facilities. The organization and activation of these units depend on full cooperation and coordination with other hospitals and community services within the area.

Additional Support Facilities

In the immediate post-disaster period, nurses will also be needed in a variety of other places. One of these is the Field Aid Points which are simple fixed or temporary facilities where the sick and injured are taken to receive initial treatment. They serve as a collecting area where patients can be held until transportation to a Principal First Aid Station or hospital can be provided. It is in these reception areas (and also in the Principal First Aid Stations) that the majority of pregnant women and infants will be cared for if there is time for evacuation. These areas may be located anywhere that is commensurate with existing conditions: homes, stores, or even street corners. The Principal First Aid Stations also may be fixed or temporary, but treatment is administered under the direction of professional doctors, nurses, and allied personnel. These stations are usually located in shelter areas, schools, churches and other substantial buildings if they are available. These units will administer to the surviving population as well as the immediate casualties.

Mass Care Centers are planned for refugees who are homeless or unable to return to their residence. Workers who are engaged in rehabilitation activities will also be allowed to share these facilities. Recuperation centers will be located on college campuses, motels or homes where simple convalescent bed and ambulatory care can be readily available without requiring the services of a full-time nursing staff. Thus, in all disasters, nurses find themselves with a dual responsibility of citizen and skilled professional. We must not only be prepared to contribute to the community's disaster preparedness but we must also enhance our own survival chances through knowledge and preparedness.

DISASTER INSURANCE FOR MOTHERS AND BABIES[2]

Insuring the lives and health of pregnant women and their newborns during national or extensive local disasters requires planning for this purpose predicated on the belief that plans and preparations prior to these events are essential and imperative.

As previously stated, protection from radioactive fallout must be provided and evacuation from expected target areas will be 20 to 50 miles distant, and some kind of care for women in labor must be provided en route. Large-scale plans are under way for evacuees to be cared for in reception areas—including pregnant women and newborn infants. As the national defenses are strengthened and increased, there is logical expectation that there may be prior warning of an attack and time to put into effect large-scale evacuation of priority groups, such as pregnant women, to predesignated reception areas. However, evacuation is cumbersome, time-consuming and requires several hours' advance warning. Provision must also be made for protection in shelters, pits, etc., to care for those who cannot be evacuated.

Although early planning for the protection of the civilian population recognized the need for pacts of mutual assistance mostly with state coordination, disaster planning now includes nationwide and continental participation. The concept is still valid that official state and community agencies, in cooperation with civil defense planners, medical and welfare, assume the major responsibility, not only for planning prior to disasters, but for the administration and operation of emergency services for expectant mothers and infants through local and regional health units.

In planning for the safeguarding of mothers and newborn infants prior to a disaster, certain

assumptions can be made and specific factors considered:

Pregnant women will be subject to all of the risks and injuries to which men and nonpregnant women will be exposed. Their general care should be in accordance with provisions made for the population at large. However, their obstetric care does require additional planning and facilities, for it should be separate from hospital and emergency facilities for casualties. Two lives are at stake, lives of particular import to the future of the country. The need for care of the pregnant woman is predictable, since sooner or later she must inevitably be delivered, and in the process will need medical attention to a greater or lesser extent. In the vast majority of instances, probably in 90 per cent of all cases, the birth process, whether it results in a viable infant or abortion, will be essentially uncomplicated. The most formidable complications to be encountered with any frequency will be hemorrhage, obstructed or prolonged labor, infection, mild and severe toxemias of pregnancy with convulsions and miscellaneous medical and surgical conditions accompanying pregnancy.

It is estimated that at any given time approximately 2 per cent of the total population will consist of women in various stages of pregnancy. In applying this prevalence rate to a given geographic area, allowance must be made for the character of the area, since the rate will, of course, be affected by the presence of large industrial plants and offices employing large numbers of males.

On the basis of the Hiroshima experience with the A-bomb, it can be anticipated that approximately one quarter of all surviving pregnant women on the periphery of the nuclear explosion will abort or deliver shortly thereafter. Furthermore, approximately 10 per cent of pregnant women within range of the effects of a nuclear explosion will have abortions or premature deliveries.

It is possible, therefore, that in the affected blast area there may be as many as 500 to 700 deliveries or abortions per 100,000 population shortly after an explosion. In areas more remote from the explosion the number of deliveries or abortions will more nearly approximate that occurring during normal times.

If the foregoing concepts are accepted and remain valid in disaster planning, what then should be the planning for minimal essential care for mothers and newborn infants in disaster situations? To the extent that it is possible, the facilities which are normally available for pregnant

---

2 Reprinted from Fetter, S. E., Whitridge, J., Jr., and Welch, J.: *The Bulletin of Material Welfare*, 49:9, 1957 with additions by the authors.

women during the antepartal, delivery and post-partal periods should be available.

However, as we have seen in the case of a thermonuclear disaster, at least, these facilities will not be functioning. Therefore adequate preparation for the care of mother and babies during a disaster, particularly a large scale one, requires that thought be given and plans made for the training of families for their own protection and survival. This is especially true for the pregnant family. As we have stressed before, a large percentage of the population ought to be trained to carry out minimal essentials of care (buddy system) to save the lives of other people.

As we have said, it can be assumed that in any major disaster, physicians, nurses and other specially trained professional personnel will be almost completely absorbed in the task of caring for casualties; normal women in labor at such times will have to rely largely on nonprofessional personnel for their needs. Just who will these nonprofessional people be? They will have to be other women who have received instruction in the procedures described. In other words, each community must contain a corps of lay women who understand the basic concepts contained in this brief review and have been given at least minimal training in providing this type of care. Preparation for civil defense is a family affair. Every citizen and every family needs to have the information necessary to protect himself, his family and his community well in advance of a disaster or an enemy attack. Those responsible for planning and implementing disaster plans have the unique responsibility for making this information available to individuals in communities in a way which they can understand and accept.

The only hope we have for the saving of lives of mothers and newborn infants depends on the family's ability to carry out the plans made with and for them.

Every expectant mother needs to know her physician's expectation of the kind of delivery she will have, so that if she needs any special facilities, she will be able to go where these are available. She needs to understand the care she and her baby will need during delivery and immediately afterward.

There are differences of opinion about how much information pregnant women should have about their own condition and the conduct and the outcome of the delivery. It is assumed that in the event of large-scale disasters, women will have to carry much of the responsibility for their own safety. Therefore, adequate information about what to do, where to go and what constitutes essential equipment will be comforting to them rather than alarming.

Essential equipment is quite minimal and is available to almost every woman in her own home. A package should be made up and kept accessible with other emergency supplies. Contents include a clean sheet, towels, washcloth and soap; blankets, clothing, a nipple and a bottle for the baby; a pair of blunt scissors; 2 pieces of clean linen tape, 6 inches long and ¼ inch wide, wrapped separately from the other articles, and a package of powdered milk for the mother. A can of powdered infant formula is also good insurance in the event that the establishment of lactation is delayed.

Those who are giving care to pregnant women need to understand that the pregnant woman's normal dependent needs may be greatly enhanced by separation from and concern for her husband and family and by increased fear for herself and her baby. Understanding in meeting this exaggerated need for mothering and providing a warm accepting environment will increase the confidence of the pregnant woman in her ability to have her baby and will comfort her and relieve some of her fear and apprehension. Every effort should be made to have someone with the patient throughout labor. The emotional support which patients in labor (who have had some preparation) derive from each other should be utilized.

There are certain preparations for impending labor and/or abortion that can be made in the immediate period of evacuation. As quickly as possible after a shelter, Field Aid Point or First Aid Station is occupied, all pregnant women should be registered and the expected date of birth recorded. As we stated previously, the nurse may be the only health professional on the scene; in that event she may want to delegate this activity to someone who appears able to carry through this activity *accurately*. The pregnant women, who will be of special concern are (1) those who are in labor or expecting at any time, (2) those who are expecting within a week or two, and (3) those who have had difficulty with previous confinements and/or who have reason to expect difficulty by reason of disease or abnormalities. *They should be appraised of these facts by their physician.*

The nurse should assign someone to assist the laboring mother. In all probability, the nurse will be too occupied with other activities to assist herself if she is the only health professional. The attendant is to be informed of the expected date of birth and any information which the mother may have learned during her prenatal care. In addition, the nurse will need to instruct the attendant in the course of labor and the activities necessary at the time of birth. A delivery area can be selected away from the general living or gathering area if space permits. It should be prepared with respect to quiet, warmth (or coolness), cleanliness, available supplies and equipment. The mother will need a clean surface to lie on for the actual delivery. Clean plastic material and/or paper can be used for padding the actual delivery bed. The mother will need clean towels or a clean garment or sheet. A warmer covering such as a sweater, jacket or blanket is also desirable. Hopefully, she will have brought these articles for the baby with her. The infant's crib can be improvised from a carton and lined with any suitable material (paper or a blanket) available. It goes without saying that the mother's confidence may be temporarily shattered; her courage may not be, however. If the nurse can convey that while conditions may be very austere, labor and delivery can progress normally, she will do much toward helping the mother mobilize her resources to proceed through labor. The nurse will instruct the mother or attendant to report the first evidence of the onset of labor. This will usually give enough time to make the immediate preparations for delivery.

Essentials of care during the first stage of labor include the maintenance of physical and emotional reserves, the interpretation of the progress of labor to the patient and the family, the provision of rest and fluids, the maintenance of cleanliness and preparation for the second stage of labor, including frequent emptying of the bladder.

There should be constant review of progress and observation of signs of complications. As the patient approaches the completion of the first stage of labor, she will need special care and encouragement and should not be left alone.

During the second stage of labor, constant observation, encouragement and interpretation are all-important. A clean delivery area should be maintained, and there should be continual observation of the patient's general condition for signs of exhaustion and other complications. The maternal pulse rate and the quality should be observed.

A progress report to the supervising physician or nurse should be made by the person giving the care. In the absence of the physician during the delivery, the nurse, the nurse-midwife or the attendant who is helping the patient can teach her

that when the baby's head is in sight to take a deep breath at the beginning of each contraction, to hold her breath and exert downward pressure, while the infant's head is controlled. As soon as the contraction is over, the patient should be encouraged to relax completely and wait for the next contraction.

Supportive care is especially important. The back can be rubbed for low back pain and the legs stretched for muscle cramps. The explanation of the progress of labor often provides the encouragement which the patient needs to complete the second stage of labor with minimal emotional stress.

When the head crowns, the perineum should be supported and protected with a clean towel if a sterile towel is not available. If there is no clean material for this purpose, it is important that the attendant be instructed *not to touch the birth canal or surrounding area of the perineum. Moreover the mother must be instructed to keep her hands away from these areas also.* If clean material is available and the *attendant has had some professional training,* then gentle pressure can be applied against the head as it emerges to prevent too rapid delivery of the head. If the attendant is not skilled and/or seems to be rather overwhelmed by events, it is wiser to allow the infant's head to deliver spontaneously and simply support it as it is born.

Immediate removal of the membranes from around the baby's head is important. If the umbilical cord is around the neck, it is slipped over the head whenever it can be done easily. The mucus should be wiped from the baby's mouth and nose. Occasionally, spontaneous rotation of the head to one side or the other will not take place within a reasonable period of time. Under such circumstances, gentle rotation of the head in the direction toward which it tends to go more easily will suffice to bring one shoulder anteriorly behind the symphysis.

If the nurse is delivering the infant, she can next deliver the anterior shoulder by gently grasping the head in both hands, and exerting gentle but steady pressure toward the floor. With this maneuver, the anterior shoulder slips under the symphysis pubis, and the upper portion of the arm can be seen. Then the direction of traction is reversed upward in order to deliver the posterior shoulder over the perineum. These maneuvers are to be carried out *slowly and carefully;* there is no need to hurry.

The baby's body is supported as it is born and is wrapped in a warm sterile towel or clean cloth and placed on the mother's abdomen with the head lower so that the mucus will drain out. Pulling on the cord should be avoided. The mother will want to know about the baby and see it as soon as it is born. If the baby does not cry immediately, or if there is mucus, the nose and the mouth should be cleared and postural drainage instituted. Gentle rubbing of the back helps to stimulate the baby's breathing. When the cord stops pulsating, it is tied in two places and cut between the two ties. After the cord is cut, the baby is warmly wrapped and placed in the mother's arms.

During the delivery of the baby and the beginning of the third stage of labor there should be constant observation of the mother's general condition and of signs indicating the separation of the placenta. If the attendant assisting with the delivery places her hand on the mother's fundus, she can report the changes to the person conducting the delivery. When the uterus rises upward in the abdomen and becomes globular and firm, and the umbilical cord extends 3 or 4 inches out of the vagina and there is a gush of blood, the patient can be asked to bear down with the next contraction. This pressure is usually sufficient to expel the placenta, which is received in a clean receptacle. In order to express the placenta, it may be necessary occasionally to apply gentle pressure on the fundus of the uterus when it is well contracted. The direction of pressure should be toward the vaginal outlet. Following the expulsion of the placenta, if the uterus tends to become soft, and bleeding occurs, the uterus should be massaged vigorously with the fingertips to promote uterine contraction, and the baby put to the breast.

The placenta and membranes should be examined to determine whether there are any missing portions.

If the uterus remains small and firm, nothing should be done other than to keep the hand on the fundus for 1 hour following the delivery of the baby. The patient should be made comfortable, given nourishment, encouraged to void and allowed to rest.

The attendant should rewash his hands before beginning care of the infant. When it is apparent that the mother can be left safely, the baby is to be identified according to the method established by the particular health department. If the usual identification tapes or bands are not available then some method is to be improvised. The infant need not be washed for 24 hours, and can wait even longer if water is in short supply. The vernix caseosa may seem unpleasant but will protect the infant much more than unclean "cleansing" materials. Baby oil can be used as a substitute for water and mild soap after 24 hours. The cord stump is to be kept clean and if at all possible, a sterile dressing is to be applied and left in place until the cord dries. The infant is to be examined for injuries and malformations.

Essentials of nursing care for the baby include gentle handling, observation of breathing, color, appearance, activity, skin and body temperature, stools, weight (if possible), and umbilical cord for bleeding and healing; provision should be made for warmth, proper food and protection from infection.

Mother and newborn baby should be considered an inseparable unit. If a mother cannot take care of her baby, full-time mothering care must be provided to enhance the baby's chances of survival and promote his well-being. Irregularities in breathing, mucus in air passages, weak sucking reflex, skin irritation and unstable temperature-regulating mechanism point to the importance of constant observation and an environment adapted to meet the needs of the individual infant.

Breast-feeding is preferable but should not be attempted at the mother's expense. The infant may be put to breast immediately after birth and at 4 to 8 hour intervals for 3 to 5 minute periods until the milk supply is established. If this regime tires the mother the intervals between nursing periods can be lengthened. Once the milk supply is sufficient to satisfy the baby, feedings can be given as often as necessary to meet his need. Artificial feedings may be necessary until the mother's milk supply is adequate or in instances in which the mother is unable to nurse. Formula may be prepared from powdered infant formula or dried skim milk immediately prior to feeding since there will be no refrigeration facilities. Diluted canned evaporated milk is also a suitable formula. (One part milk to two parts water, boiled if possible.) If a bottle and nipple are unavailable, the baby can suck on a teaspoon placed on his lower lip, or milk can be dropped on the inside of the cheek with a medicine dropper. The formula does not have to be heated. Disposable diapers are preferred, but sheets substitute nicely. Of course, any absorbent material can be used if these are not available.

The newborn is particularly susceptible to infection. Anyone with any evidence of infection, such as rash, diarrhea or upper respiratory infection, should not give infant care.

When the infant is found to be premature and in need of special care, or to have congenital malformations, the emergency facilities which have been developed for such conditions should be utilized.

When the mother and infant are to be discharged from the place where care has been given during labor and delivery, it is essential for arrangements to be made with the family and others for the mother to be relieved of responsibilities except the care of her baby and herself. The mother, the family and the attendant should know where and whom to call if she or the baby have any conditions or symptoms needing medical care.

To increase the number of people with some training in the care of pregnant women and newborn infants, the existing educational programs need to be expanded. These include mother and baby care classes, such as those given by the Red Cross and other health agencies, parent education groups, home nursing classes, first-aid training, classes for baby sitters and junior and senior high school students and the midwifery training programs. Planning for training and the achievement of the training of persons who carry this responsibility in a disaster are not easy.

During a disaster, it is assumed that it will be the responsibility of nurses, certified nurse-midwives and licensed nonprofessional midwives to carry on an intensive program of on-the-job training of whoever is available to help and to supervise the care of mothers and babies.

PSYCHOLOGICAL REACTIONS IN EMERGENCY SITUATIONS

It has been found that human behavior in disaster, like human behavior in other life situations falls into fairly predictable patterns.[3] Since the nurse's role is so vital in the event of disaster, she will need to prepare herself with knowledge of these reactions, since coping with large numbers of persons suffering massive emotional shock will become every bit as important as rendering help for physical traumas and illness. Moreover, it will help the nurse to understand better her own responses to the catastrophe.

---

[3] The following discussion is adapted from the psychology of disaster. Nurs. Clin. N. Am. 2:349-358, June, 1967.

Periods of a Disaster

For purposes of our analysis disaster can be said to have various periods. These may include a prodromal or warning period, an impact period, immediate reaction period, and finally, a delayed response period. During these segments there are characteristic modes of behavior that people may exhibit.

In the **prodromal or warning period** certain persons tend to demonstrate disorganized and/or destructive behavior. They mill around, disobey instructions, break things or lash out at anyone getting in their way. Some others, however, are able to function in the face of even grave personal danger incredibly effectively; still others become immobilized and for all practical purposes, helpless.

Some of the above individuals may respond to the warning signals as if the catastrophe had already occurred and demonstrate a penchant for ineffective action. These persons fall into two general groups. The first are those who have been through a similar experience before in which they were helpless and have developed a subsequent fear and/or helpless response to disaster or its warnings. The second group comprises those who always become helpless in any dangerous or frightening situation. These persons often present a difficult problem for helping personnel since, if left to themselves, these people often precipitate wild panic in others because of their own panicky behavior. They need to be taken aside and given definite tasks to do, no matter how simple. Clear, brief instructions and frequent reassurance help these people to regain control of their emotions.

At the **impact period,** almost everyone will experience many frightening feelings, no matter how adequate their training or drilling; thus, there will be at least some period of confusion. This is especially true in the case of an emergency in which there is no warning, such as a dam breaking, a sudden explosion or an electrical storm. Many respond with physical signs and symptoms. They may exhibit shortness of breath, rapid pulse and respiration, trembling, sweating and so on. Adequate anticipatory training and drilling has been found to shorten the period of this uncontrolled activity, thus reducing the confusion period.

The **immediate reaction period** after impact is most crucial. Non-effective behavior at this point exacts a heavy toll in terms of the life and well-being of the survivors. On the other hand, effective action will save lives, diminish disability, reduce abnormal behavior, and decrease the confusion immeasurably. It is imperative that normal behavior be resumed as quickly as possible, not only for each individual's personal safety but also to assure help for those unable to act because of an injury.

Immediately following impact, especially in a disaster of any magnitude, almost all persons will be unable to think, move or express concern, although given a reasonable length of time, most will make a tremendous effort to adjust. Some will manage this more quickly than others, and they will have to help their slower brethren in their adjustments. Help usually will be available from the relatively uninjured since professionals are often not available as we have stressed. Thus, it is wise for the less able to team with those who appear more able—the buddy system is more effective and often invaluable.

The **delayed response period** begins when the immediate danger has passed. Groups often unite for mutual protection and it is at this period that the less acutely affected psychological casualties can be salvaged. It is important to remember that minimal attention may be all that is needed, but it *must be given* and *given early* in this period. Those afflicted are often highly suggestable, and will follow almost any advice or take cues for action from the behavior of others. This can be a double-edged sword, for while they respond well to instructions and reassurance, they also tend to become infected easily with anxiety and panic, and will, in turn, precipitate panic reactions in others if not carefully watched. It is important at this time for all to realize that the menace has passed; thus, verbal reinforcement and reiteration is important. Valuable information also can be conveyed by signs and facial expressions to aid individuals in achieving some measure of security.

We have spoken of the different periods in a disaster and of some of the general behavior that might be exhibited. It would be well at this point to expand on the various types of behavior that can be demonstrated in response to danger or threat in general.

Under the heading of "normal reactions" comes apparent calmness, at least for a time. More usually seen, however, are the physical or bodily manifestations such as sweating, trembling, weakness or rapid pulse. Included here also are nausea, vomiting and diarrhea of a temporary nature. Confusion, crying and immobilization of a short duration are not uncommon and can still be classified as "normal." The ability and the length of time required to collect oneself with or without help seem to be the most likely criteria for classification in the "normal" category.

When the above reactions become prolonged and/or incapacitating, the individual condition is thought of as more serious. "Conversion hysteria" can occur in which the person unconsciously converts his massive fear into a belief that some part of his body has ceased to function. And in fact, the organ does not function in spite of the fact that no organic damage can be demonstrated. These people cannot be treated as malingerers or "fakers." Since the disability is at the level of the unconscious, the person is as truly disabled as if he had had physical injury to the limb or organ. Nausea and vomiting arising from emotional origins are also seen in prolonged and incapacitating cases. Difficulty arises in diagnosis since these symptoms are indicative of radiation sickness also. Moreover, the person may interpret his symptoms as due to radiation exposure. Problems of isolation and decontamination multiply. These cases tax both the diagnostic astuteness and the emotional reserve of those dealing with them.

Somewhere between the normal reactions and the gross abnormal reactions fall panic, and depressed and overactive responses. Panic is not expressed as frequently as one might expect, but its danger lies in its contagiousness. It can spread and cause a mass headlong flight of a crowd. Driven by a compulsion to flee, persons in the grip of this phenomenon often crush and trample one another. Purposeless uncontrolled motor behavior is indicative of a panic stage; it is evidenced by such behavior as uncontrolled weeping and running around. Sheer horror (the sight of family maimed) or the belief that avenues of escape are being blocked are the two most frequent precipitating conditions. Helping to move individuals and a crowd away from the presenting danger *in an orderly fashion* is the best preventative for this phenomenon.

Depressed reactions are characterized by a general slowing down of motor and mental processes. Persons sit and stare; they seem numbed and confused. They do not respond when spoken to or if they do, it is with monosyllables. These individuals cannot initiate action even to escape threat. Fortunately they can be salvaged if help can be given to get them moving before too long a period. Other victims respond with a flurry of overactive responses. They will chatter ceaselessly about inappropriate topics, they run back and forth and are avid rumor spreaders. If given a task, they are soon off doing something else, although to their minds, they have completed it to perfection. An unreal confidence in their abilities is their hallmark. This causes them to assume more responsibility than they can possibly discharge and to become very intolerant of other's ideas or plans. They are especially troublesome to those who are demonstrating effective leadership.

It is not possible to present a blueprint for dealing with these situations and behavior. There are some principles of behavior, however, that the nurse can utilize and which can be conveyed easily to those who will help her. First of all, she should try to accept *each person's right to his own feelings.* A quick appraisal of one's own feelings at this time makes one realize how difficult it is to make a conscious choice of their deeper feelings. An ability to make a conscious choice depends upon what we do about our feelings to relieve the tensions they create within us. Nothing is gained by trying to deny the existence of the distressed feelings in ourselves or others, simply because they appear different from what we would ordinarily expect or experience in everyday life. If we can help someone to take appropriate action, the distressed feelings may change, either quickly or gradually. Each person brings to the disaster a varied experiential background which contributes greatly to his coping with the effects of the disaster. Letting a person know that you understand *how he feels at the moment* will be the first step toward helping him. As with any patient, pity will overwhelm him; if the nurse can convey by gesture or short conversation that she is trying to see the events through his eyes, she will be helping him to find constructive outlets for his feelings and thereby aid him to rehabilitation.

A second principle involves *accepting a person's limitations.* If a person is obviously physically shattered, one does not expect him to carry on as usual. Yet, when the nurse finds herself tired, frustrated and trying to maintain her own emotional equilibrium, she is apt to resent enormously the vague "unseen" disabilities of others. This is, perhaps an understatement, for the feeling of irritability will be enhanced because others will seem to have "pulled themselves together" considering the circumstances. Again these patients, for they are patients, need understanding and patience—not resentment—because they too are laboring under a great load.

A third principle involves the *ability to assess accurately and quickly the capabilities of others.* A very upset person can easily cause the nurse to forget that he can be of real assistance; therefore it is wise to be on the lookout for skills and other assets that might be revived and utilized. The nurse can begin to help the patient reorganize his world by inquiring into what has happened to him and letting him reply in his own way. Allowing him to talk of his experiences (without letting him ramble on and/or become more upset) will greatly relieve some of his feelings of despair and helplessness. The nurse can explore briefly his concern about his family and friends, giving him an honest estimate regarding the possibility of his re-establishing contact with his dear ones. If he is too depressed to talk freely, she can talk to him about what may have happened to him and to them. This may increase his confidence in the nurse to the point where he can make conversation. Brief questions regarding his occupation will give clues to his interests and basic capabilities. The nurse can then draw conclusions as to how he can best be utilized. While this may sound exploitive, keeping someone gainfully occupied is a genuine therapeutic coup. Treating someone as a potentially valued member of the disaster team will increase his effectiveness immeasurably.

Finally, the last but perhaps the most important principle: try to *accept your own limitations in the relief role.* We have stressed the responsibility of the nurse's role to herself and others, perhaps to the detriment of the real limitations in herself that the nurse will encounter. There will be much that the nurse will want to do in a disaster; some things, however, will be beyond her strength and skill. Thus, the nurse will need to establish a set of priorities, not only with respect to what she must do for patient care but what she must undertake in the realm of responsibility generally. The first priority is to whatever emergency job that she has been assigned (or has volunteered for). In practice this job may well be more than full-time; therefore the nurse must select those activities which will be worth trying and those which would be a waste of time. While she will be pushing herself to the limits of her capacity, it is imperative that she not extend herself beyond those limits lest she become as ill as those whom she treats. If pushing herself beyond endurance is a personality characteristic, then it is wise that she acknowledge it early and pace herself accordingly. A reasonable candid self-appraisal is an important prerequisite for anyone attempting psychological first aid! If one is to deal effectively with others, then one's own concerns must be dealt with *first and promptly.* If they are, the nurse will be less likely to become bogged down when she is trying to aid others. No matter how thorough the nurse's training has been, it is important that she recognize that she will not be immune to all personal disturbance if her community is torn apart by a terrible tragedy. Her first psychological job then is to look to her own defense. If she understands herself reasonably well, she may justifiably hope to endure and control her own anxieties in the midst of a community-wide disaster and render excellent assistance to those who need her.

SUGGESTED READING

Aranow, S., et al.: The Fallen Sky, Medical Consequences of Thermonuclear War. New York, Hill and Wang, 1963.

Blakely, J.: The Care of Radiation Casualties. London, William Heinemann Medical Books, 1968.

Brown, R. K.: Disaster medicine. What is it? Can it be taught? J.A.M.A. 197:1081-1984, January 26, 1966.

Eicherly, E. E.: Nursing in thermonuclear disaster. Nurs. Clin. N. Am. 2:325-335, June, 1967.

Emergency health programs. J. S. Carolina Med. Assoc. 65:23-24, January, 1969.

Green, J. M.: Emergency care of the obstetric patient. Nurs. Outlook 6:694, 1958.

King, E. R.: Survival in Nuclear Warfare. Clinica Symposia (CIBA pamphlet) Vol. 14, No. 1, January-March, 1962.

Maryland State Department of Health, Division Public Health Nursing: Suggested Content for the Training Program in Civil Defense Nursing, Parts III and IV, Maryland State Department of Health, January, 1952.

Melber, R.: The nurse's role in obstetrical emergencies in the hospital setting. Nurs. Clin. N. Am. 2:261-269, June, 1967.

Psychology of disaster. Nurs. Clin. N. Am. 2:349-358, June, 1967.

Rayner, J. F.: How do nurses behave in disaster? Nurs. Outlook 6:572, 1958.

U.S. Department of Health, Education, and Welfare, Public Health Service, Division of Health Mobilization, Medical Care in Shelters. December, 1963.

Work Conference on Disaster Nursing: Text of addresses, Norfolk, Va., November 12-16, 1956.

History of Obstetrics* 26

Obstetrics Among Primitive Peoples • Egyptian Obstetrics • Oriental Obstetrics
Grecian Obstetrics • Byzantine, Mohammedan, Jewish and Medieval Periods
The Renaissance Period • The Seventeenth Century
The Eighteenth Century • The Nineteenth and Twentieth Centuries
Background and Development of Maternal and Infant Care in the United States
The Emergence and Development of the Maternity Nursing in the United States

In the course of one chapter it is impossible to give a detailed history of obstetrics. This account does not purport to be a complete survey of the progress of obstetrics through the ages but merely a skeletal outline on which the interested may place significant facts by additional reading. Sufficient references will be given to enable the student to obtain more complete information.

For greater simplicity and more ready understanding, the ages of obstetrics have been divided arbitrarily as set forth at the beginning of this chapter.

OBSTETRICS AMONG PRIMITIVE PEOPLES

We know little about obstetrics among the primitive races, but from careful study of the customs of the aboriginal American Indians and the African Negroes we are able to learn some of the customs which were part of the obstetric practice of the ancients. Childbirth in primitive times was a relatively simple process. The mother retired to a place apart from the tribe and there gave birth to her child without great difficulty. It is known that intertribal marriages were relatively rare; therefore, there was not the conglomeration of mingled races which exists today. A realization of this fact alone makes possible an understanding of the relative simplicity of childbirth under these circumstances. The fetal head and body were accommodated satis-

factorily within the anatomic range of the maternal pelvis. The lack of mixed marriages prevented the resultant disproportion between passenger and pelvic passages. It became customary for women who had attended other women in labor to be asked to assist or accompany more of them, and they became the primitive counterpart of our latter-day midwife. The only real danger a primitive mother faced was that of abnormal presentation, which usually terminated fatally for both mother and child. Toxemias and other complications are largely the products of more advanced civilization and were rarely if ever met among primitive peoples.

EGYPTIAN OBSTETRICS

In Egypt a highly organized state of society existed, and with it there arose a more complicated, if not more advanced, type of obstetrics. The priesthood in Egypt was interested in all the activities of society, and obstetrics was not neglected. They had a supervisory interest in it and took an active part in the care of abnormal or operative cases. They are known to have had obstetric forceps, to have performed cesarean sections on dead mothers, and podalic version was a part of their art.

ORIENTAL OBSTETRICS

Hindu medicine was probably the first authentic system of medicine to be given to the world. Among the earliest Hindus of whom there is written record was **Susrata**, one of the most prolific of

---

* By Douglas E. Cannell, M.B., B.Sc. (Med.), F.R.C.S. (C), Toronto, Canada.

Hindu writers. The exact date of his existence is still a matter of dispute, but he is variously stated to have worked and written between 600 B.C. and A.D. 500, more probably about the latter date. His knowledge of menstruation and gestation was quite modern. He knew and described intelligently the management of normal and abnormal labor. He described the use of forceps and cesarean section upon dead mothers to remove living children, and gave excellent prenatal and postpartal advice. He advised cleanliness on the part of the obstetrician; cutting the beard, the hair and the nails closely; the wearing of clean gowns; and thorough disinfection of the operating rooms prior to operation or delivery. His surgical antiseptic technique seems remarkable to modern students.

Chinese obstetrics was largely of a legendary nature until the publication of a Chinese household manual of obstetrics, *Ta Sheng P'Ien,* which, according to the author's own statement, "is correct and needs no change or addition of prescription." There were monographs on obstetrics prior to this, but none so complete. Many of his statements are unfounded; in fact, the knowledge is scanty or incorrect, but the author had the saving grace of objecting to unnecessary interference and counseled patience in the treatment of labor. He had a poor opinion of midwives in general, stating that "the majority of them are fools." The reviews of Chinese obstetrics and obstetric drugs by Maxwell are excellent and give a detailed account of an interesting phase of obstetrics, which for lack of space we are forced to dispense with in this account.

GRECIAN OBSTETRICS

Prior to Hippocrates, the Asclepiads, or followers of Aesculapius, the Father of Medicine, had a slight and largely supervisory interest in obstetrics. Abortions were not illegal. There is little definite knowledge concerning this period, but it seems probable that obstetric treatment was of a primitive nature.

The Hippocratic Period. During this age normal obstetric cases were handled by midwives under the supervision of the physicians. Abnormal labor was entirely in the hands of the medical profession. To Hippocrates is accredited the Hippocratic oath, which is still a part of the exercises for all students graduating from medical school. Treatises upon obstetrics attributed to Hippocrates are the oldest records available of the Western World's obstetric methods.

Greco-Roman Obstetrics. This period was one of progress, which was due largely to the work of Celsus, Aëtius and Soranus (second century). The last reintroduced podalic version and is responsible for the first authentic records of its use in the delivery of living children. He gave an excellent technical description of the procedure and the indications for its use.

BYZANTINE, MOHAMMEDAN, JEWISH AND MEDIEVAL PERIODS

These may be said to have been characterized by a complete absence of progress, and as a corollary, a retrogression and loss of previously known practice resulted. This was due in large part to the general failure of science in the medieval period, but the interference of the Roman Church in secular matters, particularly those of a scientific nature, must be held responsible for a large share of it. The paucity of operative treatment in difficult labor may be judged from the recommendations contained in the only textbook of the day on obstetrics and gynecology, which read as follows: "Place the patient in a sheet held at the corners by four strong men, with her head somewhat elevated. Have them shake the sheet vigorously by pulling on the opposite corners, and with God's aid she will give birth." However, hospitals and nursing services were organized in this age.

Although the ancient Jews gave very little assistance to the woman during labor and delivery, they were interested in the hygiene of pregnancy and cleanliness at the time of childbirth. Hygiene and sanitation were apparently a part of their religion. At the time of difficult deliveries, the women "were comforted until they died." The stool or obstetric chair was used at this time and continued to be used until about the 19th century A.D. Reference is made to this chair in the Bible, in the first chapter of Exodus, "when you do the office of the midwife to the Hebrew women, and see them upon the stools. . . ."

THE RENAISSANCE PERIOD

The Renaissance was characterized by advances in medicine and obstetrics commensurate with those in other fields. During this time appeared the first English text on obstetrics, the *Byrthe of Mankynde,* published by Raynalde. Both it and its German counterpart by Roesslin are copies of Soranus, and with their publication podalic version was reintroduced to obstetric practice. Many famous men were responsible for the progress in obstetrics—among them Leonardo da Vinci (who made the first accurate sketches of the fetus in utero) and Vesalius (who accurately described the pelvis for the first time).

To Ambrose Paré, the dean of French surgeons and obstetricians, must go the chief credit for making podalic version a useful and practicable procedure. Due to his skill, he preferred its use to cesarean section in difficult labor. By his careful studies of its indications and technique, he made possible the removal of obstetrics from the hands of the midwives, where it had rested since the fall of the Roman Empire, and its establishment as an independent branch of medicine. Regulations were enacted for the practice of midwives, and schools were established during this period for their training. Paré's work on version and his discouragement of cesarean section were opportune.

Sections had been practiced since antiquity upon dead mothers, but the first authentic section performed upon a living mother is credited to Trautman, of Wittenberg, in 1610. This was done upon a woman with a large ventral hernia which contained the uterus. Prior to this, Nufer, a sow gelder, is reputed to have performed the operation on his wife, after obstetricians and midwives had failed to deliver her. It has been stated that Jane Seymour was delivered by a section done by Frère, a noted surgeon of the time, at the request of Henry VIII. That she died a few days after the birth of Edward VI adds credence to the story, but no absolute confirmation is available. Due to the frightful mortality from hemorrhage, sepsis, etc., it did not become popular in spite of the advocacy of the Church. Through the following centuries it was done occasionally, but not until the advent of uterine sutures and aseptic technique did it become a practical procedure.

The origin of its name has been ascribed to Julius Caesar, but, as his mother lived many years after his birth, this seems improbable—considering the high mortality of all abdominal operations before the time of Lister. A more accurate explanation is that Numa Pompilius, one of the earlier Roman kings, passed a law making it compulsory to perform the operation upon all mothers who died while pregnant in order that the mother and the child might be buried separately. This was known as the "Lex Regis" and with the advent of the Caesars as the "Lex Caesaris"—and subsequently "cesarean section." The name has been attributed to *cedere,* the Latin verb meaning to cut, but the former explanation seems to be more reasonable.

THE SEVENTEENTH CENTURY

This century was notable for many famous obstetricians. Mauriceau, of Paris, was the first to correct the view that the pelvic bones separated in normal labor. He was also the first man to refer to epidemic puerperal fever. His description of an obstetrician, or rather of the qualities an obstetrician should possess, is both interesting and amusing. He stated:

He must be healthful, strong and robust; because this is the most laborious of all the Operations of Chirurgery; for it will make one sometimes sweat, so he shall not have a dry Thread, tho' it were the coldest Day in Winter. . . . He ought to be well shaped, at least to outward appearance, but above all, to have small hands for the easier Introduction of them into the Womb when necessary; yet strong, with the Fingers long, especially the Fore-finger, the better to reach and touch the inner orifice. He must have no Rings on his Fingers, and his Nails well pared, when he goeth about the Work, for fear of hurting the Womb. He ought to have a pleasant Countenance, and to be as neat in his Clothes as in his person, that the poor women who have need of him be not affrighted at him. Some are of the opinion, that a Practitioner of this Art ought on the contrary to be slovenly, at least very careless, wearing a great Beard, to prevent the Occasion of the Husband's Jealousy that sends for him. Truly some believe this Policy augments their Practice but 'tis fit they should be disabused; for such a Posture and Dress resembles more a Butcher than a Chirurgeon, whom the woman apprehends already too much, that he needs not such a Disguise. Above all he must be sober, no Tipler, that he may at all times have his Wits about him. . .

Van Deventer, of Holland, has been called the Father of Modern Obstetrics and is credited with the first accurate description of the pelvis, its deformities and their effect on parturition. He also shares with Ould, of Dublin, the first description of the mechanism of labor. As time passed, customs changed, and the term "accoucheur" replaced the objectionable "midman" and "man-midwife." Obstetric forceps were invented, probably about 1580, by Peter Chamberlen but were kept as a family secret until 1813 in an effort of the Chamberlens to monopolize the field. In 1699, Hugh Chamberlen sold one half of the instrument to Amsterdam but added fraud to infamy by selling the vector or worthless half. Prior to that, in 1670, he had demanded the equivalent of $7,500 for the secret and, in an attempt to show their worth, had killed a woman and baby before Mauriceau, who craftily chose for the demonstration a woman with a distorted pelvis, upon whom he previously had planned to do a cesarean section. After some hours of fruitless effort, Chamberlen failed in his attempts at delivery, with the resultant double fatality. When the Chamberlen forceps were finally revealed to the profession in 1813, their need had been met by other men, and the Chamberlens were thus justly punished for the discredit they had brought upon their calling.

This century witnessed severe population dessication due to plagues, wars and the like. In England, William Pelty realized that controlling communicable diseases and saving infant lives would prevent continued diminution of the population. To this end he recommended isolation for plague patients and maternity hospitals for unmarried pregnant women. Such ideas were too far in advance of the time, however, and hence had no immediate consequences.

THE EIGHTEENTH CENTURY

Population continued to be a great general concern to the governments of the world. Those who were concerned with general matters of health felt that governments ought to take a more active role in overseeing health matters. Between 1779 and 1817, Johan Peter Frank in Germany wrote several volumes entitled *System einer vollstandigen medicinischen Polezey*. This work is even today considered a landmark in the history of thought on the social relations of health and disease. His recommendations concerning childbirth were many and as with Pelty, farsighted for his time. He insisted that all childbirth be attended by trained persons, and further urged that a midwife be consulted prior to the expected date of confinement. In addition, he proposed legislation to enforce a reasonable period of bed rest during the puerperium and to free the mother for several weeks from any work in or outside the house which might prevent her from giving the necessary attention to her infant. When necessary, he felt that the state should support parturients for the first six weeks after delivery. He then expanded upon the above and outlined a detailed child welfare program. Acceptance of his work and ideas spread to all countries in close cultural contact with Germany.

The eighteenth century was also marked by a succession of other famous men connected with obstetrics such as Palfyne, the Hunters, Smellie, White and others. Palfyne is credited with the invention of obstetric forceps, as he presented a copy in 1770 to the Academy of Medicine of Paris.

Smellie taught obstetrics with a manikin and made improvements on the obstetric forceps in use at that time, adding a steel lock and curved blades. He also laid down the first principles for their use and differentiated by measurement between contracted and normal pelves.

William Hunter, though a pupil of Smellie, was opposed to the use of forceps, and frequently exhibited his rusted blades as evidence of their uselessness. In conjunction with his brother he laid the foundation of modern knowledge of placental anatomy.

Charles White published an obstetric thesis advocating the scrubbing of the hands and general cleanliness on the part of the accoucheur; he was the pioneer in aseptic midwifery. John Harvie, 90 years before Credé, advocated external manual expression of the placenta, and it is known that a similar procedure was in use in Dublin at that time. One of the most active and famous English obstetricians of the time, John Clarke, had his fame commemorated in this epitaph:

Beneath this stone, shut up in the dark
Lies a learned man-midwife y'clep'd Dr. Clarke.
On earth while he lived by attending men's wives,
He increased population some thousands of lives;
Thus a gain to the nation was gain to himself,
An enlarged population, enlargement of pelf.
So he toiled late and early, from morning to night,
The squalling of children his greatest delight;
Then worn out with labours, he died skin and bone
And his ladies he left all to Mansfield and Stone.

There were many famous obstetricians on the Continent in this period, chief among them being Baudelocque, who invented the pelvimeter and named and described positions and presentations. In America, prejudices against men in midwifery were carried over from Europe; as late as 1857 a demonstration before the graduating class at Buffalo roused such a storm of criticism that the American Medical Association had to intervene. Their judgment was that any physician who could not conduct labor by touch alone should not undertake midwifery.

This 18th century produced such men as Moultrie, Lloyd and Shippen. The last was a pupil of Smellie and Hunter; in 1762, he opened a school for midwifery in Philadelphia, and, since he provided convenient lodgings for the accommodation of poor women during confinement, he may be said to have established the first lying-in hospital in America. With Morgan, he founded the School of Medicine of the University of Pennsylvania, becoming its first Professor of Anatomy, Surgery and Midwifery.

THE NINETEENTH AND THE TWENTIETH CENTURIES

The increased knowledge, interest and ability which physicians brought to obstetrics were largely offset by the increased mortality due to puerperal fever. During the 17th, the 18th and the 19th centuries it became a pestilence, at times wiping out whole communities of puerperal women. The mortality rates varied in the best European clinics at Paris and Vienna from 10 to 20 per cent. The origin and the spread of the disease were little understood or studied. Obstetricians wasted futile hours on a study of minor alterations in instruments or technique and ignored the vast loss of life from puerperal fever. Oliver Wendell Holmes, of Harvard, first presented his views on the contagiousness of puerperal fever in 1843, and in 1855 he reiterated them in a monograph on *Puerperal Fever as a Private Pestilence.* This was, and still remains, a medical classic on the subject. His statements aroused great controversy in America, and he received a great deal of abuse and criticism from Meigs and Hodge, two of the foremost American obstetricians of the day. One of them stated that is was ridiculous to conceive of any gentleman carrying contamination on his hands from patient to patient.

The following is Holmes' summary of his observations on the prevention of puerperal sepsis. Written in 1843, before the discovery of any human pathologic organism, and before the adoption of disinfection in surgical procedures, it is a truly remarkable summary.[1]

1. A physician holding himself in readiness to attend cases of midwifery, should never take any active part in the postmortem examination of cases of puerperal fever.

2. If a physician is present at such autopsies, he should use thorough ablution, change every article of dress, and allow twenty-four hours or more to elapse before attending to any case of midwifery. It may be well to extend the same caution to cases of simple peritonitis.

3. Similar precautions should be taken after the autopsy or surgical treatment of cases of erysipelas, if the physician is obliged to unite such offices with his obstetrical duties, which is in the highest degree inexpedient.

4. On the occurrence of a single case of puerperal fever in his practice, the physician is bound to con-

sider the next female he attends in labor, unless some weeks, at least, have elapsed, as in danger of being infected by him, and it is his duty to take every precaution to diminish her risk of disease and death.

5. If within a short period two cases of puerperal fever happen close to each other, in the practice of the same physician, the disease not existing or prevailing in the neighborhood, he would do wisely to relinquish his obstetrical practice for at least one month, and endeavor to free himself by every available means from any noxious influence he may carry about with him.

6. The occurrence of three or more closely connected cases, in the practice of one individual, no others existing in the neighborhood, and no other sufficient causes being alleged for the coincidence, is prima facie evidence that he is the vehicle of contagion.

7. It is the duty of the physician to take every precaution that the disease shall not be introduced by nurses or other assistants, by making proper inquiries concerning them, and giving timely warning of every suspected source of danger.

8. Whatever indulgence may be granted to those who have heretofore been the ignorant causes of so much misery, the time has come when the existence of a *private pestilence* in the sphere of a single physician should be looked upon not as a misfortune but as a crime; and in the knowledge of such occurrences, the duties of the practitioner to his profession should give way to his paramount obligations to society.

While Holmes first conceived the correct idea of the nature of the disease, it is to Ignaz Philipp Semmelweiss that the glory must go of finally proving without question the nature of its source and transmission. He was an assistant in the Viennese clinic for women, and while his associates fussed with unimportant details of technic, he was studying and mourning the tremendous death rate among puerperal women in the clinic. He observed that the death rate in Clinic I, where women were delivered by medical students or physicians, was always higher than that of Clinic II, where midwives officiated or received instruction. After fruitless study and manifold changes in technique in order to follow more closely that of Clinic II, the cause of the disease was brought home to him in a desperate and startling fashion. His friend, Kalletschka, an assistant in pathology, died after performing an autopsy upon a victim of puerperal fever, during which Kalletschka had sustained a slight cut on his finger.

At postmortem the findings were identical with those of puerperal sepsis, and Semmelweiss concluded that the disease was transmitted from the dead, by contact from the physicians and the students, who often went directly from the post-

---

[1] From Abraham Levinson, Pioneers of Pediatrics.

mortem room to deliveries. Accordingly, he immediately instituted and enforced a ruling which made it obligatory that all physicians and students wash their hands in a solution of chloride of lime after attending autopsies and before examining or delivering mothers. In 7 months he had reduced the mortality in Clinic I from 12 to 3 per cent, and in the subsequent year had a mortality lower than Clinic II, a hitherto unheard-of feat. Subsequently, he observed that puerperal sepsis could be transmitted from patient to patient by contact of contaminated material, or attendants, as well as from the postmortem room, and in 1861 he published his immortal work on *The Cause, Concept and Prophylaxis of Puerperal Fever.*

Medicine provides pitiful figures in profusion, but none, it seems, met such a cruel reception and ultimate fate as Semmelweiss. His colleagues (for the most part, but with a few notable and loyal exceptions) distorted and criticized his teachings. Had they stopped there, it might have been bad enough, but they carried their distaste for his views to the stage of persecution. He was forced to leave Vienna and go to Budapest, where a similar attitude—if possible a more malignant one —awaited him. A disappointed man, he died in 1865 from a brain abscess which may have originated in an infection similar to that of his friend Kalletschka. To the tragedy of his life, his death added satire. His work, however, has lived on; Pasteur and Lister added to it; and with a more modern and tolerant age his worth has been recognized.

The organisms causing puerperal fever probably were seen by several early workers beginning with Mayrhofer, who, in 1863, described "cylindrical vibrios" or "strings of pearls" in the lochia of puerperal sepsis. In 1864, 310 deaths occurred in the 1,350 confinement cases in the Maternité hospital in Paris, and that "Vestibule of Death" had to be closed in 1865.

Pasteur, in 1879, saw "cocci in chain" in cases of puerperal sepsis and contributed definitely to our knowledge of the causal streptococci, demonstrating to doctors the "presence of the invisible foe" in a drop of blood obtained by a "simple pinprick on the finger tip of the unhappy woman doomed to die the next day" and recommending methods of aseptic technique for their control.

The 19th and the 20th centuries were largely notable for their utilization of drugs to alleviate the pains of childbirth. The use of ether as an anesthetic was first discovered in America, but it was first utilized for childbirth by Simpson in Great Britain. He brought back the lost art of version by making it a safer procedure and eventually substituted chloroform for ether. As with almost every advance in medicine, it was opposed bitterly. The opposition was loudest and most vehement from the clergy, but, in 1853, Queen Victoria accepted it for delivery and by her action silenced most of the criticism. Nitrous oxide had been used in 1880 and has continued to be popular ever since that time.

Obstetric analgesia and anesthesia have made great strides during the 20th century (see Chap. 12, Analgesia and Anesthesia in Labor).

The present century will be remembered largely for the development of antepartal clinics and the more concentrated care of the expectant mothers that came with them. The application of advances in general medicine, metabolism and public health to obstetrics has led to a marked decrease in mortality and morbidity from cardiac, pulmonic, metabolic, venereal and associated medical conditions complicating pregnancy. The consideration of adequate vitamin, mineral and caloric contents in connection with the diet of pregnant and puerperal women not only has decreased the morbidity but also has enhanced the health of all mothers and children who receive adequate obstetric care.

Many other contributions have been made and are being added constantly to the science of obstetrics, not the least of which is more intensive training and study in this specialty demanded by the public as well as the medical profession. The advent of routine external expression of the placenta, anti-bacterial prophylaxis in the eyes of the newborn, purified ergot and pituitary preparations in hemorrhage control and prevention are but a few of the methods and medications which have marked the early 20th century.

The morphologic and anthropologic studies of Naegele, Roberts, Williams, Goodwin, Caldwell, Moloy and others have done much to improve our understanding of the various types of pelves and some of their importance in labor. Roentgenologic pelvimetry, cephalometry and tokodynamometry have greatly advanced our knowledge of the probable course of labor and delivery; Thoms, Caldwell and Moloy, Hanson, Jarcho and countless others have contributed to our advances in this field (see Chap. 2).

In a necessarily brief and incomplete fashion, an endeavor has been made to touch upon some of the more interesting phases of the history of obstetrics—a delightful and fascinating subject.

BACKGROUND AND DEVELOPMENT OF MATERNAL AND INFANT CARE IN THE UNITED STATES

As we know it today, maternal and child care developed into its present status through devious avenues of investigation and many bypaths of interrelated activity and work. Individuals, both from the profession and the laity, as well as private and municipal organizations, contributed time, money and interest until, at last, Government action was obtained.

The background of our present maternity situation is of interest both as a history and a story. Antepartal care in the United States had its beginnings in the days of slavery. The intelligent slave-owners paid special attention to the diet and the care of pregnant slaves. Healthy slaves were more valuable, were worth more money and produced stronger offspring. From this beginning the chronologic efforts which led to our present-day maternal care follow.

1866. A story was written which concerned cruelty to a child. Some thoughtful person referred the case to *The Society for the Prevention of Cruelty to Animals.* Henry Bergh, a former diplomat to Russia, was the founder and director of this association and was influential in having the judgment pronounced on the ground that a child was a human animal. This incident stimulated interest in the general treatment of children.

1873. *The New York Diet Kitchen Association,* the oldest public health organization in America, was opened at the request of doctors from "de Milt Dispensary" on the lower East Side of New York City. It was first organized as a soup kitchen, and milk, gruel, beef tea and cooked rice were taken to the sick in their homes, with the idea of restoring health. In 1892, they began to make formulas for sick babies and still later dispensed free milk or sold it at 3 cents a quart. Maria L. Daniels was the first nurse director and contributed much for many years to public health progress. In 1926, this group was organized as *The Children's Health Service of New York.* The organization grew with the times, changing its program from curing the sick to preventive work—keeping well babies well. Although the organization devoted its major effort to work with babies and preschool children, it also included antepartal care in its program.

1876. The beginning of child-welfare legislation in the United States was the Act passed by the New York State Legislature, granting to *The Society for the Prevention of Cruelty to Children* a charter that gave it wide power with regard to the protection of child life. The inception of this legislation was based on the incident of the "child as a human animal" (1866).

1893. The first *Infant Milk Station* in the United States was established in New York City by Nathan Strauss. Through his persistence, milk was finally made "safe" through pasteurization; and many such stations were set up.

1900. *The United States Census Bureau* was made a permanent organization. Up to this time, *vital statistics* were considered to be of so little importance in the United States that, as soon as the population was tabulated and classified, the bureau was disbanded, to be reestablished and reorganized every 10 years.

1906. *The United States Census Bureau* published mortality statistics which drew attention to the appalling loss of life among babies and children. Up to this time, very little thought had been given to maternity and infant protection.

1907. Due to the growing interest, Mr. George H. F. Schrader was stimulated to give money to *The Association for Improving Conditions of the Poor* (now the *Community Service Society*) for the salaries of two nurses to do antepartal work. This was the first consistent effort to prevent deaths of babies by caring for the mothers *before* the babies were born. Two reasons were given as to why antepartal care would be of value: (1) nurses in convalescent homes for postpartal mothers thought that if patients had better care during pregnancy, the health of mothers would be improved; (2) social workers going into the homes felt that they were not adequately prepared to advise pregnant mothers.

1907. *The New York Milk Committee* was organized. Its object was the reduction of infant mortality through the improvement of the city's milk supply. It established milk depots which proved beyond question their great value in the reduction of infant mortality by dispensing clean pasteurized milk and by educating mothers.

1908. In this year the *Division of Child Hygiene* was established in New York City, the first in the United States, and it was important enough to be recognized nationally. Josephine Baker, M.D., was appointed chief. This was a pioneer achievement, and the methods that were evolved had no precedent.

1909 to 1914. At approximately this time, Mrs. William Lowell Putnam, of Boston, promoted a demonstration of organized antepartal care. It was called *The Prenatal Care Committee* of the Women's Municipal League. The members of this committee worked in cooperation with the Boston Lying-In Hospital through Robert L. DeNormandie, M.D., of Harvard Medical School, Dr. Ruggles, of the then Homeopathic Hospital, and the Instructive District Nurses Association. The committee functioned long enough to establish the fact that good obstetric care was not possible without antepartal care.

1909. In this year *The American Association for the Study and Prevention of Infant Mortality* was organized and held its first meeting in New Haven, Connecticut. This committee was composed of both professional and lay members and devoted itself entirely to problems connected with child life, particularly to studying and trying to correct the high mortality rate. At this time there were no records of births or deaths, and the causes of deaths were unknown. The education of physicians and nurses was shamefully unsatisfactory; there was no public health in the schools, and practically no activity on the part of municipal, state or the Federal Government to prevent infant mortality. The first president of this association was J. H. Mason Knox, M.D., and Gertrude B. Kipp was the first secretary. The committee consisted of the Honorable Herbert Hoover, Livingston Ferrand, M.D., L. Emmet Holt, M.D., Richard Bolt, M.D., and Philip Van Ingen, M.D. The work of this organization was of profound significance. In 1918, its expanding activities caused it to change its name to *The American Child Hygiene Association,* and in 1923 the name was changed to *The American Child Health Association.* In 1935, after having contributed to every angle of this pioneer work, the association was disbanded.

1909. *The First White House Conference,* on "The Dependent Child," was called by President Theodore Roosevelt. These investigations resulted in the establishment of the U. S. Children's Bureau in 1912. According to some authorities, this conference was called through the influence of a public health nurse.

1910. *The Census Bureau* published another report, this time on the mortality of infants under 1 year of age and at "special ages." As a result of this report maternity hospitals made an effort to improve the care given to infants.

1911. In New York City *the first strictly municipal baby-health stations* were organized under the jurisdiction of the Department of Health, and the full cost of the work was borne by the municipality. Soon the dispensing of milk was of minor importance, and emphasis was placed on prevention—keeping well babies well. They are now called *Child-Health Stations.*

1911. *The New York Milk Committee* (1907) made an investigation at the baby-health stations and found that 40 per cent of all infant deaths (112 per 1,000) occurred within the 1st month of life before the mothers registered their babies at the health stations. This indicated the necessity for care *before* birth. The committee then decided to carry on an experiment in antepartal work. (See 1917.) They were convinced that much could be hoped for as a result of organized antepartal care.

1912. *The Babies' Welfare Association* (formerly *The Association of Infant Milk Stations* [1893]) represents the first comprehensive and successful attempt to coordinate the various child-welfare agencies in any community. All of the organizations of this type agreed to coordinate their activities by preventing duplication and overlapping without interfering with the organizations. In 1922, the name was changed to the *Children's Welfare Federation* of New York City. It continued to act as a clearing house and, among its other activities, managed the *Mother's Milk Bureau.*

1912. The *U. S. Children's Bureau* was established. It began in the Department of Commerce and Labor; in 1913 it was made a part of the Department of Labor and, in 1946, was transferred to the Federal Security Agency. This was created by Congress through a Federal Act (Government sanction). This bureau was to set up special machinery to study and protect the child and to study all matters pertaining to the welfare of children and child life among all classes of our people, to assemble and accumulate factual information and to disseminate this information throughout the country. Miss Julia Lathrop was chosen as chief. Much of the success of this bureau is credited to Miss Lathrop's vision. Fortunately, her successor, Miss Grace Abbott, continued the work with equal zeal.

1915. *The Birth Registration Area* was established as a Federal Act. The information is compiled in a uniform manner, giving the birth and the death statistics on which are based our information on mortality rates. The New England States, New York, Pennsylvania, Michigan, Minnesota and the District of Columbia were the first states to comply. At the present time all 50 states and the District of Columbia require registration of every birth.

1915. Dr. Haven Emerson, Health Commissioner of New York City, appointed a special committee (Ralph W. Lobenstine, M.D., Clifton Edgar, M.D., and Philip Van Ingen, M.D.), in co-operation with the New York Milk Committee, to make an analysis of the facilities for maternity care in the city. The result of the survey showed that there was little antepartal work and no uniformity, and that only a very small number of pregnant mothers were receiving care. It showed also that hospitals took care of 30 per cent of the deliveries, midwives delivered 30 per cent, general practitioners delivered 30 per cent, and private doctors, who might be classified as obstetricians, delivered 10 per cent. Previous to this time little or nothing had been done to regulate or control the midwives.

1916. *The National Society for the Prevention of Blindness* was created after much pioneer work and investigation, locally and throughout the states, by Carolyn Van Blarcom, R.N. She was chosen to be the executive secretary. Through these investigations it was learned that by far the greatest cause of blindness was ophthalmia neonatorum. These findings led to the passing of a law compelling all physicians and midwives to use prophylaxis in newborn babies' eyes. Also, as a direct result of Miss Van Blarcom's surveys, a school for lay midwives was started, Belleview School for Midwives (no longer in existence). Miss Van Blarcom took out a midwife's license and was the first nurse in the United States so to register. The first obstetrical nursing textbook to be written by a nurse is to Miss Van Blarcom's credit. Her later contribution to the better care of mothers and babies was to secure for Johns Hopkins Hospital the E. Bayard Halsted Fund for medical research.

1917. The Women's City Club of New York City and the New York Milk Committee opened three antepartal centers. The one sponsored by the Women's City Club was organized as the *Maternity Service Association* and, with Frances Perkins as the first executive secretary and Miss Mabel Choate as president, provided stimulating leadership. Dr. Ralph W. Lobenstine, a famous obstetrician, gave much time, labor, authority and direction as chairman of the medical board. In 1918, this organization was incorporated as the *Maternity Center Association* and carried out the first extensive piece of organized antepartal work in the United States. Miss Anne Stevens was director. Miss Annie W. Goodrich's wise counsel, as a member of the nursing committee, gave impetus to the organization's accomplishments.

Louis I. Dublin, Ph.D., associated with this movement from the beginning, made an analysis of the first 4,000 records collected by the association. This revealed the startling fact that, through antepartal care, 50 per cent of the lives of mothers might be saved and 60 per cent of the lives of babies. Antepartal training and experience were extended to nurses throughout the world. This piece of intensive antepartal work fired increased interest in the care of mothers and babies. In 1929, the Maternity Center Association opened a school for the training of nurse midwives.

1919. *The Second White House Conference* was called by President Woodrow Wilson as a result of the activities of the U. S. Children's Bureau. It was organized in five sections. Each section was interested in a different phase of maternity and child care.

1919. *The American Committee on Maternal Welfare* was founded. The object of the committee was:

To awaken and stimulate the interest of members of the medical profession in cooperating with public and private agencies for the protection of the health of mothers and their offspring before and during pregnancy and labor and after confinement to the end that the conditions which menace and interfere with the health or life of the mother or infant may be improved or prevented, disease and disorder corrected, health promoted and life saved; to teach the principles and practices of general and personal hygiene and health to parents and to improve and generalize the standards and methods of training physicians, nurses and others dealing with the problems of maternity.

The Committee was incorporated as a nonprofit organization in 1934 for the purpose of studying the maternal mortality rate in the United States and the management of obstetric problems generally. For more recent progress, see 1957 and 1964.

This organization publishes the magazine *The Bulletin of Maternal and Child Health.* It also promoted the American Congress of Obstetrics and Gynecology, which was held every 3 years. Seven such Congresses have been held, in 1939, 1942, 1947, 1950 (the first International Congress to be held in the United States), 1952, 1954 and 1957.

1921. *The Sheppard-Towner Bill* was passed by Congress, an Act for the Promotion of the Welfare and Hygiene of Maternity and Infancy, to be administered by the Children's Bureau. This bill was introduced in the 65th Congress by Congresswoman Jeanette Rankin of New Jersey. It was reported out of committee favorably but failed to pass. A second bill was introduced in the 66th Congress. It passed in the Senate but, through delays, was not considered by the House. In the first session of the 67th Congress the bill was again introduced by Senator Sheppard and Congressman Towner and, after much agitation, finally passed— an epoch in child-welfare legislation. An appropriation of $1,240,000 per year was granted for 5 years. The Cooper Bill, passed in 1927, extended it for 2 more years. This law was accepted by all of the states except 3. This legislation gave a tremendous impetus to the education not only of laity but also of physicians. Because of this legislation there was created at once, in the states which did not already have them, departments which now are quite uniformly labeled Divisions or Bureaus of Maternity and Child Health. In 1935, the Social Security Act was passed, following the plan of the Sheppard-Towner Bill. This Act appropriated $3,800,000. In 1939, the Social Security Act was amended, increasing the appropriation to $5,820,000. The amount has been increased gradually, and by 1952 (82nd Congress), $30,000,000 was appropriated for Maternal and Child Health, Crippled Children and other Child Health Services.

1923. *The National Committee for Maternal Health* was formed with Robert L. Dickinson, M.D., as secretary and later as president. This was a clearing house and a center of information on certain medical aspects of human fertility. The object was to gather and analyze material, to stimulate research, to issue reports to the medical profession and to persuade it to take a leading part in the scientific investigations of these problems in preventive medicine. No other group existed for this purpose. It was dissolved in 1950.

1923. *The Margaret Sanger Research Bureau* came into being, an affiliation of the Planned Parenthood Federation of America, Inc., for research in the field of infertility, contraception and marriage counseling.

1923. Mary Breckinridge began her investigations in Kentucky, which led to the organization of the *Frontier Nursing Service*. With this concentrated effort of all phases of maternity and infant care, the striking results proved the value of prenatal care. Through her vision, determination and unfaltering energy, Mary Breckinridge has made this organization one of worldwide renown. In 1936, the Frontier Nursing Service opened a school for the training of nurse midwives.

1925. *The Joint Committee on Maternal Welfare* was formed. This consisted of the American Gynecological Society, the American Association of Obstetrics and Gynecology and Abdominal Surgeons and the American Child Health Association (1909). Later the section of Obstetrics, Gynecology and Abdominal Surgeons of the American Medical Association was represented. The Committee issued a pamphlet entitled *An Outline of Delivery Care*. This stimulated the Children's Bureau to publish a concise pamphlet, *Standards of Prenatal Care* (1925), an outline for the use of physicians, which did much to standardize routine procedures.

1930. *The Third White House Conference* was called by President Herbert Hoover. Mr. Hoover's interest in child welfare was very evident. The conference was very comprehensive and far-reaching and was devoted to all aspects of maternity and child care. The Children's Charter was adopted and became a Federal Act. The 45,000,000 children were analyzed in chart form to show the paramount importance of care during pregnancy and the early years.

1938. *The Conference on Better Care for Mothers and Babies* was called by the Children's Bureau. This was the first time that representatives from the states, private and public organizations, both lay and professional people, met to pool ideas.

1939. *The Maternity Consultation Service* in New York City was organized to further prenatal education and care.

1940. *The Fourth White House Conference* on Children in a Democracy was called by President Franklin D. Roosevelt. It considered the aims of our American civilization for the children in whose hands its future lies; how children can best be helped to grow into the kind of citizens who will know best how to preserve and protect our democracy. By 1940, the 48 states, the District of Columbia, Puerto Rico, Alaska and Hawaii (then Territories) were cooperating with the Children's Bureau in its administration of child-welfare services.

1940. *The Cleveland Health Museum* was opened to the public—the first health museum in the Western Hemisphere. It is significant in the maternity field because, in its workshops, it is reproducing the *Dickinson-Belskie models,* acquired in 1945. Dr. Bruno Gebhard, Director, says that, in his belief, the use of this sculptural series in professional and lay education will advance knowledge on this all-important subject more quickly and more accurately than any other visual means thus far available.

1943. *The Emergency Maternity and Infancy Care Program* was launched to care for the wives and the babies of enlisted men in the armed forces. From $17,000,000 to $45,000,000 per year was appropriated. This Act also furthered interest in prenatal and child care.

1944. *The Public Health Service Act* was signed on July 3, 1944 and brought together all existing laws affecting the Public Health Service. In addition, the act also revised existing laws, provided authority for grants and authorized expansion of the Federal-State cooperative public health programs which had bearing on maternal and child health programs. This act was to exert a great indirect impact on the care of mothers and infants because of its provisions funding research and education of personnel needed in these areas.

1946. The *World Health Organization*—an agency of the United Nations—became a reality. At the first meeting in Paris, 64 nations signed the constitution. The membership as of 1965 totaled 117 countries. The object of the organization is "the attainment of the highest possible level of health of all the peoples." So far, much has been accomplished toward that end.

1950. *The Fifth White House Conference,* with emphasis on children and youth, was called by President Harry S. Truman.

1950. *The Fred Lyman Adair Foundation* of the American Committee on Maternal Welfare was established. Its purpose is to collect funds from charitable sources to underwrite research and educational projects in this field.

1955. *The American College of Nurse-Midwifery* was established as an organization of nurse-midwives to study and evaluate the activities of nurse-midwives, to plan and develop educational programs meeting the requirements of the profession and to perform other related functions. In 1957, the College became a member of the International Confederation of Midwives, a midwifery organization with members from some 30 countries throughout the world.

1957. *The American Association for Maternal and Infant Health* (formerly the American Committee on Maternal Welfare) was activated at the Seventh American Congress held in July. Prompted by the spectacular improvements and advances in maternity care which have taken place since its founding, the Board of Directors of the Committee voted unanimously to change the name, the role and the character of the organization. The new American Association for Maternal and Infant Health provides close integration of the various disciplines which participate in providing modern maternity care, and will serve as a forum for their mutual problems related to maternal and infant health.

1960. *The Sixth White House Conference,* concerned with the nation's children and youth, was called by President Dwight D. Eisenhower. The theme of this "Golden Anniversary" Conference was "Opportunities for Children and Youth to Realize Their Full Potential for Creative Life in Freedom and Dignity."

1962. *The Conference on Maternal and Child Health Teaching in Graduate Schools of Public Health* was convened in response to the dire reports of the lack of qualified personnel with any public health background in the area of maternal and child health. The conference recommended that an MCH career development program be established to offset the existing and predicted shortages of personnel. Such a program was established at the University of California at Berkeley with financial aid from the federal government (Children's Bureau) in 1965. The objectives of early recruitment of qualified physicians and the provision of specialized training in obstetrics or pediatrics with general public health maternal and child health content has been realized.

In the same year *The National Institute of Child Health and Human Development* was authorized. The goals of this Institute were support of research and training in special health problems and needs of mothers and children. This Institute also now conducts and supports research in the basic sciences relating to the processes of human growth and development, including prenatal development. Five conferences were held in 1967, which sought to find the problems involved in maternal and infant mortality and morbidity and to establish guidelines for change towards more optimal care.

1963. *The Maternal and Child Health and Mental Retardation Planning Amendments of 1963* was enacted. This law will make it possible for the Children's Bureau to carry out some of the major recommendations of the President's Panel.

1964. *The American Association for Maternal and Child Health* (formerly the American Association for Maternal and Infant Health), as a multidisciplinary organization, is one of the most potentially valuable groups interested in matters concerning infant, child and maternal health. The Board of Directors of the Association altered the official title of the organization, not to imply any change in its proposed program but to present a more accurate definition of the organization in terms of its aims and objectives.

1964. *The Nurse Training Act,* one of the amendments of the Public Health Act, was an indirect aid to maternal and infant care. This act authorized grants for the expansion and improvement of nurse training, assistance to nursing students, scholarship grants to schools of nursing, and the establishment of a National Advisory Council on Nurse Training.

1965. *Amendments to the Social Security Act* provided for a new 5 year program of special project grants for comprehensive health care and services for school and preschool children, particularly in low income family areas. These amendments also increased the authorization for money to support maternal and child health service programs. There are now 54 such projects in existence due to this legislation.

1965. *PKU Testing* became mandatory for all infants in the states of Illinois and Michigan, thus setting a precedent for other states.

1966. *The Department of Health, Education, and Welfare* issued a policy statement on birth control which stated that the Department would support, on request, health programs making family planning information and services available. Due to this unique statement, federally supported family planning programs have since slowly begun to evolve.

The Federal Food, Drug and Cosmetic Act was instituted on June 14, 1966. This legislation required labelling of ingredients of food represented for special dietary use. Infant foods, particularly, were specified.

The Child Protection Act of 1966 banned the sale of toys and children's articles containing hazardous substances, regardless of labelling.

1967. *The Public Health Law 89-749* is considered by health authorities to be one of the most significant health measures passed by Congress since it provides for increasing flexibility at state and regional levels to attack special health problems which have regional or local impact.

The revision of the *abortion laws* began slowly. Colorado and North Carolina recognized the following justifications for terminating pregnancy (1) life and health of the mother, (2) pregnancy as the result of rape, (3) incest and (4) fetal defect. California recognized at this time the first three justifications and Mississippi the second. In 1967, new laws were pending in 7 states but had already been defeated in 20. More recently, mental health of the mother has been considered legal justification for abortion in some states.

THE EMERGENCE AND DEVELOPMENT OF MATERNITY NURSING IN THE UNITED STATES

The origins of maternity nursing derive from ancient times as we have seen from the history of obstetrics.[1] From time immemorial women have been taking care of other women during this momentous time; most cultures, both primitive and modern, have a well-developed "motherlore" which keeps alive instructions and practices to be used during the childbearing period. However, it has been only in the past 100 years that professionally trained women have shared the organized care of the mother. Yet even in this short time, and particularly in the last two decades, maternity nursing of all the speciality areas is facing a critical period. A veritable tidal wave of population is predicted. Four to five million infants are born in America every year and it is estimated that by 1975, the annual birthrate will be six million. *No corresponding increase in physicians and nurses to care for these new families is expected.*

It is true that maternity nursing along with nursing in general is slowly delineating the specific body of content through which it makes its unique contribution to patients. Yet, the anticipated shortage of personnel together with the rising birthrate threatens to hinder the forward push of these frontiers. It appears that qualified personnel barely will be able to maintain minimum safe standards, let alone engage in exploratory creative activity. Hence, the creative and innovative use of even existing facilities and personnel is also threatened.

In order to understand our predicament better, and to better prepare for the future, it is well to look at the progress of our speciality to date. Hopefully, we can then derive some guidelines for future planning to utilize and develop maternity nursing to its fullest potential.

Emergence of Professional Maternity Nursing

A variety of factors, cultural, social, and technological, have had important roles in shaping the growth and development of maternity nursing. One

---

[1] This discussion derives from the following articles: Hilliard, M. E.: The changing role of the maternity nurse. Nurs. Clin. N. Am. 3:277-288, June, 1968, and Hilliard, M. E.: The evolution of a maternity nurse. Nurs. Forum 4:6-29, 1965.

of the most important and direct of these factors was the shift from home to hospital delivery. At the turn of the century, almost all women were delivered at home by a midwife or physician. At the present time, more than 90 per cent of mothers deliver in the hospital. Two other factors, in turn, brought about this change to hospital delivery and helped shape the kind of care received there. An increase in the understanding of asepsis made physicians much more attentive to this aspect of care, particularly for maternity patients. A growing conviction developed that delivery in a hospital was mandatory. As more women began delivering in hospitals, provision had to be made for quick, efficient, aseptic care and certain time-saving devices and work simplification procedures were borrowed from industry. "Assembly-line care" soon flourished. Compliance with "time saving" techniques, performance of the somewhat ritualistic procedures called for to maintain asepsis, and the increasingly overall bureaucratic structure generated by the complex modernizing hospital all went into defining and shaping the very essence of maternity care. Hence there arose the ritualistic, rigid adherence to rules and procedures (with rather little thought to the patient) that characterizes so much of maternity care even today. It was during these early times that antepartal care was conceived and developed as an aspect of preventive medicine. Thus, women increasingly had longer contact with their physicians during the childbearing time and this, together with the still prevalent Victorian notion of dependency, served to cement the obstetric relationship. In order to do justice to this relationship, physicians even more strongly began to insist on hospital deliveries.

Maternity nursing developed as obstetrics developed and not surprisingly, was based on the medical model of obstetrics in which pathology was the main focus. Thus, the student nurse's experiences were oriented to the physical care of her patients, with emphasis on technical competence. Moreover, a good deal of the student's "patient experiences" was in reality service to the hospital. The early hospitals were, in fact, staffed largely by students. This type of service-to-the-institution, technical competence orientation produced a nurse who was efficient in organizing care for many patients. However, because of the great numbers, no in-depth nursing therapy was either attempted or possible. Little or no public health experience was offered and the nurse gradually became more "institution (i.e., hospital) oriented" and the physician's veritable right arm.

In the third and fourth decades of the century, hospitals themselves became larger and more complex and the nurse found herself having to assume more and more administrative and organizational duties. Similarly, medical science enlarged and with the new knowledge and progress, more functions, formerly in the province of the physician, were delegated to the nurse. These factors together with the acute hospital personnel shortage precipitated by World War II, combined to develop and promote impersonal routinized care for the mother and her infant. The father, incidentally, was in no way considered, except as the agent who expedited the financial matters! Another irony in the situation again lay with progress. As more became known about the transmission and control of pathogenic organisms, various sub-units were designated for the use of mothers, well newborns, sick newborns, and premature infants. Thus, restrictions and compartmentalization of nursing function (nursery nurse, postpartum nurse, etc.) proliferated in the name of "better technique" but at the expense of unity in the mother-infant relationship. Perhaps even worse was the compartmentalization of thinking and communication that also evolved. The postpartum nurse knew and cared about the progress of the particular mothers in her charge while they were on the ward. She rarely knew how they responded to their pregnancy in general. She might know something about how they had withstood their labors, but only in the physical sense, and then only in relation to their immediate postpartum course. The nursery nurse knew about the babies in her nursery, but very little about the parents who would take them home or the environment into which they would go. The author can remember one nursery nurse telling her as a young student that she liked the babies because she did not have to make conversation with them and they never talked back! Obviously, any "family centered" nursing or even much continuity of care was only a dream of the more far sighted of the nursing profession!

The end of World War II and the decade of the 1950's did bring changes, however, for the better. Dreams began to be realities because of the perseverance of dedicated nurses and physicians. Obstetrics began to realize the value and advantage of an interdisciplinary approach. Partly as a result of this cross collaboration, philosophies regarding childbearing and childrearing began to change and much more emphasis was put upon the total meaning these experiences had for the people involved, patient and practitioner alike. In addition, basic philosophies in both medical and nursing education were also becoming more fluid, turning away from the old service-to-the-institution "training" orientation to a more professional well rounded "education" focus. Thus, today it has become apparent that there exists a body of knowledge that is uniquely nursing's. Its roots lie in early day obstetric principles of safe and efficient physical care, to be sure, but the unique *enlargement* of this care to which nursing can contribute is that of assuming the responsibility for making the childbirth experience richer and more satisfying.

The potential for a rich and satisfying childbearing experience lies in helping parents to become more mature and more able to appreciate the profound significance of bringing children into the world and rearing them wisely. The interdisciplinary approach has enhanced our knowledge and understanding of these matters greatly. If the better educated maternity nurse of today would utilize this new found knowledge, we could begin to navigate the still uncharted waters of holistic care and make a genuine contribution to both nursing and society.

What Does the Future Hold?

In many ways we cannot presume to improve upon nature and the basic processes of nature have not really changed for the childbearing family. The fundamental question and problem has been and is who is going to do "what" for the mother (and family) and how is the "what" to be done. Today's modern highly technological, bureaucratic society has left our childbearing families extremely vulnerable. One fact emerges clearly, there is more than enough opportunity and work for any and all who are concerned with contributing to the well being of our basic societal unit, the family. We cannot presume to answer the above questions in this short space, but hopefully the discussion will shed light on some of the problems and give beginning direction to solutions.

It is well, at this point, to discuss some basic issues that bear on the future of maternity nursing. The first of these has to do with the traditional relationship that has existed between medicine and nursing in this country. As we said, the nurse has been regarded as "the good right arm" of the physician, but in a subordinate position, to be told what to do and how to do it. Her duties, have been delegated for the most part, those that the physician has been forced to give up. She has been a trusted helper, but only a "helper" nevertheless. It is difficult to disrupt traditional ties, but if the nurse is to make any kind of worthwhile contribution which utilizes her hard earned preparation, she is going to have to achieve a peer-type relationship. This type of relationship implies working together toward a goal, with each person contributing his skill and knowledge, assuming responsibility for his actions, and directing his actions toward helping the childbearing family. Moreover, it can only come about when both realize what each is contributing to the over-all care. It appears then that nursing must work even harder to define its area of contribution.

The second issue has to do with under-utilization of various other segments of personnel who are educated or can be educated to give maternity care. The roots of the problems encountered also arise in the traditional medicine-nursing relationship. Glaring among the under-utilization examples is that of the nurse-midwife. American nurse-midwifery has to date been misunderstood and largely misinterpreted (see Chapter 24). It is quite ironical that the group of professional nurses who are the best qualified to provide sound, effective, and meaningful care to the whole childbearing family is the group least welcomed by many of those who are loudly decrying the desperate crises in maternity care. Many American obstetricians have never accepted the nurse-midwife as a useful colleague, possibly because of an imagined threat of private competitive practice. This threat is truly imagined, however, as this competition is neither desired by the nurse-midwives nor would it fit into the framework of American maternity care. The modern nurse-midwife is prepared and qualified to guide the normal mother through all aspects of the maternity cycle. Having the experience of this type of continuity of care, she can be more sensitive to the multitude of influences which affect each family than can either the hospital based or community based nurse whose experience is often limited to seeing the family in only one phase of the childbirth cycle. The unique value of the nurse-midwife, then, lies in her ability to minister to the family throughout the reproductive cycle.

Another source of confusion and hence, under-utilization, lies with the proliferation of the various types of preparation for maternity nursing. Three levels of preparation for registered nurses exist, after which maternity specialization may be pursued on a graduate level in a university, a postgraduate level at a maternity hospital, or for a certificate of nurse-midwifery on either a graduate or undergraduate level. One only has to try to determine the commonalities and dissimilarities in the contributions of the hospital or community based maternity nurse, the maternity clinical nurse specialist and the nurse-midwife to begin to understand the dimensions of the "under-utilization—over-proliferation" problem. While all these "professional" nurse preparations are growing, there still remains the fact that all nurses are not ready to be professional persons. Nursing will grow to full stature in time, but at the present with the crises so acutely upon us, an important source of manpower should not be overlooked. The contribution of the technically well-prepared nurse is no mean one and these persons may well become the future specialists of the labor, postpartum and nursery areas. The preparation of these nurses could wisely become the focus of several of the nursing programs already extant.

The third issue has to do with current practice involving the length of hospital stay for the parturient woman. Recent tendencies to discharge the mother and infant in 3 to 5 days of delivery has compounded the joint problems of adjustment and restoration for the mother and support and teaching for the nurse. Discharge often occurs before involution has progressed very far and before lactation is either established or suppressed. If complications do arise, they often occur when the mother is literally alone (except for her infant) and certainly without prompt professional attention. Moreover her infant is still in the process of adjusting to extra-uterine existence and all of his needs must be met consciously by a mother who is still in a great period of physical and emotional adjustment herself. So much more might be accomplished during the whole maternity cycle if the required nursing supervision could be more continuous and more individualized with more emphasis on follow-through with the mother during the first weeks of the immediate postpartum period.

Maternity nurses have vital functions to perform within the institutional setting, but to do justice to these they must be freed from the constricting compartments which permit contact only with segments of the family. Moreover they may very well have to broaden their areas of activity to include the home setting. Thus, they could move easily from hospital to the community and some could be in fact home based in the latter. Hopefully, in the future, a professional maternity nurse would come to the hospital because the family she is following has need of the services of the institution *at that moment* and she would institute an individualized plan of care that would meet the needs of that par-

ticular family. The *more routine aspects* of institutional procedure can be handled easily by technicians. Professional nurses on the hospital staff might provide valuable decisions for the community based nurse and the two would work closely together. The professional maternity nurse can then fill the need that is so lacking in today's care: the need for one constant, guiding figure who can (and is qualified) to plan and support the expectant parents through all phases of the childbearing process including that so-often forgotten return-from-the-hospital period.

These possibilities together with other innovations outlined in Chapter 8 will hopefully come in time—in time to circumvent some of the crisis aspects which maternity care is facing. It will take imagination, innovation and fearlessness to break traditional bonds with the past, but the time for formulating the positive steps to be taken is already upon us. At present, maternity nursing is standing at one of the important crossroads of its development. The "trained ob. nurse" who was so desirable at the beginning of the century is no longer functional and at any rate has been replaced by a variety of "professional" maternity nurses, whose roles are, as yet, not clearly identified.

These are pressing problems requiring thoughtful answers. What is nursing's unique contribution? What can be the role of the two-year graduate, the three-year graduate, the four- and five-year graduate, the graduate of a post-graduate course, a master's program, a nurse-midwifery program? It is a critical time for us. Maternity nursing must not only look back but also ahead!

Although there is yet much to be done, many encouraging advances have been made over the years. The seemingly disconnected sequence of activities—the prevention of cruelty to children, care of the sick, maintaining babies' "good health," mortality studies, the development of antepartal clinics, federal and state funding of health related research and teaching, and finally, intra- and inter-disciplinary debate and discussion—has resulted in better health care for the childbearing family.

The credit for the advancement of this care cannot be assigned to any individual, organization or discipline. Our present somewhat improved conditions are the result of extended public health education, organized efforts through private and public agencies (national, state and local), dedicated effort of the involved health disciplines, and the intelligent interest and cooperation of the public spirited citizens (including the childbearing family) who give their time, their cooperation and their money to these efforts. Much is yet to be done and only with the continued combined cooperation can we rise to meet the crises in maternity care in this country!

SUGGESTED READING

Bookmiller, M., and Bowen, G.: Textbook of Obstetrics and Obstetric Nursing. ed. 5, Philadelphia, W. B. Saunders, 1967.

Cavanaugh, J. H.: Comprehensive health planning. Bull. N. Y. Acad. Med. 44:186-189, February, 1968.

Corbin, H.: Maternity care today and tomorrow. Am. J. Nurs. 53:201, 1953.

Egan, M. C.: Recent legislation affecting child nutrition. J. Am. Diabetic Assoc. 52:377-380, May, 1968.

Findley, P.: Priests of Lucina. Boston, Little, 1939.

Forbes, T. R.: The regulation of English midwives in the 16th and 17th centuries. Medical History 8:235-244, July, 1964.

Gordon, M.: The clinical specialist as change agent. Nurs. Outlook 17:37-39, March, 1969.

Graham, H.: Eternal Eve. Garden City, Doubleday, 1951.

Heaton, C. E.: Obstetrics and gynecology in America. N. Carolina Med. J. 8:35, 1947.

Heaton, C.: Fifty years of progress in obstetrics and gynecology. New York J. Med. 51:83, 1951.

Hellman, L. M.: Nurse-midwifery in the United States. Obstet. Gynec. 30:883-888, December, 1967.

Hershey, N.: As society's views change, law changes. Am. J. Nurs. 67:2310-2312, November, 1967.

Hilliard, M. E.: The changing role of the maternity nurse. Nurs. Clin. N. Am. 3:277-288, June, 1968.

————: The evolution of a maternity nurse. Nurs. Forum 4, No. 2:6-29, 1965.

Hingson, R. L., and Hellman, L. M.: Anesthesia for Obstetrics. Philadelphia, J. B. Lippincott, 1956.

International Digest of Health Legislation 18, No. 1:14-15, 1967.

International Digest of Health Legislation 19, No. 2:435-445, 1968.

Johnston, E. M.: When the potato was done. Nurs. Clin. N. Am. 2:373-374, June, 1967.

Kirkwood, S. B.: Twenty years of maternity care. Children 2:133, 1955.

Langor, E.: Birth control: U.S. programs off to slow start. Science 156:265-267, May 12, 1967.

Lesser, A. J.: Mental retardation and the maternal and child health amendments of 1963. Pediatrics 33:3, 1964.

Mack, H. C.: Back to Sacajawea. Am. J. Obstet. Gynec. 69:933, 1955.

Miller, D. L.: A mythologist looks at the realities of comprehensive health planning. Nurs. Outlook 17:24-27, July, 1969.

Moore, M. L.: Bright spot in the eighteenth century. Am. J. Nurs. 69:1705-1709, August, 1969.

National Institute of Child Health and Human Development: Optimal Health Care for Mothers and Children: A National Priority.

Public Health Service Act, 1944. Public Health Reports 59:916-917, July 14, 1944.

Richards, J. F.: Integrating a clinical specialist into a hospital nursing service. Nurs. Outlook 17:23-25, March, 1969.

Rosen, G.: The evolution of social medicine in Freeman, H. E., et al.: Handbook of Medical Sociology. New Jersey, Prentice-Hall, 1963.

Speert, H.: Obstetric and Gynecologic Milestones. New York, Macmillan, 1958.

U.S. Congress, Senate Committee on Labor and Public Welfare and the House Committee on Interstate and Foreign Commerce, Compilation of Selected Public Health Laws, Washington, D.C., U.S. Government Printing Office, February, 1969.

U.S. Department of Health, Education and Welfare, Welfare Administration, Research Relating to Children, Bulletin 20, Washington, D. C., U. S. Government Printing Office, October 1965—May, 1966.

Wallace, H. M., et al.: A career development program in maternal and child health. Children 15:144-146, July-August, 1968.

Ziegel, E., and Van Blarcom, C. C.: Obstetric Nursing. ed. 5, New York, Macmillan, 1964.

Appendix

Answer Key for Study Questions

UNIT ONE

1: 3
2: A
3: B
4: A. External conjugate
   B. Diagonal conjugate
   C. Intercristal
   D. Conjugata vera
   E. Intertuberous diameter.
5: A. D
   B. D
   C. C
6: C
7: A. 4
   B. 3
   C. 1
   D. 2
8: C
9: B
10: A. 2
    B. 2
    C. 3
11: B
12: C
13: C
14: D
15: 2
16: A
17: A. L.O.T.
    B. L.O.A.
    C. R.O.P.
    D. L.S.P.
    E. R.M.A.
    F. R.A.D.P.

UNIT TWO

1: 2
2: A. 3
   B. 3
3: B
4: B
5: F
6: C
7: C
8: A. 2
   B. 3
9: A. 1
   B. 3
   C. 3
10: A. 3
    B. 1
11: B
12: D
13: A

14: D
15: 1
16: 2
17: D

UNIT THREE

1: A. Full dilatation
   B. Effacement
   C. Amnesic
   D. Uterine atony
   E. Episiotomy
   F. Lightening
2: Situation No. 1: 3
   Situation No. 2: 2
   Situation No. 3: 2
3: A. 2
   B. 3
   C. 2
4: 1
5: 3
6: C
7: B
8: 4
9: 2
10: 1
11: 3
12: A. 3
    B. 2
13: A. 3
    B. 1
    C. 4
    D. 4

UNIT FOUR

1: 3
2: 2
3: 1: G
   2: D
   3: B
   4: C
   5: G
   6: G
   7: D
   8: G
4: 4
5: 2
6: 1
7: 3
8: 1

UNIT FIVE

1: 1
2: 2
3: D
4: E

5: B
6: C
7: C
8: D
9: 2
10: 3
11: 3
12: 2
13: 1
14: 1
15: 2

UNIT SIX

1: 3
2: 2
3: 2
4: 1
5: 3
6: 1

UNIT SEVEN

1: 1
2: 1
3: 3
4: 4
5: 2
6: 3
7: 1
8: 2
9: 4
10: 3
11: 3
12: 2
13: 2
14: 3
15: A. Mastitis
    B. Endometritis
    C. Pelvic cellulitis or
       parametritis
    D. Subinvolution
    E. Engorgement

UNIT EIGHT

1: 2
2: 4
3: 2
4: 4
5: 1
6: 1
7: A
8: 3
9: B
10: 2
11: 1

Glossary

Note: The pronunciations as indicated in the following paragraph in this Glossary follow Webster's Second International Dictionary.

āle, châotic, câre, ădd, ăccount, ärm, ȧsk, sofȧ; ēve, hẹre, ĕvent, ĕnd, silĕnt, makēr; īce, ĭll, charĭty; ōld, ȯbey, ôrb, ŏdd, soft, cŏnnect; fo͞od, fo͝ot; out; oil, cūbe, ûnite, ûrn, ŭp, circŭs, menü; chair; go; sing; then, thin; natûre; verdûre; k = ch in German ich or ach; bon; yet zh = z in azure

abdominal (ăb-dŏm´ĭ-nȧl). Belonging to or relating to the abdomen.
  a. delivery, delivery of the child by abdominal section. See *cesarean section.*
  a. gestation, ectopic pregnancy occurring in the cavity of the abdomen.
  a. pregnancy. See *gestation* above.

ablatio placentae. See *abruptio placentae.*

abortion. The termination of pregnancy at any time before the fetus has attained a stage of viability, i.e., before it is capable of extra-uterine existence.

abruptio placentae (ăb-rŭp´shĭ-ō plȧ-sen´-tē). Premature separation of normally implanted placenta.

acromion (ȧ-krō´mĭ-ŏn). An outward extension of the spine of the scapula, used to explain presentation of the fetus.

adnexa (ăd-nĕk´sȧ). Appendages.
  a., uterine (ū´tēr-ĭn), the fallopian tubes and ovaries.

afibrinogenemia (ȧ-fī˝brin-ō-jen-ē´mē-ȧ). Lack of fibrinogen in the blood.

after-birth (ăf´tēr-bûrth˝). The structures cast off after the expulsion of the fetus, including the membranes and the placenta with the attached umbilical cord; the secundines.

after-pains (ăf´tēr-pāns˝). Those pains, more or less severe, after expulsion of the after-birth, which result from the contractile efforts of the uterus to return to its normal condition.

agalactia (ăg´ȧ-lăk´shĭ-ȧ). Absence *or* failure of the secretion of milk.

allantois (ȧ-lăn´tȯ-ĭs). A tubular diverticulum of the posterior part of the yolk sac of the embryo; it passes into the body stalk through which it is accompanied by the allantoic (umbilical) blood vessels, thus taking part in the formation of the umbilical cord; and later, fusing with the chorion, it helps to form the placenta.

amenorrhea (ā-mĕn˝ō-rē´ȧ). Absence or suppression of the menstrual discharge.

amnesia (ăm-nē´zhĭ-ȧ). Loss of memory.

amnion (ăm´nĭ-ŏn). The most internal of the fetal membranes, containing the waters which surround the fetus in utero.

amniotic (ăm˝nĭ-ŏt´ĭk). Pertaining to the amnion.
  a. sac, the "bag of membranes" containing the fetus before delivery.

analgesia (ăn˝-ăl-jē´zĭ-a). Drug which relieves pain, used during labor.

androgen (ăn´drȯ-jĕn). Any substance which possesses masculinizing activities, such as the testis hormone.

android (ăn´droid). The term adopted for the male type of pelvis.

anencephalia (ăn-ĕn˝sḙ-fā´lĭ-ȧ). Form of monstrosity with absence of a brain.

anovular (ăn-ōv´û-lēr). Not accompanied with the discharge of an ovum; said of cyclic uterine bleeding.

anoxia (an-ox´e-ah). Oxygen deficiency; any condition of absence of tissue oxidation.

antenatal (ăn-tē-nā´tȧl). Occurring or formed before birth.

antepartal (ăn˝tḙ-pär´tal). Before labor and delivery or childbirth; prenatal.

areola (ȧ-rē´ȯ-lȧ). The ring of pigment surrounding the nipple.
  secondary a., a circle of faint color sometimes seen just outside the original areola about the 5th month of pregnancy.

articulation (är-tĭk˝û-lā´shŭn). The fastening together of the various bones of the skeleton in their natural situation; a joint. The articulations of the bones of the body are divided into two principal groups—*synarthroses,* immovable articulations, and *diarthroses,* movable articulations.

Aschheim-Zondek test (ăsh˝hīm-tsŏn´dĕk). A test for the diagnosis of pregnancy. Repeated injections of small quantities of urine voided during the first weeks of pregnancy produce in infantile mice, within 100 hours, (1) minute intrafollicular ovarian hemorrhage and (2) the development of lutein cells.

asphyxia (ăs-fĭk´sĭ-ȧ). Suspended animation; anoxia and carbon dioxide retention resulting from failure of respiration.
  a. neonatorum (nē´ȯ-nȧ-tō´rŭm), "asphyxia of the newborn," deficient respiration in newborn babies.

attitude (ăt′ĭ-tūd). A posture or position of the body. In obstetrics, the relation of the fetal members to each other in the uterus; the position of the fetus in the uterus.

axis (ăk′sĭs). 1. A line about which any revolving body turns. 2. **Pelvic a.,** the curved line which passes through the centers of all the anteroposterior diameters of the pelvis.

bag of waters. The membranes which enclose the liquor amnii of the fetus.

ballottement (bă-lŏt′měnt). Literally means tossing. A term used in an examination when the fetus can be pushed about in the pregnant uterus.

Bandl's ring (Bän′dls). A groove on the uterus at the upper level of the fully developed lower uterine segment; visible on the abdomen after hard labor as a transverse or slightly slanting depression between the umbilicus and the pubis. Shows overstretching of lower uterine segment. Resembles a full bladder.

Bartholin's glands (Bär′tô-lĭn). Glands situated one on each side of the vaginal canal opening into the groove between the hymen and the labia minora.

bicornate uterus (bī-kôr′năt). Having two horns which, in the embryo, failed to attain complete fusion.

bimanual (bī-măn′û-ăl). Performed with or relating to both hands.

    b. palpation, examination of the pelvic organs of a woman by placing one hand on the abdomen and the fingers of the other in the vagina.

blastoderm (blăs′tô-dûrm). Delicate germinal membrane of the ovum.

    b. vesicle, hollow space within the morula formed by the rearrangement of cells, and by proliferation.

Braxton Hicks sign. Painless uterine contractions occurring periodically throughout pregnancy, thereby enlarging the uterus to accommodate the growing fetus.

    B.H. version, one of the types of operation designed to turn the baby from an undesirable position to a desirable one.

breech (brēch). Nates or buttocks.

    b. delivery, labor and delivery marked by breech presentations.

bregma (brĕg′mă). The point on the surface of the skull at the junction of the coronal and sagittal sutures.

brim (brĭm). The edge of the superior strait or inlet of the pelvis.

caked breast. See *engorgement.*

caput (kā′pŭt). 1. The head, consisting of the cranium, or skull, and the face. 2. Any prominent object, such as the head.

    c. succedaneum (sŭk″sē-dā′nê-ŭm), a dropsical swelling which sometimes appears on the presenting head of the fetus during labor.

catamenia (kăt-a-mē′nĭ-a). See *menses.*

caudal (kô′dăl). The term applied to analgesia or anesthesia resulting from the introduction of the suitable analgesic or anesthetic solution into the caudal canal (nonclosure of the laminae of the last sacral vertebra).

caul (kôl). A portion of the amniotic sac which occasionally envelops the child's head at birth.

cephalhematoma (sĕf″ăl-hē″mă-tō′mă). A tumor or swelling between the bone and the periosteum caused by an effusion of blood.

cephalic (sê-făl′ĭk). Belonging to the head.

    c. presentation, presentation of any part of the fetal head in labor.

cervix (sûr′vĭks). Necklike part; the lower and narrow end of the uterus, between the os and the body of the organ.

cesarean section (sê-zâ′rê-ăn). Delivery of the fetus by an incision through the abdominal wall and the wall of the uterus.

Chadwick's sign (tshăd′wĭks). The violet color on the mucous membrane of the vagina just below the urethral orifice, seen after the 4th week of pregnancy.

change of life. See *climacteric.*

chloasma (klô-ăz′mă). Pl. *chloasmata.* A cutaneous affection exhibiting spots and patches of a yellowish-brown color. The term chloasma is a vague one and is applied to various kinds of pigmentary discoloration of the skin.

    c. gravidarum, c. uterinum, chloasma occurring during pregnancy.

chorioepithelioma (kō′rĭ-ō-ĕp-ĭ-thē-lĭ-ō′-mă). Chorionic carcinoma; a tumor formed by malignant proliferation of the epithelium of the chorionic villi.

chorion (kō′rĭ-ŏn). The outermost membrane of the growing zygote, or fertilized ovum, which serves as a protective and nutritive covering.

chromosome (kro′mo-sōm). One of several small, dark-staining and more or less rod-shaped bodies which appear in the nucleus of the cell at the time of cell division and particularly in mitosis.

circumcision (sûr″kŭm-sĭzh′ŭn). The removal of all or part of the prepuce, or foreskin of the penis.

cleft palate (klĕft păl′ĭt). Congenital fissure of the palate and the roof of the mouth.

climacteric (klī-măk-tēr′ĭk). A particular epoch of the ordinary term of life at which the body undergoes a considerable change; especially, the menopause or "change of life."

clitoris (klī′tô-rĭs). A small, elongated, erectile body, situated at the anterior part of the vulva. An organ of the female homologous with the penis of the male.

coitus (kō′ĭt-ŭs). Sexual intercourse; copulation.

colostrum (kô-lŏs′trŭm). A substance in the first milk after delivery, giving to it a yellowish color.

    c. corpuscles, large granular cells found in colostrum.

colporrhaphy (kŏl-pōr′a-fē). 1. The operation of suturing the vagina. 2. The operation of denuding and suturing the vaginal wall for the purpose of narrowing the vagina.

colpotomy (kŏl-pŏt′o-mē). Any surgical cutting operation upon the vagina.

conception (kŏn-sĕp′shŭn). The impregnation of the female ovum by the spermatozoon of the male, whence results a new being.

condyloma (con-dil-o′mah). Pl. *condylomata.* A wartlike excrescence near the anus or the vulva; the flat, moist papule of secondary syphilis.

confinement (kŏn-fīn′mĕnt). Term applied to childbirth and the lying-in period.

congenital (kŏn-jĕn′ĭ-tĕl). Born with a person; existing from or from before birth, as, for example, congenital disease, a disease originating in the fetus before birth.

conjugate (kŏn′jōō-gât). The anteroposterior diameter of the pelvic inlet.

contraception (kŏn″tra-sĕp′shŭn). The prevention of conception or impregnation.

coronal (kŏr′ô-năl). Belonging to, or relating to, the crown of the head.

    c. suture, the suture formed by the union of the frontal bone with the two parietal bones.

corpus luteum (kôr′pŭs lū′tê-ŭm). The yellow mass found in the graafian follicle after the ovum has been expelled.

cotyledon (kŏt″ĭ-lē′dŭn). Any one of the subdivisions of the uterine surface of the placenta.

cul-de-sac (kōōl′dê-săk′) **of Douglas.** A pouch between the anterior wall of the rectum and the uterus.

cyesis (sī-ē′sĭs). Pregnancy.

decrement (dĕk′rē-mĕnt). Decrease; also the stage of decline.

delivery (dê-lĭv′ĕr-ĭ). [French, *délivrer,* to free, to deliver.] 1. The expulsion of a child by the mother, or its extraction by the obstetric practitioner. 2. The removal of a part from the body; as *delivery* of the placenta.

dizygotic (dī″zī-gŏt′ĭk). Pertaining to or proceeding from two zygotes (ova).

Döderlein's bacillus (dĕd′er-līnz). The large grampositive bacterium occurring in the normal vaginal secretion.

Douglas' cul-de-sac (kōōl′dê-săk′). A sac or recess formed by a fold of the peritoneum dipping down between the rectum and the uterus. Also called *pouch of Douglas* and *recto-uterine pouch.*

ductus (dŭk′tŭs). A duct.

    d. arteriosus (är-tē″rĭ-ō′sŭs), "arterial duct," a blood vessel peculiar to the fetus, communicating directly between the pulmonary artery and the aorta.

    d. venosus (vĕ-nō′sŭs), "venous duct," a blood vessel peculiar to the fetus, establishing a direct communication between the umbilical vein and the inferior vena cava.

Duncan (dŭng′kăn) **mechanism.** The position of the placenta, with the maternal surface outermost; to be born edgewise.

dystocia (dĭs-tō′shĭ-a). Difficult, slow or painful birth or delivery. It is distinguished as *maternal* or *fetal* according as the difficulty is due to some deformity on the part of the mother or on the part of the child.

    d., placental, difficulty in delivering the placenta.

eclampsia (ĕk-lămp′sĭ-a). Acute "toxemia of pregnancy" characterized by convulsions and coma which may occur during pregnancy, labor or the puerperium.

ectoderm (ĕk′tô-dûrm). The outer layer of cells of the primitive embryo.

ectopic (ĕk-tŏp′ĭk). Out of place.

    e. gestation, gestation in which the fetus is out of its normal place in the cavity of the uterus. It includes gestations in the interstitial portion of the tube, in a rudimentary horn of the uterus (cornual pregnancy) and cervical pregnancy as well as tubal, abdominal and ovarian pregnancies. See also *extrauterine pregnancy.*

    e. pregnancy, same as *ectopic gestation.*

effacement (ĕ-fās′mĕnt). Obliteration. In obstetrics, refers to thinning and shortening of the cervix.

ejaculation (ĕ-jăk″ŭ-lā′shŭn). A sudden act of expulsion, as of semen.

embryo (ĕm′brĭ-ō). The product of conception in utero from the 3rd through the 5th week of gestation; after that length of time it is called the fetus.

empathy (ĕm′pa-thĭ). The projection of one's own consciousness into that of another. Empathy may be distinguished from sympathy in that the former state includes relative freedom from emotional involvement.

endocervical (ĕn′dô-sûr′vĭ-kăl). Pertaining to the interior of the cervix of the uterus.

endometrium (ĕn″dô-mē′trĭ-ŭm). The mucous membrane which lines the uterus.

engagement (ĕn-gāj′mĕnt). In obstetrics, applies to the entrance of the presenting part into the superior pelvic strait and the beginning of the descent through the pelvic canal.

engorgement (ĕn-gôrj′mĕnt). Hyperemia; local congestion; excessive fullness of any organ or passage.

In obstetrics, refers to an exaggeration of normal venous and lymph stasis of the breasts which occurs in relation to lactation.

entoderm (ĕn′tō-dûrm). The innermost layer of cells of the primitive embryo.

enzygotic (ĕn-zī-gŏt′ĭk). Developed from the same fertilized ovum.

episiotomy (ĕp″ĭs-ĭ-ot′ō-mĭ). Surgical incision of the vulvar orifice for obstetric purposes.

Erb's paralysis. Partial paralysis of the brachial plexus, affecting various muscles of the arm and the chest wall.

ergot (ûr′gŏt). A drug having the remarkable property of exciting powerfully the contractile force of the uterus, and chiefly used for this purpose, but its long-continued use is highly dangerous. Usually given in the fluid extract.

erythroblastosis fetalis (ĕ-rĭth″rō-blăs-tō′sĭs). A severe hemolytic disease of the newborn usually due to Rh incompatibility.

estrogen (ĕs′trō-jĕn). A hormone secreted by the ovary and the placenta.

extraperitoneal (ĕks″trȧ-pĕr-ĭ-tō-nē′ȧl). Situated or occurring outside of the peritoneal cavity.

extra-uterine (ĕks″trȧ-ū′tēr-ĭn). Outside of the uterus.
> **e. pregnancy,** pregnancy in which the fetus is contained in some organ outside of the uterus, i.e., tubal, abdominal and ovarian pregnancies.

fallopian (fȧ-lō′pĭ-ȧn). [Relating to G. *Fallopius*, a celebrated Italian anatomist of the 16th century.]
> **f. tubes,** the oviducts—two canals extending from the sides of the fundus uteri.

fecundation (fē″kŭn-dā′shŭn). The act of impregnating or the state of being impregnated; the fertilization of the ovum by means of the male seminal element.

fertility (fĕr-tĭl′ĭ-tĭ). The ability to produce offspring; power of reproduction.

fertilization (fûr-tĭ-lĭ-zā′shŭn). The fusion of the spermatozoon with the ovum; it marks the beginning of pregnancy.

fetus (fē′tŭs). The baby in utero from the end of the 5th week of gestation until birth.

fimbria (fĭm′brĭ-ȧ). A fringe; especially the fringe-like end of the fallopian tube.

fontanel (fŏn″tȧ-nĕl′). The diamond-shaped space between the frontal and two parietal bones in very young infants. This is called the *anterior f.* and is the familiar "soft spot" just above a baby's forehead. A small, triangular one (*posterior f.*) is between the occipital and parietal bones.

foramen (fō-rā′mĕn). A hole, opening, aperture or orifice—especially one through a bone.
> **f. ovale** (ō-vā′lē), an opening situated in the partition which separates the right and left auricles of the heart in the fetus.

foreskin (fōr′skĭn). The prepuce—the fold of skin covering the glans penis.

fornix (fôr′nĭks). Pl. **fornices** (fôr′nĭ-sēz). An arch; any vaulted surface.
> **f. of the vagina,** the angle of reflection of the vaginal mucous membrane onto the cervix uteri.

fourchette (foor-shĕt′). [French, "fork."] The posterior angle or commissure of the labia majora.

frenum (frē′nŭm). Lingual fold of integument or of mucous membrane that checks, curbs or limits the movements of the tongue (ankyloglossia). Congenital shortening.

Friedman's test (frēd′mȧn). A modification of the Aschheim-Zondek test for pregnancy; the urine of early pregnancy is injected in 4-cc. doses intravenously twice daily for 2 days into an unmated mature rabbit. If, at the end of this time, the ovaries of the rabbit contain fresh corpora lutea or hemorrhagic corpora, the test is positive.

F.S.H., FSH. Abbreviation for follicle-stimulating hormone.

fundus (fŭn′dŭs). The upper rounded portion of the uterus between the points of insertion of the fallopian tubes.

funic souffle (fū′nĭc soo′f'l). A soft, blowing sound, synchronous with the fetal heart sounds and supposed to be produced in the umbilical cord.

funis (fū′nĭs). A cord—especially the umbilical cord.

galactagogue (gȧ-lăk′tȧ-gŏg). 1. Causing the flow of milk. 2. Any drug which causes the flow of milk to increase.

galactorrhea (gȧ-lak-tō-re′ȧ). Excessive flow of milk.

gamete (găm′ēt). A sexual cell; a mature germ cell, as an unfertilized egg or a mature sperm cell.

gastrula (găs′troo-lȧ). The early embryonic stage which follows the blastula.

gene (jēn). An hereditary germinal factor in the chromosome which carries on an hereditary transmissible character.

genitalia (jĕn-ĭtăl′ĭ-ȧ). The reproductive organs.

gestation (jĕs-tā-shŭn). The condition of pregnancy; pregnancy; gravidity.

gonad (gŏn′ăd). A gamete-producing gland; an ovary or testis.

gonadotropin (gŏn″ăd-ō-trō′pĭn). A substance having an affinity for or a stimulating effect on the gonads.

Goodell's sign (good′elz). Softening of the cervix, a presumptive sign of pregnancy.

graafian follices or **vesicles** (grāf′ĭ-ăn). Small spherical bodies in the ovaries, each containing an ovum.

gravida (grăv′ĭd-ä). A pregnant woman.

habitus (hăb′ĭt-ŭs). Attitude, disposition or tendency; to act in a certain way; position acquired by frequent repetition.

Hegar's sign (hā′gärz). Softening of the lower uterine segment; a sign of pregnancy.

homologous (hŏ-mŏl′ŏ-gŭs). Corresponding in structure or origin; derived from the same source.

hormone (hôr′mōn). A chemical substance produced in an organ, which, being carried to an associated organ by the blood stream, excites in the latter organ a functional activity.

hydatidiform (hi″dah-tid′ĭ-form) **mole.** Cystic proliferation of chorionic villi, resembling a bunch of grapes.

hydramnios (hī-drăm′nĭ-ŏs). An excessive amount of amniotic fluid.

hymen (hī′mĕn). A membranous fold which partially or wholly occludes the external orifice of the vagina, especially in the virgin.

hypofibrinogenemia (hī″pŏ-fī-brĭn″ō-jen-ē′mē-ă). Deficiency of fibrinogen in the blood.

hypogalactia (hī″pŏ-gă-lăk′she-ă). Deficiency in the secretion of milk.

hypoxia (hī-pŏks′ī-a). Insufficient oxygen to support normal metabolic requirements.

iliopectineal line (ĭl″ĭ-ŏ-pĕk-tĭn′ē-ăl). The linea terminalis.

impregnation (ĭm″prĕg-nā′shŭn). See *fertilization.*

increment (ĭn′krĕ-mĕnt). That by which anything is increased.

inertia (in-ûr′shĭ-ă). Inactivity; inability to move spontaneously. Sluggishness of uterine contractions during labor.

infant (ĭn′fănt). A baby; a child under 2 years of age.

infertility (ĭn-fûr-tĭl′ĭ-tĭ). The condition of being unfruitful or barren; sterility.

inlet (ĭn′lĕt). The upper limit of the pelvic cavity (brim).

introitis (ĭn-trō′ĭ-tŭs). A term applied to the opening of the vagina.

in utero. Inside the uterus.

inversion (ĭn-vûr′shŭn). A turning upside down, inside out, or end for end.
   i. of the uterus, the state of the womb being turned inside out, caused by violently drawing away the placenta before it is detached by the natural process of labor.

involution (ĭn″vŏ-lū′shŭn). 1. A rolling or pushing inward. 2. A retrograde process of change which is the reverse of evolution: particularly applied to the return of the uterus to its normal size and condition after parturition.

ischium (ĭs′kĭ-ŭm). The posterior and inferior bone of the pelvis, distinct and separate in the fetus or the infant, or the corresponding part of the innominate bone in the adult.

jelly (jĕl′ĭ). A soft substance which is coherent, tremulous and more or less transparent.

j. of Wharton, the soft, pulpy, connective tissue that constitutes the matrix of the umbilical cord.

labia (ā′bĭ-ă). The nominative plural of *labium.* Lips or liplike structures.
   l. majora (mă-jō′ră), the folds of skin containing fat and covered with hair which form each side of the vulva.
   l. minora (mĭ-nō′ră), the nymphae, or folds of delicate skin inside of the labia majora.

labor (lā′bēr). Parturition; the series of processes by which the products of conception are expelled from the mother's body.

lactation (lăk-tā′shŭn). The act or period of giving milk; the secretion of milk; the time or period of secreting milk.

lambdoid (lăm′doid). Having the shape of the Greek letter λ (lambda).
   l. suture, the suture between the occipital and two parietal bones.

lanugo (lă-nū′gō). The fine hair on the body of the fetus. The fine, downy hair found on nearly all parts of the body except the palms of the hands and the soles of the feet.

leukorrhea (lū″kŏ-rē′ă). A whitish discharge from the female genital organs.

L.H. Abbreviation for luteinizing hormone.

lightening (līt′n-ĭng). The sensation of decreased abdominal distention produced by the descent of the uterus into the pelvic cavity, which occurs from 2 to 3 weeks before the onset of labor.

linea (lĭn′ē-ă). Pl. *lineae* (lĭn′ē-ē). A line or thread.
   l. alba (ăl′bă), the central tendinous line extending from the pubic bone to the ensiform cartilage.
   l. nigra (nī′grä). A dark line appearing on the abdomen and extending from the pubis toward the umbilicus—considered one of the signs of pregnancy.
   l. terminalis. The oblique ridge on the inner surface of the ilium, continued on the pubis, which separates the true from the false pelvis. Formerly called the iliopectineal line.

lingua (lĭng′gwĭ). Tongue.
   l. frenum, tonguetie.

liquor (lĭk′ēr). A liquid.
   l. amnii (lī′kwôr ăm′nĭ-ī), the fluid contained within the amnion in which the fetus floats.

lochia (lō′kĭ-ă). The discharge from the genital canal during several days subsequent to delivery.

mask (măsk) **of pregnancy.** See *chloasma.*

maturation (măt″ŭ-rā′shŭn). In biology, a process of cell division during which the number of chromosomes in the germ cells is reduced to one half the number characteristic of the species.

meatus (mē-ā'tŭs). A passage; an opening leading to a canal, duct or cavity.

    m. urinarius (ū″-rĭ-nā′rĭ-ŭs), the external orifice of the urethra.

mechanism (mĕk′ȧ-niz'm). The manner of combinations which subserve a common function. In obstetrics refers to labor and delivery.

meconium (mē-kō′nĭ-ŭm). The dark-green or black substance found in the large intestine of the fetus or newly born infant.

menarche (mē-när′kē). The establishment or the beginning of the menstrual function.

menopause (mĕn′ō-pôz). The period at which menstruation ceases; the "change of life."

menorrhagia (mĕn′ō-rā′jĭ-ȧ). An abnormally profuse menstrual flow.

menses (mĕn′sēz). [Pl. of Latin *mensis,* month.] The periodic monthly discharge of blood from the uterus; the catamenia.

menstruation (mĕn″stroo-ā′shŭn). The cyclic, physiologic uterine bleeding which normally recurs at approximately 4-week intervals, in the absence of pregnancy, during the reproductive period.

mentum (mĕn′tŭm). The chin.

mesoderm (mĕs′ō-dûrm). The middle layer of cells derived from the primitive embryo.

metrorrhagia (mē-trō-rā′jĭ-ȧ). Abnormal uterine bleeding.

migration (mī-grā′shŭn). In obstetrics refers to the passage of the ovum from the ovary to the uterus.

milia (mĭl′ē-ȧ). Plural of *milium.*

milium (mĭl′ē-ŭm). A small white nodule of the skin, usually caused by clogged sebaceous glands or hair follicles.

milk-leg. See *phlegmasia alba dolens.*

miscarriage (mĭs-kăr′ĭj). Abortion.

molding (mōld′ĭng). The shaping of the baby's head so as to adjust itself to the size and shape of the birth canal.

monozygotic (mŏn″ō-zī-gō′tĭk). Pertaining to or derived from one zygote.

    m. twins (mŏn″ō-zī-gō′tĭk). Pertaining to or derived from one zygote.

mons veneris (mŏnz vĕn′ĕ-rĭs). The eminence in the upper and anterior part of the pubes of women.

Montgomery's tubercles (mŭnt-gŭm′ēr-ĭz). Small, nodular follicles or glands on the areolae around the nipples.

multigravida (mŭl″tĭ-grăv′ĭ-dȧ). A woman who has been pregnant several times, or many times.

multipara (mŭl-tĭp′ȧ-rȧ). A woman who has borne several, or many, children.

navel (nāv′ĕl). The umbilicus.

neonatal (nē″ō-nā′tăl). Pertaining to the newborn, usually considered the first 4 weeks of life.

nevus (nē′vŭs). A natural mark or blemish; a mole, a circumscribed deposit of pigmentary matter in the skin present at birth (birthmark).

nidation (nĭ-dā′shŭn). The implantation of the fertilized ovum in the endometrium of the pregnant uterus.

nullipara (nŭ-lĭp′ȧ-rȧ). A woman who has not borne children.

occipitobregmatic (ŏk-sĭp″ĭt-ō-brĕg-măt′-ik). Pertaining to the occiput (the back part of the head) and the bregma (junction of the coronal and sagittal sutures).

oligohydramnios (ŏl″ĭ-gō-hī-drăm′nĭ-ŏs). Deficiency of amniotic fluid.

omphalic (ŏm-făl′ĭk). Pertaining to the umbilicus.

oocyesis (ō′ō-sī-ē′sĭs). Ovarian pregnancy.

ophthalmia neonatorum (ŏf-thăl′mĭ-ȧ). Acute purulent conjunctivitis of the newborn usually due to gonorrheal infection.

os (ŏs). Pl. **ora** (ō′rȧ). Mouth.

    o. externum (*external os*), the external opening of the canal of the cervix.

    o. internum (*internal os*), internal opening of canal of cervix.

    o. uteri, "mouth of the uterus."

ova. Plural of ovum.

ovary (ō′vȧ-rī). The sexual gland of the female in which the ova are developed. There are two ovaries, one at each side of the pelvis.

ovulation (ō-vŭ-lā′shŭn). The growth and discharge of an unimpregnated ovum, usually coincident with the menstrual period.

ovum (ō′vŭm). The female reproductive cell. The human ovum is a round cell about $\frac{1}{120}$ of an inch in diameter, developed in the ovary.

oxytocic (ŏk″sĭ-tō′sĭk). 1. Accelerating parturition. 2. A medicine which accelerates parturition.

oxytocin (ŏk-sĭ-tō-sĭn). One of the two hormones secreted by the posterior pituitary.

palsy (pôl′zĭ). A synonym for paralysis, used in connection with certain special forms.

    Bell's p., peripheral facial paralysis due to lesion of the facial nerve, resulting characteristic distortion of the face.

    Erb's p. the upper-arm type of brachial birth palsy.

para (păr′ä). The term used to refer to past pregnancies which have produced an infant which has been viable, whether or not the infant is dead or alive at birth.

parametrium (păr-ȧ-mē′trĭ-ŭm). The fibrous subserous coat of the supravaginal portion of the uterus, extending laterally between the layers of the broad ligaments.

parity (păr′ĭ-tĭ). The condition of a woman with respect to her having borne children.

parovarian (pär-ô-vâr′ĭ-ăn). Pertaining to the residual structure in the broad ligament between the ovary and the fallopian tube.

parturient (pär-tŭ′rĭ-ĕnt). Bringing forth; pertaining to child-bearing. A woman in childbirth.

parturition (pär″tŭ-rĭsh′ŭn). The act or process of giving birth to a child.

patulous (păt′ŭ-lŭs). Spreading somewhat widely apart; open.

pelvimeter (pĕl-vĭm′ĕ-tĕr). An instrument for measuring the diameters and capacity of the pelvis.

pelvimetry (pĕl-vĭm′ĕ-trĭ). The measurement of the dimensions and capacity of the pelvis.

penis (pē′nĭs). The male organ of copulation.

perineorrhaphy (pĕr″ĭ-nē-ŏr′a-fĭ). Suture of the perineum; the operation for the repair of lacerations of the perineum.

perineotomy (pĕr″ĭ-nē-ŏt′ō-mĭ). A surgical incision through the perineum.

perineum (pĕr″ĭ-nē′ŭm.) The area between the vagina and the rectum.

periotoneum (pĕr″ĭ-tŏ-nē′ŭm). A strong serous membrane investing the inner surface of the abdominal walls and the viscera of the abdomen.

phimosis (fī-mō′sĭs). Tightness of the foreskin.

phlegmasia alba dolens (flĕg-mā′zhĭ′a ăl′ba dō′lĕnz). Phlebitis of the femoral vein, occasionally following delivery.

Pitocin (pī-tŏ′sĭn). A proprietary solution of oxytocin.

placenta (pla-sĕn′ta). The circular flat, vascular structure in the impregnated uterus forming the principal medium of communication between the mother and the fetus.

    ablatio p. See *abruptio placentae.*

    abruptio p., premature separation of the normally implanted placenta.

        previa p., a placenta which is implanted in the lower uterine segment so that it adjoins or covers the internal os of the cervix.

polygalactia (pŏl″ē-ga-lăk′shē-a). Excessive secretion of milk.

polyhydramnios (pŏl″ĭ-hī-drăm′nĭ-ŏs). Hydramnios.

position (pô-zĭsh′ŭn). The situation of the fetus in the pelvis; determined by the relation of some arbitrarily chosen portion of the fetus to the right or the left side of the mother's pelvis.

postnatal (pōst-nā′tăl). Occurring after birth.

postpartal (pōst-pär′tal). After delivery or childbirth.

preeclampsia (prē-ĕk-lămp′sĭ-a). A disorder encountered during pregnancy or early in the puerperium, characterized by hypertension, edema and albuminuria.

pregnancy (prĕg′năn-sĭ). [Latin, *praeg′nans,* literally "previous to bringing forth."] The state of being with young or with child. The normal duratión of pregnancy in the human female is 280 days, or 10 lunar months, or 9 calendar months.

premature infant. An infant which weighs 2,500 Gm. or less at birth.

prepuce (prē′pūs). The fold of skin which covers the glans penis in the male.

    p. of the clitoris, the fold of mucous membrane which covers the glans clitoris.

presentation (prē″zĕn-tā′shŭn). Term used to designate that part of the fetus nearest the internal os; or that part which is felt by the physician's examining finger when introduced into the cervix.

primigravida (prī″mĭ-grăv′ĭ-da). Pl. *primigravidae* (prī″mĭ-grăv′ĭ-dē). A woman who is pregnant for the first time.

primipara (prī-mĭp′a-ra). Pl. *primiparae* (prī-mĭp′a-rē). A woman who has given birth to her first child.

primordial (prī-môr′dĭ-ăl). Original or primitive; of the simplest and most undeveloped character.

prodromal (prŏ-drô′măl). Premonitory; indicating the approach of a disease.

progesterone (prô-jĕs′tĕr-ōn). The pure hormone contained in the corpora lutea whose function is to prepare the endometrium for the reception and development of the fertilized ovum.

prolactin (prô-lăk′tĭn). A proteohormone from the anterior pituitary which stimulates lactation in the mammary glands.

prolan (prô′lăn). Zondek's term for the gonadotropic principle of human-pregnancy urine, responsible for the biologic pregnancy tests.

promontory (prŏm′ŭn-tō″rĭ). A small projection; a prominence.

    p. of the sacrum, the superior or projecting portion of the sacrum when in situ in the pelvis, at the junction of the sacrum and the last lumbar vertebra.

pseudocyesis (sū″dō-sī-ē′sĭs). An apparent condition of pregnancy; the woman really believes she is pregnant when, as a matter of fact, she is not.

puberty (pū′bĕr-tĭ). The age at which the generative organs become functionally active.

pubic (pū′bĭk). Belonging to the pubis.

pubiotomy (pū′bī-ŏt′ô-mĭ). The operation of cutting through the pubic bone lateral to the median line.

pubis (pū′bĭs). The os pubis or pubic bone forming the front of the pelvis.

pudendal (pū-dĕn′dăl). Relating to the pudenda.

pudendum (pū-dĕn′dŭm). [Latin, *pude′re,* to have shame or modesty.] The external genital parts of either sex, but especially of the female.

puerperium (pū″ĕr-pē′rĭ-ŭm). The period elapsing between the termination of labor and the return of the uterus to its normal condition, about 6 weeks.

quickening (kwĭk′ĕn-ĭng). The mother's first perception of the movements of the fetus.

rabbit test. See *Friedman's test*.

Rh. Abbreviation for *Rhesus*, a type of monkey. This term is used for a property of human blood cells, because of its relationship to a similar property in the blood cells of *Rhesus* monkeys.

Rh factor. A term applied to an inherited antigen in the human blood.

Ritgen maneuver (rĭt′gĕn). Delivery of the infant's head by lifting the head upward and forward through the vulva, between contractions, by pressing with the tips of the fingers upon the perineum behind the anus.

Schultze's mechanism (sho͞olt′sĕz). The expulsion of the placenta with the fetal surfaces presenting.

secundine (sĕk′ŭn-dīn). The afterbirth; the placenta and membranes expelled after the birth of a child.

segmentation (sĕg″mĕn-tā′shŭn). The process of division by which the fertilized ovum multiplies before differentiation into layers occurs.

semen (sē′mĕn). 1. A seed. 2. The fluid secreted by the male reproductive organs.

show (shō). 1. Popularly, the blood-tinged mucus discharged from the vagina before or during labor.

Skene's gland. Two glands just within the meatus of the female urethra; regarded as homologues of the prostate gland in the male.

smegma. A thick cheesy secretion found under the prepuce and in the region of the clitoris and the labia minora.

souffle (so͞of′f'l). A soft, blowing, auscultatory sound.

    funic s., a hissing souffle synchronous with the fetal heart sounds and supposed to be produced in the umbilical cord.

    placental s., a souffle supposed to be produced by the blood current in the placenta.

spermatozoon (spûr″ma-tŏ-zō′ŏn). Pl. *spermatozoa* (spûr″ma-tŏ-zō′a). The motile microscopic sexual element of the male, resembling in shape an elongated tadpole. The male reproductive cell.

stillborn (stĭl′bôrn″). Born without life; born dead.

stria (strī′a). Pl. *striae* (strī′ē). A Latin word signifying a "groove," "furrow" or "crease."

    striae gravidarum (grăv-ĭ-där′ŭm), shining, reddish lines upon the abdomen, thighs and breasts during pregnancy.

subinvolution (sŭb″ĭn-vŏ-lū′shŭn). Failure of a part to return to its normal size and condition after enlargement from functional activity, as subinvolution of the uterus which exists when normal involution of the puerperal uterus is retarded.

succedaneum (sŭk′sĕ-dā′nĕ-ŭm). See *caput*.

superfecundation (sū′pĕr-fē-kŭn-dā′shŭn). The fertilization at about the same time of two different ova by sperm from different males.

superfetation (sū′pĕr-fĕ-tā′shŭn). The fecundation of a woman already pregnant.

symphysis (sĭm′fĭ-sĭs). The union of bones by means of an intervening substance; a variety of synarthrosis.

    s. pubis (pū′bĭs), "symphysis of the pubis," the pubic articulation or union of the pubic bones which are connected with each other by interarticular cartilage.

synchondrosis (sĭng″kŏn-drō′sĭs). A union of bones by means of a fibrous or elastic cartilage.

testicle (tĕs′tĭ-k'l). One of the two glands contained in the male scrotum.

thrush. An infection caused by the fungus *Candida albicans*, characterized by whitish plaques in the mouth.

tonguetie. See *lingua frenum*.

toxemia (tŏks-ē′mĭ-a). The toxemias of pregnancy are disorders encountered during gestation, or early in the puerperium, which are characterized by one or more of the following signs: hypertension, edema, albuminuria, and in severe cases, convulsions and coma.

trichomonas (trĭk-ŏm′ŏ-nas). A genus of parasitic flagellate protozoa.

    t. vaginalis, a species sometimes found in the vagina.

trophectoderm (trŏf-ĕk′tŏ-dûrm). The outer layer of cells of the early blastodermic vesicle; it develops the trophoderm—the feeding layer.

umbilical (ŭm-bĭl′ĭ-kăl). Pertaining to the umbilicus.

    u. arteries, the arteries which accompany and form part of the umbilical cord.

    u. cord [Latin, *funis umbilicalis*], the cord *con*-necting the placenta with the umbilicus of the fetus, and at the close of gestation principally made up of the two umbilical arteries and the umbilical vein, encased in a mass of gelatinous tissue called "Wharton's jelly."

    u. hernia, hernia at or near the umbilicus.

    u. vein, forms a part of the umbilical cord.

uterus (ū′tēr-ŭs). The hollow muscular organ in the female designed for the lodgement and nourishment of the fetus during its development until birth.

vagina (va-jī′na). [Latin, a sheath.] The canal in the female, extending from the vulva to the cervix of the uterus.

vernix caseosa (vûr′nĭks kā″sĕ-ō′sa). "Cheesy varnish." The layer of fatty matter which covers the skin of the fetus.

version (vûr′shŭn). The act of turning; specifically, a turning of the fetus in the uterus so as to change the presenting part and bring it into more favorable position for delivery.

vertex (vûr′tĕks). The summit or top of anything. In anatomy, the top or crown of the head.

v. presentation, presentation of the vertex of the fetus in labor.

vestibule (vĕs′tĭ-būl). A triangular space between the labia minora; the urinary meatus and the vagina open into it.

viable (vī′a̤-b'l). A term in medical jurisprudence signifying "able or likely to live"; applied to the condition of the child at birth.

villus (vĭl′ŭs). A small vascular process or protrusion growing on a mucous surface, such as the chorionic villi seen in tufts on the chorion of the early embryo.

vulva (vŭl′va̤). The external genitals of the female.

Wharton's jelly (hwôr′tŭnz). [Thomas *Wharton,* English anatomist, died 1673.] The jellylike mucous tissue composing the bulk of the umbilical cord.

witches' milk (wĭch′ĕz). A milky fluid secreted from the breast of the newly born.

womb (wo͝om). See *uterus.*

zona pellucida (zō′na̤ pĕll-ū′sĭd-ä). A transparent belt; translucent or shining through.

zygote (zī′gōt). A cell resulting from the fusion of two gametes.

Conversion Table for Weights of Newborn

(Gram equivalents for pounds and ounces)

For example, to find weight in pounds and ounces of baby weighing 3315 grams, glance down columns to figure nearest 3315 = 3317. Refer to number at top of column for pounds and number to far left for ounces = 7 pounds, 5 ounces.

POUNDS→ OUNCES↓	3	4	5	6	7	8	9	10
0	1361	1814	2268	2722	3175	3629	4082	4536
1	1389	1843	2296	2750	3203	3657	4111	4564
2	1417	1871	2325	2778	3232	3685	4139	4593
3	1446	1899	2353	2807	3260	3714	4167	4621
4	1474	1928	2381	2835	3289	3742	4196	4649
5	1503	1956	2410	2863	3317	3770	4224	4678
6	1531	1984	2438	2892	3345	3799	4252	4706
7	1559	2013	2466	2920	3374	3827	4281	4734
8	1588	2041	2495	2948	3402	3856	4309	4763
9	1616	2070	2523	2977	3430	3884	4338	4791
10	1644	2098	2551	3005	3459	3912	4366	4819
11	1673	2126	2580	3033	3487	3941	4394	4848
12	1701	2155	2608	3062	3515	3969	4423	4876
13	1729	2183	2637	3090	3544	3997	4451	4904
14	1758	2211	2665	3118	3572	4026	4479	4933
15	1786	2240	2693	3147	3600	4054	4508	4961

Or, to convert grams into pounds and *decimals* of a pound, multiply weight in grams by .0022. Thus, 3317 × .0022 = 7.2974, i.e., 7.3 pounds, or 7 pounds, 5 ounces.

To convert pounds and ounces into grams, multiply the pounds by 453.6 and the ounces by 28.4 and add the two products. Thus, to convert 7 pounds, 5 ounces, 7 × 453.6 = 3175; 5 × 28.4 = 142; 3175 + 142 = 3317 grams.

Aid for Visualization

of Cervical Dilatation

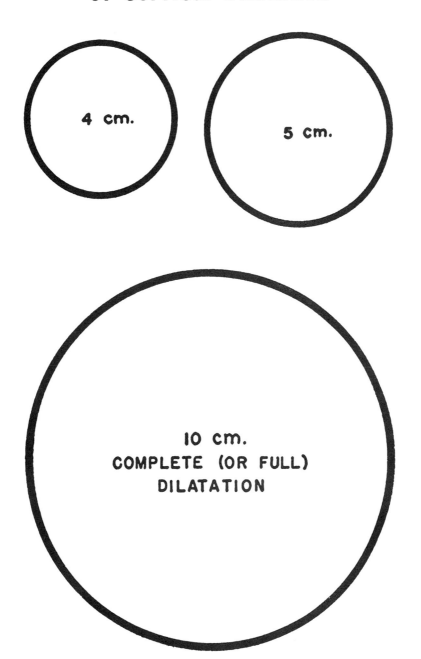

Index